Please insure that this Book is returned on
or before the last date stamped below

MM01978

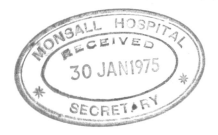
OCCUPATIONAL
LUNG DISORDERS

OCCUPATIONAL LUNG DISORDERS

W. RAYMOND PARKES
M.D., M.R.C.P., D.I.H.

Pneumoconiosis Medical Panel,
Department of Health and Social Security, London;
Honorary Clinical Lecturer, Cardiothoracic Institute
(Brompton Hospital), London

with a foreword by
MARGARET TURNER-WARWICK
D.M., Ph.D., F.R.C.P.

Professor of Medicine (Thoracic Medicine)
Cardiothoracic Institute, London

ERRATA

Page 3: Table 1.2. In some copies the characters in lines 5 and 6 of the column headed '1971' have been poorly impressed. They should read '16' and '30' respectively

Page 40: Table 2.1, Column 1. For 'Quintz' read 'Quartz'

BUTTERWORTHS

ENGLAND: BUTTERWORTH & CO. (PUBLISHERS) LTD.
                LONDON: 88 Kingsway, WC2B 6AB

AUSTRALIA: BUTTERWORTHS PTY. LTD.
                SYDNEY: 586 Pacific Highway, NSW 2067
                MELBOURNE: 343 Little Collins Street, 3000
                BRISBANE, 204 Queen Street, 4000

CANADA: BUTTERWORTH & CO. (CANADA) LTD.
                TORONTO: 14 Curity Avenue, 374

NEW ZEALAND: BUTTERWORTHS OF NEW ZEALAND LTD.
                WELLINGTON: 26-28 Waring Taylor Street, 1

SOUTH AFRICA: BUTTERWORTH & CO. (SOUTH AFRICA) (PTY.) LTD.
                DURBAN: 152-154 Gale Street

Contents

Quidem enim tanti operis vtilitatem temptaui tractare et ordine certo doctorum precedencium sententias sub compendio redigere desideraui, plus fuit ex desiderio simplicioribus mihi similibus proficiendi quam ex cupiditate alicuius inanis iactancie procurande. Que circa prouidus lector simplicitati compilatoris parcat corrigendo. Et discat potius deliberata ratione emendare.

(My object, in wishing to reduce the opinions of the most distinguished teachers into one abridgement, was more the desire of assisting simpletons such as myself, than any passion to indulge in empty-headed ostentation. Wherefore, let the prudent reader spare the simpleness of the compiler by correcting the book and let him learn to amend its faults with mature deliberation.)

From *Breviarium Bartholomei* by Johannes de Mirfeld of St. Bartholomew's Priory, Smithfield. Medical Austin friar, died 1407. (*His Life and Works*. By Percival Horton-Smith Hartley and Harold Richard Alridge (1936), Cambridge University Press.)

Foreword

The hazard of inhaling silicious material into the lungs has existed so long as man has required stone for building. The industrial revolution triggered an explosion in the demand for coal and steel and the hazard to health of those providing the raw materials and the manufactured products which transformed the world in the nineteenth century, was accepted at first with fatalism. The plight of many of these workers was gradually appreciated as the nation's social conscience was roused towards the end of the century.

The study of industrial diseases has always presented special difficulties and these have tended to isolate this branch from the common run of general medicine. Not only has detection of the exact nature of the damaging agents often proved extremely difficult when complex industrial processes involve multiple exposures, but conflicting pressures from both management and workers have often hindered and complicated scientific investigation. These understandable attitudes have not been eased by the additional pressures introduced by legislation and compensation.

Lack of understanding about occupational disease cannot, however, be excused entirely on these grounds and it is certainly due in large part to the complexity of the scientific problems themselves.

Understanding occupational medicine involves knowledge far beyond the training of most medical graduates and includes the study of geology, chemistry, and biochemistry, and a detailed understanding of a very wide range of industrial and engineering processes. Even within the field of medicine the range of skills is great and requires expert knowledge of radiology, pathology, epidemiology, physiology and immunology.

In the face of these far-reaching demands it is not surprising that the subject of occupational medicine has been left to the experts and the gulf between them and the general clinician has remained wide. The situation has been aggravated by the dearth of readable textbooks.

Against this background, it is particularly valuable to have a succinct and up-to-date account of occupational lung disease which is relevant to present-day industrial processes, which summarizes selectively the basic information necessary for intelligent understanding and at the same time approaches the problem from the viewpoint of the practising physician.

Dr Raymond Parkes has had first-hand experience both as clinician and in the special field of pneumoconiosis with the Pneumoconiosis Medical Panels in Cardiff and London: with this he has been able to bring together successfully the mysteries of industrial pulmonary disease and the clinical manifestations and natural history as it affects the patient.

He discusses in detail many of the newer conditions now being recognized, with the increasing use of new materials the hazards of which are only just being realized. He has also included a discussion of the increasing number of lung diseases relating to organic dusts as well as those relating to noxious fumes and gases: the pathogenesis of these, depending so often on immunological factors, is opening up a new era in occupational medicine.

Disorders relating to environmental factors are perhaps above all others susceptible to control and prevention. An authoritative but readable account of occupational pulmonary disease is therefore of extremely practical importance to doctors in all branches of medicine who have to deal with the working population of our industrialized island.

Cardiothoracic Institute, London   M. TURNER-WARWICK

Preface

This book aims to be a reasonably comprehensive and up-to-date study of occupational disorders of the lung. It has been designed principally with the general, chest and industrial physician, and the postgraduate student of occupational medicine in mind; but I hope it will also be of value to the radiologist, pathologist, thoracic surgeon and to the general medical practitioner in industrial areas. Although the contents of Chapters 1, 4 and 5 will be known to readers in some of these categories I believe that they may be of value to others as they include many of the basic facts necessary to a proper understanding of the disorders described in the rest of the book.

Occupational lung disorders are important not only because they may give rise to respiratory disability but because of the diagnostic difficulties they often cause (especially when a worker has moved out of the area or from the country where the occupational exposure occurred), prognostic and therapeutic uncertainties, and because the increasing complexity of the materials and methods of modern technology multiplies potential risks—a point which has relevance to developing as well as to old-established industrial countries. Furthermore, in recent years, a heightened interest in these problems has been occurring throughout the world.

All these disorders can be conceived of as a confrontation between the lungs and all their resources, on the one hand, and inhaled mineral, chemical or organic aerosols, on the other; accordingly they should be regarded as being within, and not outside, the fold of thoracic and general medicine. Therefore, the book is concerned primarily with their medical features *vis-à-vis* the relevant occupational hazards some of which, indeed, have ceased to exist in recent years—although many folk who bear their stigmata survive—while *pari passu* new risks have arisen and increased. But for an accurate diagnostic assessment of individual cases or the study of groups of workers exposed to a particular hazard the physician may need to seek the expert knowledge of the geologist, geochemist, physicist, chemist, immunologist, engineer, occupational hygienist, factory manager or epidemiologist; in short, interdisciplinary collaboration is invaluable, if not essential. However, the techniques of dust sampling and control, ventilation, protective clothing, codes of practice and other aspects of hygiene are only briefly discussed in these pages as they not only lie outside my competence but constitute a book in themselves. Reference is made in the appropriate places to sources of this information. Important extrapulmonary disease in the form of the tumour malignant mesothelioma of the parietal pleura and peritoneum is necessarily included in Chapter 9.

Many national and international experts—who are acknowledged in a later page—in various fields have given me their unstinted and invaluable help in the preparation of the book but if it contains any shortcomings or inaccuracies these are to be attributed to me and not to them.

At this point it is fitting to pay tribute to Dr Anthony Caplan—with whom I have been privileged to be associated for some years both as colleague and friend—who unmasked the association of atypical behaviour and unusual radiographic appearances of coal pneumoconiosis in coal-miners with rheumatoid arthritis; for this observation and his subsequent elaboration of it has undoubtedly given a strong impetus to the recognition and investigation of the part which may be played by immunological reactions to inhaled agents which has implications far beyond his original discovery, not only in regard to other types of pneumoconiosis, but in lung disease unrelated to occupation. As Parkes Weber wrote some years ago, 'For one common disease or syndrome there are several rare ones, the study of any one of which can help scientific progress as much as the study of a common one.'* The full fruits of Caplan's observations still remain to be harvested.

Finally, I wish to express my gratitude to Professor Margaret Turner-Warwick for contributing the Foreword; and also to Dr J. Watkins-Pitchford, Chief Medical Adviser (Social Security) Department of Health and Social Security, for encouraging this work to go forward to publication, although I should make it clear that opinions expressed throughout the book do not necessarily reflect the views of the Department.

* Parkes Weber, F. (1946). *Rare Diseases and Some Debatable Subjects*, p. 7. London; Staples Press.

London   W. RAYMOND PARKES

Acknowledgements

I owe a great debt of gratitude to the following medical colleagues and to others in various non-medical disciplines—both in this country and from overseas—all of whom have given me the invaluable benefit of their advice and criticism with unfailing generosity and patience, some having read and re-read different parts of the typescript:

Dr A. C. Allison, National Institute of Medical Research, London: Dr N. F. Astbury, Director of Research, The British Ceramic Research Association: Dr L. C. F. Blackman, Director General, British Coal Utilisation Association: Dr P. M. Bretland: Dr W. D. Buchanan, Department of Employment and Productivity: Dr J. D. Cameron, Medical Advisor, Pilkington Brothers Limited: Mr W. A. Campbell, M.Sc., Mineral Resources Division, Institute of Geological Sciences, London: Dr J. E. Cotes: Mr B. T. Commins, Medical Research Council Air Pollution Unit, St Bartholomew's Hospital Medical College, London: Mr A. A. Cross, The Cape Asbestos Company Limited, London: Dr C. N. Davies: Dr M. Greenberg: Dr Harriet L. Hardy: Dr N. H. Hartshorne: Dr B. E. Heard: Mr D. E. Highley, B.Sc., Mineral Resources Division, Institute of Geological Sciences, London: Dr Marion Hildick-Smith: Dr K. F. W. Hinson: Dr A. A. Hodgson, Cape Asbestos Fibres Limited, Uxbridge: Mr M. W. Jesson, National Institute of Agricultural Engineering, Silsoe, Bedfordshire: Dr W. Jones Williams: Dr John Lacey, Rothamsted Experimental Station, Harpenden: Dr R. M. McGowan, Department of Health and Social Security: the late Dr C. B. McKerrow: Dr C. L. Mantell, Manhasset, New York: Dr W. Marshall, F.R.S., Atomic Energy Research Establishment, Harwell: Dr D. C. F. Muir: Dr S. B. Osborn, Department of Medical Physics, King's College Hospital, London: Dr F. D. Pooley, Department of Mineral Exploitation, University College, Cardiff: Professor Lynne Reid: Dr Ralph L. Sadler: Dr Roger M. E. Seal: Dr W. J. Smither: Dr Sidney Speil, Johns-Manville Research and Engineering Center, New Jersey: Professor Margaret Turner-Warwick: Dr J. C. Wagner: Dr R. G. B. Williamson (Department of Health and Social Security).

I am grateful to the American Conference of Governmental Hygienists for permission to reproduce some of its Threshold Limit Values for airborne contaminants and physical agents.

ACKNOWLEDGEMENTS

My thanks are also due to Mr K. G. Moreman (Chester Beatty Institute, London) for his excellent photomicrographs in *Figures 7.3, 7.4, 7.12, 7.14, 7.16, 8.6, 8.14, 9.4, 9.22* and *9.23*; to Miss L. Pegus and Mrs J. Muskett of the Medical Art and Photographic Departments of the Royal Marsden Hospital, London; to Mr R. T. Harris of the Pneumoconiosis Research Unit, Cardiff, for some of the whole-lung section photographs; the staff of Butterworths for their guidance and help; and to Mrs N. H. Murray for much secretarial assistance.

I am grateful, too, to Weidenfeld (Publishers) Ltd. (London) for permission to reproduce a short excerpt from *The Origin of Life* by the late Professor J. D. Bernal (1967). Acknowledgements accompany the tables and figures derived from the work of other authors.

Lastly, I am especially thankful to my wife for her forbearance during the long gestation of the book and for much typing and other help in its preparation.

W. R. P.

Abbreviations

ACGIH American Conference of Governmental Hygienists
ANF antinuclear factor
DAT differential agglutination test
FEV forced expiratory volume
FEV_1 forced expiratory volume in one minute
FRC functional residual capacity
FVC forced ventilatory capacity
HDI hexamethylene diisocyanate
IgA (E, G, M) immunoglobulin A (E, G, M)
MAC maximum allowable concentration
MDI diphenylmethane diisocyanate
NDI naphthalene diisocyanate
PEFR peak expiratory flow rate
PVP polyvinyl-pyrollidone
RF rheumatic factor
RV residual volume
SCAT sheep-cell agglutination test
TDI toluene diisocyanate
T_L lung gas transfer
TLC total lung capacity
TLV threshold limit value
UDS unit density sphere

VC vital capacity
WL working level
WLM working level month

Units and quantities

Å ångström(s) (10^{-10} m)
g gramme(s)
in inch(es)
kg kilogramme(s)
l litre(s)
m metre(s)
m² square metre(s)
m³ cubic metre(s)
(*similarly mm² and mm³, square and cubic mm*)
MeV mega electron volt(s)
mmHg millimetres of mercury pressure (torr)
mppcf million particles per cubic foot
*nm nanometre(s) (10^{-9} m)
*μm micrometre(s) (10^{-6} m)
ppm parts per million

* The use of the terms 'mμ' and 'milli-micro' is discouraged by the BSI and other bodies as is that of the terms 'μ' and 'micron' for micrometre.

1—Introductory Considerations

I. TERMINOLOGY

To begin with, it is necessary to have a clear idea of what we mean by 'pneumoconiosis' because a variety of general definitions and descriptions have been current—and still are—since Zenker coined the term in 1867. In some cases their form has been conditioned by the compensation standards of various countries and is then rarely scientifically adequate. There are some authorities today who advocate outright rejection of the term but, as it has been in use for more than a century, this is hardly practical and the necessity of defining and classifying pneumoconiosis from the medical standpoint, cannot be avoided. As Card (1967) has written: 'That the concept of disease is a mental construct and belongs logically to the class of useful fictions should not blind us to its practical utility. If we accept this mode of analysis of our experience and we wish to diagnose, that is, assign a group of data to a particular disease, we must be able to define the disease.'

'Pneumoconiosis'—Proust's (1874) modification of Zenker's term 'pneumonokoniosis' ($\pi\nu\epsilon\acute{\upsilon}\mu\omega\nu$, lungs; $\kappa\omega\eta\grave{\iota}os$, dust; $\acute{o}\sigma\iota s$, state of)—just means 'dusty lung'. Thus, semantically, any dust-ridden state of the lungs or disease process resulting from it may legitimately be called pneumoconiosis. Now, while it is true that classification may be done in a variety of ways according to the purpose for which it is intended, the most appropriate method of definition and classification for medical purposes (having in mind the meaning of the word 'pneumoconiosis') rests upon morbid anatomical changes.

In this light, therefore, pneumoconiosis can be defined simply as *the presence of inhaled dust in the lungs and their non-neoplastic tissue reaction to it*. There are three key words here; dust, lungs, and reaction.

Dust

Dusts consist of solid particles of mineral or organic origin dispersed in air and, as such, are distinct from vapours, fumes and smoke (these terms are defined in Chapter 3), although all these categories are commonly embraced by the general term *aerosol*. Hence, by definition, pneumoconiosis does not include lung disorders due to inhaled aerosols other than dusts.

Lung

Strictly anatomically, 'lung' does not include the pulmonary (visceral) or

B   1

parietal pleura which is of different embryological origin from the lung; and so, primary pleural disease due to inhaled dust (for example, hyaline plaque formation and malignant mesothelial tumours attributed to asbestos dusts) should not be classified as pneumoconiosis.

Reaction

The lungs react to inhaled dust in a variety of ways which are discussed in Chapter 4 but, briefly, the reaction may be transient as, for example, in the case of the acute 'interstitial pneumonia' or granuloma formation of farmers' lung, or give rise to permanent reticulin proliferation or collagenous fibrosis.

To avoid misunderstanding at the outset it is important to emphasize that, by common consent among pathologists, 'fibrosis' means excessive production of collagen fibres (or scarring) and not an excess of reticulin fibres (*see* Chapter 4). Dusts which cause fibrosis are termed fibrogenic.

Both inorganic (mineral) and organic dusts may be classified according to the type of reactions they produce and individual diseases placed into these categories (Table 1.1).

TABLE 1.1

A Classification of Pneumoconiosis with some Examples

Type of dust	Lung reaction	Examples
Inorganic (mineral)	No fibrosis—'inert' Local macrophage accumulation; little structural change; mild reticulin proliferation	Soot Iron (siderosis) Tin (stannosis) Barium (baritosis) Early stages of coal pneumoconiosis
	Sarcoid-like granuloma Foreign body granuloma	Beryllium disease Talc
	Collagenous fibrosis	Quartz and certain other forms of free silica (silicosis) 'Mixed dust' fibrosis Later stages of coal pneumoconiosis Asbestos (asbestosis) 'Talc' pneumoconiosis Beryllium disease
Organic (non-mineral) (e.g. antinomycete spores, avian and animal proteins	No fibrosis Transient 'interstitial pneumonia' or granuloma formation (acute extrinsic allergic alveolitis')	Farmers' lung Mushroom workers' lung Bagassosis Bird fanciers' lung
	Fibrosis Collagenous fibrosis (fibrosing 'alveolitis')	Farmers' lung Bagassosis Bird fanciers' lung

2

The foregoing definition of pneumoconiosis, it should be noted, embraces harmless as well as harmful changes in the lungs and in this book it refers both to dust accumulation and to dust-induced disease confined to the gas exchanging region of the lungs (that is, the acini—q.v. page 5) but which, in some instances (for example, farmers' lung), may also involve non-respiratory bronchioles.

Beryllium disease is a special case for, in addition to being a pneumoconiosis, it is also a systemic disorder and may be caused by fumes as well as dusts.

Because acute and chronic functional changes in the larger airways of the lungs caused by the inhalation of cotton and certain other vegetable dusts (that is, the 'byssinosis' group of diseases) are not associated with any characteristic morbid anatomical features, it is probably better not to classify them as 'pneumoconiosis' and, in accordance with common usage, this group is considered separately.

TABLE 1.2

NUMBERS OF NEW CASES OF MAJOR TYPES OF PNEUMOCONIOSIS AND BYSSINOSIS IN SELECTED ATTRIBUTABLE INDUSTRIES DIAGNOSED IN THE UNITED KINGDOM BY THE PNEUMOCONIOSIS MEDICAL PANELS

Industry	1951	1954	1957	1960	1963	1964	1966	1967	1968	1969	1970	1971
Coal mining	3035	4449	3456	3279	2268	1213	937	741	765	624	773	623
Asbestos	15	31	56	29	67	83	114	168	128	134	153	145
Refractories	20	26	51	16	24	13	14	18	10	16	11	17
Pottery	135	345	233	50	76	65	27	31	30	31	29	25
Slate mining and splitting	34	21	27	43	38	69	51	23	42	38	40	16
All foundries	156	256	259	99	86	72	55	44	52	40	48	30
Cotton (byssinosis)	43	73	160	403	354	271	149	146	126	78	110	
Flax (byssinosis)	–	–	–	–	–	–	9	14	3	–	–	

From H.M. Department of Health and Social Security Annual Reports. London: H.M.S.O. Every third year selected up to 1963.

Improper terminology, which is sometimes encountered and should be avoided at all costs, is exemplified by the use of 'silicosis' as a general term for all forms of pneumoconiosis, and 'pneumoconiosis' as a synonym for coal pneumoconiosis.

During the past hundred years the incidence of silicosis and the pneumoconiosis of coal miners steadily increased in most major industrial countries until the 1950s, since when it has undergone a downward trend, while asbestosis has become increasingly more frequent, and disorders of the extrinsic allergic 'alveolitis' type (for example, farmers' lung) have only recently been properly recognized. These trends are reflected in Table 1.2 which shows newly diagnosed compensation cases in Britain. Figures such as these, of course, are crude in that they are selective. The Report of the Katowice Symposium (1968), however, indicates that similar trends are occurring in other major industrial countries. But in newly developing countries the hazards which cause some of these diseases have only recently arisen and, if not properly controlled, will lead to new endemic areas of pneumoconiosis.

3

In short, pneumoconiosis and other dust-induced diseases are an important medical problem from the standpoint of differential diagnosis, and in causing respiratory disability and, sometimes, premature death in certain occupations.

II. ANATOMY

Some familiarity with the basic features of lung anatomy and cytology is necessary for an understanding of the pathogenesis and behaviour of the different types of pneumoconiosis and other occupational lung diseases.

Lung airways

From the trachea downwards each branch of the airways divides progressively into two daughter branches the length and diameter of which are not necessarily uniform. The average diameter of daughter branches is smaller than

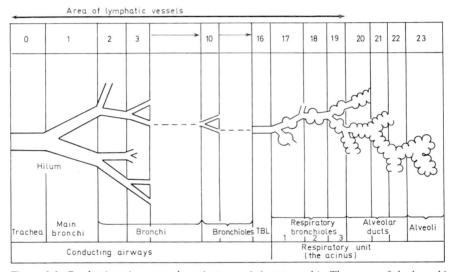

Figure 1.1. Conducting airways and respiratory unit (not to scale). The zones of the bronchi and bronchioles are truncated. The relative size of the respiratory unit is greatly enlarged; this is in fact about one-sixth of the distance from hilum to distal alveoli. Figures at the heads of the columns indicate the approximate number of generations from trachea to alveoli. (Modified, with permission, from Weibel, 1963)

that of the parent branch but, over the complete number of some twenty-three generations, the total cross-section and volume of the airways system increase progressively while the individual airways become smaller.

   Bronchi are characterized by the presence of variable amounts of cartilage in their walls; the continuations of these airways without cartilage to the alveolar areas of the lung constitute the *bronchioles*. The last three or four (rarely, up to eight) generations of bronchioles which carry a variable number of *alveoli* (alveolus, a little hollow) in their walls are named *respiratory bronchioles* because they are capable of gas exchange. The *terminal bronchiole* is the last airway without alveoli before the first respiratory bronchiole (*Figure 1.1*). This diagram is not drawn to scale, the airways of the respiratory unit being shown disproportionally large by comparison with the conducting

4

airways, and the distance between generations 4 and 17 spans the greater length of the lung.

The lining of the airways as far as the terminal bronchiole consists of epithelial cells which are of pseudo-stratified, columnar and ciliated type; situated irregularly between them are mucus-secreting *goblet cells* opening to the surface. Goblet cells are plentiful proximally but become progressively fewer in number distally until, in the bronchioles, they are extremely scanty— at least in health.

Mucous glands are found only in bronchi and lie between the epithelium and cartilage. Their total volume is substantially greater than that of the goblet cells and it is likely that they produce the greater part of mucus secretion in health and disease (Reid, 1960). Increased activity is expressed by hypertrophy. This hypertrophy is the structural basis of chronic bronchitis, and the comparison of gland thickness to bronchial wall thickness is a valuable practical index of its presence and degree of severity (Reid, 1960). (Section V, this chapter.)

Secreted mucus spreads as an uneven layer on the cilia which possess an auto-rhythmic stroke directed proximally and advancing the layer in that direction; this process is often referred to as the 'ciliary escalator'. Although this is an efficient arrangement for removal of inhaled foreign particles it may be impaired or destroyed by some noxious agents, and excess mucus in chronic bronchitis may sometimes impose an undue burden upon the cilia.

The respiratory unit

The most distal respiratory bronchioles end in *alveolar ducts* which open into the *alveolar sacs* with clusters of alveoli (*Figure 1.1*). *Alveoli*, and their contained gas, are so closely in contact with the alveolar capillaries as to be integral with them.

The respiratory bronchioles, alveolar ducts and alveoli, therefore, comprise a respiratory unit—the *acinus* (a berry) (*Figure 1.1*). The size and shape of acini vary but they are from 0·5 to 1·0 cm in length.

Lobules consist of a variable number of respiratory units (from three to five) which may be partly bound by connective tissue; their shape and size are very variable.

Alveoli are, on average, about 0·15 mm in diameter, approximately 300 million in number (possibly more) and their total surface area, which is proportional to lung volume, of the order of 70 to 80 square metres (Weibel, 1968). This area is estimated to vary by about one-third between full expiration and inspiration with a range of values from approximately 30 to 100 square metres respectively (von Hayek, 1960). Obviously, therefore, the lungs possess great respiratory reserve. It appears that about 40 per cent of alveoli are located on the respiratory bronchioles and alveolar ducts (Pump, 1969).

There are small tubular communications—the accessory bronchiolo-alveolar communications of Lambert (1955)—between some terminal and respiratory bronchioles and neighbouring alveoli. These accessory air inlets, as they appear to be, probably contribute to collateral ventilation, and dust particles or dust-containing macrophages may be found in them and in contiguous alveoli.

Alveolar walls are composed of a number of differing cell types which are variously responsible for gas exchange, disposal of inhaled foreign material, and immunological activity within the lung. Their appearance, distribution and relationships have been established by electron microscopy and six groups of cells can be distinguished morphologically in human lungs (Brooks, 1966). This is shown diagrammatically in *Figure 1.2*.

(1) *Type I Pneumocytes.*—Flat and extremely thin epithelial cells which form a continuous layer (about 0·2 μm thick away from their nuclei and invisible by light microscopy) over the alveolus apart from sporadic interruption by Type II pneumocytes. Both types of cell rest on a tenuous, but

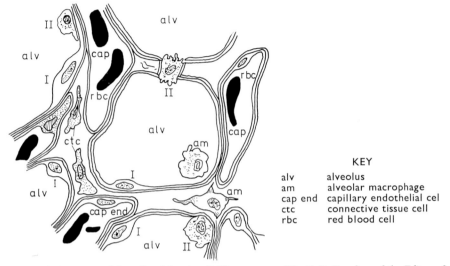

KEY

alv	alveolus
am	alveolar macrophage
cap end	capillary endothelial cel
ctc	connective tissue cell
rbc	red blood cell

Figure 1.2. Diagram of the cells of the alveoli. (By courtesy of Dr R. E. Brooks and the Editor of American Review of Respiratory Diseases)

continuous, basement membrane composed of reticulin fibres (*see* Chapter 4). These cells are generally regarded as non-phagocytic but some doubt concerning this has been expressed (*see* Chapter 3).

(2) *Type II pneumocytes.*—Rounded or cuboidal epithelial cells set here and there in the alveolar walls; they are characterized by lamellated inclusions and may have mild phagocytic properties. They appear to develop from Type I cells, and most probably secrete surfactant.

(3) *Alveolar macrophages.*—These lie in contact with Type I cells or in small groups within the alveolus but are distinct from Type II cells. They contain a variable number of phagosomes (*see* Chapter 4) with ingested material. They apparently originate outside the lungs from precursor cells (promonocytes) in the bone marrow and from peripheral blood monocytes (that is, promonocyte→monocyte→macrophage) thus forming a distinct cell line (van Furth, 1970) to which the term 'mononuclear phagocyte system' has been given. They are actively mobile and phagocytic and the chief protagonists in the reaction of lungs to inhaled particles (*see* Chapter 4).

(4) *Endothelial cells.*—In the capillaries these rest on a basement membrane of reticulin. The capillaries, of course, contain the cellular elements of the blood.

(5) *Connective tissue cells.*—Fibroblasts.

(6) *Leucocytes and lymphocytes in the interalveolar septa.*—These are infrequent in the normal lung.

This arrangement—shown in the electron micrograph (*Figure 1.3*) of rat lung which is similar to human lung—provides intimate proximity of alveolar gas and capillary blood (gas/blood 'interface') and the opportunity for macrophages and, possibly to some extent, Type II pneumocytes to ingest exogenous and endogenous material (*see* Chapters 3 and 4). Cells containing dust migrate from the alveoli to the ciliary 'escalator' and are subsequently expelled in the sputum or into the bronchiolar lymph vessels from which they pass to regional lymph nodes (*see* Chapter 3).

Lung framework

The cellular elements of the lung are supported mainly by reticulin, elastic and collagen fibres. Reticulin fibres are the main support of alveolar walls which are reinforced by elastic fibres with collagen less well represented. As already stated, both basement membranes consist of reticulin fibres which are also found in the ground substance of the alveolar septa between the capillary and pulmonary epithelial cells.

The rest of the lung also has a framework of reticulin, collagen and elastic fibres.

Surface active agent (surfactant)

A substance which may be produced (at least in part) by Type II cells (Corrin, 1970) and reduces surface tension has been demonstrated in the alveoli (Pattle, 1955). It is a lipoprotein containing saturated dipalmitoyl lecithin which, *in vitro*, is one of the most stable surface active agents known; it has the unusual property of its surface tension rising when it is stretched and falling nearly to zero when compressed. Almost certainly this prevents the lung collapsing when its transpleural pressure is reduced (as in expiration) and allows alveoli of different sizes to remain open at the same transpleural pressure (Pattle, 1968).

There is as yet no evidence that alteration in its properties is involved in the pathogenesis of pneumoconiosis.

Blood supply

Pulmonary arteries conveying venous blood and bronchial arteries conveying arterial blood into the lungs are closely associated with the bronchi and all are enveloped by a common connective tissue sheath the *broncho-arterial bundle*.

Pulmonary arteries accompany the bronchi—although they branch more frequently—and do not become capillaries until they reach the respiratory bronchioles, at which point they form an increasingly rich plexus in intimate proximity to the alveolar epithelium so that only the thickness of the pulmonary epithelial cells, the two basement membranes and a fine tissue space separate alveolar gas from capillary blood (*Figure 1.3*). This thickness away from cell nuclei may be as little as 0·2 μm. The capillary surface area is equal to that of the alveoli, that is, some 70 to 80 square metres (Weibel, 1963).

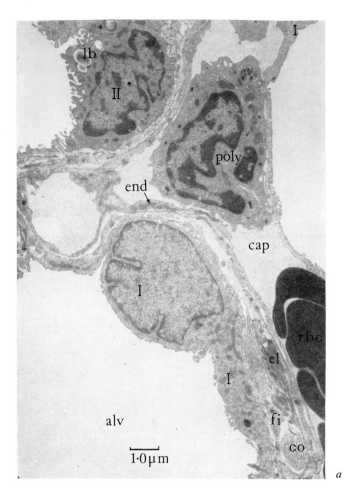

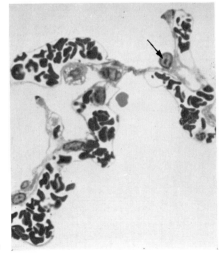

Figure 1.3. (a) Electron micrograph of part of rat alveolar wall showing a polymorph and red blood cells (rbc) in a capillary (cap) lined by endothelial cell (end). The majority of the alveolus (alv) is lined by processes from the Type I pneumocyte (I). The top left of the picture shows a Type II pneumocyte (II) characterized by its lamellated bodies (lb). The interstitium contains collagen (co) and elastin (el); a fibroblast (fi) can be seen. (Original magnification × 15,000, reproduced at × 7,500; fixation, glutamic acid and osmium tetroxide; stain, uranyl acetate and lead hydroxide). (b) Part of a rat alveolar wall showing red blood cells in a capillary. A type II pneumocyte can be recognized by its vacuolated cytoplasm and a Type I pneumocyte is arrowed. (1 μm section; magnification × 675; stained toluidine blue.) Note: the morphology of rat and human lung is similar. (By courtesy of Professor Lynne Reid)

Lymphatics

These are evident in the vicinity of respiratory bronchioles and there are lymph capillaries between the alveolar walls and interlobular, pleural, peribronchiolar and perivascular connective tissue, but not in the alveolar walls (Lauweryns, 1970); these are important channels for elimination of particles from the lungs. Anastomoses exist between lymph vessels in the walls of blood vessels and those in bronchial walls (Trapnell, 1963, 1964).

Lymph moves in the interstitial tissue 'spaces' which are under sub-atmospheric pressure and so enters lymph vessels situated at the periphery of lobules or in the walls of blood vessels and bronchi. Because of the arrangement of valves in these vessels most of the lymph flows centrally to the hilar lymph nodes, but numerous small lymph nodes sited throughout the lung at or near the bifurcation of bronchioles and bronchi intercept its flow. Minute collections of lymphoid tissue which contain both phagocytic and immunologically active cells form cuffs around respiratory bronchioles and their arteries (von Hayek, 1960), and are undoubtedly important in the lung's reaction to inhaled particles which often accumulate at these sites.

The relationship of the lymphatic vessels to the A and B lines of Kerley sometimes seen on chest radiographs is referred to in Chapter 5.

III. PHYSIOLOGY

A detailed discussion of the principles, definitions and techniques of lung function tests is out of place here. (There are some excellent books available on the subject, for example, Comroe *et al.*, 1962; Campbell, 1968; Cotes, 1968.) But as the performance and appraisal of lung function tests is commonly an integral part of the diagnosis and follow-up of suspected and known cases of pneumoconiosis, a brief summary of the patterns of abnormal function and reference to a few important practical points is, perhaps, indicated.

Before doing this, however, it is worth recalling that *dyspnoea* is a subjective sensation of discomfort caused by the necessity for increased respiratory effort to a point beyond which it is obtrudes unpleasantly into consciousness, and that it has causes other than diseases of the lungs and pleura. For example, anaemia and obesity; congenital and acquired heart diseases; metabolic disturbances such as hyperthyroidism and the acidosis of diabetes mellitus and uraemia; and severe kyphoscoliosis. Sometimes one or other of these disorders may be overlooked as the cause of dyspnoea in a patient who also happens to have a pneumoconiosis. In which case dyspnoea may be wrongly attributed to the pneumoconiosis and not to the true cause which thus remains untreated. Indeed the dramatic nature of abnormal radiographic appearances in some pneumoconiosis cases may be an effective distraction in this respect.

PATTERNS OF DISORDERED LUNG FUNCTION

Obstructive syndrome

Chronic non-specific lung disease—by which is meant asthma, emphysema and chronic bronchitis with or without emphysema—usually causes a greater or lesser degree of obstruction to air flow in the airways due to narrowing of the smaller bronchi. It may be reversible, as in the case of asthma, or irreversible, as in chronic obstructive bronchitis and some types of emphysema.

Obstruction to air flow occurs chiefly on expiration—but to some extent on inspiration—and in emphysema of panlobular type (Section IV, this Chapter) it may exist only during expiration. Resistance to air flow in the airways is increased and the degree of obstruction is easily and practically determined by measuring the proportion of the *forced vital capacity* (FVC) which can be expelled during a fixed period of time—that is, the *forced expiratory volume* (FEV). The time interval most commonly used is one second (FEV_1). The FEV_1/FVC percentage varies widely in normal subjects according to age and height, the range being about 55 to 99 per cent in males and 64 to 98 per cent in females.

Normally FVC and *vital capacity* (VC) have closely similar values but, in the presence of obstruction to air flow, VC may be substantially larger than FVC because forced expiration increases airway narrowing more than unforced expiration.

Air flow obstruction frequently gives rise to uneven distribution of inspired air which results in an increase in the inequality of the ratio of ventilation to blood flow which normally exists in the lungs. In normal lungs ventilation and blood flow (perfusion) are, for the greater part, not equally matched and either one is greater than the other in different positions in the lungs. Regional differences of the ratio of ventilation to perfusion are the chief reason why normal oxygen tension of arterial blood is not 100 mmHg, but varies from 95 to 97 mmHg mercury. Hence, lung disease which impairs ventilation or causes a local or general reduction in perfusion will give rise to arterial oxygen desaturation. When emphysema is the cause of air flow obstruction—'air trapping'—the normal elastic recoil tendency of the lungs is reduced and *residual volume* (RV) increased, thereby occupying a greater percentage of *total lung capacity* (TLC) than normal; and TLC is also increased. This increase in RV is not specific for emphysema as it also occurs in other forms of chronic non-specific lung disease.

Restrictive syndrome
This consists in the inability of the lungs to expand as fully as they should from any cause, such as: the effects of left ventricular failure, impairment of full movement of the chest wall (as for example, the sequelae of haemothorax), and by diffuse interstitial fibrosis ('fibrosing alveolitis') of the lungs from whatever origin, including asbestosis.

VC and FVC are reduced but FEV_1/FVC per cent remains normal (or is increased), provided there is no co-existent obstructive airways disease. The VC is, in fact a most valuable, simple, discriminating test of the presence of parenchymal lung disease in asbestos workers (*see* Chapter 9). TLC is reduced because the distensibility of the lungs is diminished and, in the case of diffuse interstitial fibrosis, the elastic recoil is greater than normal and its reciprocal, *compliance*, reduced.

Impairment of gas exchange
Exchange of gases across the alveolar-capillary interface is impaired when ventilation is reduced in relation to blood flow either locally or generally.

This may occur in diseases causing the 'restrictive' or 'obstructive' patterns of functional disorder, or when blood flow is reduced relative to ventilation. The appearance of diffuse interstitial fibrosis (from whatever cause) under the light microscope may give the impression that resistance to diffusion of gases across the interface would unfailingly result, but this is often not so to any significant degree.

However, although impairment of gas diffusion due to increased interface resistance alone is unusual, in the early stages of diffuse interstitial fibrosis and granulomatous lung diseases the diffusing capacity of the alveolar capillary membrane (D_m) and arterial oxygen saturation, while normal at rest, may be reduced during exercise and associated with hyperventilation, without any abnormality of other parameters of lung function. This may be encountered, for example, in asbestosis, chronic beryllium disease and chronic extrinsic allergic 'alveolitis'. Although interpretation of the results of the D_m test has often been uncertain due to a high coefficient of variation, recent work has shown that when the conditions of its measurement are properly controlled it is a reliable test (Cotes and Hall, 1970).

Apart from inequality of the ventilation-perfusion ratio, arterial hypoxaemia is also caused by loss of diffusing surface and reduction of the capillary bed (Burrows, 1967) which may occur in some aged lungs and in panlobular emphysema.

The effects of impaired gas diffusing capacity are the same irrespective of the underlying cause and can be summarized as follows.

(1) Increased frequency of ventilation on effort; that is, the minute ventilation is increased relative to oxygen uptake.

(2) Diminished diffusion of gas across the alveolar–capillary interface either at rest or on exercise, or under both conditions.

(3) Hypoxaemia on exercise.

The misleading term 'alveolar capillary block syndrome', is best avoided, and the exchange of gases by the lungs should be referred to as either 'lung diffusing capacity' or *gas transfer factor* (Cotes, 1968). This emphasizes that impairment of gas diffusion occurs for reasons other than abnormality of interface.

It is worth noting that molecular diffusion is the primary factor governing the distribution of inhaled gases in the acinar airways, mechanical mixing being of minor importance (Muir, 1967).

Hyperventilation

Anxiety, disease of the lung parenchyma, panlobular emphysema (rarely chronic obstructive bronchitis) and skeletal diseases which restrict thoracic movement, if sufficiently severe, cause hyperventilation on exercise or at rest. Hyperventilation may be present at rest as well as on effort in persons with the granulomatous (or 'proliferative') stages of 'farmers' lung' type disease, beryllium disease and sarcoidosis. It is out of proportion to reduction in VC and may be of reflex origin mediated by the vagus nerve and due to involvement of lung receptors—possibly the 'deflation receptors' of Paintal (1970) —by the disease process. Some support for this is given by the fact that the breathlessness is reduced by vagus nerve block (Guz *et al.*, 1970) and steroid therapy (Cotes, Johnson and McDonald, 1970). It is important to recognize this possibility in order that dyspnoea from this cause is not dismissed as psychoneurotic. By contrast, this effect does not occur with established fibrosis, for example, asbestosis.

Hypoventilation
Reduction in the volume of ventilation per minute impairs alveolar ventilation which in turn leads to hypoxaemia due to ventilation-perfusion imbalance, and also to carbon dioxide accumulation (hypercapnia) in the arterial blood. It may be caused by depression of activity of the respiratory control centre in the reticular formation of the medulla oblongata due to local lesions or the action of inhibiting drugs, by pronounced weakness of the respiratory muscles (e.g. old age and myopathies), and by excessive obesity and severe kyphoscoliosis or ankylosing spondylitis which also impair chest movement. The lungs themselves may be free of disease or be the seat of unrelated disease.

Mixed patterns
Disturbance of lung function usually consists of more than one of the foregoing categories.

PRACTICAL POINTS RELATING TO ROUTINE LUNG FUNCTION TESTS

The simpler tests of ventilatory function can be done in the consulting room, chest clinic, home, factory, or the hospital ward side-room; the more elaborate can only be done in the laboratory. The most valuable of all simple tests for routine use are FEV_1, FVC and VC. Of these FEV_1, which fulfils all the criteria for choice of lung function tests (Cotes, 1968) provides the best single test there is for assessment of respiratory disability, and the presence and severity of airway obstruction is given by its percentage of the FVC.

There are various instruments available for the performance of these tests but it is important that the one employed is robust, has a good capacity, as low a resistance to air flow as possible, and an accurate automatic timing device; and furthermore, that its maintenance and calibration should be simple and carried out regularly.

Because these tests are frequently done by non-physiologists (including physicians, nursing and non-medical personnel) it is important that every detail of their performance is properly carried out. The subject must remove heavy or tight clothing, lumbar belts and loose dentures; be comfortably seated before the apparatus; make the deepest possible inspiration and then close his mouth firmly round the mouthpiece, taking care not to obstruct it with his tongue. He must blow without hesitation as forcefully as possible down the tube; make two or three preliminary attempts before recording some three or four blows, of which the mean is taken as the result; and rest for about thirty seconds between each blow. It is not necessary to blow much beyond one second until the last blow when FVC is tested and then forceful expiration must be pressed to the utmost. This is best done last as it is more exhausting and sometimes provokes a paroxysm of coughing. VC is performed in the same way but with a slow expiratory effort. Clipping of the nose, which is not otherwise necessary when performing these tests, is required in persons with cleft palate.

One observer, rather than a number, should do the tests and it is advisable that checks are made to establish that his results have consistent agreement with those of a known reliable observer or laboratory.

The other commonly used single breath test which reflects ventilatory capacity is the *peak expiratory flow rate (PEFR)*. This varies with the interval of time during which it is recorded, but it is usually taken as the maximum expiratory flow that can be sustained for a period of 10 ms. To perform the test the deepest possible inspiration is taken followed by a sudden forceful expiration. Used alone, it is less informative than FEV_1 and FVC. Portable instruments for its measurements (such as the Wright peak flow meter) tend to vary in their characteristics so that comparison of results from different instruments is likely to be unsatisfactory. The test should never be used as an equivalent of FEV_1 and FVC or by itself, other than to furnish a serial index of, say, the effect of treatment with a bronchodilator drug.

Records of all tests should include the subject's age, height, sex, ethnic group and smoking habit. Prediction of 'normal' values is related to the first four of these. The importance of smoking is referred to later.

Prediction formulas or nomograms should be derived from data from the same ethnic group as the subject tested and, as far as possible, from a kindred population. When recording the results, the source of the predicted normal should be stated; this applies equally to all lung function tests. Acceptable prediction indices and tables are available for the United Kingdom (Cotes, 1968), the United States (Kory *et al.*, 1961; Boren, Kory and Syner, 1966; these do not distinguish racial groups) and India (Rao *et al.*, 1961; Cotes, 1968). Normal values for the gas transfer factor are reviewed by Cotes and Hall (1970).

Inter-laboratory variation of 'normal' values, especially for gas transfer, are often very large and may invalidate comparison of physiological data at different times in the same subject.

Standardization

Not only must apparatus used outside the laboratory be generally acceptable but it must be frequently calibrated against a known standard. This means that the timing units of direct reading spirometers should be calibrated daily, as should the technical features of other apparatus.

The temperature of the room where tests are performed must be kept at a reasonably constant level in keeping with that of the country in which they are being performed, and at least one hour should have elapsed between the subject's last smoking or receiving bronchodilator drugs and performance of the test and two hours between a main meal and the test.

INFLUENCE OF AGE ON LUNG FUNCTION

There is evidence that from the fifth decade onward, alveolar volume decreases and airway volume increases—both significantly. In other words there is 'a shift in pulmonary air-space volume from alveoli to ducts which is often called "ageing emphysema" if the shift is marked enough' (Weibel, 1968). This is likely to explain certain of the changes of values in lung function tests associated with age, although weakness of the respiratory muscles contributes.

The elastic recoil of the lungs gradually becomes reduced. In men RV

13

increases but TLC does not increase significantly. In women, however, TLC is apt to decline; and in both sexes the RV/TLC percentage gradually increases. The values of VC and FEV_1 fall with increasing age; in Caucasian males without respiratory disease FEV_1 falls by about 0·03 litre per year (Cotes, 1968) if they are non-smokers.

The capacity for transfer of gases across the alveolar-capillary interface is reduced by about 33 per cent between the ages of 20 and 60 years due primarily to some loss of interface and to a decrease in alveolar capillary blood vessel volume which is also responsible for a less progressive reduction in the diffusing capacity (or transfer factor, T_L) of the lungs (Cotes, 1968).

Most parameters of lung function are closely related to age throughout life; a fact which must always be taken into account when the possible effects of lung disease upon function are assessed.

INFLUENCE OF SMOKING ON LUNG FUNCTION

Tobacco smoke has a significantly deleterious effect on lung function which is most pronounced with cigarette smoking.

First, there is increased airways resistance which is observed as an acute effect lasting for about an hour after smoking both in habitual smokers and non-smokers (McDermott and Collins, 1965; Stirling, 1967) and second, there is a chronic effect characterized by a high correlation of airways obstruction with cigarette smoking in both sexes and all age groups.

Therefore, FEV_1/FVC per cent and FVC are, on average, lower in smokers than non-smokers; it has been shown that the mean annual decline of FEV_1 in a United Kingdom population is between 0·05 and 0·10 litre per year in smokers (Higgins and Oldham, 1962) compared with approximately 0·03 litre in non-smokers.

Airways obstruction in smokers, however, is not always accompanied by symptoms (Franklin and Lowell, 1961) even though chronic obstructive bronchitis is very much more prevalent among smokers than non-smokers.

Vital capacity, TLC and compliance (that is, 1/elastic recoil) are lower, and RV_1 RV/TLC percentage, gas mixing index and non-elastic resistance higher in smokers than in non-smokers (Zwi et al., 1963; Krumholz, Chevalier and Ross, 1964); and, by comparison with non-smokers, gas transfer factor is reduced at rest and on effort in smokers (Krumholz, Chevalier and Ross, 1964; Van Ganse, Ferris and Cotes, 1972) and the coefficient of diffusion for carbon monoxide is impaired. It is believed that the reduction in the transfer factor may be due to a change in the volume of blood in the pulmonary capillaries (Van Ganse, Ferris and Cotes, 1972). All these changes of function are found in both sexes and are of significant order; they tend to be greater the larger the cigarette consumption and are well established after ten years of smoking. Furthermore, impairment of gas transfer occurs even in seemingly healthy smokers who have no evident impairment of ventilatory function or airways abnormality (Martt, 1962; Rankin, Gee and Chosy, 1965).

Stopping smoking, however, results in a decrease of airways obstruction and resistance, both inspiratory and expiratory, but not in improvement of VC (Wilhelmsen, 1967). Even so, return to functional levels equal to those of persons who have never smoked is unusual.

Women smokers are affected in the same way as men but less severely. Pipe and cigar smoking causes a similar pattern of functional impairment to that of cigarettes although of significantly less severity.

It is clear, then, that because of the profound effect smoking has upon the lungs, a detailed history of smoking habits must never be omitted. This should show whether a person is a non-smoker (that is, has never smoked), a smoker, or an ex-smoker and the duration of smoking in years and the number of cigarettes or grammes of tobacco smoked; if an ex-smoker, the year of stopping should be ascertained. Cigarette, pipe and cigar smoking should be shown separately. And, finally, smoking history and its effects must always be considered when interpreting the results of lung function tests.

APPLICATION OF LUNG FUNCTION TESTS IN OCCUPATIONAL LUNG DISEASE

Diagnosis

Lung function tests themselves are not diagnostic of any particular disease, but in many cases they form a necessary part of diagnostic criteria.

Whereas the standard tests of lung volumes, ventilation, gas distribution and transfer are not required in every case or at each examination, the basic ventilatory tests are indispensable in all.

Function tests may provide some guide to prognosis in cases (for example) of asbestosis, chronic beryllium disease and chronic obstructive bronchitis; they evaluate the response to treatment of reversible disorders, such as acute extrinsic allergic 'alveolitis' from any cause, and those which are present coincidently with a pneumoconiosis. When the effects of increasing age are allowed for, periodic tests are helpful in establishing whether or not disease has progressed and, if so, to what extent.

Prevention of disease

Determination of FEV_1 and FVC when a worker is about to enter any industry which may be hazardous to the lungs is essential in establishing a point of reference for later similar tests, and subsequently to detect the onset of incipient lung disease as early as possible. Data of this sort from a large number of individuals in an industry can be related to conditions of their work and exposure to dust or to physical or chemical agents. This not only provides essential prospective data about the health of a working population, but is a valuable contribution to the health of the individual worker.

More comprehensive tests may be indicated in workers in some industries (for example, those where there is exposure to asbestos or beryllium compounds) whose FVC or FEV_1 show an unexpected fall.

The application of physiological tests to industrial lung disease is surveyed in detail by Cotes in the International Labour Office publication *Respiratory Function Tests in Pneumoconiosis* (1966).

IV. EMPHYSEMA

The term emphysema—$\dot{\epsilon}\mu\phi\nu\sigma\hat{a}\nu$, to inflate or puff up—is descriptive of altered form without implying the cause or pathogenesis of this alteration. Like anaemia, emphysema of the lungs is a morphological complex comprising not one disease process but a number.

15

The terminology of emphysema was much confused until the definitions of the Ciba Foundation Guest Symposium (1959) in the United Kingdom and the American Thoracic Society (1962) were proposed, since when there has been fairly good, if not complete, agreement.

The definition of emphysema given by Reid (1967), which rests on structural and not functional abnormality, has the merit of simplicity and avoids implication of pathogenesis:

> Emphysema is a condition of the lung characterized by increase beyond the normal in the size of air spaces distal to the terminal bronchiolus, i.e. the acinus.

As a general rule air spaces are said to be emphysematous if they measure 1 mm or more in diameter.

Although dilated air spaces are found in some cases of diffuse interstitial pulmonary fibrosis (fibrosing alveolitis) as 'honeycomb lung' and might, therefore, be classed as emphysema, the lesions are distinguished by commonly involving terminal and non-respiratory bronchioles as well as acini, and by gross and microscopical features which are referred to briefly on page 26.

Only those types of emphysema which are common in adult life are briefly described as they are most likely to be associated with a pneumoconiosis or other occupational lung disorders. The classification used throughout is that of the Ciba Foundation Guest Symposium and much of what follows rests on the work of Reid (1967).

The unit of description used by Reid (1967) is the acinus, but some other pathologists (e.g., Wyatt, Fletcher and Sweet, 1961; Gough, 1968; Heard, 1969) prefer to employ the lobule for this purpose as it can usually be seen with the unaided eye in lung slices, partly delineated by fibrous septa. Hence the terms 'centriacinar' and 'panacinar' are taken as equivalent, respectively, to 'centrilobular' and panlobular' Although the acinus cannot be distinguished by the unaided eye its use is more consistent with the accepted definition of emphysema. However, as the terminology based on the lobule is so widely current it will be used throughout this book, but with this reservation continually in mind.

The types of pathological changes which may be found are described, according to their dominant position in the lobule or acinus, as follows (*Figure 1.4*).

(1) Enlargement of alveoli in or near the centre of the lobule or acinus: *centrilobular* (*centriacinar*) *emphysema.*

(2) Enlargement of alveoli throughout the lobule or acinus: *panlobular* (*panacinar*) *emphysema.*

(3) Enlargement of alveoli at the periphery of the acinus only and contiguous with connective tissue septa or sheaths: *paraseptal* (*periacinar*) *emphysema.*

(4) Enlargement of alveoli which does not involve the acinus universally, is not characteristically located in one part of it, and is associated with scars; *scar, paracicatricial or irregular emphysema.*

Each of these types may be localized or widespread, of slight or severe degree, and more than one type may be found in the same lung. The characteristic appearances of centrilobular and panlobular emphysema are shown in

16

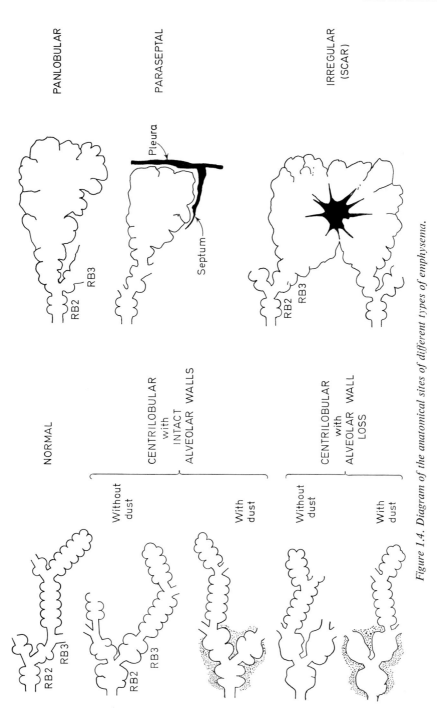

Figure 1.4. Diagram of the anatomical sites of different types of emphysema.

C

17

the accompanying illustrations compared with normal lung (*Figures 1.5 to 1.10*). *Figures 1.5 to 1.7* are natural-size photographs of lung sections and *Figures 1.8 to 1.10* are slightly magnified photomicrographs of the same types of emphysema.

Abnormal enlargement of alveoli may be caused by:

(*a*) Atrophy of their walls due to causes which are not understood.

(*b*) Destruction of their walls may sometimes result from inflammatory disease, although in most cases the cause is obscure. However, some cases of panlobular emphysema which has a predilection for the lower parts of the

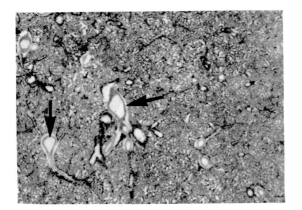

Figure 1.5. Normal lung. Alveolar spaces are less than 1 mm in diameter. Arrows indicate bronchi. (From paper-mounted section, natural size)

lungs, and is usually accompanied by chronic bronchitis and the onset of dyspnoea on exertion before the fifth decade are now known to be associated with an inherited deficiency of the enzyme α_1-antitrypsin carried by an autosomal recessive gene. The incidence of homozygous deficiency in these cases may be as much as 18 per cent (Leading Article, 1971) or even higher (Hutchinson *et al.*, 1971). The pathogenesis of the emphysema remains to be explained but cigarette smoking appears to have an important contributory effect (Leading Article, 1971). Immunological processes may be of importance in other types.

It is possible to separate types of emphysema into those with 'air trapping' (or airways obstruction) and those without. Air trapping is revealed by physiological tests during life and observations of the lungs at operation or post-mortem examination when they fail to deflate normally in whole or in part. It is a common and important cause of functional impairment.

Centrilobular (centriacinar) emphysema
This consists of a localized enlargement of the alveoli of respiratory bronchioles and, to some extent, of the walls of these bronchioles. The walls of the distended alveoli either remain intact, though distorted, or are lost to a variable degree. These two states can be referred to respectively as '*distensive*' *and* '*destructive*' *centrilobular emphysema* (Heard, 1969), but it is to be understood that 'distensive' and 'destructive' are used here in a descriptive sense and do not imply pathogenesis. When the walls are intact ('distensive'

centrilobular emphysema) the lesions appear to the naked eye as small
isolated holes across which tenuous strands of the walls of enlarged alveoli

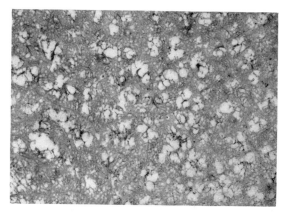

(*a*) *Slight to moderate without
dust pigmentation*

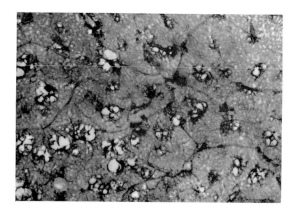

(*b*) *Slight to moderate with dust
pigmentation*

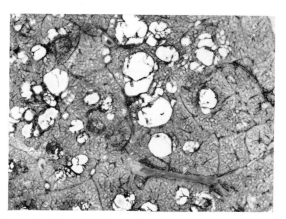

(*c*) *Moderately severe with very
slight pigmentation*

*Figure 1.6. Examples of centrilobular emphysema.
(From paper-mounted sections, natural size)*

are visible, but the basic alveolar structure persists. The holes vary from 1 mm to 4 mm diameter and the surrounding alveoli are normal (*Figure 1.6*a, b). When the walls are lost ('destructive' centrilobular emphysema) the holes are

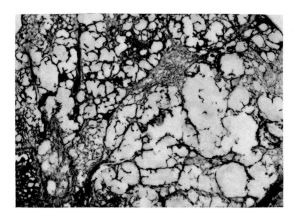

Figure 1.7. Moderate to severe panlobular emphysema. Little normal lung remains. (From paper-mounted section, natural size)

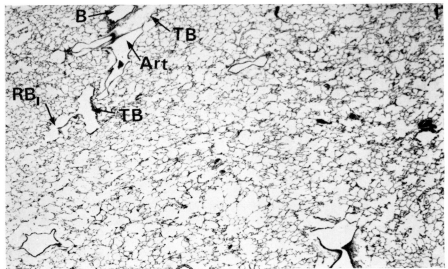

Figure 1.8. Microsection of normal lung: (art) pulmonary artery; (b) bronchiole; (tb) terminal bronchiole; (rb_1) first respiratory bronchiole. (Magnification × 10; by courtesy of Dr David Lamb)

larger and may reach 1 cm or more in diameter (*Figure 1.6*c and *Figure 1.9*). Traversing strands are absent or very few, but small arteries may be seen coursing across them (*Figure 1.11*). Alveoli immediately surrounding these holes tend to be flattened and form a thin encircling wall; otherwise the neighbouring lung appears normal.

Both types of lesion may be present in the one lung and both may contain pigment or inhaled dust particles (for example, soot, coal, carbon, hematite and foundry dust according to the nature of past exposure) and, in these circumstances and especially when the dust is coal, the 'distensive' type with intact alveolar walls has been referred to as 'focal emphysema' (Heppleston, 1947). The lesions of centrilobular emphysema, therefore, may be of distensive type with or without dust, or of destructive type with or without dust. The

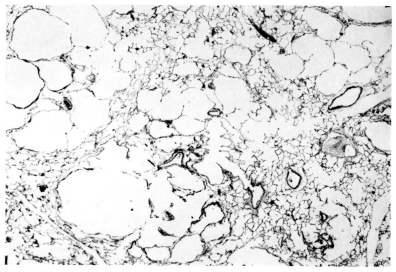

Figure 1.9. Microsection of centrilobular emphysema; normal lung between the lesions. (Magnification × 10; by courtesy of Dr David Lamb)

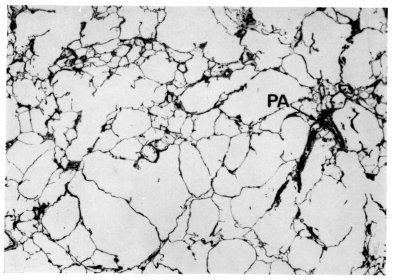

Figure 1.10. Microsection of panlobular emphysema; (pa) pulmonary artery. (Magnification × 10; by courtesy of Dr David Lamb)

quantity of pigment in the lungs of urban smokers appears to be significantly greater than in those of urban non-smokers (Pratt and Kilburn, 1971).

Centrilobular emphysema of both types is characteristically distributed in the upper two-thirds of the lungs, particularly in the posterior apical segments, but may be scattered throughout the lungs. It does not appear to be associated with air trapping (Reid, 1967).

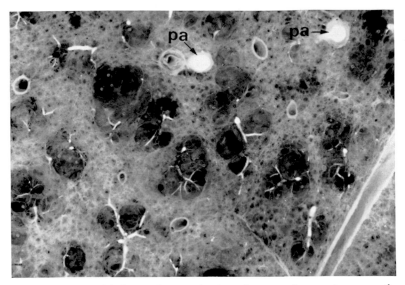

Figure 1.11. Centrilobular emphysema showing minute arteries coursing across the emphysema spaces which appear dark because of their depth; (pa) pulmonary arteries. (Barium-gelatin preparation; magnification ×3; by courtesy of Dr B. E. Heard and the Editor of Thorax)

Pathogenesis

(1) Both the 'distensive' and 'destructive' forms are found throughout the world. They have been observed in Jamaica, where there is virtually no air pollution, in at least 45 per cent of male autopsies (Hayes and Summerell, 1969) and in association with soot and pigment in the lungs of male Londoners (Heard and Izukawa, 1963). Centrilobular emphysema is found in the lungs of persons with no known history of chronic respiratory diseases during life and who die of other causes (Snider, Brody and Doctor, 1962), as well as in those of persons known to have had chronic respiratory disease. It is more common in men that in women and is not found in children.

(2) There is a strong correlation between centrilobular emphysema and cigarette smoking (e.g. Anderson *et al.*, 1966); indeed, by observing this type of emphysema in whole lung sections (*see* Appendix), and without other information, it has been found possible to distinguish those of smokers from those of non-smokers with statistically significant accuracy (Anderson and Foraker, 1967). Cigarette smoke inhaled by experimental animals lowers the surface tension and increases the surface compressibility of surfactant (Webb *et al.*, 1967) which may diminish the stability of alveoli and thus render them likely to dilate (Miller and Bondurant, 1962).

(3) Chronic bronchitis, being a common disorder, is often present in lungs with 'distensive' or 'destructive' centrilobular emphysema—with or without

dust. It has been suggested that bronchitis is the cause of 'destructive' centrilobular emphysema (Leopold and Gough, 1957), but this is open to doubt for the following reasons. This form of emphysema is often found in the lungs of persons who did not have chronic respiratory disease. Chronic obstructive bronchitis, like centrilobular emphysema, is closely correlated with cigarette smoking, but either may exist independently of the other. And chronic bronchitis, determined by the Reid gland/wall ratio (q.v.), is present uniformly throughout the lungs whereas centrilobular emphysema is distributed in sporadic fashion mostly in the upper halves of the lungs (Greenburg, Bousby and Jenkins, 1967). Furthermore, Reid and Millard (1964) were unable to find any significant correlation between severe chronic bronchitis and this type of emphysema. In short, chronic bronchitis does not appear to be the predominant cause.

However, bronchiolitis in the form of inflammatory changes and some loss of muscle and elastic fibres in the bronchioles leading into affected acini have been reported (Leopold and Gough, 1957; Heard, 1969), though complete obliteration rarely occurs. But it has not been shown that these changes are characteristically associated with 'destructive' centrilobular emphysema.

(4) 'Focal emphysema' is 'distensive' centrilobular emphysema with pigment and dust and, particularly in the case of coal dust, has been causally attributed to this (Heppleston, 1953, 1968). It is postulated that accumulation of dust in respiratory bronchioles weakens their walls and allows them to dilate. But the existence of focal emphysema as a separate entity is controversial and the possibility that dusts may be preferentially deposited in already existing emphysema lesions rather than in normal lungs has not been excluded. This question is discussed in more detail in Chapter 8.

(5) 'Destructive' centrilobular emphysema has also been attributed to the inhalation of high concentrations of cadmium fumes. This is considered in Chapter 12.

Clinical features

'Distensive' centrilobular emphysema is not responsible for any respiratory symptoms nor for any detectable impairment of lung function. This is not surprising when it is recalled that the lesions involve only a small fraction of the total alveolar surface, and do not cause air trapping.

'Destructive' centrilobular emphysema cannot be identified as such during life by physiological tests. But it has been suggested on theoretical grounds that abnormal enlargement of respiratory bronchioles may cause impairment of gas diffusion to the acini they supply (Staub, 1965; Horsfield, Cumming and Hicken, 1966), although the presence of this type of emphysema *post-mortem* in individuals with no respiratory symptoms or physiological abnormality during life suggests that in many cases at least it does not cause significant functional deficiency. However, when the lesions are numerous and large, reduction of effective alveolar ventilation with increased ventilation-perfusion inequality may result. Dyspnoea and impaired lung function are most likely to be due to co-existent chronic obstructive bronchitis.

This type of emphysema even when extensive cannot be detected on standard chest radiographs although it may be demonstrated by bronchography (*see* Chapter 5).

Panlobular (panacinar) emphysema

This is the commonest type of emphysema associated with the retention or 'trapping' of air within the acinus. It occurs in any part of the lungs, the lower halves as much as the upper, but with a preferential tendency for the anterior and basal regions; it may be local or general, and vary from a slight to gross order of severity. The affected parts of the lungs do not deflate normally when the thorax is opened at necropsy, and the lung substance may be so attenuated that when cut it sags away from blood vessels and airways. To

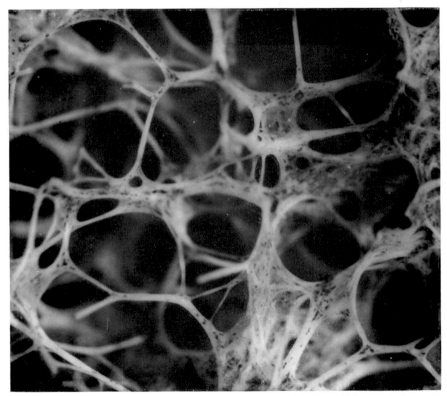

Figure 1.12. Severe panlobular emphysema with extensive alveolar wall loss and pigment in the surviving walls; city dweller's lung. (Magnification ×22·4; courtesy of Dr B. E. Heard)

the naked eye the earliest stage reveals enlarged air spaces in part or all of the lobule anywhere in the lung; the most severe stage shows extensive loss of structure and dilatation of lung parenchyma (*Figure 1.7*). Microscopy (*Figure 1.10*) shows breakdown of alveolar walls which are consequently much reduced in number throughout the acinus and, in the more severe grades, respiratory bronchioles are also involved (*Figure 1.4*). Pigment or dust apparently deposited after formation of the emphysema may be present in surviving alveolar walls (*Figure 1.12*). Centrilobular and panlobular emphysema may both occur in the same lung.

Pathogenesis

(1) Panlobular emphysema is not causally related to any form of pneumoconiosis.

(2) In adult life it is commonly found in association with chronic bronchitis and is, therefore, a disease of the second half of life. The frequency of this association is significantly higher than can be explained by chance. But panlobular emphysema may occur in the absence of chronic bronchitis in this age group and, rarely, in young men and women when it is known as *primary emphysema*, the cause of which is obscure (Reid, 1967). Contrawise, chronic obstructive bronchitis is often present in the absence of this type of emphysema.

(3) Deficiency of the enzyme α_1-antitrypsin.

Clinical features

There is gradually increasing breathlessness on effort and, ultimately, at rest. There are no abnormal physical signs until the disease is fairly advanced; before it reaches this stage it cannot be detected in chest radiographs, but it presents a characteristic appearance when widespread and severe (*see* Chapter 5). Its effect on lung function is referred to in Section III, this chapter.

Paraseptal (periacinar) emphysema

This takes the form of rows of small bullae typically distributed along the margins of the lungs; the anterior margins of the upper and middle lobes and lingula, and the costophrenic margin of the lower. It is also contiguous with connective tissue septa, blood vessels and bronchi. The lesions are characterized by loss of the walls of alveoli at the periphery of the acinus and they contain little or no lung tissue; neighbouring alveoli and the rest of the lung are normal. Bullae may become very large (Edge, Simon and Reid, 1966; Reid, 1967).

Important features are:

(1) It does not cause airways obstruction and is, therefore, symptomless and rarely associated with impairment of respiratory function.

(2) It can often be clearly recognized on chest radiographs.

(3) It tends to cause spontaneous pneumothorax or enlarging bullae. Although large bullae may cause impairment of ventilation and blood flow of adjacent lung, resulting in dyspnoea, this does not necessarily occur (Davies, Simon and Reid, 1966); lung function may be nearly normal with disease advanced enough to be seen on the radiograph.

(4) It is not causally related to any type of pneumoconiosis, but may contain dust and pigment.

Irregular (or scar) emphysema

In the United States of America this is referred to as *paracicatricial emphysema* (cicatrix, a scar). It has two possible primary causes in adult life:

(1) Complete or partial destruction of alveoli by an inflammatory process with subsequent resolution and the formation either of a central, contracted, collagenous scar surrounded by enlarged and distorted alveoli, or of an area of interstitial scarring between alveoli. Some loss of capillary blood vessels is apt to occur in the lesions.

25

(2) Over-inflation of the alveoli on a large scale may be caused by retraction of a scar in neighbouring lung tissue (as is seen, for example, in healed tuberculosis). When severe, many alveoli are lost with consequent reduction in alveolar surface.

It is not to be confused with *compensatory emphysema* which is characterized by over-inflation of otherwise normal lung to occupy an adjacent area from which lung tissue has been lost due, for example, to segmental or lobar collapse or resection.

Irregular emphysema may be associated with the fibrotic nodules and confluent fibrotic lesions of some types of pneumoconiosis, especially coal pneumoconiosis (Chapter 8) when it is sometimes incorrectly referred to as 'focal emphysema'.

Irreversible airways obstruction may be present, but not always, and the disease is often detectable in chest radiographs.

Before leaving the question of emphysema in general, Heard's (1966) practical interpretation of the morbid anatomical appearances should be noted:

> We believe that emphysema should, like atherosclerosis, be accepted as a common and, in small amounts, unimportant necropsy finding. . . . There is a danger that too much importance be attached to small amounts of emphysema in problematical cases, forgetting the commonness of emphysema at necropsy anyway. There is a great reserve of activity in lungs, and a patient is not necessarily disabled by the surgical removal of the whole of one lung. On these grounds it would seem unwise to attribute pulmonary insufficiency to emphysema that involves less than half the area of a slice of prepared lung.
>
> (From Heard, B. E. (1966). In *Recent Advances in Pathology*, 8th edition. London, Churchill)

Diffuse interstitial fibrosis with 'honeycomb' cysts ('honeycomb lung') should not, as a rule, be confused with emphysema. It represents an end-point of many different pathological processes most of which are poorly understood (for example, systemic lupus erythematosus, scleroderma, Sjögren's disease and rheumatoid disease) or not known (cryptogenic), although immunological reactivity is associated with many of them. It tends to be distributed beneath the pleura in the posterior and diaphragmatic regions of the lower lobes but may be observed in the depths of these lobes and, in some cases, subpleurally in the upper lobes. The walls of the air spaces and cysts are thick, no strands cross the spaces and there is dense fibrous tissue between them. Microscopically, these lesions are distinguished from emphysema by the presence of inflammatory exudate within the spaces, the density of mural fibrosis and, occasionally, a significant increase in smooth muscle.

It is important at this point to emphasize that, in order to make an accurate post-mortem assessment of the type, distribution and extent of emphysema, lungs should be perfused with fixative until their size is equivalent to their position in full inflation during life, after which they can be cut in sections for inspection (*see* Appendix).

V. CHRONIC BRONCHITIS

Chronic bronchitis, once regarded as pre-eminently the 'English Disease', is recognized today as common in many parts of the world thanks to the standardization of terminology and examination techniques exemplified by Fletcher *et al.* (1964). It is important in the present context because of the widespread belief that, in some cases, it may be caused by occupational air-pollution.

Definition

In the United Kingdom the Medical Research Council Committee on the Aetiology of Chronic Bronchitis (1965) has defined three types of chronic bronchitis:

(1) *Simple chronic bronchitis*: chronic or recurrent increase in the volume of mucoid bronchial secretion sufficient to cause expectoration.

(2) *Chronic mucopurulent bronchitis*: chronic bronchitis in which the sputum is persistently or intermittently mucopurulent when this is not due to localized broncho-pulmonary disease.

(3) *Chronic obstructive bronchitis*: chronic bronchitis in which there is persistent widespread narrowing of the intrapulmonary airways, at least on expiration, causing increased resistance to air flow.

The American Thoracic Society (1962) defined chronic bronchitis as

> A clinical disorder characterized by excessive mucus secretion in the bronchial tree. It is manifested by chronic or recurrent productive cough. Arbitrally, these manifestations should be present on most days, for a minimum of three months in the year and not less than two consecutive years.

As these are clinical definitions they assume that other broncho-pulmonary diseases productive of sputum, such as bronchiectasis or tuberculosis, or the expectoration of 'postnasal drip' mucus from disorders of the nasal cavities are excluded. And it should also be remembered that simple chronic bronchitis is not necessarily accompanied by cough but only by throat-clearing efforts, and that, although it causes no disability, a proportion of persons with this stage of the disease show some evidence of mild airways obstruction (Gregg, 1967). By contrast, chronic obstructive bronchitis usually gives rise to a greater or lesser degree of disability with substantial airways obstruction.

The fundamental disorder in chronic bronchitis is excessive production of mucus and a useful morbid anatomical criterion of over-activity of bronchial mucous glands is Reid's gland/bronchial wall ratio in which 'wall' is the distance between the bronchial epithelium and cartilage, and 'gland' is the depth of the mucous gland layer at the same point (Reid, 1967). It is necessary to take the mean of several measurements. The average value of the index in normal lungs is 0·26, and in those with chronic bronchitis, 0·59 (Reid, 1960). But in addition to gland hypertrophy there is thickening of the bronchial walls and a direct measurement of this expressed as a ratio of wall thickness (internal to cartilage) to the lumen radius correlates well with ante-mortem evidence of airways obstruction (McKenzie, Glick and Outhred, 1969) and appears to be a good index of the severity of bronchitis. However, evidence has been offered to suggest that the technique of weighing paper cut-outs upon which projected magnified images of the separate bronchial components have been sketched, offers a more accurate index of mucous gland hypertrophy (Bedrossian, Anderson and Foraker, 1971).

27

Prevalence

Assessment of comparative prevalence in different countries and even in different parts of the same country is fraught with difficulty caused by the varying criteria which are often used for diagnosis during life and for death certification from which mortality rates are calculated. It is certain that 'chronic bronchitis' on some death certificates—especially in countries where the diagnosis is fashionable—may have many meanings other than the true one.

Therefore, the use of the definitions given in association with a standardized method of questioning by the physician (such as that of the Medical Research Council Committee, 1966) is an essential part of diagnosis during life.

Comparison between surveys of chronic bronchitis in the United States of America and Scandinavia has revealed a higher prevalence of symptoms in the former which were partly attributable to cigarette smoking and partly to air pollution (Olsen and Gilson, 1960; Mork, 1962). All surveys have demonstrated the dominant role of cigarette smoking and the influence of air pollution both in the United Kingdom and in the United States. Reid *et al.* (1964) showed that, after differences in age and smoking habits of persons in these two countries had been taken into account, chronic obstructive bronchitis was equally common in British rural areas as in United States cities, although it was more prevalent in British towns. There was little difference in the prevalence of simple chronic bronchitis between American towns and rural and urban areas in the United Kingdom, and it was clearly related to cigarette smoking in both countries.

Pathogenesis

There is little doubt that the dominant cause of chronic bronchitis is cigarette smoking which has greatly increased in most Western countries since 1920 (Table 1.3), although general air pollution appears to play a part (Lawther, 1967). The correlation between smoking and chronic bronchitis and bronchial mucous gland hypertrophy is confirmed, but atmospheric pollution is less well correlated.

TABLE 1.3

CIGARETTE CONSUMPTION PER ADULT PER ANNUM IN SELECTED YEARS IN FIVE COUNTRIES

(Data by courtesy of TOBACCO RESEARCH COUNCIL)

Year	U.K.	U.S.A.	S. Africa	Australia	Germany
1920	1080	610	380	610	NA
1930	1380	1370	520	610	680
					West Germany
1940	2020	1820	720	640	NA
1950	2180	3250	1170	1280	630
1960	2760	3810	1080	2440	1630
1966	2810	3850	1140	2760	2210
1967	2840	3830	1200	2650	2150
1968	2900	3730	1290	2780	2280
1969	2970	3580	1330	2860	2410
1970	3050	3670	1360	2910	2500

NA—No information available.

The chief polluting substances in the atmosphere are smoke and sulphur dioxide, but noxious organic substances are sometimes produced by unusual photochemical meteorological conditions. It is not clear, however, what role air pollution plays in pathogenesis.

The prevalence of chronic bronchitis increases as social class declines. The College of General Practitioners' Survey (1961) showed that this applies to non-smokers as well as to smokers.

There is also the possibility, which requires some attention, that occupational exposure to dust and fumes might be important in pathogenesis.

Chronic bronchitis and occupation

It might be thought most probable that dusts or fumes are an important cause of chronic bronchitis and, indeed, this is often assumed to be the case

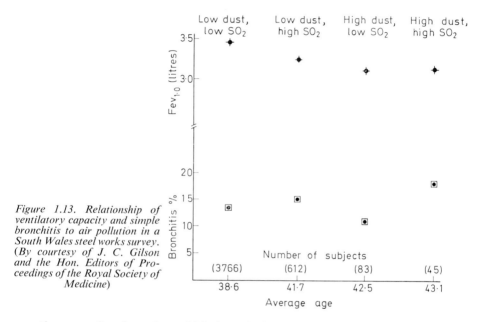

Figure 1.13. Relationship of ventilatory capacity and simple bronchitis to air pollution in a South Wales steel works survey. (By courtesy of J. C. Gilson and the Hon. Editors of Proceedings of the Royal Society of Medicine)

as the mortality from bronchitis in Britain and the United States is above average in dusty occupations (Gilson, 1970).

However, the problem of chronic bronchitis is complicated by the fact that many different influences may operate, and the relative significance of these has not yet been clarified. The great effect of smoking tends to overwhelm other possible causes.

It is known that the immediate effects of inhalation of coal dust are cough, increased secretion of mucus and airways resistance which are both acute and transient (McDermott, 1962). The degree of the airways reaction is the same irrespective of whether an individual has been occupationally exposed to the dust in the past (Ulmer, 1967).

Investigation of 20,000 steel foundry workers (Warner *et al.*, 1969; Lowe *et al.*, 1970) failed to reveal a relationship between bronchitis and exposure to dust and sulphur dioxide either alone or in combination (*Figure 1.13*), although the influence of smoking clearly emerged. Other studies of foundry workers (Brinkman and Coates, 1962; Cole, 1967; Ulmer, Reichel and Werner, 1968) have not, in general, demonstrated a correlation between occupation and bronchitis. However, a recent survey of iron, steel and non-ferrous foundries involving 1780 men and an almost equal number of control subjects has shown that there is a significant excess of chronic bronchitis (that is, the production of sputum for more than 3 months a year and one or more attacks of chest illness in the previous 2 years) among the foundry workers, but that, when smoking habits in the different foundry occupations are taken into account, this is slight. The effect of smoking and working in a foundry atmosphere appeared to be additive. Airways obstruction was associated with chronic bronchitis and not with exposure to foundry environment (Lloyd Davies, 1971).

A significant excess of chronic bronchitis among South African gold-miners exposed to rock dust compared with controls was found only in those who smoked (Sluis-Cremer, Walters and Sichel, 1967a; b). A study of metal ore miners in the United States (U.S. Public Health Service, 1963) showed no association between dust exposure and chronic bronchitis, and Paul (1961) made a similar observation in Northern Rhodesian copper-miners and confirmed the role of smoking.

In South Wales coal-miners no evident trend of prevalence of bronchitis in relation to years of dust exposure has been found (Cochrane and Higgins, 1961). Miners of bituminous coal in West Virginia (excluding those in the sixth decade) do not have a higher rate of chronic obstructive bronchitis or a lower ventilatory capacity than non-miners in the same population (Higgins *et al.*, 1968); and a study of coal-miners in Western Germany indicates that dust exposure is not a factor in the development of bronchitis or obstructive airways disease (Ulmer, Reichel and Werner, 1968). Again, although coal-miners in New Zealand tend to produce more sputum than compatriot non-miners, irrespective of smoking habits, diminution in their ventilatory capacity is attributed to cigarette smoking rather than coal-mine dust (de Hamel, 1961). And the Medical Research Council Special Committee (1966) set up to review this problem concluded that 'on present evidence intensity of dust exposure does not appear to be a very significant factor in determining the prevalence of bronchitis'.

Although, in Britain, the prevalence of chronic bronchitis has been found to be higher in coal miners and foundry workers than in agricultural workers a similar trend to that observed in the men in these groups was also found in their wives (Higgins *et al.*, 1959); and comparable observations have been made in the United States (Enterline, 1967). It has been argued from the higher death rates for bronchitis which exist among miners and their wives compared with agricultural workers and their wives that the difference must be due to occupation (Lowe, 1968). But analysis of the same data by another method failed to demonstrate that a factor additional to that of socio-economic class is responsible for this difference (Gilson, 1970).

If occupation were an important cause of chronic bronchitis it might be expected that the prevalence of bronchitic symptoms and decline in ventilatory capacity would be related to the number of years in the work after age and smoking habits have been duly taken into account. But this has been shown not to be the case (Gilson, 1970) (*see Figure 8.19*). There is no significant relationship (*see* Chapter 8) between the amount of coal dust in the lungs (as shown by the radiographic category of discrete ('simple') pneumoconiosis) and impairment of ventilatory capacity. This fact and the apparent lack of an effect of duration of exposure constitute, in the words of Gilson (1970), 'one of the more compelling reasons for believing that factors other than exposure to dust are more important in producing respiratory disability'.

To summarize: despite morbidity and mortality statistics and the suggestion that smoking might obscure the effects of dust or fumes there is little evidence that chronic obstructive bronchitis is causally related to past exposure to dusts or that occupational exposure to sulphur dioxide is significant. A synergistic relationship between smoking and inhaled dust has been postulated but not proven, although, in Britain, it appears that smokers are more likely to suffer from the effects of air pollution than non-smokers (Royal College of Physicians Report, 1970). There is some evidence in experimental animals that such an effect may exist (Boren, 1964).

The question of chronic obstructive bronchitis and exposure to 'nitrous fumes' is discussed briefly in Chapter 12.

VI. SOME PRACTICAL POINTS IN MEDICAL EXAMINATION

HISTORY TAKING

Occupational history

An inscription on a bell in an old Suffolk church which reads *Ars Incognita Imperitus Contemnitur* (an unknown art is considered unimportant by those who do not practise it) is relevant to the taking of an occupational history. For, although this is an essential part of the medical examination, it is commonly inadequately done or, worse, omitted altogether.

It cannot be too strongly emphasized that a carefully detailed history of the patient's present and previous occupations is the means by which, on the one hand, attention may be directed to the occupational nature of his lung disease or, on the other, to the fact that the disease in question cannot be occupational because it can be shown that he never worked in a relevant occupation or its immediate environment.

The work history must be taken in strictly chronological order starting with details of the first job on leaving school and progressing step by step to the present job or retirement. As far as possible no gaps or uncertainties should exist when it is complete and the nature of the materials to which a worker has been exposed must be established. When a man has done a number of jobs which sound innocuous it is easy to accept this at face value with the result that a hazardous process remains unidentified; equally, not all processes which are imagined to be dangerous are so. It is also necessary to form some idea of the intensity of a man's exposure to a hazard (that is, whether dust or fume concentrations were in general high or low) as well as the duration of this exposure.

The description of a job or the name given to it by the worker may conceal its true nature and, therefore, an unexpected hazard. For example, a *bricklayer* may have worked with refractory bricks (not house bricks) containing high concentrations of free silica and, furthermore, may have used asbestos fibre or rope for grouting; a *stoker* may not only have stoked a factory, power station or hospital boiler but may also have been exposed to free silica dust produced when cleaning ('scaling') its tubes, or to an intermittent asbestos risk during the stripping, mixing and reapplication of lagging materials around the boiler and neighbouring pipes by laggers working in his immediate vicinity; a *labourer* in a factory producing poultry meal may have worked for years at a flint crushing mill and so have been exposed to the risk of silicosis; a man may describe himself as a *scrap-metal worker* but only on further enquiry does it become clear that his work involved the melting down of beryllium alloys; *a welder* may be exposed to cadmium fumes from cadmium-plated metals; and a *clerk* or a *housewife* may have been an asbestos worker many years previously.

Exposure of a worker to a hazardous aerosol from a nearby process and the disease which may result from it is often referred to as being *para-occupational*.

The popular description of a job may give no clue to its identity or to the nature of the work involved. It should be a rule, therefore, to establish precisely what the job entails and the materials used if these are not self-evident. The possibility of multiple risks operating in the one work process, or of a man having worked in different hazardous industries must be kept in mind.

The worker should also be asked whether, in what way and over what period of time, protective measures were used: in particular, local exhaust and general ventilation and the wearing of respirators and protective clothing. This enables the physician to obtain some impression of the concentrations of dust to which the man may have been exposed.

Environmental history
Due to contamination outside the factory by harmful industrial materials, lung disease has sometimes been caused in persons who have never worked in the industry concerned. Non-occupational exposure has resulted from the discharge of dusts (such as beryllium and asbestos) by exhaust ventilation systems and smoke stacks into the atmosphere around a factory, and by the dumping in the open air of dangerous materials. Sources such as these are now generally controlled (*see* Chapter 3), but may still occur from time to time. Under these circumstances both sexes of all ages may have been potentially at risk in the past. Hence, some present-day adults may have been subjected to such exposures in childhood or adolescence. Disease contracted in this way is referred to as *neighbourhood disease*.

Domestic History
Potentially hazardous dusts shaken from a worker's overalls at home during cleaning or preparation for laundering, may be (or may have been in the past) a possible source of disease risk to his family. Asbestos and beryllium compounds have chiefly been indicted.

Delayed (Type III) allergic reactions (*see* Chapter 4) to the serum proteins and droppings of certain birds—notably pigeons and budgerigars—are recognized as a cause of acute and chronic lung disease (Chapter 11). Eliciting a history of bird fancying is especially important in those cases in which there has been repeated exposure to small amounts of antigen for, under these conditions, the disease is apt to be of slow and insidious onset and its relationship with the cause most likely to be unsuspected.

Smoking habits

Accurate information about past and present smoking habits must always be obtained and recorded. People fall into one of three groups: smokers, ex-smokers and non-smokers. Cigarette, cigar and pipe smoking must be distinguished and its duration and the question of inhaling established.

It is usual to record cigarette consumption as the number smoked per day, but for comparison with other types of smoking it is helpful to note that one manufactured cigarette is approximately equivalent to 1 gramme of tobacco and that 1 oz (28 grammes) of tobacco per week, therefore, equals 4 grammes daily, whether smoked in a pipe or hand-rolled cigarettes (Higgins, 1959).

PHYSICAL SIGNS

There are no physical signs which are pathognomonic of any one form of pneumoconiosis. Certain fibrogenic types of pneumoconiosis (silicosis and coal pneumoconiosis, for example) may reach an advanced stage and yet present no abnormal physical signs in the lungs.

Adventitious sounds in the lungs

Throughout this book the term 'crepitations' rather than 'rales' is used for the crackling sounds which may be heard. Crepitations are of particular importance in asbestosis and other forms of diffuse interstitial fibrosis (fibrosing 'alveolitis'). They must be sought meticulously over the lungs anteriorly, laterally and posteriorly while the subject inhales and exhales as deeply as possible, otherwise this important sign may be missed. In general, crepitations due to these diseases are crisp and sharp in quality, persistent, and are predominant during the inspiratory phase.

BIOPSY

Examinations of a scalene node may help to resolve a difficult diagnosis especially in the presence of generalized systemic disease. Sarcoid-like granulomas of beryllium disease and silicotic nodules may sometimes be identified.

Sampling of lung or pleura by any technique must always be fully justified on the grounds of being essential either to diagnosis (and this usually means exclusion of non-occupational disease) or to the control of treatment and never solely for research or other interests. All available methods have a roughly similar incidence of complications to which the patient should not be unnecessarily exposed. In general, thoracotomy is preferable to drill and needle methods (although more unpleasant for the patient) because the most appropriate site for sampling can be selected by inspection and palpation of lung or pleura, and a larger and more representative sample of tissue obtained.

As a rule, it can be said that if the occupational and medical history, physical examination and appropriate investigations are carefully carried out and their results accurately and logically analysed, sampling of the intrathoracic tissues in suspected cases of any type of pneumoconiosis should rarely be necessary. It is axiomatic that inspection of earlier chest radiographs is an integral part of investigation, and this alone may often prevent embarrassing mistakes.

ROUTINE MEDICAL EXAMINATIONS

Before entering work in an industry with a known dust hazard the prospective employee should have a clinical examination, chest radiograph and assessment of FEV_1 and FVC. A basic reference point for future examination is thus established. Persons with chest disease should, in most cases, be excluded from a risky process.

Established workers exposed to a pneumoconiosis risk should be examined regularly; an interval of two years is probably most satisfactory for the majority of industries, but, in the case of possible exposure to asbestos or beryllium, a shorter interval is desirable. In some industries, such as those with a 'silica' risk, a chest radiograph is all that is required; but in others, in particular those involving asbestos, clinical, radiographic and physiological examination is mandatory.

Details of examinations must be fully recorded and the records kept readily available. To have maximal prospective value, each worker's record must include a description of his job and the nature of materials used (that is, their analysis and origin) and, whenever possible, the concentration of the relevant dust or fume in his environment. Changes in his work must also be noted. This demands close co-operation between medical, engineering and production departments and safety personnel. It is clear that such co-operation not only ensures the best information upon the incidence and behaviour of disease in the factory population, but also confers the greatest long-term advantage on the worker.

The necessity for these examinations should always be explained to the workers concerned. If this is done few will fail to understand that they are done for their benefit and will co-operate accordingly.

REFERENCES

American Thoracic Society (1962). 'Statement on definitions and classification of chronic bronchitis, asthma and pulmonary emphysema.' *Am. Rev. resp. Dis.* **85**, 762–768

Anderson, A. E. Jr. and Foraker, A. G. (1967). 'Predictability of smoking habits, sex and age in urbanists from their macroscopic lung morphology.' *Am. Rev. resp. Dis.* **96**, 1255–1258

— Hernandez, J. A., Holmes, W. L. and Foraker, A. G. (1966). 'Pulmonary emphysema. Prevalence, severity and anatomical patterns in macrosections with respect to smoking habits.' *Archs envir. Hlth* **12**, 569–577

Bedrossian, C. W. M., Anderson, A. E. Jr., and Foraker, A. G. (1971). 'Comparison of methods of quantitating bronchial morphology.' *Thorax* **26**, 406–408

Boren, H. G. (1964). 'Carbon as a carrier mechanism for irritant gases.' *Archs envir. Hlth* **8**, 119–124

Boren, H. G., Kory, R. C. and Syner, J. C. (1966). 'The Veterans Administration—Army cooperative study of pulmonary function II. The lung volume and its subdivisions in normal men.' *Am. J. Med.* **41**, 96–114

Brinkman, G. L. and Coates, E. O. Jr. (1962). 'The prevalence of chronic bronchitis in an industrial population.' *Am. Rev. resp. Dis.* **86**, 47–54

Brooks, R. E. (1966). 'Concerning the nomenclature of the cellular elements in respiratory tissue.' *Am. Rev. resp. Dis.* **94**, 112–113

Burrows, B. (1967). 'Pulmonary diffusion and alveolar capillary block.' *Med. Clin. N. Am.* **51**, 427–438

Campbell, E. J. M. (1968). In *Clinical Physiology*, pp. 93–148. Ed. by E. J. M. Campbell, C. J. Dickinson and D. J. H. Slater. Oxford and Edinburgh; Blackwell

Card, W. (1967). 'Towards a calculus of medicine. In *Medical Annual*, pp. 9–21. Bristol; Wright

Ciba Foundation Guest Symposium (1959). 'Terminology, definitions and classification of chronic pulmonary emphysema and related conditions.' *Thorax* **14**, 286–299

Cochrane, A. L. and Higgins, I. T. T. (1961). 'Pulmonary ventilatory functions of coal miners in various areas in relation to the X-ray category of pneumoconiosis.' *Br. J. prev. soc. Med.* **15**, 1–11

Cole, C. (1967). 'Bronchitis in foundry men—an analytical description of some clinical experience.' *Ann. occup. Hyg.* **3**, 277–282

College of General Practitioners (1961). 'Chronic bronchitis in Great Britain: a national survey.' *Br. med. J.* **2**, 973–979

Comroe, J. H. Jr., Forster, R. E., Dubois, A. B., Briscoe, W. A. and Carlsen, E. (1962). *The Lung, Clinical Physiology and Pulmonary Function Tests.* 2nd Ed. Chicago; Year Book Publishers

Corrin, B. (1970). 'Phagocytic potential of pulmonary alveolar epithelium with particular reference to surfactant metabolism.' *Thorax* **24**, 110–115

Cotes, J. E. (1966). 'Tests of lung function in current use; proposals for their standardisation.' In *Respiratory Function Tests in Pneumoconiosis*, pp. 93–140. Occupational Safety and Health Series, No 6. Geneva; I.L.O.

— (1968). *Lung Function.* 2nd Ed. Oxford; Blackwell

— and Hall, A. M. (1970). 'The transfer factor for the lung; normal values in adults.' *Panminerva med.* 327–343

— Johnson, G. R. and McDonald, A. (1970). 'Breathing frequency and tidal volume; relationship to breathlessness.' In *Breathing: Hering-Breuer Centenary Symposium*', pp. 297–314. Ed. by R. Porter. London; Churchill

Davies, G. M., Simon, G. and Reid, L. (1966). 'Pre- and post-operative assessment of emphysema.' *Br. J. Dis. Chest.* **60**, 120–128

Edge, J., Simon, G. and Reid, L. (1966). 'Periacinar (paraseptal) emphysema: its clinical, radiological and physiological features.' *Br. J. Dis. Chest* **60**, 10–18

Enterline, P. E. (1967). 'The effects of occupation on chronic respiratory disease.' *Archs envir. Hlth* **14**, 189–198

Fletcher, C. M., Jones, N. L., Burrows, B. and Niden, A. H. (1964). 'American emphysema and British bronchitis.' *Am. Rev. resp. Dis.* **90**, 1–13

Franklin, W. and Lowell, F. C. (1961). 'Unrecognised airway obstruction associated with smoking: a probable forerunner of obstructive pulmonary emphysema.' *Ann. intern. Med.* **54**, 379–386

Gilson, J. C. (1970). 'Occupational bronchitis.' *Proc. R. Soc. Med.* **63**, 857–864

Greenburg, S. D., Bousby, S. F. and Jenkins, D. E. (1967). 'Chronic bronchitis and emphysema: correlation of pathologic findings.' *Am. Rev. resp. Dis.* **96**, 918–928

Gregg, I. (1967). 'Chronic bronchitis.' In *The Encyclopaedia of General Practice.* Ed. by G. F. Abercrombie and E. M. S. McConaghey. Service Volume, pp. 15–30. London; Butterworths

Guz, A., Noble, N. I. M., Eisele, J. H. and Trenchard, D. (1970). 'Experimental results of vagal block in cardio-pulmonary disease.' In *Breathing; Hering-Breuer Centenary Symposium.* Ed. by R. Porter, pp. 315–336. London; Churchill

Hamel, F. A. de (1961). *The Grey Valley Survey. Smoking, Lung Function and the Effects of Dust in Coal miners in New Zealand* (Special Report Series No. 3). Wellington, N.Z.; Department of Health

Hayes, J. A. and Summerell, J. M. (1969). 'Emphysema in a non-industrialised tropical island.' *Thorax* **24**, 623–625

Heard, B. E. (1966). 'Diseases of the Lungs.' In *Recent Advances in Pathology*, 8th Edition, p. 363. Ed. by C. V. Harrison. London; Churchill

— (1969). *Pathology of Chronic Bronchitis and Emphysema*. London; Churchill

— and Izukawa, T. (1963). Dust pigmentation of the lungs and emphysema in Londoners. Fortschr. der Staublungen forschung. Ed. by H. Reploh and W. Klosterkötter. Dislaken pp. 249–255

Heppleston, A. G. (1947). 'The essential lesion of pneumoniosis in Welsh coal miners.' *J. Path. Bact.* **59**, 453–460

— (1953). 'The pathological anatomy of simple pneumoniosis in coal workers.' *J. Path. Bact.* **66**, 235–246

— (1968). 'Lung architecture in emphysema.' In *Form and Function in the Human Lung*, pp. 6–19. Ed. by G. Cumming and L. B. Hunt. Edinburgh and London; Livingstone

Higgins, I. T. T. (1959). 'Tobacco smoking, respiratory symptoms and ventilatory capacity.' *Br. med. J.* **1**, 325–329

— and Oldham, P. D. (1962). 'Ventilatory capacity in miners: a five-year follow up study.' *Br. J. ind. Med.* **19**, 65–76

— Cochrane, A. L., Gilson, J. C. and Wood, C. H. (1959). 'Population studies of chronic respiratory disease. A comparison of miners, foundry workers and others in Stavely, Derbyshire.' *Br. J. ind. Med.* **16**, 155–268

— Higgins, M. W., Lockshin, M. D., and Canale, N. (1968). 'Chronic respiratory disease in mining communities in Marion County, West Virginia.' *Br. J. ind. Med.* **25**, 165–175

Horsfield, K., Cumming, G. and Hicken, P. (1966). 'A morphologic study of airway disease using bronchial casts.' *Am. Rev. resp. Dis.* **93** 900–906

Hutchinson, D. C. S., Cook, P. J. L., Barter, C. E., Harris, H. and Hugh-Jones P. (1971). 'Pulmonary emphysema and α_1-antitrypsin deficiency.' *Br. med. J.* **1**, 689–694

Kory, R. C., Callahan, R., Boren, H. G. and Syner, J. C. (1961). 'The Veterans Administration–Army Cooperative Study of Pulmonary Function. 1. Clinical spirometry in normal men.' *Am. J. Med.* **30**, 243–258

Krumholz, R. A., Chevalier, R. B., and Ross, J. C. (1964). 'Cardio-pulmonary function in young smokers.' *Ann. Intern. Med.* **60**, 603–610

Lambert, M. W. (1955). 'Accessory bronchiolo-alveolar communications.' *J. Path. Bact.* **70**, 311–314

Lauweryns, J. M. (1970). 'The juxta-alveolar lymphatics in the human adult lung.' *Am. Rev. resp. Dis.* **102**, 877–885

Lawther, P. J. (1967). 'Air pollution and chronic bronchitis.' *Medna thorac.* **24**, 44–52

Leading Article (1971). 'Enzyme deficiency and emphysema.' *Br. med. J.* **3**, 655–656

Leopold, J. C. and Gough, J. (1957). 'The centrilobular form of hypertrophic emphysema and its relation to chronic bronchitis.' *Thorax* **12**, 219–235

Lloyd Davies, T. A. (1971). *Respiratory Disease in Foundrymen. Report of a Survey*, Dept. of Employment. London; H.M.S.O.

Lowe, C. R. (1968). 'Chronic bronchitis and occupation.' *Proc. R. Soc. Med.* **61**, 98–102

— Campbell, H. and Khosla, T. (1970). 'Bronchitis in two integrated steel works. III. Respiratory symptoms and ventilatory capacity related to atmospheric pollution.' *Br. J. ind. Med.* **27**, 121–129

Martt, J. M. (1962). 'Pulmonary diffusing capacity in cigarette smokers.' *Ann. intern. Med.* **56**, 39–45

McDermott, M. (1962). 'Acute respiratory effects of the inhalation of coal dust particles.' *J. Physiol. Lond.* **162**, 53P.

— and Collins, M. M. (1965). 'Acute effects of smoking on lung airways resistance in normal and bronchitic 'subjects.' *Thorax* **20**, 562–569

McKenzie, H. I., Glick, M. and Outhred, K. G. (1969). 'Chronic bronchitis in coal miners: antemortem/post-mortem comparisons. *Thorax* **24**, 527–535

Medical Research Council Committee on the Aetiology of Chronic Bronchitis (1965). 'Definition and classification of chronic bronchitis for clinical and epidemiological purposes.' *Lancet* **1**, 775–779

— (1966). 'Questionnaire on respiratory symptoms and instructions for use.' Dawlish; Holman

Medical Research Council Special Committee (1966). 'Chronic bronchitis and occupation.' *Br. med. J.* **1**, 101–102

Miller, D. and Bondurant, S. (1962). Effects of cigarette smoke on the surface characteristics of lung extracts.' *Am. Rev. resp. Dis.* **85**, 692–696

Mork, T. (1962). 'A comparative study of respiratory disease in England and Wales and Norway.' *Acta med. scand.* **172**, Suppl. 384

Muir, D. C. F. (1967). 'Distribution of aerosol particles in exhaled air.' *J. appl. Physiol.* **23**, 210–214

Olsen, H. C. and Gilson, J. C. (1960). 'Respiratory symptoms, bronchitis and ventilatory capacity in men: an Anglo-Danish comparison with special reference to difference in smoking habits.' *Br. med. J.* **1**, 450–456

Paintal, A. S. (1970). 'The mechanism of excitation of Type J receptors and the J reflex.' In *Breathing: Herring-Breuer Centenary Symposium*, pp. 59–76. Ed. by R. Porter. London; Churchill

Pattle, R. E. (1955). 'Properties, function and origin of the alveolar lining layer.' *Nature, Lond.* **175**, 1125–1126

— (1968). 'The surface active lining of the lung.' *J. R. Coll. Physns* **2**, 137–140

Paul, R. (1961). 'Chronic bronchitis in African miners and non-miners in Northern Rhodesia.' *Br. J. Dis. Chest* **55**, 30–34

Pratt, P. C. and Kilburn, K. H. (1971). 'Extent of pulmonary pigmentation as an indicator of particulate environmental air pollution.' In *Inhaled Particles, 3,* pp. 661–669. Ed. by W. H. Walton. Woking; Unwin

Proust, A. (1874). *Bull. Acad. Méd.*, Ser. 2, **3**, 624

Pump, K. K. (1969). 'Morphology of the acinus of the human lung.' *Dis. Chest* **56**, 126–134

Rankin, J., Gee, J. B. L. and Chosy, L. W. (1965). 'The influence of age and smoking on pulmonary diffusing capacity in healthy subjects.' *Medna thorac.* **22**, 366–374

Rao, M. N., Sen Gupta, A., Saha, P. N. and Sita, Davi, A. (1961). *Physiological norms in Indians.* New Delhi; India Colonial Medical Research Spec. Rep. Ser. 38

Reid, D. D., Anderson, D. O., Ferris, B. G. and Fletcher, C. M. (1964). 'An Anglo-American comparison of the prevalence of bronchitis.' *Br. med. J.* **2**, 1487–1491

Reid, L. (1960). 'Measurement of bronchial mucous gland layer; a diagnostic yardstick in chronic bronchitis.' *Thorax* **15**, 132–141

— (1967). *The Pathology of Emphysema.* London; Lloyd Luke

— and Millard, F. J. C. (1964). 'Correlation between radiological diagnosis and structural lung changes in emphysema.' *Clin. Radiol.* **15**, 307–311

Report on a Symposium (1968). *Pneumoconiosis, Katowice,* 1967. Copenhagen; W.H.O.

Royal College of Physicians Report (1970). *Air Pollution and Health.* London; Royal College of Physicians

Sluis-Cremer, S. K., Walters, K. G. and Sichel, H. B. (1967a). 'Chronic bronchitis in miners and non-miners; an epidemiological survey of a community in the gold mining area in the Transvaal.' *Br. J. ind. Med.* **24**, 1–12

— — — (1967b). 'Ventilatory function in relation to mining experience and smoking in a random sample of miners and non-miners in a Witwatersrand town.' *Br. J. ind. Med.* **24**, 13–25

Snider, G. L., Brody, J. S. and Doctor L. (1962). 'Subclinical pulmonary emphysema.' *Am. Rev. resp. Dis.* **85**, 666–683

Staub, N. C. (1965). 'Time dependent factors in pulmonary gas exchange.' *Medna thorac.* **22**, 132–145

37

Stirling, G. M. (1967). 'Mechanisms of bronchoconstriction caused by cigarette smoking.' *Br. med. J.* **2**, 275–277

Tobacco Research Council (1968). Personal communication

— (1972). *Tobacco Consumption in Various Countries.* Research Paper No. 6. 3rd Ed. Ed. by G. F. Todd. To be published

Trapnell, D. H. (1963). 'The peripheral lymphatics of the lung.' *Br. J. Radiol.* **36**, 660–672

— (1964). 'Radiological appearances of lymphangitis carcinomatosa of the lung.' *Thorax* **19**, 251–260

Ulmer, W. T. (1967). 'Reaction of the lungs to various broncho-irritating substances.' In *Inhaled Particles and Vapours.* Vol. 2, pp. 87–91. Ed. by C. N. Davies. Oxford; Pergamon

— Reichel, G. and Werner, U. (1968). 'Die chronisch obstruktive Bronchitis des Bergannes. Untersuchungen zur Haufigkeit bei der Normalbevelkerung und bei Bergleuten. Die Bedentung der Staubbeslasitung und der Einfluss des Rauchens.' *Int. Arch. Gewerbepathol. Gewerbehyg.* **25**, 75–98

United States Public Health Service Publications (1963). No. 1076. *Silicosis in the Metal Mining Industry: a Revaluation 1958–1961.* Washington; U.S. Government Printing Office

Van Furth, R. (1970). 'Origin and kinetics of monocytes and macrophages.' *Semin. Hematol.* **7**, 125–141

Van Ganse, W. F., Ferris, B. G., Jr. and Cotes, J. E. (1972). 'Cigarette smoking and pulmonary diffusing capacity (transfer factor).' *Am. Rev. resp. Dis.* **105**, 30–41

von Hayek, H. (1960). *The Human Lung.* Trans. by V. E. Krahl. New York; Hafner

Warner, C. G., Davies, G. H., Jones, J. G. and Lowe, C. R. (1969). 'Bronchitis in two integrated steel works. II. Sulphur dioxide and particulate atmospheric pollution in and around the two works.' *Ann. occup. Hyg.* **12**, 151–170

Webb, W. R., Cook, W. A., Lannis, J. W. and Shaw, R. R. (1967). Cigarette smoke and surfactant. *Am. Rev. resp. Dis.* **95**, 244–247

Weibel, E. R. (1963). *Morphometry of the Lung.* New York; Academic Press

— (1968). 'Airways and respiratory surface.' In *The Lung.* Ed. by A. A. Liebow and D. E. Smith. Baltimore; Williams and Wilkins

Wilhelmsen, L. (1967). 'Effects of broncho-pulmonary symptoms, ventilation and lung mechanics of abstinence from tobacco smoking.' *Scand. J. Resp. Dis.* **48**, 407–414

Wyatt, J. P., Fischer, V. W. and Sweet, H. (1961). 'Centrilobular emphysema.' *Lab. Invest.* **10**, 159–177

Zenker, F. A. (1866). *Staubinhalations Krankheiten der Lungen*

Zwi, S., Goldman, H. I. and Levin, A. (1964). 'Cigarette smoking and pulmonary function in healthy young adults.' *Am. Rev. resp. Dis.* **89**, 73–81

2—Elements of Geology and Geochemistry

The medical worker in the field of industrial lung disease often encounters mineral and rock names with which he may not be familiar, or he may be unaware of the composition of some well-known substance. A basic knowledge of geology should enable him to decide what the nature and composition of a particular natural mineral or rock is likely to be. This not only saves time and points further enquiry in the right direction but also helps to establish rational thinking about pathogenesis and to avoid mistaken diagnosis.

According to the theory of the formation of the Earth put forward by Urey (1952) oxygen actively combined with silicon, aluminium, magnesium, iron, calcium and potassium atoms (themselves forged by thermonuclear processes) within nebulous gas to form complex silicates, and with hydrogen to form water. Hydrogen combined with nitrogen and carbon to form fundamental units of organic structure.

The Earth consists of a superficial *Crust* a few miles thick which rests on a denser mass, the *Mantle*, nearly 2000 miles thick, and a central *Core* which is probably solid but behaves in some respects as if in a molten state. Molten rock material, or *Magma* (which contains gases and steam) also exists as pockets within the crust and mantle or is extruded on to its surface as volcanic lava.

Chemically, the 'average' composition of the crust consists of about 27·7 per cent silicon, 46·6 per cent oxygen, 8 per cent aluminium and 16·2 per cent in aggregate of calcium, iron, magnesium, potassium and sodium. This gives a total of 98·5 per cent, the remainder consisting of all the other elements.

In our present context it is the crust and its rocks which are of importance. The crust is considered to have an upper and lower zone; the upper zone, which is confined to continents, is composed largely of *si*lica and *a*lumina (SIAL); and the lower zone, which is present beneath both continents and oceans, is predominantly *si*lica and *ma*gnesia (SIMA).

Rock means 'any mass or aggregate of one or more kinds of mineral or of organic matter, whether hard and consolidated or soft and incoherent, which owes its origin to the operation of natural causes. Thus granite, basalt,

39

limestone, clay, sand, silt and peat are all equally termed rocks' (Geikie, 1908).

The ingredients available for rock formation are known as *minerals*. A mineral is probably best defined as an inorganic homogeneous substance which occurs naturally and has definite chemical composition and physical properties.

Silicon and oxygen are the two most important elements in the crust and form a fundamental SiO_4 tetrahedral unit consisting of a central silicon ion with oxygen ions attached three-dimensionally at the four 'corners' of a tetrahedron. All forms of 'silica'—that is, silicon dioxide $(SiO_2)_x$—are composed of these tetrahedra joined by common oxygen atoms so that each crystal consists of a giant molecule with an average stoicheiometric formula of SiO_2. Being uncombined they are referred to as 'free silica'. The tetrahedra are linked in various ways by $-Si-O-Si-$ chains, and the manner in which metallic cations are included in this linkage decides their form and characteristics.

TABLE 2.1

TYPES OF SILICON DIOXIDE AND INFLUENCE OF HIGH TEMPERATURES
C = crystalline   CC = cryptocrystalline   A = amorphous

Initial form	Resulting form after exposure to temperatures of		
	800 to 1000°C (approx.)	1100 to 1400°C (approx.)	1700°C (approx.)
Quintz (C) Flint (CC) Chert (CC) Opal (CC) Chalcedony (CC) Diatomite (A)	Tridymite (C)→	Cristobalite (C)	→Melts

Free silica occurs in *polymorphic crystalline, cryptocrystalline* (that is, consisting of minute crystals) and *amorphous* (that is, non-crystalline) forms.

The distinction between 'free' and 'combined' silica is important. *Combined silica* is SiO_2 in combination with various cations as silicates. *Free silica* is the most widespread substance in nature with a fibrogenic potential for the lungs, but examples of combined silica which are fibrogenic (mainly and most importantly the asbestos group of minerals) are of more restricted distribution. It should be noted that reported chemical analyses of rocks frequently make no distinction between 'combined' and 'free' silica and only the total SiO_2 content may be shown. Under these conditions the quantity of 'free' silica remains unknown.

Crystalline forms of free silica are *quartz, tridymite* and *cristobalite* which are structurally different, although chemically identical; that is, they are allotropes. Cryptocrystalline forms are *flint, chert, opal* and *chalcedony* (agate) in which the crystal size is about 400 Å (Å = Ångstrom Unit = 10^{-10} metre) (Drenk, 1959). They are often referred to as 'amorphous silica', but this is incorrect. The most important examples of amorphous silica from the standpoint of lung disease is *diatomite*.

Quartz is transformed into its other allotropic forms under the influence of high temperature or pressure and the presence of certain metallic ions. Quartz subjected to a temperature of about 1000°C is converted into tridymite and at higher temperatures (about 1400°C), into cristobalite. Quartz is stable at temperatures below 870°C, tridymite between 870°C and 1470°C, and cristobalite between 1470°C and 1710°C at which temperature it melts (Holt, 1957). Furthermore, both cryptocrystalline and amorphous forms are also changed to tridymite and cristobalite under the same temperature conditions. As will be seen later (Chapter 7) these metamorphoses (summarized in Table 2.1) are of practical importance whenever quartz and the other types of silicon dioxide are subjected to high temperatures in certain industrial processes or conditions.

TYPES OF ROCK

Silicon does not exist free in nature. Free silica, therefore, is the principal rock-forming constituent and the proportions in which it is present determines the nature of many rocks.

There are three principal types of rocks:

1 - IGNEOUS ROCKS

These are the primary rocks of the crust which were formed from magma either by rapid extrusion of magma on to the Earth's surface or by intrusion of magma within the crust (igneous = fiery); in the first case cooling occurred quickly and in the second, slowly. The rate of cooling determined the size of the rock crystals: the quicker the cooling, the smaller the crystals; and the slower the process, the larger the crystals.

2 - SEDIMENTARY ROCKS

Sedimentary rocks are formed in two ways:

(1) By the gradual breakdown of igneous or older sedimentary and metamorphic rocks (*see* next section) by the action of wind, sun, water, frost and ice in weathering and corrosion processes to form deposits of debris such as sand and mud.

(2) By the deposition in former seas or swamps of the shells of marine organisms, rotting vegetation and chemical substance.

Slow or cataclysmic earth movements altered the levels of both types of accumulation and new sediments were deposited on top of them squeezing out their water and compressing them into rocks such as sandstone, limestone and coal.

3. METAMORPHIC ROCKS

Metamorphism implies change of form, structure and constitution in already existing igneous and sedimentary rocks. This change is brought about in four ways:

41

(1) By a local and substantial rise in temperature caused by the intrusion of magma which bakes the neighbouring rocks (thermal metamorphism).

(2) By movement of the crust which applies shearing or thrusting forces to the rocks and so distorts them that the formation of new minerals results (dynamic metamorphism).

(3) By percolation of hot water through rocks, and steam and gases through the magma which causes important chemical changes (hydrothermal metamorphism).

(4) By a combination of thermal and dynamic metamorphism (regional metamorphism).

Composition

For the most part all such rocks are composed of silicate minerals.

The proportion of silica which was available in the original magma determined the form which igneous rocks were to take and it varied from approximately 30 to 75 per cent.

Where the percentage of silicon dioxide was very low, iron and magnesium, which have a strong affinity for it, combined with all that was available, especially if they were predominant among the cations. This gave rise to the 'ferro-magnesian' group of minerals (such as the olivine group). When a large quantity of uncombined iron remained, this was deposited as iron ore; when the percentage of silica was of intermediate order, iron and magnesium again combined with it, but, if their concentration was low, aluminium, potassium, sodium and calcium combined with the available remaining silica to produce the *feldspar group* of minerals. Where the percentage of silicon was high, all available cations were absorbed and an excess of silica left which crystallized as quartz.

Acid and basic rocks

Silica-rich magmas are termed 'acid' and those having little silica but large quantities of bases, such as aluminium, iron and magnesium, are termed 'basic'. Four magma types are distinguished according to their total or 'combined' silica content.

Ultrabasic	from 30 to 44 per cent silica
Basic	from 45 to 54 per cent silica
Intermediate	from 55 to 64 per cent silica
Acid	from 65 to 75 per cent silica

The more acid the rock, therefore, the more free silica it contains. The proportions of free silica in any rock can only be expressed in general terms. It is practically impossible to give numerical values which are valid for a given rock type found in any one area or globally. Rocks which contain no quartz do not contain free (uncombined) silica.

Among the igneous rocks the quartz content of the acid group (chiefly the granite family) may be as much as 30 per cent; in some rocks of the intermediate group, the content is negligible, while in others it may be up to 5 per cent. Quartz is absent from rocks of the basic and ultrabasic groups.

CLASSIFICATION OF IGNEOUS ROCKS

The common igneous rocks can be classified in seven groups:

Olivine group

These have the lowest proportion of silica and are, therefore, generally confined to ultrabasic and basic rocks. They are iron and magnesium silicates and contain no aluminium.

Pyroxene group

The most important member is *augite* which possesses more silica than the previous group and is a calcium magnesium iron aluminium silicate. It has a single chain structure.

Amphibole group

The silica content is not substantially different from the pyroxene group. *Hornblende* is the commonest member and is a complex calcium magnesium iron and sodium silicate, and like *tremolite* (calcium magnesium silicate), it has a double chain structure which lends itself to the formation of long fibres. *Actinolite* differs from tremolite in containing a considerable quantity of iron but it, too, is usually of fibrous habit. *Amosite* and *crocidolite* asbestos also belong to this group.

Micas and clay group

This group is generally associated with acid rocks such as granite. The structure of micas is of the sheet lattice type which gives them their well-known characteristic of cleavage into layers. Important members of the group are *biotite*, a complex silicate of magnesium, aluminium, potassium and iron found in many igneous and metamorphic rocks; and *muscovite* (potassium aluminium silicate), the common white mica. *Sericite*, once thought to be important in the pathogenesis of coal pneumoconiosis, is a secondary muscovite which may be produced by the alteration of orthoclase feldspar.

The clay group of minerals contributes to the majority of the sedimentary rocks and is produced by the breakdown of feldspar and ferro-magnesium minerals. They are hydrous aluminium silicates of sheet lattice type.

Feldspar group

Members of this group are the most common of all the rock-forming minerals and the most important constituents of igneous rocks. Chemically they are silicates of aluminium with either potassium, sodium or calcium, or a combination of these three. They fall into two main series:

(1) *Orthoclase feldspars* which are potassium rich and usually occur in 'acid' rocks with a high percentage of quartz.

(2) *Plagioclase feldspars* which contain variable proportions of sodium and calcium. Sodium plagioclases occur in more 'acid' rocks and are, therefore, frequently associated with orthoclase, whereas calcium plagioclases are found in the 'basic' rocks.

Feldspathoid group

Members of this group are composed of the same elements as the feldspars but in different proportions and they play a similar, though subordinate, part in rock formation. Their proportion of free silica is very low and that of alkalis, such as sodium and potassium, high.

Quartz group

As already stated, when silica is present in abundance and all other substances have entered into combination with it a variable amount remains and crystallizes as quartz. This almost pure free silica is found in such important igneous rocks as *quartz-porphyry*, *rhyolite* and *granite*. The sedimentary and metamorphic rocks which were subsequently formed from them also have a high silica content.

Crystalline structure

The order of crystallization of these rocks depended primarily on the composition of the magma: for example, in a magma rich in silicon dioxide, quartz tended to crystallize first—hence, quartz-porphyries. Similarly, in basic rocks, feldspar often crystallized before pyroxene. Within the ferromagnesian and feldspar groups therefore, fairly well-defined sequences are observed. For example:

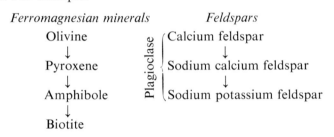

It is worth noting, as a general principle, that some minerals cannot occur together in rocks. In particular, quartz is not present in rocks of the olivine group (other than those which are almost pure iron-olivine) or in the feldspathoid group. Rocks which contain quartz are often classified as 'oversaturated'; those with little or no quartz but which contain olivine and feldspathoids, as 'undersaturated'.

NON-SILICATE ROCKS

Non-silicate minerals are also rock-forming and are important constituents of certain sedimentary and metamorphic rock types. They fall into the following groups:

Carbonates

These are the predominant non-silicates and they consist of *calcite* ($CaCO_3$—the chief constituent of limestone) *dolomite* ($MgCO_3.CaCO_3$—which constitutes dolomite limestone) and *siderite* ($FeCO_3$). Marbles are metamorphosed calcite or dolomite. Siderite occurs in some coal measures.

Haloids and sulphates

Rock salt (NaCl), *anhydrite* ($CaSO_4$), and *gypsum* ($CaSO_4.2H_2O$) which were deposited by evaporation of lakes and land-locked sea, and *fluorspar* (CaF_2) contain no free silica unless by contamination.

Oxides and sulphides

These are mainly iron minerals and their most important representatives are *magnetite* (Fe_3O_4 and *iron pyrites* (FeS_2). The principal rocks can now be briefly described.

IGNEOUS ROCKS

The rate at which the original magma cooled determined the degree and form of its crystallization and, therefore, the 'texture' or fundamental structure of the igneous rock. Magma which solidified within the crust is called 'intrusive'.

Three primary categories of igneous rocks are recognized:

Extrusive or volcanic which are glassy or fine grained ('grain' refers to crystal size) because they cooled very rapidly.

Minor intrusive or hypabyssal which, being fairly near the surface of the crust, cooled rather more slowly and are medium grained.

Major intrusive or plutonic (after Pluto, the god of the Underworld) are deep below the surface, cooled very slowly and are medium to coarse grained.

Intrusive rocks reach the surface of the crust through the action of earth movements and the erosion and disruption of overlying rocks.

SEDIMENTARY ROCKS

Sedimentary rocks fall broadly into three categories:

(1) *Fragmental rocks*

As the chief ingredients of these were produced mechanically by attrition and erosion they are classed according to the nature and size of the fragments.

(a) *Rudaceous (that is, rubbly) rocks.*—These are composed of granules, pebbles or boulders which, when rounded by wear produce *conglomerates*; but if angular, are called *breccias*. The fragments are cemented together by a mineral such as secondary silica, leached out from elsewhere, or by mud.

(b) *Arenaceous (arena = sand) rocks.*—The raw materials of these are sands and silts cemented by siliceous and clay substances. The chief members of this group are the *sandstones* and they are composed predominantly of quartz grains.

(c) *Argillaceous (argilla = clay) rocks.*—These consist essentially of clay minerals but may contain very finely divided free silica derived from older quartz-bearing rocks. They are laid down as clays and when consolidated become rocks. They are an important group because they include the black (or carbonaceous) shales, fireclays, china clay, and fuller's earth, some of which contain finely divided quartz often in high concentrations (*see* Table 2.3). The combined silica content of fireclays varies from about 50 to 76 per cent and that of alumina, from about 16 to 36 per cent.

(2) *Organic rocks*

(a) *Limestones.* These are chiefly of organic origin and consist mostly of calcium carbonate. Small amounts of magnesium carbonate are often present but when this reaches significant proportions the rock is referred to as dolomite limestone or *dolomite.* Many different types of organism have contributed to their formation including among others corals, crustacea, foraminifera, molluscs and algae. The calcium carbonate of some limestones, however, is entirely of chemical origin. In general they do not contain any free silica but small amounts are sometimes present as an impurity. However, flint occurs as nodules in some chalk deposits, and chert in some limestone deposits.

Rottenstone and wollastonite are found in association with limestone and are used in industrial processes.

Rottenstone is a siliceous-argillaceous limestone from which calcium carbonate has been removed in solution. It contains up to 15 per cent quartz and 85 per cent alumina, and has been used in industry as a refractory material and as a filler.

Wollastonite is a naturally occurring calcium metasilicate ($CaSiO_3$) formed mainly by contact metamorphism of quartz-bearing limestone and by silica-bearing emanations from igneous intrusions (often granite) reacting with pure or impure limestone. It is used in some countries as a substitute for flint, quartz sand, feldspar and china clay (*see* page 54) in ceramic-bonded abrasives, and in other industries (Andrews, 1970).

(b) *Carbonaceous rocks.*—Lignite and coals were mostly formed (in the British Isles) some 200 to 300 million years ago from the accumulation of rotting vegetation (trees, ferns, giant club mosses) in swampy conditions and subsequent inundation by sediment and solute-bearing river, lake or sea waters which overlaid it with deposits destined later to become sandstone, shale or limestone. The subsequent raising of the area or drop in sea level caused by earth movements allowed forest vegetation to take root once again, so that the cycle was repeated, not once but many times in succession.

Most plant tissues possessed a high proportion of carbohydrates and many hydrocarbons in the form of resins, waxes, oils and fats together with mineral salts originally absorbed from the soil. Their residue, therefore, contains at least 50 per cent carbon, not more than 44 per cent oxygen and 6 per cent hydrogen.

Where dead vegetation accumulated in stagnant water in conditions of poor oxygen supply, decomposition was slow and plant structure remains clearly distinguishable. In this way *peat* was formed. When organisms such as unicellular algae, spores and pollen grains petrified in deeper waters and mingled with inorganic muds a jelly-like carbonaceous slime, *sapropel,* resulted.

Peat and sapropel are the basis of all coals.

As earlier layers of peat and sediment subsided and were successively overlain by new layers, so they became subjected to increasing pressure and temperature as well as to chemical changes. These processes gave rise to the gradual change of peat first to *brown coal* and *lignite* which, by comparison with peat, have a slight increase in carbon and loss of oxygen; then to *bituminous coal* well known as house and gas coals which are much richer in carbon content but poorer in oxygen and volatiles (*sub-bituminous coals* are intermediate between these two); and, finally, to *anthracite coals* which contain some 95 per cent carbon and less than 5 per cent oxygen and volatile materials (Table 2.2).

Coals formed from sapropel, known as *cannel and boghead coals* are less important. Their content of carbon is high, being about 85 per cent and that of volatiles fairly high.

The progression of the lignite–anthracite series of coals from low carbon

TABLE 2.2

Coal type	Rank	Composition (%) (*dry mineral matter-free basis*)		
		Carbon	*Hydrogen*	*Oxygen*
Peat		50–65	5–7	30–40
Lignite	(Low)	60–75	5–6	20–30
Sub-bituminous		75–80	5–6	13–20
Bituminous	(Intermediate)	80–90	4·9–5·7	5–15
Semi-bituminous		90–92	4·5–4·9	4–5
Anthracite	(High)	92–95	2–4	2–4

and high oxygen content and volatile residue at the one end of the scale to high carbon and low oxygen and volatile contents at the other defines the '*rank*' of coal; the former being classed as low rank and the latter, high. The rank of coal may have some bearing on the pathogenesis of coal pneumoconiosis (*see* Chapter 8).

It will be seen from the process by which coal series (or coal measures) were formed that strata of sedimentary rocks (sandstones, mudstones, siltstones, and shales) lie between the coal-seams.

Arenaceous rocks, the *ganisters*, of high quartz content, are found directly beneath many coal-seams and are mined for the manufacture of refractory materials—some of the best quality being found in Britain near Sheffield and in County Durham. Such strata, often folded and faulted, are responsible for the varying composition of dusts in different coal-mines and in different parts of the same mine. The coals themselves contain no free or combined silica.

(c) *Siliceous earths.*—These consist of the fossilized remains of myriads of diatoms deposited in fresh-water or marine conditions of unusual purity. Organisms such as diatoms, radiolaria, and siliceous sponges secreted the silica of their skeletons which has, seemingly, unique and distinctive physical properties and, as already stated, is amorphous.

The degree of consolidation of these deposits which are known as diatomite, diatomaceous earth or kieselguhr is variable. The term '*tripolite*', which has also been applied to diatomite, is no longer in general use and must be distinguished from *tripoli* which is a chalecodonic quartz and contains no diatoms.

TABLE 2.3

CLASSIFICATION OF SOME COMMON SEDIMENTARY ROCKS

Group character	Type	Main features of composition
Mechanical origin		
Rudaceous	Conglomerate	Quartz content similar to parent rock; iron oxides (e.g. limonite, hematite); sometimes calcite or dolomite.
	Breccia	Mixed rock fragments; calcite and limonite with fine silt or mud in matrix
Arenaceous	Sandstone	Quartz, muscovite, and feldspar rock particles cemented by siliceous, ferruginous, calcareous, argillaceous and carbonaceous matter
	Gritstone	Similar to sandstone. Particles slightly different in shape
	Arkose	Sandstone or gritstone with about 25 per cent feldspars of various sorts. Siliceous and ferruginous content
	Quartzite	Sandstone or gritstone with detrital quartz cemented by secondary silica
	Ganister	Highly siliceous. Quartz, chert, orthoclase, feldspar, clay minerals such as kaolinite ($Al_2Si_2O_5(OH)_4$). Hematite and limonite are accessory minerals
	Siltstone	Fine-grained, compact detritus from river, lakes and glacial action. Quartz, muscovite, feldspars and iron ores with siliceous, ferruginous and calcareous cementing material
Argillaceous	Clay	Fine-grained, earthy material, plastic when wet; hard when dry. Consists of orthoclase and plagioclase feldspars, muscovite and occasionally a little quartz (*see note*)
	Fuller's earth	Mainly montmorillonite[$(Mg, Ca)O . Al_2O_3 . 5SiO_2(5-8)H_2O$] but also mica, glauconite and variable slight quartz content
	Residual clay	Formed *in situ* from rock decomposition. Very finely divided: for example, bauxite (hydrous aluminium oxides) and china clay (kaolin) (*see note*)
	Mudstone Fireclay	Consolidated, non-fissile clay with similar constituents. Usually from beneath coal seams ('seat-earths'). Contain quartz, feldspars, mica, secondary silica and iron compounds. Quartz content high
	Shale	Indurated, laminated, fine-grained clay mineral matter; contains quartz, mica, iron ores, secondary silica, calcite and iron oxides. Quartz content moderate
Calcareous-argillaceous	Marl	Unconsolidated, non-laminated calcareous clay. Composition as clays but more calcareous materials as matrix. Quartz content small and variable
	Calcareous shale	Consolidated, laminated clay with such calcareous material, i.e. consolidated marl with similar composition

Origin	Group	Rock	Description
Organic origin	Calcareous	Limestone	CaCO₃ mainly of organic origin (e.g. corals, crustacea, molluscs, algae, foraminifera), occasionally iron ores. Very small quantities of free silica may be present
		Dolomite	Limestone with large quantity of Ca.Mg(CO₃)₂, much of organic origin; also variable hematite
		Oolitic and pisolitic limestone	Limestone, more chemical than sedimentary in origin, with large characteristic grains of CaCO₃ found in successive layers round nucleus of shell fragments or quartz grains. ('Grains' resemble fishroe or peas.) Small and variable amounts of free silica
	Siliceous	Chalk	Almost pure CaCO₃. No free silica, but nodules of flint found in some chalk deposits
		Chert and flint	Crystalline and cryptocrystalline silica (microcrystalline quartz) often aggregated into 'nodules' in chalk. Very high free silica content with traces of limonite
		Siliceous earth	Group of siliceous deposits of organic origin. Total silica content (amorphous only) of diatomite ranges from 58 to 90 per cent. Some iron salts and calcareous matter. No crystalline or cryptocrystalline free silica
	Carbonaceous	Carbonaceous rocks	Peat, lignite, coal, anthracite, and cannel. Variable but usually small amounts of iron ore (pyrite, siderite, limonite) and clays (e.g. kaolinite). No free silica
Chemical origin	Calcareous	Calcium carbonate (calcite)	CaCO₃ but some impurity such as limonite. Traces of free silica are rare and accessory
		Dolomite (partly)	Occurring as mineral, not limestone replacement. Ca.Mg(CO₃)₂ with some iron impurities
	Ferrugineous	Bedded iron ores	From aqueous solutions in mudstones, limestones, primary hematite, magnesite. Variable quartz content
		Bog iron ores	Negligible quartz
	Saline	Chlorides	Mainly rock salt (NaCl) with many other salt impurities but negligible quartz
		Sulphates	Gypsum, anhydrite, barytes (BaSO₄), celestine (SrSO₄). Rarely free of rock impurity from slight mineral contamination due to variable amounts of sands, marls, clays, shales and limestones: therefore, small quantities of free silica may be present

NOTE: The majority of true clays contain very little free silica and what there is depends upon the nature of the parent rock. Clays with particle size greater than 2 μm (μm = 1/1000 millimetre) may contain a small quantity (occasionally up to 10 per cent) but those of smaller particle size contain an insignificant quantity.
'Free silica' refers to crystalline or cryptocrystalline forms unless otherwise stated.
Table freely adapted, by permission of the publishers, from Milner, H. B. (1962). *Sedimentary Petrography*, Vol. 2. London; Allen and Unwin.

E

The amorphous silica content of the siliceous earths is very high ranging from about 58 to 90 per cent. Examples from North America are especially high.

(3) Non-fragmental rocks of chemical origin

These include 'evaporites' which are, for the most part, precipitates of desiccated seas and lakes; they include *calcite, rock salt, anhydrite, gypsum,* and a form of calcium carbonate known as *aragonite*.

Iron from aqueous solutions or iron-storing bacteria is found in two main forms:

(a) Bedded iron ore (bedded ironstones) in which iron was deposited in mudstones and limestones in the form of *glauconite* (hydrated silicate of iron and potassium), *hematite* (Fe_2O_3) and *limonite* ($2Fe_2O_3.3H_2O$). Hematite is, in addition, probably formed by processes other than sedimentation, namely hydrothermal, in areas such as Cumberland. These ores are sometimes intimately associated with beds of chert, so that a high concentration of free silica may be encountered when they are mined.

(b) *Bog iron ores* which consist mostly of limonite deposited in swampy ground and underlaid by clay; free silica is absent. Siderite forms the clay-ironstone of many coal measures, in Britain, notably those of South Wales and Durham.

The more important sedimentary rocks relevant to this study are shown with their main compositional characteristics in Table 2.3.

METAMORPHIC ROCKS

Examples of metamorphic rocks which are encountered in industry are:

(1) *The asbestos group.*—'Asbestos' includes minerals of different origins. Firstly, crystals of ultrabasic rocks such as *peridotite* (an intrusive igneous rock composed mainly of olivine) and of *serpentine* (hydrous magnesium silicate often containing iron) which is itself a derivative of such ferromagnesian minerals as olivine, pyroxenes and amphiboles, were altered by enormous forces of hydrothermal and dynamic metamorphism to fibrous magnesium silicate or *chrysotile*, the commonest form of asbestos.

Secondly, minerals of the amphibole and pyroxene groups were transformed by the same forces into *crocidolite* (hydrous iron sodium silicate) and *amosite* (hydrous iron magnesium silicate)—their host rock usually being a sedimentary ironstone—also *tremolite* (hydrous calcium magnesium silicate), *actinolite* (hydrous calcium magnesium iron silicate) and *anthophyllite* (magnesium iron silicate). The host rock of these three is sedimentary as well as igneous by virtue of hydrothermal metamorphism of impure dolomite (magnesium-rich) limestones.

All forms of asbestos are usually of fibrous habit.

Talc (*see* next section) and serpentine share a common origin from metamorphosed ultrabasic rocks but, in the majority of talc deposits, talc has replaced serpentine; hence, chrysotile is rarely found as an accessory mineral.

Chrysotile and crocidolite are the most important forms of asbestos in industry; the others are employed to a more limited extent.

(2) *Talc (french chalk).*—This is a hydrous magnesium silicate which was formed by the same metamorphic processes applied to dolomite limestones and ultrabasic igneous rocks rich in magnesium carbonate. It may take the form of flat, flaky plates, granules or fibres (chiefly talcose anthophyllite). The process was closely akin to that of the production of asbestos minerals and, in fact, actinolite, anthophyllite and tremolite may be present as accessory minerals with talc which is then often referred to as *asbestine*; and, in addition to these, dolomite, magnesite, magnetite, pyrite, pyrophyllite (*see* next section) and quartz may be present. The amount of quartz varies from negligible to about 20 per cent in some deposits (Weiss and Boetner, 1967).

Some so-called 'talcs', therefore, consist mainly of tremolite or talcose anthophyllite and others may contain substantial quantities of quartz.

This variation in the identity and quantity of accessory minerals according to the origin of talc deposits is undoubtedly important in the pathogenesis and variable characteristics of 'talc' pneumoconiosis (*see* Chapter 9).

Neither the flaky nor the fibrous habit of talc is lost by grinding.

The term *steatite* (*soapstone*) has long been applied to an impure, massive form of talc which can be quarried in large blocks, but it is now often used to designate especially pure forms of talc for industry.

Pyrophyllite (*hydrous aluminium silicate*) is closely similar in origin, structure and properties and is commercially included with, and defined as, talc. However, aluminium replaces magnesium in its composition and, unlike talc, it does not fuse when fired.

(3) *Kaolin* (*china-clay*).—This is finely divided aluminium silicate derived from the feldspars of igneous rocks by weathering and sedimentation (as in Georgia and South Carolina, U.S.A.) or by hydrothermal attack (as in Cornwall and Devon). Therefore, most of the commercial china clay of the U.S.A. is not metamorphic in origin.

In the most advanced stage of the hydrothermal process only quartz may remain unaltered in powdery feldspar so that it is found in variable, but significant quantities. This is the form of china clay most suitable to the ceramic industry.

(4) *Quartzites.*—These are the result of thermal or dynamic metamorphism cementing sandstones. They, therefore, consist of a mosaic of quartz crystals and their free content is consequently very high.

(5) *Slates.*—Slates, shales and mudstones (which contain quartz grains and clay minerals) compressed by lateral forces so that re-orientation of their crystalline structure allows of easy and fine cleavage. Their quartz content is usually high; for example, about 20 per cent in Cornish slate and 30 per cent in Blaenau Ffestiniog (North Wales) slate.

(6) *Schists.*—These resulted from the effects of regional metamorphism upon argillaceous and certain metamorphic rocks and include mica-schists and talc.

(7) *Marbles.*—These were produced by thermal and dynamic metamorphism on limestone. If the limestone was pure (dolomite, for example) a pure marble with negligible free silica content resulted, but if it were impure, marbles with variable silicate composition were produced; for example, *forsterite* (magnesium silicate of the olivine group).

(8) *Mineral ores.*—Mineral ores originated in a number of ways; early

crystallization from magma and then separation (for example, *chromite* ($FeCr_2O_4$); percolation and subsequent solidification of magmatic gas or liquid in pockets within native rock which was frequently of igneous type (for example, *beryl, copper, gold, lead, silver, zinc*); and by subterranean waters dissolving scattered minerals and depositing these elsewhere in increased concentration.

It is evident, therefore, that mineral ores are apt to be found deposited in 'pockets' and 'veins' among rocks of widely differing type and composition.

(9) *Graphite*, a soft black form of carbon, is found disseminated mostly in mica-schists, micaceous quartzites, and occasionally in various igneous rocks. For this reason, although some graphite is pure carbon and, therefore, lacks combined and free silica, it may contain various impurities derived from the associated rock minerals, especially in the mined material. These include feldspars, pyrites, iron oxides, muscovite and quartz; their amount varies according to the origin of the graphite deposit. The amount of quartz is usually low, but may be about 2 per cent and an example as high as 11 per cent has been reported (Parmeggiani, 1950).

EARTH MOVEMENTS

The various rock types have not remained in the order in which they were formed. The effects of weathering and enormous pressures due to earth movements caused by earthquakes and volcanic activity folded, dislocated and fractured the crust. The effects of movements are exemplified by simple folds, overfolds, faults and thrusts of sedimentary rocks, the original strata of which were thereby extensively displaced and intermingled.

This means that in tunnelling and mining or quarrying for a mineral in a particular stratum, a variety of different and unrelated materials may be encountered, from which it is evident that the composition of dusts produced by these processes will vary from locality to locality.

ROCK NAMES

The local names attached to similar rocks in different regions of the British Isles vary greatly and are sometimes the cause of confusion; a valuable key to the meanings is provided by Arkel and Tomkeieff (1953).

SOME COMMON USES OF ROCKS AND MINERALS

The following, presented in brief note form, is not intended to be comprehensive but to give some indication of the range of use of these materials.

Abrasives

Diamond, corundum (natural, crystallized Al_2O_3), emery (corundum with iron oxides); garnet, quartz, tripoli, quartzite and sandstone; pumice, diatomite, iron oxides (e.g. jeweller's rouge, 'crocus' and black rouge), talc and zircon ($ZrSiO_4$). Corundum, garnet, quartzose sands and flint grains are used for sandblasting of building stones and concrete, for etching glass and cleaning metal castings (*see* Chapter 7). Feldspar has been recently used in abrasive soap powders.

Building Materials

Gravels and crushed flint or chert for concrete; sand for cement mortar and plaster; marl for cement; limestones for lime, Portland cement, and plaster. There are many different types of cements but, for the most part, they consist of limestones and clay or slate; gypsum is added to retard the setting time of the cement.

Aggregates (that is, crushed rocks of various types or blast furnace slag) are mixed with sand and cement to make concrete.

Gypsum is widely used for plaster (plaster of Paris) and to manufacture plaster board.

Of separate but great importance is asbestos (of one type or another) which, when added as a lightweight aggregate produces a cement from which corrugated roofing, pipes, wall sheets and sections of pipe-covering materials are moulded or pressed; it is also used in millboards and putties, as fillers in floor tiles and sprayed in suspension on to walls and ceilings.

Building and monumental stones (dimension stone)

Granite (and other igneous rocks), sandstones, limestone, dolomite, and marble.

Roofing materials

Materials crushed into granular form and applied as fillers in asphaltic or bituminous mixtures include: limestone, calcined flint, chert, mica, slate dust, quartzite, gravels, asbestos, talc and diatomite. These are used in the manufacture of damp course materials as well as roofing felts, and finely ground slate (slate flour may also be added to the rubber mix to provide 'body').

Talc powder is also employed in the manufacture of roofing felt to prevent its adhesion when rolled.

Slates cut into blocks by circular saws and split to desired thickness by chisel and mallet.

Road construction materials

Some igneous rocks, limestone dolomite, most members of the rudaceous and arenaceous sedimentary rock groups, chert, flint, ganister and quartzite crushed to size are used to fill or aggregate asphalt and concrete for highways, pavements, airfield runways and the like. Asbestos has also been used as a filler for asphalt.

Ceramics

There are three ceramic groups: (1) refractory and technical; (2) earthenware, chinaware and stoneware; (3) structural clay products.

Refractory and technical

(a) *A refractory ceramic* is a substance possessing the ability to resist high temperatures and changes of temperature without loss of physical or chemical identity.

Bricks and cements for the lining of furnaces and kilns may have to withstand temperatures of 1500°C or more and mortars and crucibles may be required to resist temperatures of in excess of 3000°C.

Materials used are: fireclays; ganisters; quartz, and chert; graphite; magnesite; olivine rock as 'forsterite'; chromite; alumina (bauxite); sillimanite minerals (anhydrous aluminium silicate), and zircon.

(b) *Technical ceramics* are employed in the electronic and other specialized industries, for example, metallurgy, atomic reactors and other forms of nuclear engineering, electrical and radio engineering, cutting tools, aircraft, missiles and spaceships.

The materials used are selected for their special dielectric, thermal conductivity and low neutron absorption properties according to their required purpose; refractory properties are secondary. Examples are: alumina which has great toughness, and excellent thermal conductivity and qualities of electrical insulation; Carborundum (a synthetic compound, silicon carbide); beryllium oxide, widely used in nuclear engineering, thorium oxide and zirconium dioxide; uranium and plutonium oxides for ceramic fuels; a mixture of talc (or pyrophyllite), china clay or ball clay and a flux, usually barium carbonate, is fired at about 1400°C and used extensively for valve holders, insulators and condenser plates in the radio and television industry. Beryllium oxide (beryllia) possesses all the necessary properties in high degree and is increasingly important in modern technology (*see* Chapter 10).

Earthenware, chinaware and stoneware

Both non-plastic and plastic materials are required. Non-plastic materials include quartz, flint and feldspar; plastic materials include china clay, ball clay, fire clay and red clay.

Enamel glazes are prepared from sands and sandstones of very high quartz content.

Wollastonite is used extensively in the U.S.A., Finland and Denmark as a substitute for these ingredients in the ceramic mix and in glazes.

Structural clay products

Those include building and engineering bricks of all sorts, floor and roof tiles, drain pipes and chimney pots. Clays and shales are the chief ingredients but silica sand, and wollastonite are used in various combinations in the manufacture of wall tiles. The use of wollastonite without flint, or with a small quantity only, has reduced the risk of silicosis (Andrews, 1970). Talc or pyrophyllite is the main ingredient in some body formulas, but not in the United Kingdom.

Fillers

Fillers are substances which are used to fill the voids within a material and to modify its chemical or physical properties (for example, its viscosity) and also to lower the cost. According to their function, therefore, they are also referred to as *extenders* when they aid even spreading of paint pigments without impoverishing their colour. In general, they require to be finely divided so that a substantial proportion of their particles are less than 10 μm in size.

Some important materials in which they are used are as follows.

Asphalt and concrete.—Limestones, clays, silica, mica, slate dusts, asbestos (in some countries), diatomite and talc.

Gramophone records (before 1948 in U.K.).—Rottenstone, finely ground slate and barytes.

Paints.—Barium sulphate (barytes), calcined diatomite, gypsum, china-clay, mica, pyrophyllite, crystalline silica and talc are used as extenders.

Paper.—China clay, natural and calcined diatomite, gypsum and talc may be added at the stage of the beater process. Diatomite also functions as an extender of white pigment.

Pesticides.—A 'carrier' is needed to sustain the physical properties and efficiency of the active chemical agent; clays, fuller's earth, diatomite, pyrophyllite and talc are among those used.

Plastics.—Asbestos, mica or talc are added to some thermosetting and amino-resins; asbestos only to laminated and some polyvinyl chloride plastics. Diatomite, crystalline silica and alumina are constituents of silicone resins.

Rubber (natural and synthetic).—Fillers have two functions here. Apart from increasing bulk for the sake of cheapness, they also improve one or more of the physical properties of the rubber. Carbon black is most commonly used but others of importance are china clay (the particles of which are usually less than 2 μm diameter), other clay powders, slate powder, barytes, graphite, gypsum, diatomite, ground mica, talc (both as a filler and extender in heat-resistant mixes) and asbestos.

Textiles.—Fillers are often added to the starch, glue or synthetic sizes and include clays, gypsum and talc.

Moulding and foundry sands

Quartzose sands of high quartz content are bonded with clays such as halloysite ($Al_2O_3 . 2SiO_2 . 2H_2O$), illite (a mica-like clay), kaolinite and montmorillonite. Zircon sand bonded with oil is now used because of its high resistance to thermal shock and to reduce the 'silica' risk, and there is an increasing use of olivine sand.

Glass

Quartz sands of exceptionally high purity and uniform grain size are employed with lime in glass manufacture. For special glasses there is a wide range of other materials such as lithium, boron and strontium.

Pigments

Hematite and limonite, iron-stained clays (ochres, sienna and umbers) and shales, frequently found in areas of fracture and fault of rocks such as limestone and quartzite, are widely used. They contain iron or aluminium oxides. Their free silica content is rarely significant.

Graphite is used in paints and pigments. Carbon black (a synthetic substance) is the chief pigment in printing ink and is also used in gramophone records (*see* Chapter 8).

Cosmetics

Talc, mainly from France and Italy and purified by elutriation or acid treatment, is used in 'talcum' and baby powders. Despite purification, significant quantities of 'free silica' are occasionally found in some samples (Cralley *et al.*, 1968).

Dusting agents

Talc is used to prevent adhesion of material, in the manufacture of rubber roofing felts, linoleum, leather, corks and chewing gum, and apparently to produce a polished surface on chocolate bars so that adhesion to the wrapping does not occur.

Heat insulation materials

Mixes of various compositions for application to boilers, pipes and joints, bulkheads and other parts of ships include asbestos of various types, diatomite, kaolinite, magnesite, and mineral wools (*see* Chapter 9).

Other uses of asbestos materials

As the asbestos minerals are known to be of great medical importance, reference to some uses other than those already mentioned should be made:

(1) Spinning and weaving fibres for textiles such as fireproof suits and ropes. Chrysotile and, to a lesser extent, crocidolite are used.

(2) In gaskets, brake linings, clutch facings, insulating blocks, welding rod coatings and cooking mats. Again, mainly chrysotile and occasionally crocidolite are employed.

(3) Filters for beer, fruit juices, plasma, wine, pharmaceutical and other liquids. Chrysotile is most commonly used and diatomite is sometimes added. Anthophyllite and tremolite are also, but less often, employed.

(4) Mixes of chrysotile, amosite or anthophyllite in an adhesive medium are sprayed under pressure on to walls and ceilings in buildings for fire protection and modification of acoustics. The method is also used in ships. Asbestos is a frequent ingredient of coloured dressings for the outside of houses and other buildings.

(5) Chrysotile, crocidolite and amosite are (or have been) compounded with resins to impregnate paper or millboard for use in aeroplane wings, motor-car bodies, small boats and missile nose cones; and with waterproofing resins and other materials to make caulking compounds.

Crocidolite seems to have been used in cigarette filters in the U.S.A. but not in the United Kingdom (Tobacco Research Council, 1968).

REFERENCES

Andrews, R. W. (1970). *Wollastonite*. Institute Geol. Sc. London; H.M.S.O.
Arkel, W. J. and Tomkeieff S. I. (1953). *English Rock Terms*. London; Oxford University Press
Cralley, L. J., Key, M. M., Gorth, D. H., Leinhart, W. S. and Ligo, R. M. (1968). 'Fibrous and mineral content of cosmetic talcum products.' *Am. ind. Hyg. Ass. J.* **29**, 350–354
Drenk, K. (1959). *X-ray Particle Size Determination and its Application to Flint*. Pennsylvania State University; X-ray and Crystal Structure Laboratory
Geikie, J. (1908). *Structural and Field Geology*, 2nd Ed., p. 32. London; Oliver and Boyd
Holt, P. F. (1957). *Pneumoconiosis*, p. 14. London; Arnold
Parmeggiani, L. (1950). 'Graphite pneumoconiosis.' *Br. J. ind. Med.* **7**, 42–45
Tobacco Research Council (1968). Personal communication
Urey, H. C. (1952). *The Planets; Their Origin and Development*. New Haven, Conn.; Yale University Press
Weiss, B. and Boettner, E. A. (1967). 'Commercial talc and talcosis.' *Archs envir. Hlth* **14**, 304–308

3—Inhaled Particles and their Fate in the Lungs

A detailed discussion of this highly technical subject is beyond the scope and purpose of this book. Nevertheless some basic knowledge of the behaviour of inhaled particles is necessary to appreciate the sizes at which they are likely to reach the depths of the lungs (and hence require detection and control in the work environment), and the forces which govern their deposition and retention in the lungs, and subsequent elimination.

Substances of diverse nature and physical form, once airborne, may reach the upper and lower airways of the lungs in inspired air. Their ability to do this depends on their physical properties. The more a material (such as rock) is broken down, finely divided and dispersed the more likely are its particles to be airborne and, therefore, capable of inhalation. But there are types of particulate clouds, other than those produced by attrition of rock, which have a wide range of particle size; everyday language speaks of 'dusts', 'fumes', 'smokes' and 'mists', and it is important that these should be distinguished.

Dust, in daily speech, means tiny particles which have settled on a surface, can be readily disturbed and are visible in a shaft of sunlight. It is more properly defined as consisting of solid particles dispersed in air (or other gaseous media) due to mechanical disintegration of rocks, minerals and other materials by such impulsive forces as drilling, blasting, crushing, grinding, milling, sawing and polishing; or to the agitation or breaking down of organic materials such as cotton fibres, pollens and fungal spores.

The approximate size ranges of some different types of particles are shown for comparison in Table 3.1.

Rock dusts vary greatly in size depending upon the sort of material worked, the process involved, the magnitude of the sample of dust taken and the time for which a dust cloud has been airborne. The majority of asbestos particles are fibrous and are produced by handling, disintegrating, carding (that is, combing out or disentangling) and weaving of amosite, chrysotile and crocidolite, their length usually ranging from 5 μm to 100 μm; but, in addition, a substantial proportion are non-fibrous, small and compact. (*See* page 59 for the distinction between 'fibrous' and 'compact' particles.)

Fumes consist of metal oxides formed by heating metals to their melting points. Particle size ranges from 0·1 μm to 1 μm diameter at source, but aggregation of these particles readily occurs and, although these aggregations are often of large diameter, they have very low densities. This term is often used to refer to clouds of acid droplets but strictly speaking these should be classed as *vapours*.

Mists are liquid droplets formed by the condensation of vapours or the 'atomization' of liquids around appropriate nuclei. Many particles are less than 0·1 μm diameter and therapeutic mists are usually less than 10 μm, but some droplets may be up to 500 μm diameter.

The term *aerosol* is now commonly used to embrace all of these categories and so includes both dispersed particles and droplets.

Potentially dangerous particles, therefore, vary in size from those just small enough to enter the upper respiratory tract down to gas molecules.

TABLE 3.1

COMPARISON OF PARTICLE SIZES

Material	Dimension range
Sand grains	200–2000 μm dia.
Cement dusts	4– 100 μm dia.
Grass pollen	26– 35 μm dia.
Fungal spores	{ 2– 100 μm length { 0·5– 7 μm dia.
Actinomycete spores	0·6– 2·5 μm length
*Rock dusts	1– 10 μm dia.
Tobacco smoke	0·2– 2 μm dia.
Viruses	28 nm– 0·2 μm dia.

* Particles of flint, sandstone, shale, coal and other rock dusts produced by such processes as drilling, blasting shovelling, chiselling and milling.

PROPERTIES OF DUSTS

The majority of dust particles are not spherical but of irregular shape and, according to their composition, exist either individually or as aggregations. All particles have a small but independent motion of their own and their primary characteristic, when airborne, is a tendency to settle under the influence of gravity. The gravitational force exerted on a particle is equal to its mass multiplied by the gravitational constant. Against this is opposed the force of the viscosity of air and, although this is greater for large than for small particles, its effect is overwhelmed by the mass of larger particles. Other things being equal, the terminal velocity of a particle is proportional to the square of its density. Hence, a spherical particle of unit density and 50 μm diameter falls through air at speed of 73 mm/s whereas one of 5 μm diameter falls through air at a speed of about 1 mm/s. This settling tendency —*free-falling speed*—is an important determinant of the aerodynamic behaviour of particles in the airways of the lungs and is related to their shape, surface characteristics and density. It is not their apparent microscopic size which decides the manner in which particles behave, but their aero-dynamic properties; the particle sizes of importance in pneumoconiosis are those which behave as if they were *unit density spheres* (UDS) of 1 to 10 μm diameter. Hence, an aggregation of dust particles with a total microscopic diameter of (say) 20 μm may have a terminal velocity equivalent to a UDS of 5 μm diameter which will enable it to penetrate deeply into the lung.

Particles which approximate to a sphere (for example, quartz, coal, clays and some spores) are referred to as *compact* and those whose length exceeds their diameter by a factor of 3 to 1 or more (for example, chrysotile and crocidolite asbestos), as *fibrous*. (However, a fibrous particle is usually regarded by geologists as one whose length/diameter ratio is 10/1 or more.) The tendency of either type of particle to be deposited in the lung is largely governed by their falling speeds.

Particles smaller than 1 μm diameter are referred to as *submicron particles* and are apt to remain airborne for long periods of time; hence they may present a special hazard if their concentration is sufficiently high.

BEHAVIOUR OF INHALED PARTICLES

Aerosols inhaled into the respiratory tract closely follow the movement of the air in which they are suspended, and the depth to which they penetrate into the lung depends not only upon their physical characteristics (size,

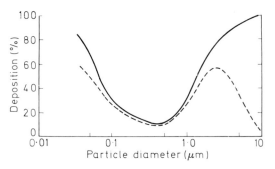

Figure 3.1. Deposition curves of compact particles during mouth breathing. The dotted curve represents particle deposition in the alveolar region of the respiratory tract (alveolar deposition); maximum deposition is seen to lie in the 2 μm to 5 μm range. The continuous curve represents deposition throughout the respiratory tract from nose to alveoli (total deposition). Below 0·1 μm diameter there is again some tendency for alveolar deposition to increase. (From Clinical Aspects of Inhaled Particles, by courtesy of Dr D. C. F. Muir and the publishers, Heinemann)

density, shape and aerodynamic properties) but also upon the volume of each respiration. Once a particle comes in contact with the wall of an airway or an alveolus it cannot again become airborne, and it is then said to be *deposited*. Because the majority of inhaled particles less than 1 μm diameter are expelled in exhaled air (*Figure 3.1*) their concentration in the inhaled air must be high to enable some to be deposited in the lungs.

The composition of particles, whether in the solid or liquid state, does not influence their deposition.

There are four ways in which solid particles are deposited—sedimentation, inertial impaction, interception and diffusion.

Sedimentation

Sedimentation is settlement influenced by gravity. It is determined by the density and diameter of particles (density × diameter^2). Under some circumstances the form of airflow in a tube may influence sedimentation but, for practical purposes, it has no effect upon particle sedimentation in the lungs which occurs predominantly at low velocities. Particles deposited in this way have aerodynamic sizes of about 2 μm or less. Deposition in the larger airways is chiefly due to sedimentation.

The free-falling speed of fibrous particles is determined by the square of their diameter and is little influenced by their shape or length. Gravitational settlement of fibres occurs only in large airways and it limits the diameter of fibres which can penetrate to small airways to less than 3 μm (Timbrell, 1970). In small airways, therefore, deposition of fibres is not determined by their falling speed, but by their length and shape (see Interception).

Inertial impaction

When an airstream carrying fairly large particles has its direction changed by the curving or branching of airways (as in nasal cavities and large airways of the lungs) the particles tend to follow their original path in the airstream and, in consequence, impinge upon the walls. Impaction of particles in this way is related to their density × diameter^2, the diameter and change of direction of the tube, and the rate of air flow in the tube.

This is the primary mechanism of deposition in the nose and is important in large airways for compact particles larger than 10 μm. Particles smaller than this are able to penetrate to the small airways and alveoli.

Interception

This concerns particles of irregular shape (for example, mica plates) or of fibrous habit (such as asbestos) in which the length and shape of the particles is more important than their falling speed.

The lower the length/diameter ratio of a fibrous particle the closer its behaviour resembles that of a compact particle, but the longer a fibre the less likely it is to behave in this way. Hence, long fibres of small diameter (less than 3 μm), unlike compact particles, avoid sedimentation and impaction in larger airways and are intercepted by collision with the walls of terminal and respiratory bronchioles particularly at their bifurcations. This explains the fact that asbestos fibres as long as 200 μm may be found in this region.

Chrysotile fibres are invariably curled, a property which increases their likelihood of collision with the walls of narrow airways, mainly at their bifurcations. Amphibole fibres, on the other hand, are always straight, and this favours their orientation parallel to the axis of the airways by the aerodynamic forces so that they penetrate deeper into the lung. Crocidolite (blue asbestos) fibres reach the periphery of the lung having suffered little sedimentation en route (Timbrell, Pooley and Wagner, 1970).

The variable depth of penetration by different types of asbestos fibre may be significant in determining which types are likely to cause disease (*see* Chapter 9).

Diffusion

This effect, which is exhibited by very small particles (less than 0·1 μm diameter) and which is independent of their density, influences their deposition significantly in the region beyond the terminal bronchioles and also upon the wall of the trachea; indeed, it may be responsible for their complete deposition (*Figure 3.1*). It does not affect the behaviour of larger particles.

Because the diffusion forces of oxygen and carbon dioxide operate in opposite directions and are almost equal they are unlikely to have any effect on the movement and deposition of particles in the region beyond the terminal bronchiole (Davies, 1967).

Deposition for a given particle size shows great variation from subject to subject and, in cigarette smoking, appears to occur more proximally than distally due, possibly, to the bronchoconstrictive effect of tobacco smoke (Lippman, Albert and Peterson, 1971). There is some evidence that significantly fewer particles smaller than 5 μm are deposited beyond terminal bronchioles in cigarette smokers compared with non-smokers (Sanchis et al., 1971).

INFLUENCE ON DEPOSITION OF AERODYNAMIC SIZE AND PATTERNS OF RESPIRATION

The size of particles is a decisive factor in determining how far they can penetrate into the respiratory tract and the probability of their deposition. When breathing is through the nose the majority of particles with a diameter greater than 10 μm UDS equivalent are trapped in the nose and pharynx. Precise knowledge of the size range of compact particles which reach the alveoli is lacking and the size at which maximum alveolar deposition occurs is a subject of controversy but it is clear that, in addition to size, tidal volume plays an important role.

Experimental work on human adults breathing through the mouth suggests that alveolar deposition occurs at a size greater than 2 μm (Altshuler, Palmas and Nelson, 1967), but less than 4 μm (Lippman and Albert, 1969). On theoretical grounds, however, Davies (1967) believes that the size of maximal deposition is probably in excess of 0·5 μm but not greater than 1 μm; this view has not received general acceptance.

The tidal volume of each respiration and the frequency of the respiratory cycle profoundly influence the behaviour of particles in the airways. The greater the tidal volume the deeper the mass flow of transporting air penetrates into the lungs, whereas with increasing frequency of respiration the deposition of compact particles decreases (Muir and Davies, 1967). Both tidal volume and respiration frequency are increased by effort, and it is the *minute volume* (that is, the product of tidal volume and number of breaths per minute) which is the most important factor determining the *total volume* of particles deposited. In short, the increase in minute volume which accompanies heavy physical effort results in a greater deposition of particles than

61

occurs when the subject is at rest or performing light work. It has been calculated (Report, 1966) that during nose breathing, maximal deposition should occur for particles of approximately 2·2 μm, 2·0 μm and 1·9 μm (UDS) at tidal volumes of 750, 1450 and 2150 cm³ respectively. Lippmann and Albert (1969) re-examined these results for mouth breathing and predicted that maximal deposition would then occur at approximately 3·3 μm, 2·3 μm and 2·5 μm (UDS) at the same respective tidal volumes.

Different breathing patterns also probably impose significant individual variations in deposition.

Dust particles recovered after death from the lungs of coal-miners have a wide range of sizes but the majority are about 1 μm (Cartwright, 1967; Leiteritz, Einbrodt and Klosterkötter, 1967). This is due largely to the breakdown of aggregations of particles which individually are approximately 1 μm diameter.

For practical purposes then, and on the grounds of present knowledge, it appears that maximal alveolar deposition of compact particles occurs between 2 μm and 5 μm UDS (*Figure 3.1*) and *Figure 3.2* shows the percentage of inhaled particles which is calculated to penetrate beyond the terminal

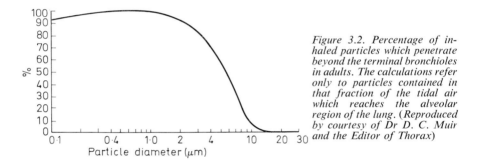

Figure 3.2. Percentage of inhaled particles which penetrate beyond the terminal bronchioles in adults. The calculations refer only to particles contained in that fraction of the tidal air which reaches the alveolar region of the lung. (Reproduced by courtesy of Dr D. C. Muir and the Editor of Thorax)

bronchioles in adults (Hislop *et al.*, 1972). These size ranges and the size-selecting characteristics of the respiratory tract have particular significance in the design specification of dust sampling instruments and in deciding the maximum allowable concentrations of specified dusts (*see* Threshold Limit Values) in a work environment.

Experiments in man (admittedly artificial in that they analysed only a single inspiration followed by breath holding) have shown that 30 to 50 per cent of 5 μm particles are deposited beyond the ciliated airways during mouth breathing (Thompson and Short, 1969). During breathing through the nose there is a significant, though lesser, deposition of these particles in the alveolar region at tidal volumes of 500 to 600 cm³ (Booker *et al.*, 1967). The importance of these observations is that they indicate that fungal spores (such as those responsible for the various forms of extrinsic allergic 'alveolitis') can reach the gas-exchanging region of the lungs (*see* Chapter 11).

The distribution in the lungs of inhaled air carrying dust particles is of particular interest in relation to the zonal preference of certain types of pneumoconiosis. Although it is virtually simultaneous in all zones during normal breathing, the lower zones are ventilated more than the upper when breathing from FRC but, at lung volumes approaching RV, ventilation of the upper zones is greater than the lower (Milic-Emili, Henderson and Kaneko, 1968). It is not known to what extent these events at the extremes of tidal volumes determine the zonal distribution of deposited particles.

Other mechanisms which have been suggested as influencing particle deposition are turbulence in the upper airways and surges of air flow in the lower airways synchronous with the heart beat (West, 1961). There is little evidence to support or refute these contentions.

CLEARANCE OF PARTICLES FROM THE LUNGS

Both inert and cytotoxic insoluble particles which are deposited in the conducting airways above the terminal bronchioles are eliminated either in a free (that is, extracellular) state or within macrophages via the mucociliary 'escalator' and are expectorated in sputum or swallowed usually about 12 hours after inhalation. However, in the gas-exchanging region distal to the terminal bronchioles the behaviour of inert and cytotoxic particles appears to be different.

Inert particles deposited in alveoli tend to remain in the alveolar area and to be eliminated mainly by the bronchial route. They are engulfed by macrophages which migrate from the alveoli over the non-ciliated zone of the respiratory bronchioles to the mucociliary 'escalator' in the terminal bronchioles. It is not understood how they are able to bridge this gap but it has been suggested (Kilburn, 1968) that a proximal movement of surfactant may be responsible. Particles lodged in the interstitium may be carried by macrophages in tissue fluids to the lymphatics whence they travel to intrapulmonary and hilar lymph nodes, but others are retained, or 'stored', in the interstitial site for years.

Cytotoxic dusts, for example, free silica dusts, behave differently. Their lethal effect upon macrophages (*see* Chapter 4) appears to be decisive so that particles deposited distal to the terminal bronchioles have a greatly limited chance of being transported by these cells to the mucociliary 'escalator' and eliminated. Most of them, therefore, penetrate into the interstitium whence some are removed by the lymphatic system (possibly mainly in an extracellular state) to the regional lymph nodes but many are carried only a limited distance from their point of entry where they provoke local fibrogenesis. Those particles which reach the 'escalator' are probably transported and removed in the extracellular state.

It appears that if a small quantity of quartz (3 to 4 per cent) is intermingled with inert dusts their penetration into the interstitium is facilitated and their bronchial elimination reduced (Klosterkötter and Bünemann, 1961).

Smaller insoluble particles tend to travel to hilar lymph nodes more quickly than larger ones (Nagelschmidt *et al.*, 1957), but quartz particles reach the lymphatics more rapidly than non-toxic particles, such as titanium oxide, of similar size (Klosterkötter and Bünemann, 1961). Furthermore, some small particles may pass into the blood stream; this explains the occasional presence of silicotic lesions in the liver and spleen and other organs.

The efficiency with which insoluble dusts are removed from the lungs varies, therefore, according to whether they are inert or cytotoxic as well as upon the load or concentration of particles imposed upon the elimination routes. Soluble particles dissolve readily and pass into the capillary blood or, possibly, are bound to lung tissue proteins; hence, if they are toxic they may cause damage either systemically or locally (*Figure 3.3*).

The process by which inert and cytotoxic dusts pass from the alveolar lumen into the alveolar wall or its adjacent interstitum is obscure. Breaching of the wall by damage to Type I pneumocytes is thought to occur by some workers (Spencer, 1968) but is denied by others. There is experimental evidence to show that particles may penetrate into the alveolar wall without

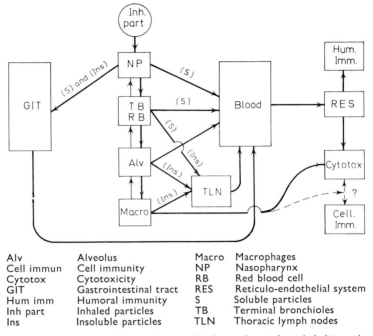

Alv	Alveolus	Macro	Macrophages
Cell immun	Cell immunity	NP	Nasopharynx
Cytotox	Cytotoxicity	RB	Red blood cell
GIT	Gastrointestinal tract	RES	Reticulo-endothelial system
Hum imm	Humoral immunity	S	Soluble particles
Inh part	Inhaled particles	TB	Terminal bronchioles
Ins	Insoluble particles	TLN	Thoracic lymph nodes

Figure 3.3. Diagram showing the possible fates of particles inhaled into the lungs. (After Kilburn, 1968; by courtesy of the Editor of American Review of Respiratory Diseases)

the mediation of phagocytic cells (Gross and Westrick, 1954) and that this tends to occur where alveoli are in opposition to bronchiolo-vascular bundles. Type I pneumocytes have always been regarded as lacking phagocytic potential but evidence has been offered (Casarett and Milley, 1964; Hapke and Pedersen, 1968) to suggest that this may not be true and that in fact they may be capable of ingesting particles and of migrating either into the alveolar lumen or into its wall (Casarett and Milley, 1964). This suggestion, which if true, is obviously important, has not been confirmed and requires further study.

Elimination of particles from the lungs occurs in rapid and slow phases. The rapid phase is usually complete in about 24 hours and is accounted for by the clearance of particles which have been recently deposited in the bronchi and bronchioles either by their transportation up the airways or their solution and subsequent passage into the blood stream. The slow phase takes months—up to 300 days in the case of 5 μm particles (Booker *et al.*, 1967). Inert particles which are not removed within months appear as if stored in the lungs although, in fact, they are slowly eliminated over a period of many years; indeed, the appearance of coal or hematite dusts, for example, in the sputum of men who have been away from dust exposure for years is well known both to them and to their physicians.

There is, however, large individual variation in the rate mucociliary clearance of particles (Albert, Lippmann and Briscoe, 1969) but there appears to be uncertainty as to whether or not smoking influences the efficiency of clearance; some investigators have found evidence that it does impair clearance (Albert, Lippmann and Briscoe, 1969) and others that it does not (Pavia, Short and Thomson, 1970). But there seems little doubt that cigarette smoke is ciliatoxic (Kennedy and Elliot, 1970) and it appears that the normally rapid first phase of clearance in man is slowed down and the slow phase accelerated by cigarette smoking (Sanchis *et al.*, 1971).

It is possible that particles deposited upon ciliated respiratory epithelium may remain *in situ* for a significantly longer period than has previously been thought. If this is so it is of particular importance in the case of radioactive particles.

THRESHOLD LIMIT VALUES

In industry (especially where there are processes using potentially dangerous materials) it is important to know if an inhalable aerosol is generated and exists in the ambient air, and if so in what concentration. If such an aerosol cannot be completely eradicated at source it is necessary to devise a method capable of defining a concentration level in the atmosphere which should not be exceeded if health is not be be endangered.

Clinical and epidemiological experience and animal experiments have shown that some aerosols have greater disease-producing potential than others; and some individuals a greater susceptibility to them (and, therefore, greater liability, to disease) than others. That is, a more dangerous dust may provoke disease at very low concentrations in a short period of time whereas another, less dangerous, may require fairly high concentrations over a long period. It is possible from such studies to find an approximate empirical level of concentration of a potentially hazardous airborne aerosol which will cause no lung disease—or very little—in workers exposed to it over a period of a working life. This empirical level is the *Threshold Limit Value* (TLV) or *Maximum Allowable Concentration* (MAC) of the aerosol. Concentration is expressed either as particles/cm³ or as millions of particles per cubic foot (mppcf).

In the United Kingdom and the United States TLVs for the majority of airborne contaminants are related to the time that a worker is exposed to a particular risk and they refer to *time-weighted* concentrations during a 7 or 8 hour 'Working Day' and a 5 day (40 hour) 'Working Week'. In some countries—for example, the U.S.S.R.—continuous exposure is measured. Although time-weighted average concentration is the most practical method of controlling most hazardous materials, substances which have a rapid action (for example, nitrogen dioxide and toluene diisocyanate (*see* Chapter 12) are best controlled by a *Ceiling Limit* which should not be exceeded at any time.

Threshold limit values of all hazardous substances are reviewed and published annually by the Committee on Threshold Standards of the American Conference of Governmental Industrial Hygienists (ACGIH) and by the Department of Employment and Productivity in the United Kingdom, but other countries also issue their own standards referring either to general lists of substances or to individual materials. For example, the British National Coal Board (1966) has laid down its own standards for coal and rock dusts in collieries, and the Committee on Hygiene Standards of the British Occupational Hygiene Society (1968) has similarly defined standards for chrysotile asbestos dust. The International Labour Office (1970) has also published TLVs employed in most countries of the world. Unless otherwise stated the TLVs quoted in this book are those of the ACGIH (1971) and are reproduced with the Conference's permission.

It should be understood that a TLV does not indicate a definitive dust concentration to which it is *safe* to be exposed, and above which it is not. Obviously, freedom from the effects of a dangerous dust is certain only when it is absent from the environment. But the TLV assumes that, if individual hazardous materials can be prevented from exceeding a certain empirically determined level at any time, then below this level it is unlikely to cause disease during the period of a working life; in the majority of cases this has been well borne out by experience. As far as possible concentrations of dusts or fumes should at all times be kept below their TLVs.

The question arises as to whether it is preferable to measure average or 'peak' dust concentrations in the worker's environment. Whereas average concentrations can be readily related to the period of a working life there is much evidence to suggest that 'peak' measurements of some substances (especially certain harmful dusts) are more significantly correlated with risk to health. For example, it has been urged (Roach, 1966) that sampling time should be related to the biological half-life in the body of the sampled particles so that in the case of soluble or radioactive particles, absolute—not average —'peak' values should be determined. Nevertheless, because cumulative deposition appears to be roughly the same with both high and low concentrations of environmental dust when the values of 'dust concentration × time of exposure' are similar (Klosterkötter, 1968), determination of average exposure should give a satisfactory indication of cumulative deposition (and hence the risk of certain types of pneumoconiosis) which may be expected to occur in the lungs.

The naturally-occurring gases radon and thoron constitute an important potential hazard to the lungs; radon and radon 'daughters' are found in uranium mines, some other types of mine and, occasionally, in tunnelling works (*see* Chapter 12). Decay of the unstable atoms of these gases releases α particles and the remaining decay product, which has the property of a solid, may adhere to aerosol (dust) particles. Radioactive aerosols are the most hazardous of all and they have the lowest concentration which can be tolerated indefinitely.

Alpha particles have low energy and when deposited in the airways or alveoli are absorbed within a few micrometres distance from their source; that is, in neighbouring cells. Gamma particles possess much greater energy and so pass through the tissues to leave the body, and hence are less damaging to cells. The TLV for α-emitters, therefore, is lower than that for γ-emitters.

Of non-radioactive aerosols beryllium is the most toxic and other substances fall into a scale of decreasing toxicity.

Inert substances

Particles of inert substances are sometimes referred to as 'Nuisance Particulates' mainly because they may have an irritant effect in the upper respiratory tract. They do not cause fibrotic pneumoconiosis, although this may occur if fibrogenic or radioactive contaminants are associated with them. Some inorganic examples are chalk, Portland cement, corundum, emery, gypsum, iron oxides, limestone and silicon carbide, and because of their nuisance potential they are subject to a TLV of 10 mg/m³ over the period of a 'Working Day' (*see* Chapters 6 and 7).

Sampling

The frequency of sampling required differs according to whether the potential hazard is subject to a 'ceiling' or 'time-weighted' limit: a single short period of sampling is sufficient in the former case, but a number of samples taken throughout the period of the work shift are necessary in the latter.

The underlying principles of instruments for sampling atmospheric dusts varies according to the nature and TLV of the dust to be analysed: whether particle counting or compositional analysis is required; the siting of instruments in the work environment, and the duration of sampling planned. Hence, there are many different types of instrument, both portable and static. Samples may be obtained from the workers' immediate environment ('breathing zone'), from the locality of the work process ('source zone'), or from the general factory atmosphere ('background zone'); and they can be either of very brief duration and taken at random ('grab samples') or of prolonged duration.

Identification of radioactive gases and aerosols and the assessment of the degree of their radioactivity requires instruments of special design to separate dust particles, radioactive particles and gas.

The prospective as well as the immediate value of analyses of sampling data is apparent in the protection afforded the worker, in the identification of faulty methods of dust suppression and in computation of the worker's possible total exposure to a specific dust hazard over his working life.

The complexities of sampling instruments and sampling strategy and of the details of the many techniques for protecting the worker and for the disposal of dusts and fumes are beyond the scope and competence of this book. A comprehensive account of sampling instruments is given by the American Conference of Government Industrial Hygienists (1972). A shorter, but useful, account of the formation and elimination of industrial dusts has been given by Lasserre (1967) and of dust sampling methods and dust suppression, by Lawrie (1967). Lippmann (1970) has given a critical review of the techniques of and equipment for aerosol sampling in relation to field conditions and their ability to satisfy the standards of the Threshold Limits Committee of the ACGIH and the Medical Research Council in the United Kingdom, and there is a recent valuable summary of the measurement of airborne dust by Walton and Hamilton (1972). In addition, there are authoritative recent handbooks, *Guide to Prevention and Suppression of Dust in Mining, Tunnelling and Quarrying* (1965) and *Dust Sampling in Mines* (1967) produced by the ILO. The same office publishes consolidated international reports on the subject from time to time.

The basic principles of protection can be briefly summarized.

(1) Substitution of the hazardous material by another without hazard, or a modification of the process designed to render the material innocuous. If neither of these is possible one or more of the following is employed.

(2) Complete enclosure of the process from the work atmosphere.

(3) Partial enclosure of the process with exhaust ventilation applied locally and to the 'background' air of the factory.

(4) High-velocity exhaust ventilation applied to the source of fume and dust.

(5) Suppression of dust by wet processes.

(6) Protective clothing and respirators. Respirators are, however, a last line of defence and, for the most part, unsatisfactory in that their use depends upon workers' co-operation; the protection given by some designs is inadequate.

(7) Good factory 'housekeeping' to prevent, by appropriate cleaning and disposal methods, accumulation of dust about workrooms and its dispersal in the atmosphere.

(8) Efficient storage and transport methods of dangerous materials (for example, asbestos fibres) so that accidental spilling and leakage does not occur.

(9) Controlled disposal of potentially dangerous waste substances.

REFERENCES

Albert, R. E., Lippmann, M. and Briscoe, W. (1969). 'The characteristics of bronchial clearance in humans and the effects of cigarette smoking.' *Archs envir. Hlth* **18**, 738–755

Altshuler, B., Palmas, E. D. and Nelson, D. (1967). 'Regional aerosol deposition in the human respiratory tract.' In *Inhaled Particles and Vapours*, Vol. 2, pp. 323–355. Ed. by C. N. Davies. Oxford; Pergamon

American Conference of Government Industrial Hygienists (1972). *Air Sampling Instruments*. 4th Ed. Cincinnati; A.C.G.I.H.

— (1971). *Threshold Limit Values of Airborne Contaminants and Physica· Agents with Intended changes adopted by ACGIH for 1971*. Cincinnati; A.C.G.I.H.

Booker, D. V., Chamberlain, A. C., Rundo, J., Muir, D. C. F. and Thomson, M. L. (1967). 'Elimination of 5 μ particles from the human lung.' *Nature, Lond.* **215**, 30–33

Cartwright, J. (1967). Airborne dust in coal miners: the particle-size—selection characteristics of the lung and the desirable characteristics of dust sampling instruments.' In *Inhaled Particles and Vapours*, Vol. 2, pp. 393–406. Ed. by C. N. Davies. Oxford; Pergamon

Casarett, L. J. and Milley, P. S. (1964). 'Alveolar reactivity following inhalation of particles.' *Hlth Phys.* **10**, 1003–1011

Committee on Hygiene Standards of the British Occupational Hygiene Society (1968). 'Hygiene standards for chrysotile asbestos dust.' *Ann. Occup. Hyg.* **11**, 47–69

Committee on Threshold Standards (1968). *Documentation of Threshold Limit Values.* Cincinnati; A.C.G.I.H.

Davies, C. N. (1967). 'Aerosol sampling related to inhalation.' In *Assessment of Airborne Radioactivity*, pp. 3–20. Vienna; International Atomic Energy Agency

Department of Employment and Productivity (1969). *Dust and Fumes in Factory Atmosphere, 1968.* New Series No. 8. London; H.M.S.O.

Gross, P. and Westwick, M. (1954). 'The permeability of lung parenchyma to particulate matter.' *Am. J. Path.* **30**, 195–213

Hapke, E. J. and Pederson, H. J. (1968). 'Cytoplasmic activity in Type 1 pulmonary epithelial cells induced by macroaggregated albumin.' *Science* **161**, 380–382

Hislop, A., Muir, D. C. F., Jacobsen, M., Simon, G. and Reid, L. (1972). 'Postnatal growth and function of pre-acinar airways.' *Thorax* **27**, 265–274

International Labour Office (1965). *Guide to the Prevention and Suppression of Dust in Mining, Tunnelling and Quarrying.* Geneva; I.L.O.

— (1967). *Dust Sampling in Mines.* Occup. Safety and Hlth Ser. No. 9. Geneva; I.L.O.

— (1970). *Permissible Levels of Toxic Substances in the Working Environment.* Occup. Safety and Hlth Ser. No. 20. Geneva; I.L.O.

Kennedy, J. R. and Elliott, A. M. (1970). 'Cigarette smoke: the effect of residue on mitochondrial structures.' *Science* **168**, 1097–1098

Kilburn, K. H. (1968). 'A hypothesis for pulmonary clearance and its implications.' *Am. Rev. resp. Dis.* **98**, 449–463

Klosterkötter, W. (1968). 'Pneumoconiosis of coalworkers: results, problems and practical consequences of recent research.' In *Pneumoconiosis.* Report on a Symposium at Katowice, pp. 99–109. Copenhagen; World Health Organization

— and Bünemann, G. (1961). 'Animal experiments on the elimination of inhaled dust.' In *Inhaled Particles and Vapours*, Vol. 1, pp. 327–341. Ed. by C. N. Davies. Oxford; Pergamon

Lassere, P. (1967). 'The formation and elimination of dust in industry.' In *Course on Dust Prevention in Industry*, pp. 45–101. Occ. Safety and Hlth Ser. No. 8. Geneva; I.L.O.

Lawrie, W. B. (1967). 'Some aspects of dust, dust sampling the interpretation of results, and an approach to the methods of suppressing dust clouds.' In *Course on Dust Prevention in Industry*, pp. 4–45. Occ. Safety and Hlth Ser. No. 8. Geneva; I.L.O.

Leiteritz, H., Einbrodt, H. J. and Klosterkötter, W. (1967). 'Grain sizes and mineral content of lung dust of coal miners compared with mine dusts.' In *Inhaled Particles and Vapours*, pp. 381–390. Vol. 2. Ed. by C. N. Davies. Oxford; Pergamon

Lippman, M. (1970). 'Respirable dust sampling.' *Am. ind. Hyg. Ass. J.* **31**, 138–159

— and Albert, R. E. (1969). 'The effect of particle size on the regional deposition of inhaled aerosols in the human respiratory tract.' *Am. ind. Hyg. Ass. J.* **30**, 257–275

— Albert, R. E. and Paterson, H. T. (1971). 'The regional deposition of inhaled aerosols in man.' In *Inhaled Particles III*, pp. 105–120. Ed. by W. H. Walton. Woking; Unwin

Milic-Emili, J., Henderson, J. A. M. and Kaneko, H. (1968). 'Regional distribution of pulmonary ventilation.' In *Form and Function in the Human Lung*, pp. 66–75. Ed. by G. Cumming and L. B. Hunt. London; Livingstone

Muir, D. C. F. and Davies, C. N. (1967). 'The deposition of 0·5 μ diameter aerosols in the lungs of Man.' *Ann. occup. Hyg.* **3**, 161–173

Nagelschmidt, G., Nelson, E. S., King, E. J., Attygalle, D. and Yoganathan M. (1967). 'The recovery of quartz and other minerals from the lungs of rats; a study in experimental silicosis.' *Archs Industr. Hlth* **16**, 188–202

National Coal Board (1966). *The Sampling of Airborne Dust for the Testing of 'Approved Dust Conditions'* (F4000). London; N.C.B.

Pavia, D., Short M. D. and Thomson, M. L. (1970). 'No demonstrable long-term effects of cigarette smoking on the muco-ciliary mechanism of the lung.' *Nature, Lond.* **226**, 1228–1231

Report (1966). 'Deposition and retention models for internal dosimetry of the human respiratory tract.' (Task Group on Lung Dynamics to ICRP Committee 2.) *Hlth Phys.* **12**, 173–207

Roach, S. A. (1966). 'A more rational basis for air sampling programmes.' *Am. ind. Hyg. Ass. J.* **27**, 1–12

Sanchis, J., Dolovich, M., Chalmers, R. and Newhouse, M. T. (1971). 'Regional distribution and lung clearance mechanisms in smokers and non-smokers.' In *Inhaled Particles III*, pp. 183–188. Ed. by W. H. Walton. Woking; Unwin

Spencer, H. (1968). 'Chronic interstitial pneumonia.' In *The lung*, pp. 134–150. Ed. by A. A. Liebow and D. E. Smith. Baltimore; Williams and Wilkins

Thompson, M. L. and Short, M. D. (1969). 'Mucociliary function in health, chronic obstructive airway disease, and asbestosis.' *J. appl. Physiol.* **26**, 535–539

Timbrell, V. (1970). 'The inhalation of fibres.' In *Pneumoconiosis. Proceedings of the International Conference, Johannesburg, 1969*, pp. 3–9. Ed. by H. A. Shapiro. London and Capetown; Oxford University Press

— Pooley, F. D. and Wagner, J. C. (1970). 'Characteristics of respirable asbestos fibres.' In *Pneumoconiosis. Proceedings of the International Conference, Johannesburg, 1969*, pp. 120–125. Ed. by H. A. Shapiro. London and Capetown; Oxford University Press

Walton, W. H. and Hamilton, R. J. (1972). 'The measurement of airborne dust.' In *Medicine in the Mining Industries*, pp. 145–165. Ed. by J. M. Rogan. London; Heinemann

West, J. B. (1961). 'Observations on gas flow in the human bronchial tree.' In *Inhaled Particles and Vapours*, Vol. 1, pp. 3–7. Ed. by C. N. Davies. Oxford; Pergamon

4—Fundamentals of Pathogenesis and Pathology

We are too much accustomed to attribute to a single cause that which is the product of several and the majority of our controversies come from that.

Baron Justus von Liebig (1803–1873)

INTRODUCTION

Human lungs and those of experimental animals react in a variety of ways to retained dust particles, from a trivial local aggregation of cells at one end of the scale to striking and often progressive collagenous fibrosis or widespread, but resolvable, cell accumulations or granulomas at the other. The character and severity of reactions are determined by at least three basic factors:

(1) The nature and properties of the dust.
(2) The amount of dust retained in the lungs and the duration of exposure to it; that is, a dose/time relationship.
(3) Individual idiosyncrasy and immunological reactivity of the subject.

Each of these poses complex problems. Whereas the identity and physicochemical characteristics of inhaled dusts are usually known, the reasons for the differing patterns of events which follow their retention are not completely understood. In a general way it can be said that the extent of disease likely to be produced by a dust of fibrogenic potential is proportional to the amount of dust and the period of time over which it is inhaled; a large dose over a short period and a small dose continued over a long period are both liable to cause disease.

The possible end-results of reactions caused by different dusts have been broadly distinguished in Chapter 1. Inorganic (mineral) dusts either have or do not have an intrinsic fibrogenic potential and organic dusts may be fibrogenic in the lungs of hypersensitive subjects (*see* Chapter 9). Obviously, a simple, all-embracing concept of the pathogenesis of the different types of pneumoconiosis cannot be expected because, on the one hand, the composition of inhaled and potentially noxious substances, and, on the other, the reaction of the body to them, differ both qualitatively and quantitatively.

71

In the encounter between extraneous materials and the lungs the pulmonary cells are of crucial importance, not only because they remove dust particles, but because of their positive role in pathogenesis. Immunological reactions are responsible for diseases caused by inhaled fungal spores and other foreign proteins, and are found in association with some cases of inorganic pneumoconiosis—an association which, although not yet properly understood, is undoubtedly important. For these reasons a brief outline of basic cytological and immunological principles is indicated.

Non-fibrotic pneumoconiosis is described as 'inert', or 'benign', because it does not damage the structure of the lungs nor cause progressive disease as may pneumoconiosis due to a fibrogenic dust.

RELEVANT CYTOLOGICAL FEATURES

The different types of pulmonary cells have been enumerated in Chapter 1.

It appears that the intracellular lysosomal system of macrophages plays a fundamental role in pathogenesis.

Lysosomes (lytic bodies) belong to the group of minute units known collectively as 'organelles' which, among their other activities, produce catalytic

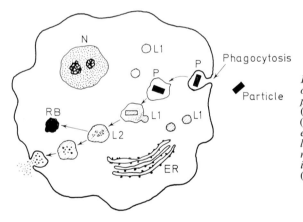

Figure 4.1. Simplified diagram of a macrophage ingesting a particle. A primary lysosome (L$_1$) is attached to phagosome (P) and is discharging its enzymes into it. The secondary lysosome (L$_2$) either forms a residual body (RB) or discharges its contents outside the cell. (ER, endoplasmic reticulum with ribosomes; N, nucleus)

enzymes, ribonucleic acid and the structural protein precursors of tropocollagen (q.v.). They are also referred to as *storage granules* or *primary lysosomes*, and are tiny vesicles bounded by membranes of lipoprotein.

Macrophages ingest foreign materials (such as dust particles) by invagination of their boundary membrane (phagocytosis) and the vesicle formed is known as a *phagosome* (*Figure 4.1*). Primary lysosomes then migrate on to its wall and discharge their enzymes within; it is now referred to as a *secondary lysosome* or *digestive vacuole*. These events resemble those of a rudimentary intestinal tract in that the contents are ingested, digested and the residue subsequently extruded from the cell. But in other instances digestion of particles is incomplete and they remain within the cell as a *residual body*. Normally the membrane of secondary lysosomes remains intact until the contents are extruded from the cell and escape of enzymes into the cytoplasm, which would result in auto-digestion and consequent cell death, does not occur.

Ingested foreign particles may be innocuous to the membranes of secondary lysosomes in which case they either pass harmlessly through the cell or remain within it as 'residual bodies' until the natural death of the cell releases these bodies and they are engulfed once again by other cells or survive as fragmentary extracellular 'residual bodies'. But if they have noxious properties (such as quartz possesses in high degree) the membrane structure is damaged and the secondary lysosome ruptures, releasing its enzymes into the cytoplasm. Death and disruption of the cell then follow and the released particles are taken up again by other cells and the cycle repeated.

Alveolar macrophages (*see* Chapter 1) are normally found in the alveolar spaces and to a lesser degree within the walls. Apart from their phagocytic activity they produce a variety of enzymes and other substances.

Ribosomes are the organelles related to endoplasmic reticulum which synthesize antibody (*see* next Section) in addition to other proteins, and they are particularly abundant in plasma cells and their precursors the plasmablasts. These cells are the main source of circulating antibody (Nossal, 1964) and their presence in a lesion in large numbers implies significant local antibody activity.

Tropocollagen is the elementary unit which synthesizes all collagen structures and it is elaborated by the organelles of fibroblasts.

IMMUNOLOGICAL CONSIDERATIONS

. . . the greatest development of purely biochemical activity is shown by cells, particularly by cells of the latest developed class in the Phylum Chordata, *the vertebrates. This is the development of the mechanisms of immunity, the capacity which these organisms have for dealing with foreign and harmful substances, inanimate and animate, which have found their way into their bodies. This seems to be the latest and most successful application of biochemical evolution in organisms. It is demonstrated by the extraordinary capacity which cells of these organisms have for dealing with foreign chemical substances.*

J. D. Bernal,
The Origin of Life.

(Courtesy; Weidenfeld and Nicolson)

It has become increasingly clear that immunological reactions underlie certain types of occupational lung disease either directly and causally (for example, in the extrinsic allergic group of disorders—Chapter 11) or indirectly (as is the case in some types of diffuse interstitial fibrosis and the rheumatoid variants of pneumoconiosis—*see* later in this Chapter).

Terms and concepts

On entering the body, micro-organisms and some alien substances act as *antigens* (or *allergens*) and stimulate the production of specific immunoglobulins—*antibodies*—which react with them in several different ways and play a prime role in the protection of the host from foreign invasion. The antigen-antibody reaction is commonly termed the *immune reaction* (immunis = free, exempt) because it frees the body of noxious agents. But although many antibodies are protective in that they aid the neutralization or destruction of foreign antigens, others react with antigens in such a way as to give rise to hypersensitivity diseases such as hay fever, eczema and asthma; and yet others play no active role in the destruction of antigen nor in pathogenesis, and are merely 'markers' of the underlying events. For this reason the term *allergy* ($\mathring{\alpha}\lambda\lambda o\varsigma$ = other; $\mathring{\epsilon}\rho\gamma o\nu$ = work), coined originally by von Pirquet to indicate an increased tissue response dependent upon an interaction between antigens and antibodies and including reactions which are harmful as well as protective to the host, appears preferable to 'immune reaction'; and, in fact, an effort has been made in recent years to reinstate it as originally defined (Gell and Coombes, 1968).

Antibodies are γ globulins which have been classified by electrophoretic and ultracentrifuge analysis. Electrophoresis reveals two overlapping fractions: one which moves rapidly in an electric field—γ1; and the other, slowly—γ2. The ultracentrifuge determines their sedimentation coefficient (designated 'S' for Svedberg units of measurements). Hence, the different γ globulins are distinguished in the following way and, in accordance with the World Health Organization nomenclature (1964), referred to as *immunoglobulins* (Ig):

(1) *7S in the γ2 fraction* (or IgG) which has a molecular weight of about 150,000 and makes up about 78 per cent of normal immunoglobulins.

(2) *7S in the γ1 fraction* (or IgA) which has the same molecular weight but contributes less—about 16·6 per cent—to antibody globulins. It is designated as γ 1A to distinguish it from 19S globulins. This fraction may also contain polymers with higher sedimentation coefficients—from 9 to 13S.

(3) *19S in the γ1 fraction* (or IgM) which has a molecular weight of about 900,000 and constitutes about 2 to 5 per cent of total serum immuno-globulins.

IgE is a more recently discovered γ1 (8·2S) globulin (molecular weight about 200,000) which forms only a minute fraction of serum immunoglobulins in normal individuals.

An antigen provokes appropriate cells to manufacture and release anti-body. But antigen is not always of extrinsic origin and, under certain circum-stances, the body's own cellular components may provoke the production of antibodies. Antigens, whether extrinsic or 'intrinsic', do not necessarily *react* with antibody and they may do no more than stimulate its production. Under normal circumstances antibodies are not directed against the body's own cells and proteins which are 'recognized' as 'self'; that is, their antigenic potential is tolerated or ignored. But under abnormal conditions antibodies may be directed against 'self' cells or proteins resulting in an *auto-allergic* reaction; the reacting antibodies are then referred to as *auto-antibodies*. There are various hypotheses to explain the underlying mechanism of auto-immune reactions; one of these is that the body's tolerance of its own antigens fails. This (suggested) failure of *antigen* (or *immune*) tolerance may be causally related to at least some of the manifestations of so-called auto-immune diseases, and it is now thought possible that it may be involved in the pathogenesis of some forms of pneumoconiosis.

There are two fundamental modes of allergic (or immune) reaction:

(1) *Humoral immunity.*—In response to antigen antibody, globulins are produced by plasma cells and circulate freely in body fluids and, on reacting with antigen, may produce tissue damage in a variety of ways. In the respiratory secretions, IgA elaborated by plasma cells around mucous glands and in the lamina propria in the respiratory tract is the main protective antibody, and IgA-containing plasma cells are found in large numbers in the lymphoid tissue of the upper respiratory tract (Tomasi *et al.*, 1965).

(2) *Specific cell-mediated immunity.*—Circulating lymphocytes also perform an antibody-like function which appears to be dependent upon the integrity of the thymus during embryonic and early neonatal life. It is directed against extraneous antigens such as microbial proteins (the most notable example of which is tuberculin), simple chemicals and homografts which are consequently 'rejected'. The response produced is called *'delayed hypersensitivity'*.

Allergic (immune) reactions with tissue damaging potential
When antigen reacts with humoral or cell-mediated antibody, damage to host tissues is apt to occur. Four types of reaction are recognized and have been classified as follows (Gell and Coombes, 1968).

Immediate, anaphylactic and reagin-dependent reaction (Type I)
The antibodies, known as *reagins*, which are believed to be responsible, belong to the IgE group of immunoglobulins and differ from the 'conventional' IgG, IgA and IgM antibodies in that they are thought to become attached to certain cell surfaces on which the antigen-antibody reaction occurs provoking the release of pharmacologically vaso-active substances (such as histamine and serotonin) which, in turn, give rise to the common clinical disorders—urticaria, hay fever and 'extrinsic' asthma.

Cytolitic or cytotoxic reaction (Type II)
Antibody reacts with antigen which is either a component of tissue cells which the body fails to recognize as 'self' (that is, a *complete antigen*) or is formed by *haptens* (that is, protein-free chemicals of low molecular weight) which are capable of binding on to cell or other body protein to form an antigen complex. A hapten, therefore, is also referred to as an *incomplete antigen*.

Examples of Type II responses are blood transfusion reactions, drug-induced purpura and haemolytic anaemia. But although there is no evidence at present that it participates in the pathogenesis of lung disease, immunoglobulins and complement have, in fact, been demonstrated on the basement membrane of alveoli and the glomeruli of the kidneys in cases of Goodpasture's syndrome (that is, glomerulonephritis with lung haemorrhage and haemoptysis); basement membrane antibodies present in the serum have been shown to react with lung and kidney.

Arthus type reaction (Type III)
Circulating precipitating antibodies react with antigen in varying proportions.

When this happens with antigen in tissue spaces, microprecipitins are frequently formed in and around small blood vessels. In other circumstances an excess of *circulating* antigen is exposed to antibody so that soluble antigen-antibody complexes are precipitated in the walls of blood vessels.

Hence, both types of reaction are associated with vasculitis. The precipitating antibodies are of the IgG or IgM class. Complement, which has a number of components, is activated in the course of the reaction and is an important factor in the local assembly of polymorphonuclear leucocytes and the resulting cell death. Typically the Arthus reaction occurs in from four to twelve hours after injection of antigen.

The typical example of disease due to the Type III reaction is serum sickness, but the importance of this reaction in the present context is that it plays an important part in the pathogenesis of the extrinsic allergic type of lung diseases following inhalation of foreign protein antigens (*see* Chapter 11). In such cases the Arthus reaction can be produced in the patient's skin by intradermal injection of the antigen.

Type I, Type II and Type III reactions are all examples of *humoral immunity*.

Cell-mediated reaction; delayed hypersensitivity (*Type IV*)

Some types of antigen, such as the vaccinia virus, tuberculin, histoplasmin and certain chemical substances, evoke a response which is slow to develop (24 to 48 hours) and consists mainly of the mobilization and infiltration of immunologically competent lymphocytes into the antigen-bearing region. This is a cell-mediated reaction and circulating antibodies do not appear to take part. It is possible that it may operate in some lung diseases in which circulating antibodies cannot be demonstrated against the relevant antigens. For example, the lesions of tuberculosis and other microbial infections which are characterized by a delayed skin reaction or challenge may be due to cell-mediated tissue damage.

From the clinical point of view it is important to appreciate that an antigen may provoke more than one type of tissue-damaging immunological response.

Because of the possibility that auto-allergy may play a part in the pathogenesis of some forms of pneumoconiosis this concept is briefly considered.

Auto-allergy (*auto-immunity*)

Antigen tolerance is established in a short period before and just after birth. This is exemplified experimentally by the effect of injecting bovine serum albumin as antigen into newborn rabbits which do not thereafter produce antibody to the same antigen when it is again injected in later life. In order to be tolerated, therefore, antigen must be in contact with the antibody-producing system at this critical period, otherwise antibodies will be produced against it.

Alteration or denaturation of host antigen by chemical, physical or biological means, or the presence of foreign antigens which bear a close structural resemblance to the host antigen, but are not identical with it, may weaken or destroy antigen tolerance. Similarly, complex antigens produced by the combination of host haptens with exogenous materials may have the same effect.

Tissue-damaging antibodies resulting from these changes are of two types (Hijmans *et al.*, 1961):

(1) those reacting with a specific tissue component of a particular organ or system of organs—*organ-specific antibodies.*

(2) those reacting with cellular components which are common to many organs—*non-organ-specific antibodies.*

Examples of organ-specific auto-allergic diseases include thyroglobulin antigens in Hashimoto's thyroiditis and gastric parietal cell antigens in pernicious anaemia. Examples of diseases associated with non-organ-specific antibodies are connective tissue disorders such as systemic lupus erythematosus and Sjögren's syndrome in which antibody to cell nuclei is especially common and is referred to as *antinuclear factor* (ANF); and rheumatoid arthritis in which the antigen is denatured γ globulin and the antibody is known as *rheumatoid factor* (RF).

Rheumatoid factor is found in association with coal pneumoconiosis, silicosis and asbestosis in a proportion of cases and, although ANF is similarly associated with asbestosis, its occurrence with other types of pneumoconiosis has not yet been recorded. This matter is considered later in the appropriate chapters.

Organ-specific antibodies have not so far been shown to be responsible for any form of lung disease, although this is theoretically possible (*see* section on Lung Reactive Antibodies); but non-organ-specific antibodies are present in a proportion of patients with diffuse interstitial fibrosis ('fibrosing alveolitis') of various types.

There is some evidence that both cell-mediated mechanisms and circulating antibodies may co-operate in organ-specific reactions and it may be that immunologically active cells inflict increased permeability on the cells of the organ attacked so that circulating antibodies are able to enter them and cause a damaging reaction.

The type of cells found in auto-allergic lesions varies but, as a rule, lymphocytes or plasma cells predominate.

Both organ-specific and non-organ-specific antibodies are usually readily detectable by standard immunological techniques.

Antinuclear factor (ANF)

In systemic lupus erythematosus many different organs of the body are involved and antibodies are directed against a variety of cytoplasmic and nuclear antigens. Some of these antigens are located in the nuclei of different cells and the IgG, IgM or IgA antibodies—ANF—which react with them can be detected within nuclei by an immunofluorescent technique.

Antinuclear factor in titres of 1 : 10 and over has been observed in about 5 per cent of a large number of men and women in a control population in the United Kingdom, and of 1 : 16 and over in 2 per cent of men over 40 years of age (Beck, 1963).

Although antinuclear factor is usually found in association with LE cells in systemic lupus erythematosus, it is present in a proportion of persons with rheumatoid arthritis (Ward, Johnson and Holborrow, 1964), systemic sclerosis and Sjögren's syndrome (Bunim, 1961) in the absence of LE cells. In systemic lupus erythematosus it is composed predominantly of IgG but in the connective tissue diseases it consists of IgM and IgG. It has been observed in titres of 1 : 40 or more in some 37 per cent of patients with cryptogenic diffuse interstitial fibrosis, and mainly as IgM in 25 per cent of persons with the diffuse interstitial fibrosis of asbestosis (Turner Warwick and Haslam, 1971) (Chapter 9).

Recent work (Hughes and Rowell, 1970) has shown that certain types of antinuclear factor can worsen an experimental inflammatory lesion in rats. This offers some support for the possibility that antinuclear factor may be actively involved in the pathogenesis of human connective tissue disease, not as a primary agent, but as an auto-immune response to tissue or cell components already damaged by some immunological or other process.

Rheumatoid factor (RF)

Many patients with rheumatoid arthritis are found to have circulating antibodies directed against slightly altered (that is, denatured) γ globulins. These are detected by their ability to agglutinate sheep cells coated with a subagglutinating dose of anti-sheep-cell antiserum (that is, γ globulin) prepared in the rabbit. They are mainly IgM produced by plasma cells and they appear to develop against IgG complexes (and, therefore, denatured) with unidentified antigen. There are many reasons for believing that rheumatoid factor is not directly related to the pathogenesis of the rheumatoid syndrome; for instance, the presence of rheumatoid arthritis in some patients with hypogammaglobulinaemia in whom rheumatoid factor cannot be demonstrated (Gitlin et al., 1959; Good and Rotstein, 1960).

In rheumatoid arthritis and other disorders such as systemic lupus erythematosus, Sjögren's disease and cryptogenic diffuse interstitial fibrosis in which rheumatoid factor is often found whether or not there is polyarthritis, it has been suggested that normal tissue globulins become denatured in some way so that antigen is formed. Experimentally, globulin degraded by proteolytic enzymes becomes antigenic and provokes the production of rheumatoid factor in animals (Williams and Kunkel, 1962).

Circulating rheumatoid factor cannot always be detected by the standard differential agglutination test (DAT) which employs sheep red cells coated with rabbit IgG γ globulins but can by newly developed techniques (Torrigiani et al., 1970). The prevalence of circulating rheumatoid factor in different types of pneumoconiosis may, therefore, be higher than it appears at present (see Chapters 8 and 9).

Although antinuclear factor and rheumatoid factor can be regarded as antibodies directed against entirely different antigens, they are not uncommonly present in the same clinical disorders and may be found in the same serum sample.

The prevalence of rheumatoid factor with or without rheumatoid arthritis is higher in members of urban populations than in those of rural populations (Miall, Ball and Kellgren, 1958; Ball and Lawrence, 1961; Lawrence, 1967), but the significance of this is not clear. Rheumatoid factor is present in some 5 per cent of men and women in random populations (Ball and Lawrence, 1961). In general, titres are higher in the older age groups; those with high titres are more likely to have rheumatoid arthritis than those without, and rheumatoid factor is found more often among the offspring of parents whose serum also contains this factor compared with unrelated persons of the same age in the same populations (Lawrence, 1967). Clinical rheumatoid arthritis is present in only about one-quarter of rheumatoid-factor-positive Caucasians (Lawrence, 1965).

All these facts emphasize that rheumatoid factor may result from several different stimuli of uncertain nature. But, it is known that rheumatoid factor is present in some 31 per cent of patients with cryptogenic diffuse interstitial fibrosis ('fibrosing alveolitis') which is not accounted for at present by any known extraneous agency (Turner Warwick and Haslam, 1971). This is in agreement with an earlier observation (Doctor and Snider, 1962) that one in five patients with diffuse interstitial fibrosis has rheumatoid disease. It is of interest, therefore, that preliminary studies have shown rheumatoid factor to be present in 22·6 per cent of persons with the diffuse interstitial fibrosis of asbestosis (Turner Warwick and Haslam, 1971) (*see* Chapter 9). It has been known for some years that when coal pneumoconiosis or silicosis are associated with rheumatoid factor (with or without rheumatoid arthritis) their course and radiographic features are atypical and their pathological appearances differ from those which are characteristic of these types of pneumoconiosis (*see* Chapters 7 and 8). By contrast, neither antinuclear factor nor rheumatoid factor are associated with the diffuse interstitial fibrosis of farmers' lung, bird fanciers' lung and similar diseases (*see* Chapter 11) in which their prevalence (3 per cent) is comparable with that in the general population (Turner Warwick and Haslam, 1971).

Although rheumatoid factor is commonly found in rheumatoid arthritis, in a proportion of cases of non-occupational diffuse interstitial fibrosis, and in certain cases of pneumoconiosis it is not yet known whether it plays any part in pathogenesis.

Pleural effusion (Berger and Seckler, 1966) or pulmonary nodules, with or without necrosis and cavitation, may occur in association with rheumatoid arthritis in individuals who have been exposed to industrial dusts (Price and Skelton, 1958; Panettiere, Chandler and Libeke, 1968). Such nodules are histologically identical with rheumatoid subcutaneous nodules and have also been found in other viscera including the dura mater (Maher, 1954). It is of importance that both pleural effusion and somewhat similar nodules may also occur in some types of pneumoconiosis (such as coal pneumoconiosis and silicosis) in association with circulating rheumatoid factor.

Lung reactive antibodies
Hagadorn and Burrell (1968) reported having found 'lung reactive' antibodies in IgA fractions in a majority of subjects with confluent (that is, massive) coal pneumoconiosis and that antibody reacts with collagen. However, the same authors (1966) also showed that these antibodies were cross-reactive with other tissues. Nevertheless, an important histological feature of some cases of coal and other types of pneumoconiosis which undergo rapid progress and have atypical radiographic appearances during life, is the presence of abundant plasma cells in the lesions. This suggests an allergic process even though its nature and that of the antigen involved has not been specified.

To summarize, the fact that both antinuclear factor and rheumatoid factor are often found in individuals with certain types of non-occupational and occupational fibrosis of the lungs and not in others suggests that these non-organ-specific antibodies do not arise simply as a consequence of destructive lung disease. They may occur for a number of different, and as yet unidentified, reasons under different circumstances. This prompts speculation as to whether certain inhaled mineral dusts when retained in the lungs might, by virtue of their cytotoxic effects and resultant fibrogenesis, cause the formation of these antibodies which, under some conditions, accelerate or modify the disease process. An adjuvant effect is probably the most likely mechanism. Organ-specific anti-lung antibodies do not appear to have been demonstrated so far (1972) in human lung disease either of occupational or non-occupational origin.

RETICULIN AND COLLAGEN

The distinction between these connective tissue components and their significance is important in the study of pneumoconiosis and the difference between them must be recognized when interpreting their place in lung micro-anatomy both normal and abnormal.

All connective tissues consist of fibres, cells and matrix or ground substance. There are three types of fibre: collagen, reticulin and elastin. Elastic fibres do not concern us here and are not discussed. The cells associated with collagen and reticulin (reticulin fibres) are fibroblasts and fibrocytes which are scattered between the fibres and their matrix.

Light microscopy reveals obvious differences between collagen and reticulin:

Collagen, which appears to the naked eye as white fibrous tissue, consists microscopically of bundles of fibres of uniform diameter, non-branching, and staining bright red with van Gieson's connective tissue stain, slightly pink with periodic acid Schiff (that is, a negative reaction), and yellow or brown with silver impregnation methods. Mature collagen is refringent under polarized light.

Reticulin consists of delicate, randomly arranged fibres of varying thickness which branch and anastomose; they stain only faintly red with van Gieson's stain, magenta with periodic acid Schiff (a strong reaction) and black with silver impregnation, and are isotropic under polarized light.

There is a continuous network of connective tissue fibres composed mainly of collagen extending from the pulmonary pleura to the peribronchial and peritracheal regions; by contrast, reticulin fibres form the basement membranes to the cells of alveoli and capillaries and are present in small quantity in the alveolar walls.

In spite of these differences in morphological and staining characteristics both types of fibre show a similar cross-striated structure under the electron microscope and their protein analysis is identical (Chvapil, 1967). Fibres of either type and the matrix between them appear to be structurally indistinguishable and it is the composition of the matrix which is responsible for their different functional and staining properties. The collagen matrix is scanty and contains fewer polysaccharides than reticulin, whereas the reticulin matrix is abundant, rich in polysaccharides and also contains lipids. It is believed that the reticulin matrix, under the influence of unknown stimuli, transforms reticulin fibres into collagen fibres—a transformation, nevertheless, which need not and does not necessarily take place.

The term 'reticulin', incidentally, was originally introduced by Siegfried (1893) to refer to the matrix extract and not to the fibres themselves and, although reticulin fibres are certainly better referred to explicitly, it is unlikely that the custom of using 'reticulin' to include both fibres and matrix will change.

The molecular precursors of both types of fibre are synthesized chiefly by fibroblasts and become *tropocollagen* which contains the amino acids proline and hydroxyproline. Tropocollagen appears outside the cells and polymerizes into reticulin or collagen fibres. Fibroblasts originate primarily from fibrocytes and appear to have a different lineage from macrophages. The stimuli causing fibroblasts to function in this way in health or disease are not known. It appears that the closer fibroblasts are grouped together, the more likely they are to produce increased amounts of collagen, and that in some circumstances macrophage disruption may release an intermediary substance which stimulates fibroblasts to fibrogenic activity.

Collagen, therefore, is formed either directly by fibroblasts or indirectly, and subsequently, from reticulin when an appropriate stimulus is applied.

Both reticulin and collagen are antigenically active, but in different ways. This fact presents a new and important field of study. There is experimental evidence which suggests that cross-immunity may occur as a result of antibodies to an exogenous antigen reacting with similar connective tissue components of a variety of organs, and basement membranes may be an important component of such reactions (Hammerman and Sandson, 1970). No doubt future work will determine whether or not this has any relevance to the pathogenesis of fibrotic types of pneumoconiosis.

The hyaline change which may occur in connective tissue is normally composed almost entirely of collagen (Letterer, Gerok and Schneider, 1955) but that commonly found in silicotic nodules is strikingly deficient in collagen, although rich in γ globulins (Vigliani and Pernis, 1959). The question as to whether this is indicative of an antigen-antibody reaction is considered later with theories of the pathogenesis of silicosis.

It is clear, therefore, that whereas there are fundamental similarities in the chemical structure of reticulin and collagen, there are important differences between them in their function, behaviour in health and disease, appearance under the light-microscope and in their antigenic properties. To a large extent the quantity of these fibres depends upon whether the local stimuli acting upon them are negligible, provoke proliferation of reticulin alone, or give rise to collagenous fibrosis.

The confusion to which the word 'reticulation' may give rise if used, as is sometimes done, to indicate proliferation of reticulin fibres (reticulin) is discussed in Chapter 5. It should also be understood that *fibrosis*, by general agreement, means collagenous fibrosis and not proliferation of reticulin fibres.

In order to indicate the microscopic degree of fibrosis present in human lungs, a modification of the system suggested by Belt and King (1945) for grading in experimental animals can be used.

Grade 1. Cellular lesions; loose reticulin; no collagen.

Grade 2. Cellular lesions; compact reticulin with or without a few collagen fibres.

Grade 3. Lesions somewhat cellular, but mostly collagenous.

Grade 4. Acellular collagen.

Using this scale, Grade 2 when collagen is present, indicates very slight or negligible fibrosis; Grade 3, moderate fibrosis, and Grade 4, severe fibrosis. This grading, of course, expresses the *degree* of fibrosis and not the *extent* of its distribution.

BASIC REACTIONS OF THE LUNGS TO INHALED PARTICLES

The major site of deposition of both mineral and organic particles is, as described in the last chapter, in the alveoli of respiratory bronchioles and more distal alveoli (the gas-exchanging region of the lungs) though deposition of some spores and other organic particles in non-respiratory bronchioles is of importance in the 'farmers' lung' group of diseases.

Mineral dusts

Mineral dusts (such as iron, coal, quartz and asbestos) become plastered on to alveolar walls, especially those adjacent to bronchiolo-vascular bundles (Duguid and Lambert, 1964). Many particles find their way into the interstitium of the walls, although how this occurs is not properly understood; alveolar macrophages play an active part and it is possible that Type II and even Type I pneumocytes may also participate. The integrity of the surface layer of Type I cells may be breached in places and the alveolar septum exposed.

Within the alveolar walls, macrophages rapidly converge upon extracellular particles and engulf them. If the number of particles is large the elimination mechanisms described in Chapter 3 may fail, and dust particles and dust-containing macrophages collect in the interstitium—especially in perivascular and peribronchiolar regions. If these aggregations remain *in situ*, Type I pneumocytes grow over them so that they become enclosed and completely interstitial in position but, in the case of inert dusts and coal and quartz dusts, they are strictly localized in these regions. According to the amount of dust and cell accumulation the alveolar walls either protrude to a greater or lesser degree into the alveolar spaces or obliterate them altogether. Meanwhile, a delicate supporting framework of fine reticulin fibres develops between the cells, but in the case of dusts with fibrogenic potential, proliferation of collagen fibres subsequently occurs.

Inert dusts, such as carbon, iron and tin, remain within macrophages in these lesions until they die at the end of their normal life span when the particles are released and reingested by other macrophages; secondary lysosomes are unharmed in the process. But the lesions are not static and some dust-laden macrophages continually migrate to lymphatics or to bronchioles whence they are eliminated; migration is increased by infection or oedema of the lung.

Some fibrogenic dusts, most notably quartz, cause rapid destruction of the macrophages by which they are engulfed, and when these cells die, fibroblasts appear and, later, collagen fibres form and proliferate, resulting in local fibrous lesions. Although asbestos dusts apparently have little cyto-toxicity (*see* page 94) their ingestion by macrophages is also followed by fibroblast production and collagenous fibrosis in the walls of terminal and respiratory bronchioles which, by contrast with silicotic lesions, spreads *diffusely* in alveolar walls; that is, a diffuse interstitial fibrosing or 'fibrosing alveolitis'.

To summarize, there are four different basic types of lesion caused by the alveolar deposition of inorganic (mineral) dusts.

(1) Plastering of the walls of the alveoli of respiratory bronchioles to a greater or lesser degree by dust particles.

(2) A small, *localized* interstitial—that is, mainly peribronchiolar—lesion consisting of accumulations of dust, macrophages and a mild proliferation of reticulin without collagenous fibrosis. This is caused by inert dusts, for example, iron (siderosis); many of the discrete lesions of coal pneumo-coniosis are of this sort.

(3) A localized, *nodular*, peribronchiolar interstitial lesion of collagenous fibrosis caused by particles of quartz, flint and certain other fibrogenic dusts.

(4) A *diffuse* interstitial fibrosis of bronchiolar and alveolar walls, the most important example of which is asbestosis.

The chief characteristics of 2, 3 and 4 are described in more detail in Chapters 6, 7 and 9 respectively.

Organic dusts

The foreign proteins of *organic dusts*, such as the spores of the thermophylic actinomycete *Micropolyspora faeni* from mouldy hay or the droppings and serum of certain birds, may act as antigens which, in sensitized subjects, provoke an Arthus (Type III) allergic reaction in alveolar and bronchiolar walls. This may result in an acute (reversible) interstitial pneumonia, sarcoid-like granuloma formation or (irreversible) diffuse interstitial fibrosis; in other words, the *extrinsic allergic 'alveolitis'*, or *'farmers' lung'* group of diseases (*see* Chapter 11). Similar type lesions, however, are also produced by beryl-lium compounds but their pathogenesis is different (*see* Chapter 10). By contrast, the organic dusts of cotton, flax, and hemp do not give rise to any distinctive histopathological lesions.

DIFFUSE INTERSTITIAL FIBROSIS AND FIBROSING 'ALVEOLITIS'

In addition to the diffuse interstitial fibrosis of asbestosis, the chronic stage of the 'farmers' lung' group of diseases and some other occupational diseases, pulmonary fibrosis, in which inhaled aerosols apparently play no part, also occurs for unknown (cryptogenic) reasons or as a result of only partly understood causes (for example, 'rheumatoid lung', systemic lupus ery-thematosus, Sjögren's syndrome, and scleroderma). Acute and subacute 'interstitial pneumonia' (that is, cellular infiltration of alveolar walls and spaces often accompanied by vascular changes) is also known to occur for reasons which are not understood. The terms employed to designate these various lesions are confusing and this is an appropriate point at which to explain them and the way in which they are used in this book.

In 1944 Hammon and Rich described some cases of 'acute' diffuse interstitial fibrosis of unknown cause to which, at first, the name of 'Hammon-Rich lung' was applied, but later this became known as diffuse idiopathic (or cryptogenic) interstitial fibrosis. 'Chronic' diffuse interstitial fibrosis then came into general use to describe 'end-point' diffuse fibrosis whether of unknown or of partly understood cause.

In 1964, Scadding proposed that 'fibrosing alveolitis' might be a more appropriate term in that it could include the earlier dynamic and cellular stage of the disease process in addition to the final irreversible fibrosis, and he termed disease of unknown cause 'cryptogenic fibrosing alveolitis'. Since when 'fibrosing alveolitis' has also been increasingly employed in Britain as a synonym for 'diffuse interstitial fibrosis'. Subsequently, it was proposed that allergic disease in the peripheral parts of the lungs caused by inhaled organic antigens should be called 'extrinsic allergic alveolitis' (Pepys, 1969), a term which is now widely used to embrace both its acute (pneumonic) and chronic stages—that is, 'acute' and 'chronic' extrinsic allergic alveolitis (see Chapter 11).

Following the classification of interstitial pneumonias given by Liebow, Steer and Billingsley (1965), Scadding and Hinson (1967) described the essential pathological features of 'diffuse fibrosing alveolitis' as 'cellular thickening of alveolar walls showing a tendency to fibrosis, and the presence of large mononuclear cells, presumably of alveolar origin, within alveolar spaces'. They stated that the degree of thickening of alveolar walls correlated inversely with the number of mononuclear cells in the alveolar spaces. They distinguished two main types of lesion:

(1) At one extreme alveolar walls are little, if at all, thickened by fibrosis, but numerous mononuclear cells, either Type II pneumocytes or macrophages, occupy the air spaces; they called this the 'desquamative' type of fibrosing alveolitis and it is distributed uniformly in the lung.

(2) At the other extreme, alveolar walls are greatly thickened by fibrosis and intra-alveolar cells are few; this they called the 'mural' type which is irregularly distributed. There are many intermediate patterns between these two extremes. The 'mural' type, therefore, corresponds to 'diffuse interstitial fibrosis'. As Hinson (1970) has pointed out, the following terms appear to have been used synonymously:

Hammon-Rich disease.

Diffuse idiopathic interstitial fibrosis.

Usual or 'classic' interstitial pneumonia (Liebow, Steer and Billingsley, 1965).

Diffuse fibrosing alveolitis.

Diffuse cryptogenic fibrosing alveolitis—desquamative and mural.

'Alveolitis' is not a wholly satisfactory term because asbestosis (a diffuse interstitial fibrosis) and extrinsic allergic disease due to organic dusts commonly commence in the walls of terminal and respiratory bronchioles (see Chapters 9 and 11 respectively), Arthus (Type III) reactions of extrinsic allergic lesions frequently involve small pulmonary blood vessels, and sarcoid-like granulomas occur in both bronchiolar and alveolar walls in acute and chronic extrinsic allergic disease.

Both 'diffuse interstitial fibrosis' and 'fibrosing alveolitis' are used in this book: the former for 'end-point' fibrosis which may be accompanied by 'honeycomb' formation (*see Figure 5.14*), and the latter for 'desquamative' disease and disease of extrinsic allergic type. 'Alveolitis' is placed in inverted commas to remind the reader that the term is not limited to lesions in alveolar walls.

SOME THEORIES OF THE PATHOGENESIS OF INORGANIC PNEUMOCONIOSIS AND EXPERIMENTAL OBSERVATIONS

Precisely why inhaled particles of one material provoke collagenous fibrosis or other disease processes whereas those of another do not is poorly understood, but one thing is clear: the form that the lesions of each type of pneumoconiosis takes is primarily determined by particular attributes of the inhaled particles and by the response of the body to them; possibly, concomitant infection in the lung may sometimes play a part. Cytological, immunological and enzymatic activities, therefore, may all be involved, and observation of the accompanying intracellular events by electron microscopy has proved invaluable in the elucidation of some fundamental mechanisms of pathogenesis.

Many theories to explain the pathogenesis of different types of pneumoconiosis have been elaborated, but only those which have some bearing upon contemporary conceptions are referred to here.

SILICOSIS

Theory of mechanical injury

The sharp or jagged nature of free silica particles was believed to cause fibrosis by irritation, and the same attribute was at one time supposed to be exhibited by the mica mineral, sericite, which is widely distributed in many of the world's mines. These suggestions were discarded when animal experiments showed that materials such as diamond and Carborundum (silicon carbide), which are harder and sharper than either quartz or sericite, did not produce collagen fibrosis.

Theory of piezoelectric effect

This suggested that minute electrical currents produced by mechanical stresses on some crystals may damage tissue cells (quite how does not seem to have been made clear). But substances other than quartz which also possess piezoelectric activity have been shown to be non-fibrogenic to animals whereas tridymite, which has no piezoelectric effect, is strongly fibrogenic.

Theory of protein adsorption

This theory proposed that the known capacity of free silica to adsorb proteins on to its surface might initiate collagen fibrogenesis. Other substances with equal potential for protein adsorption, however, do not cause fibrosis in experimental animals. Nevertheless, adsorption on to quartz particles alters or denatures protein (Scheel *et al.*, 1954)—a fact which features in the immunological theories of silicosis to be discussed.

The solubility theory

Kettle (1926) postulated that free silica in passing slowly into solution in tissue fluids produces silicic acid which in some way gives rise to collagen

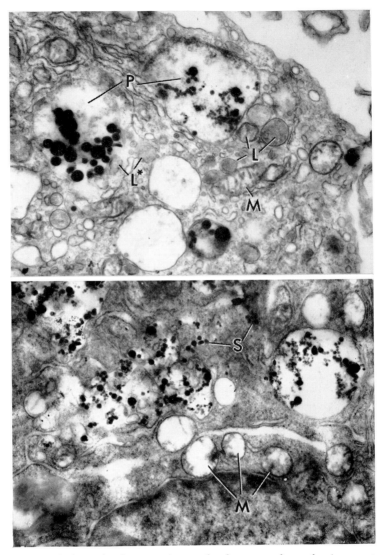

Figure 4.2. (Upper) Electron micrograph of a macrophage showing quartz particles in phagosomes (P). There are numerous lysosomes (L) some of which are apparently attached to a phagosome (L*). The structure of the cytoplasm and mitochondria (M) is well preserved. (Lower) Phagosomes in the centre of the field have disrupted, releasing the quartz particles (S) into the cytoplasm, the detail of which is becoming obscured. The phagosome on the right of the field is still intact. Mitochondria (M) above the nucleus are swollen and degenerating. (Original magnification ×24,000, reproduced at ×19,200; by courtesy of Dr A. C. Allison)

fibrosis. After holding a commanding place for some years this theory was shown to be untenable because different forms of free silica, though all of equal solubility, nevertheless have different fibrogenic potential in experimental animals. This potential increases progressively and significantly in order from quartz glass (vitreous silica), to quartz, to cristobalite and to tridymite (King *et al.*, 1953; Stöber, 1968). Quartz etched with hydrofluoric acid is much less soluble than unetched quartz, yet it is more fibrogenic (Englebrecht *et al.*, 1958). The recently discovered dense, crystalline, high temperature and pressure variant of silicon dioxide, stishovite, in which the basic structural unit has an octahedral, not a tetrahedral, configuration (Chao, Fahey and Littler, 1962), has the same solubility as quartz glass and quartz but causes no fibrosis whatsoever in experimental animals (Brieger and Gross, 1967). Furthermore, in experiments such as those of Curran and Rowsell (1958) in which quartz is enclosed in a semi-permeable collodion diffusion chamber in the peritoneal cavity of an animal, no fibrosis results although silicic acid diffuses freely into the tissues while the quartz is excluded from them.

A modification of this theory, often referred to as the Extended Solubility Theory, was suggested by Holt (1957). Silicic acid is presumed to be adsorbed on to the protein of collagen precursors, causing their polymerization into collagen. However, no satisfactory evidence has been found to support this.

It appears, then, that the ability of free silica to cause fibrosis depends fundamentally on two conditions: a particular type of crystal structure, and intimate contact with cells.

In spite of the failure of the solubility theories, they provided the most useful guide-lines to research into pathogenesis until recent times. But with increased knowledge of cell structure and chemistry a fresh approach to the problem became possible. It had long been realized that the ingestion of free silica particles by macrophages was a prerequisite for the development of the silicotic lesion, and the discovery that these particles cause destruction of macrophages (in turn an essential precursor of fibrogenesis) together with the suggestion that immunological processes may also be involved at some stage in the development of silicotic nodules, has led to two new theories.

Theory based on destruction of lung macrophages

Non-cytotoxic particles (such as diamond and amorphous carbon) and cytotoxic particles of quartz coated with serum proteins when added to a culture of macrophages are quickly ingested by these cells and enclosed in their phagosomes (*Figure 4.2*). The subsequently formed digestive vacuoles which contain diamond or carbon particles remain intact and the cell itself undamaged, whereas those containing quartz soon rupture (or become permeable) and discharge their contents, particles and enzymes into the cytoplasm (*Figure 4.2*). The macrophages then become round and immobile and disintegrate, liberating the particles and enzymes (*Figure 4.3*). The particles are reingested by other macrophages and the process repeated (Allison, Harington and Birbeck, 1966; Nadler and Goldfischer, 1970). A similar train of events occurs in experimental animals after inhalation of quartz dust (Bruch, 1967), and there is no reason to doubt that this also occurs in man.

Macrophages, therefore, are affected in differing ways by different materials. Inert particles, after phagocytosis, apparently do not interfere with the normal activities or life span of the cells, whereas particles of quartz, on the other hand, appear repeatedly to destroy macrophages until they (the particles) are successfully incarcerated by the development of collagenous tissue which presumably prevents an infinitely self-perpetuating state of cell destruction. It is for this reason that macrophages probably play a minor role in eliminating quartz and other forms of fibrogenic free silica particles from the lungs.

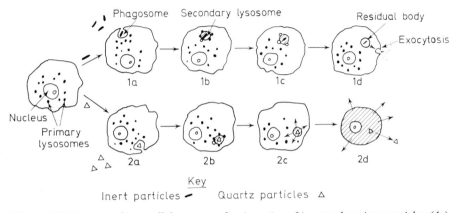

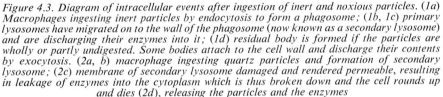

Figure 4.3. Diagram of intracellular events after ingestion of inert and noxious particles. (1a) Macrophages ingesting inert particles by endocytosis to form a phagosome; (1b, 1c) primary lysosomes have migrated on to the wall of the phagosome (now known as a secondary lysosome) and are discharging their enzymes into it; (1d) residual body is formed if the particles are wholly or partly undigested. Some bodies attach to the cell wall and discharge their contents by exocytosis. (2a, b) macrophage ingesting quartz particles and formation of secondary lysosome; (2c) membrane of secondary lysosome damaged and rendered permeable, resulting in leakage of enzymes into the cytoplasm which is thus broken down and the cell rounds up and dies (2d), releasing the particles and the enzymes

The mechanism by which quartz particles cause cell destruction appears to depend upon their breaching the integrity of the membrane of the digestive vacuole because this damage can be prevented, or at least greatly reduced, if the cells are first treated with poly-2-vinyl-pyridine-N-oxide (PVPNO) before they ingest the particles (Allison, Harington and Birbeck, 1966), or if the particles themselves are coated with aluminium. Polyvinylpyridino-acetic acid (polybetaine) has an even stronger inhibitory effect than PVPNO (Nash, Allison and Harington, 1966; Sakabe and Koshi, 1967). The fibrogenic effect of tridymite (which is greater than that of quartz) is also suppressed by PVPNO (Cavagna and Nichelatti, 1963).

These observations are the basis of a 'macrophage theory' to explain the cytotoxicity of free silica which can be summarized as follows.

(1) Free silica reacts chemically with proteins and phospholipids but inert substances exhibit little or no activity. This is exemplified by the experimental observation that particles of crystalline silica (with the exception of

stishovite) cause haemolysis of red cells whereas most inert particles have a negligible effect (Stalder and Stöber, 1965). Free silica particles coated with PVPNO do not cause haemolysis, but when cells only and not the particles are coated, lysis still occurs (Nash, Allison and Harington, 1966). It appears, therefore, that the essential first stage in the silicotic process involves damage to the membranes of the digestive vacuoles (secondary lysosomes) of macrophages which is blocked by PVPNO, polybetaine and aluminium. Silica particles are more cytotoxic than silicic acid in solution even though the acid possesses many hydrogen bonding groups. Allison (1971) has suggested that the rigid structure of crystalline silica, which has many regularly arranged hydrogen-bonding groups on its surface, may be particularly injurious to lysosomal membranes.

Macrophages are protected from harm if they ingest free silica particles coated with PVPNO or if the particles and PVPNO are ingested separately. The reason for this may be that the numerous strong hydroxyl groups of silicic acid on the particle surfaces act as hydrogen donors in hydrogen-bonding reactions with the membrane of the digestive vacuole which is thereby injured; but, in the presence of PVPNO, this injurious effect is prevented probably because of preferential formation of strong hydrogen bonds with the hydroxyl groups of silicic acid before these can damage the membrane (Allison, 1968).

PVPNO administered to experimental animals also inhibits fibrogenesis due to quartz (Klosterkötter, 1968) and other fibrogenic substances.

(2) Given that macrophage destruction by free silica is crucial to fibrogenesis it still remains to be explained how this is brought about. Heppleston (1971) has offered evidence that some 'factor' (or 'factors') released from disrupted macrophages stimulates fibroblasts to fibrogenesis. Fallon (1937) showed experimentally that the cellular reaction in the lungs associated with quartz particles was accompanied by increased amounts of phospholipids and that these (or a 'factor' accompanying them) when reinjected into the lungs without quartz produced lesions resembling experimental silicosis. But quartz inhaled by 'standard pathogen-free' rats may fail to cause silicotic nodules and give rise instead to extensive consolidation by an intra-alveolar amorphous granular material containing quartz particles which consists chiefly of phospholipid, protein and muco-substances and closely resembles human alveolar lipoproteinosis (Corrin and King, 1970; Heppleston, Wright and Stewart, 1970). The absence of silicotic nodules is explained on the grounds that quartz particles are enmeshed in the granular material and are thus out of reach of macrophages.

In this light the following hypothesis has been offered by Heppleston (1971).

(1) Disruption of quartz-containing macrophages releases a non-lipid 'fibrogenic factor' which provokes fibroblastic activity.

(2) Simultaneously, a 'lipid factor' is released and stimulates augmentation of the macrophage population in the lungs and, on the assumption that fibroblasts are derived from macrophages, furnishes increased numbers of fibroblasts for fibrogenesis.

Against this it must be said that radioactive labelling of cells does not support this origin of fibroblasts. Nevertheless, the possibility of a macrophage 'lipid factor' acting directly upon fibroblasts is not discounted.

It should also be noted that quartz (in common with other forms of free silica) does not appear to have a direct effect upon fibroblasts. The problem is still under investigation.

Theory based on immunological reactions

There are three possible ways in which free silica particles might cause immunological reactions.

(1) *By acting as an antigen.*—Unlike organic dusts (Chapter 11) which may provoke an Arthus (Type III) reaction, mineral dusts—including free silica—do not act in this way. Theoretically, they may function as a hapten to produce a Type II allergic response, but no satisfactory evidence to support this has been produced. Although some workers, notably Kashimura (1959), have apparently demonstrated antibodies against quartz in experimental animals, this observation has not been confirmed (Collet *et al.*, 1961; Voison *et al.*, 1964), so the results of the earlier experiments may have been due to bacterial contamination of quartz particles.

(2) *By producing an auto-antigen.*—They may modify the structure of some body protein and thereby produce antigen. As already noted, proteins adsorbed on to the surface of quartz are denatured and, by virtue of this, may develop antigenic potential. Gamma globulins are most likely to be involved and it has been shown that when denatured in various ways they produce antibodies in experimental animals (Milgrom and Witebsky, 1960; McClusky, Miller and Benacerraf, 1962). But there is no conclusive evidence that this occurs in man.

(3) *By acting as an adjuvant.*—They may, like Freund's adjuvant, facilitate an allergic reaction which might not otherwise occur. In experimental animals the induction of hypersensitivity causes larger and more clearly demarcated silicotic lesions (due to powdered quartz) than in control animals (Powell and Gough, 1959).

Although experimental work (Thiart and Engelbrecht, 1967) has indicated that the ground substance of silicotic nodules in rats consists, not of γ globulins but of β globulins derived from macrophages killed by quartz, human silicotic nodules (*see* Chapter 7) apparently contain IgG and IgM which are found among collagen fibres and may be bound to them (Pernis, 1968). Plasma cells around the periphery of actively developing lesions are believed to be the source of the immune globulins. These features vary widely in lesions from different subjects and in different lesions in the same subject; and in some they cannot be identified at all. They appear to be most prominent in actively evolving lesions and absent from old inactive lesions. The nodules contain a variable amount of hyaline in which there is no more than about 40 per cent collagen (Vigliani and Pernis, 1963).

Proof that auto-allergic reactions are involved in the pathogenesis of silicotic lesions has, therefore, not been confirmed; but it is of interest that amyloid lesions, in which auto-immune phenomena are thought to play a part, also contain variable amounts of IgG (Schultz *et al.*, 1966) and complement, and there are similarities in the hyaline of both types of lesion (Pernis, 1968). However, it seems probable that the presence of globulins may be due to permeation of serum proteins which remain sequestered in the lesions (Heppleston, 1969). In view of the lack of agreement in reported observations a possible adjuvant effect of quartz or other types of free silica is, at present, speculative.

To summarize: although silicotic lesions are not likely to be *initiated* by an allergic reaction, such a reaction might subsequently occur in some cases of silicosis as a result of an adjuvant effect especially in the genesis of rapidly developing and progressing massive, or conglomerate lesions, often long after dust exposure has ceased (*see* Chapter 7). But there appears, in fact, to be little satisfactory evidence to suggest that a secondary immunological process is involved (Heppleston, 1969).

COAL PNEUMOCONIOSIS AND 'MIXED DUST FIBROSIS'

Fibrogenesis in coal pneumoconiosis, unlike silicosis, appears to be determined in some way by the amount of total dust in the lungs. Whether or not the small quantities of quartz which may be associated with coal dust contribute to this is controversial and the problem is discussed further in Chapter 8. Certainly, experimentally, coal particles are not cytotoxic and cause little evident change in macrophages (Collet *et al.*, 1967).

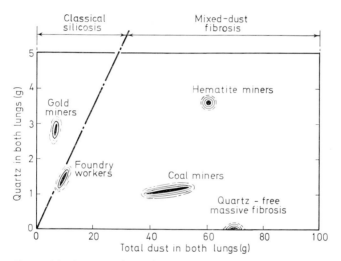

Figure 4.4. Average values of total dust and quartz in lungs with advanced forms of different dust diseases. (From Nagelschmidt (1960). Br. J. ind. Med. **17**, 247 by courtesy of H.M.S.O.)

On the basis of mineralogical examination of human lungs Nagelschmidt (1960) has suggested that smaller amounts of relatively insoluble dusts, such as coal, are required for a given severity of fibrosis the more quartz they contain; and, conversely, larger amounts of dust, the less quartz they contain. This is illustrated in *Figure 4.4.*

An additional feature which may have pathogenic importance in both silicosis and coal pneumoconiosis is that organic iron (as ferritin) is taken up by macrophages in the same way as quartz and shortens their life span.

Collagen-stimulating substances may be released when these cells disrupt after death (Chvapil and Hurych, 1968). Indeed, accumulation of organic iron occurs in both silicotic lesions (Otto and Moran, 1959) and those of coal pneumoconiosis. The source of this non-haem iron is probably mainly endogenous; experimentally, iron accumulates in macrophages which have ingested a mixture of carbon and 2 per cent quartz (Collet et al., 1967) or mucoid substances, and it is thought likely to originate from plasma trans-ferrin (McCarthy, Reid and Gibbons, 1964). Iron in this form is not identified by routine iron stains. Whether or not it influences collagen synthesis in these and in any of the pneumoconioses, it has a significant effect upon determin-ing their appearances on the chest radiograph (see Chapter 5). Inorganic iron, by contrast, when mixed with quartz inhibits its fibrogenic potential (see Chapter 7).

Coal dust may act as an adsorbing surface for abnormal antigens and it has been suggested that, in this way, it may localize antigen-antibody re-actions. But the evidence is conflicting and its relevance to the pathogenesis of 'rheumatoid' and 'non-rheumatoid' coal pneumoconiosis is referred to in Chapter 8.

Influence of coexisting tuberculosis

For years past it has been believed that tuberculosis enhances the progress of lesions of silicosis and coal pneumoconiosis and this has been demon-strated in experimental animals. It is possible that, if such an effect exists in man, it may be caused by an adjuvant influence of live or dead tubercle bacilli upon the production of non-specific antibody which becomes localized, not only where the bacilli are situated, but also in the pneumoconiotic lesion. On the other hand, the growth of tubercle bacilli is only increased by free silica through the intermediary of macrophages (Allison and Hart, 1968) and cell-mediated (Type IV) allergic responses are apparently potentiated in animals exposed to quartz (Pernis and Paronetto, 1962).

A direct influence of the tuberculous inflammatory process in causing the development of the confluent masses ('progressive massive fibrosis') of coal and carbon pneumoconiosis in man has been suggested for years but not convincingly demonstrated, although it is possible that it may initiate these lesions in a proportion of cases and subsequently die out. The problem is discussed in more detail in Chapter 8.

'Opportunist' mycobacteria, distinct from tubercle bacilli, are found in some cases of fibrotic pneumoconiosis which seems to favour their growth. *M. avium* is probably the most important of these and, as it is poorly sensitive to antituberculous agents, it carries a poor prognosis (Marks, 1970). *M. kansasii*, a photochromogen, is also pathogenic for man, and work with guinea-pigs has shown that its pathogenicity is enhanced by quartz and coal dusts (Policard et al., 1967). No evidence has been forthcoming to show that these organisms play any part in the formation of pneumoconiotic lesions.

ASBESTOSIS

The pathogenesis of asbestosis appears different again from that of silicosis or coal pneumoconiosis, although experimental work on macrophages and other cells in culture has not, so far, shown the consistent results observed with quartz and carbon. But all observers seem to be agreed that short asbestos fibres are taken up by the phagosomes of macrophages (*Figure 4.5*) although there is disagreement about the toxicity of different fibre types. The types of asbestos are distinguished in Chapters 2 and 9. Some investigators have found chrysotile to be cytotoxic (Allison, 1968; Koshi, Hayashi and Sakabe, 1968) and others record it as showing a lack of toxicity in striking contrast to the effects of quartz (Davis, 1967). Long chrysotile fibres which are incompletely ingested by the cells and remain partly extracellular increase

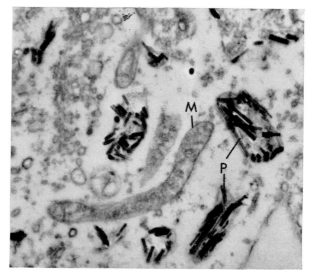

Figure 4.5. Electron micrograph of a segment of a macrophage that has ingested asbestos particles. These are grouped in phagosomes (P) which remain intact; mitochondria (M) are still well preserved. (By courtesy of Dr A. C. Allison)

the permeability of the cell membrane (Beck, Holt and Manojlović, 1972). Crocidolite is said to be non-cytotoxic by some observers (Sakabe, Koshi and Hayashi, 1971) whereas others have reported it to be highly cytotoxic (Parazzi *et al.*, 1968). Chrysotile has a similar haemolytic effect to quartz (McNab and Harington, 1967), but is much less sensitive than quartz to the inhibiting effect of PVPNO. Crocidolite, anthophyllite and amosite are only feebly haemolytic.

These discrepancies are probably due to varying experimental conditions (for example, lack of standardization of asbestos samples used) and, in particular, the nature of the medium in which they have been performed.

When chrysotile fibres are added to macrophages in a saline medium (that is, without serum) severe cytotoxic effects rapidly occur; these are probably determined in a similar way to haemolysis. This early cytotoxicity is most pronounced for chrysotile and then, in descending order, for crocidolite, amosite and anthophyllite (Allison, 1971). However, because these experiments were not done in a serum medium (that is, one which contains proteins similar to those in body fluids) they are not physiological and are unlikely to be relevant to *in vivo* events. But when they are repeated in a serum medium all these types of asbestos are much less toxic to macrophages than quartz, and this comparatively mild effect is demonstrated by the fact that only a proportion of cells die while others exhibit pyknosis of their nuclei and cytoplasm (Allison, 1971). By contrast, Pernis and Castano (1971) have reported that neither chrysotile nor crocidolite are cytotoxic (but they used higher serum concentrations), and Sakabe, Koshi and Hayashi (1971) also found that chrysotile was not cytotoxic in a protein medium. Evidently a physiological level of serum protein is of critical importance in these experiments.

A significant feature revealed by electron microscopy is the appearance of an electron-dense matrix around asbestos particles in secondary lysosomes; this may protect the lysosomal membranes from damage and account for the difference between the comparatively mild cytotoxicity, on the one hand, and strong haemolytic effect, on the other (Allison, 1971). Iron-containing pigment collects in the vacuoles and is important *in vivo* in the formation of 'asbestos bodies' (q.v.). There is evidence that chrysotile increases the membrane permeability of alveolar macrophages (Beck *et al.*, 1971).

Although macrophages readily ingest fibres less than 5 μm in length they cannot ingest long fibres (that is, longer than about 10 μm) completely, but individual cells may envelop one end of a fibre so that part of it remains extracellular, and a number of cells may attach themselves to very long fibres (Allison, 1971). This situation is very different from the effect of quartz particles, and the mild, or possible lack, of cytotoxicity of chrysotile and crocidolite under physiological conditions suggest that fibrosis in both animal and human asbestosis is produced without significant damage to macrophages. That the mechanism of fibrogenesis is different from that of silicosis is supported by the contrasting results in experimental animals when aluminium is mixed with quartz and with crocidolite: the fibrogenic effect of quartz, on the one hand, is reduced but that of crocidolite, on the other, is enhanced (Engelbrecht and Bester, 1969). Nevertheless, PVPNO inhibits the cytotoxic effects of chrysotile (Koshi, Hayashi and Sakabe, 1968).

Much work remains to be done to solve the enigma of fibrogenesis in asbestosis. The possibility that an immunological role may have an adjuvant effect in pathogenesis is discussed in Chapter 9.

BERYLLIUM DISEASE

Immunological reactions may be involved in the chronic form of this disease and beryllium is a powerful adjuvant to antibody production in experimental animals (*see* Chapter 10).

CONCLUSIONS

The occurrence, evolution and characteristics of lung diseases caused by the inhalation of extraneous particles depend not only upon the nature of the particles and the dose and duration of their inhalation, but also their crucial effect on macrophages and the intermediate events which may or may not follow upon this, and probably upon subsequent humoral responses— that is, the 'host response'. The end-result of the inhalation of some fibrogenic dusts in many cases of pneumoconiosis is likely to depend as much upon complex reactions to them by the body as upon the inherent fibrogenic potential of the dust. The patterns of these reactions appear to vary qualitatively and quantitatively in different subjects. The relevance of immunological reactions to the development of pneumoconiotic lesions, therefore, can be summarized in this way.

(1) Non-organ-specific auto-antibody activity may occur at some stage, and to a varying degree during the course of the pathogenesis of silicosis, coal pneumoconiosis and asbestosis, but its significance is not yet understood.

(2) Immunological reactions may be involved in the development of chronic beryllium disease.

(3) An Arthus (Type III) antigen-antibody reaction appears to be largely responsible for acute extrinsic allergic 'alveolitis' provoked by certain organic dusts and for the diffuse interstitial fibrosis which may follow.

POST-MORTEM EXAMINATION OF LUNGS

Sound practical knowledge of the various types of pneumoconiosis is achieved only by correlating, whenever possible, observations made during life with the morbid anatomical features of the lungs after death. As Morgagni wrote two centuries ago: 'those who have dissected many bodies, have at least learned to doubt when the others, who are ignorant of anatomy and do not take the trouble to attend to it, are in no doubt at all'. No opportunity, therefore, should be lost to study lungs removed after death and relate the findings to the industrial history, symptomatology and clinical, physiological, radiological and other data obtained during life. Modern techniques for preparing lungs and making paper-mounted whole sections for permanent record contribute greatly to this end. These and some other technical considerations, including polarized light microscopy, are referred to in the Appendix.

REFERENCES

Allison, A. C. (1968). 'Lysosomes and the responses of cells to toxic materials.' In *Scientific Basis of Medicine Annual Reviews*, pp. 18–30. (Br. Postgrad. Med. Fed.) London; Athlone Press
— (1971). 'Effects of silica and asbestos on cells in culture.' In *Inhaled Particles 3*, pp. 437–441. Ed. by W. H. Walton. Woking; Unwin
— and Hart, P. D. (1968). 'Potentiation by silica of the growth of *Mycobacterium tuberculosis* in macrophage cultures.' *Br. J. exp. Path.* **49**, 465–476
— Harington, J. S. and Birbeck (1966). 'An examination of the cytotoxic effects of silica on macrophages.' *J. exp. Med.* **124**, 141–154
Ball, T. and Lawrence, J. S. (1961). 'Epidemiology of the sheep cell agglutination test.' *Ann. rheum. Dis.* **20**, 235–245
Beck, E. G., Holt, P. F. and Nasrallah, E. T. (1971). 'Effects of chrysotile and acid-treated chrysotile on macrophage cultures.' *Br. J. ind. Med.* **28**, 179–185
— — and Manojlović, N. (1972). 'Comparison of effects on macrophage cultures of glass fibre, glass powder and chrysotile asbestos.' *Br. J. ind. Med.* **29**, 280–286
Beck, J. S. (1963). 'Auto-antibodies to cell nuclei.' *Scott. med. J.* **8**, 373–388
Belt, T. and King, E. J. (1945). *Chronic Pulmonary Disease in South Wales Coal Miners.* III. Experimental Studies. MRC. SRS. No. 250. London; H.M.S.O.
Berger, H. W. and Speckler, S. G. (1966). Pleural and pericardial effusions in rheumatoid disease.' *Ann. Inter. Med.* **64**, 1291–1297

Bernal, J. D. (1967). *The Origin of Life*, p. 93. London; Weidenfeld and Nicolson

Brieger, H. and Gross, P. (1967). 'On the theory of silicosis III.' *Archs envir. Hlth* **15**, 751–757

Bruch, J. (1967). 'Ein elektronenmikroscopische Beitrag zum Frühstadium der Silikose.' In *Fortschritte der Staublungenforschung*, Vol. 2, pp. 249–255. Ed. by H. Reploh and H. J. Einbrodt. Dinslaken; Niederrheinische Druckerie

Bunim, J. J. (1961). 'A broader spectrum of Sjögren's syndrome and its pathogenic implications.' *Ann. rheum. Dis.* **20**, 1–9

Cavagna, G. and Nichelatti, T. (1963). 'The protective influence of polyvinyl-pyridine-N-oxide in experimental silicosis.' *Medna Lav.* **54**, 621–627

Chao, E. C. T., Fahey, J. J. and Littler, J. (1962). 'Stishovite, SiO$_2$, a very high pressure new mineral from Meteor Crater, Arizona.' *J. geophys. Res.* **67**, 419–421

Chvapil, M. (1967). *Physiology of Connective Tissue*, p. 230. London; Butterworths

— and Hurych, J. (1968). 'Control of collagen biosynthesis.' In *International Review of Connective Tissue Research*, Vol. 4, p. 97. Ed. by D. A. Hall. New York and London; Academic Press

Collet, A., Voisin, G. A., Daniel-Moussard, H. and Toullet, F. (1961). 'Production of antibodies by quartz and beryllium oxide.' *Archs envir. Hlth* **2**, 409–417

— Martin, J. C., Normand-Renet, C. and Policard, A. (1967). 'Recherches infra-structurales sur l'évolution des macrophages alvéolaires et leurs réactions aux poussières minérales.' In *Inhaled Particles and Vapours*, II, pp. 155–163. Ed. by C. N. Davies. Oxford; Pergamon

Corrin, B. and King, E. (1970). 'Pathogenesis of experimental pulmonary alveolar proteinosis.' *Thorax* **25**, 230–236

Curran, R. C. and Rowsell, E. V. (1958). The application of the diffusion-chamber techniques to the study of silicosis.' *J. Path. Bact.* **76**, 561–568

Davis, J. M. G. (1967). 'The effects of chrysotile asbestos dust on lung macrophages maintained in organ culture.' *Br. J. exp. Path.* **48**, 379–385

Doctor, L. and Snider, G. L. (1962). 'Diffuse interstitial pulmonary fibrosis associated with arthritis.' *Am. Rev. resp. Dis.* **85**, 413–422

Duguid, J. B. and Lambert, M. W. (1964). 'The pathogenesis of coal miner's pneumoconiosis.' *J. Path. Bact.* **88**, 389–403

Engelbrecht, F. M. and Bester, J. C. P. (1969). 'The mechanism of aluminium in the prevention of pneumoconiosis.' *S. Afr. med. J.* **43**, 203–205

Englebrecht, F. R., Yoganathan, M., King, E. J. and Nagelschmidt, G. (1958). 'Fibrosis and collagen in rat's lungs produced by etched and unetched free silica dusts.' *A.M.A. Archs ind. Hlth* **17**, 287–294

Fallon, J. T. (1937). 'Specific tissue reaction to phospholipids: a suggested explana-tion for the similarity of the lesions of silicosis and pulmonary tuberculosis.' *Canad. med. J.* **36**, 223–228

Gell, P. G. H. and Coombs, R. R. A. (1968). *Clinical Aspects of Immunology*, 2nd Ed., pp. 575–596. Oxford; Blackwell

Gitlin, D., Janeway, C. A., Apt, R. and Craig, J. M. (1959). In *Cellular and Humoral Aspects of Hypersensitive States*. (New York Academy of Medicine Symposium No. 9), p. 425. Ed. by H. S. Lawrence. London; Cassell

Good, R. A. and Rotstein, J. (1960). 'Rheumatoid arthritis and agammaglobulin-aemia.' *Bull. rheum. Dis.* **10**, 203–206

Hagadorn, J. E. and Burrell, R. (1968). 'Lung reactive antibodies in IgA fractions of sera from patients with pneumoconiosis.' *Clin. exp. Immunol.* **3**, 263–267

Hammerman, D. and Sandson, J. (1970). 'Antigenicity of Connective Tissue Components.' *Mount Sinai J. Med.* **37**, 453–465

Hammon, L. and Rich, A. R. (1944). 'Acute diffuse interstitial fibrosis of the lungs.' *Bull. Johns Hopkins Hosp.* **74**, 117–212

Heppleston, A. G. (1969). 'Pigmentation and disorders of the lung.' In *Pigments in Pathology*, pp. 33–73. Ed. by M. Wolman, New York and London; Academic Press

— Wright, N. A. and Stewart, J. A. (1970). 'Experimental alveolar lipo-proteinosis following the inhalation of silica.' *J. Path.* **101**, 293-307

Heppleston, A. G. (1971). 'Observations on the mechanism of silicotic fibrogenesis.' In *Inhaled Particles and Vapours, III*, pp. 357–369. Ed. by W. H. Walton. Woking; Unwin.

Hijmans, W., Doniach, D., Roitt, M. and Holborrow, E. J. (1961). 'Serological overlap between lupus erythematosus, rheumatoid arthritis and thyroid auto-immune disease.' *Br. med. J.* **2**, 909–914

Hinson, K. F. W. (1970). 'Diffuse pulmonary fibrosis.' *Hum. Path.* **1**, 275–288

Holt, P. F. (1957). *Pneumoconiosis. Industrial Diseases of the Lung caused by Dust*, pp. 138–141. London; Edward Arnold

Hughes, P. and Rowell, N. R. (1970). 'Aggravation of turpentine-induced pleurisy in rats by "homogenous" and "speckled" anti-nuclear antibodies.' *J. Path.* **101**, 141–155

Kashimura, M. (1959). 'A study of the antibody produced after intravenous administration of particulate silicic acid in suspension.' *Bull. Hyg., Lond.* **34**, 636–637

Kettle, E. H. (1926). 'Experimental silicosis.' *J. ind. Hyg. Toxicol.* **8**, 491–495

King, E. J., Mohanty, G. P., Harrison, C. V. and Nagelschmidt, G. (1953). 'The action of different forms of pure silica on the lungs of rats.' *Br. J. ind. Med.* **10**, 9–17

Klosterkötter, W. (1968). 'Pneumoconiosis of coal workers: results, problems and practical consequences of recent research.' In *Pneumoconiosis*. (Report of Symposium at Katowice, June 1967, pp. 99–109.) Copenhagen; W.H.O.

Koshi, K., Hayashi, H. and Sakabe, H. (1968). 'Cell toxicity and haemolytic action of asbestos dust.' *Ind. Hlth* **6**, 69–79

Lawrence, J. S. (1965). 'Surveys of rheumatic complaints in the population.' In *Progress in Clinical Rheumatology*. Ed. by A. St J. Dixon. London; Churchill

— (1967). 'Genetics of rheumatoid factor and rheumatoid arthritis.' *Clin. exp. Immunol.* **2**, 769–783

Letterer, E., Gerok, W. and Schneider, G. (1955). 'Vergleichende Untersuchungen uber den Aminosauerenbestand von Serum-Eweiss, Leberweiss, Amyloid, Hyalin und Kollagen.' *Virchows Arch. Path. Anat. Physiol.*, 327–342

Liebow, A. A., Steer, A. and Billingsley, J. G. (1965). 'Desquamative interstitial pneumonia.' *Am. J. Med.* **39**, 369–404

McCarthy, C., Reid, L. and Gibbons, R. A. (1964). 'Intra-alveolar mucus—removal by macrophages: with iron accumulation.' *J. Path. Bact.* **87**, 39–47

McClusky, R. T., Miller, F. and Benacerraf, B. (1962), 'Sensitisation to denatured autologuous gammaglobulin.' *J. exp. Med.* **115**, 153–273

McNab, G. and Harington, J. S. (1967). 'Haemolytic activity of asbestos and other mineral dusts.' *Nature, Lond.* **214**, 522–523

Maher, J. A. (1954). 'Dural nodules in rheumatoid arthritis.' *A.M.A. Archs Path.* **58**, 354–359

Marks, J. (1970). 'New mycobacteria.' *Hlth Trends* **2**, 68–69

Miall, W. E., Ball, J. and Kellgren, J. H. (1958). 'Prevalence of rheumatoid arthritis in urban and rural populations in South Wales.' *Ann. rheum. Dis.* **17**, 263-272

Milgrom, F. and Witebsky, E. (1960). 'Studies on the rheumatoid and related serum factors.' *J. Am. med. Ass.* **174**, 56–63

Morgagni, G. B. (1769). *De Sedibus et Causis Morborum*, Vol. 1. Book 2, p. 396. Letter 16. Trans. by B. Alexander

Nadler, S. and Goldfischer, S. (1970). The intracellular release of lysosomal con-tents in macrophages that have ingested silica.' *J. Histochem. Cytochem.* **18**, 368–371

Nagelschmidt, G. (1960). 'The relationship between lung dust and lung pathology in pneumoconiosis.' *Br. J. ind. Med.* **17**, 247–259

Nash, T., Allison, A. C. and Harington, J. S. (1966). 'Physio-chemical properties of silica in relation to its toxicity.' *Nature, Lond.* **210**, 259–261

Nossal, G. J. V. (1964). 'How cells make antibodies.' *Scient. Am.* **211**, 106–115

Otto, H. and Moran, R. (1959). 'Zur Histologie der Eisenablagerungen bei Por-zellinersilikoson.' *Arch. Gewerbepath. Gewerbehyg.* **17**, 117–126

Panettiere, F., Chandler, B. F. and Libeke, J. H. (1968). 'Pulmonary cavitation in rheumatoid disease.' *Am. Rev. resp. Dis.* **97**, 89–95

Parazzi, E., Pernis, B., Secchi, G. C. and Vigliani, E. C. (1968). 'Studies on *in vivo* cytotoxicity of asbestos dusts.' *Medna Lav.* **59**, 561–576

Pepys, J. (1969). *Hypersensitivity Diseases of the Lungs due to Fungi and Organic Dusts.* Basel and New York; Karger

Pernis, B. (1968). 'Silicosis.' In *Textbook of Immunopathology*, Vol I, pp. 293–301. Ed. by P. A. Miescher and H. J. Muller-Eberhard. New York and London; Grune and Stratton

— and Castano, P. (1971). 'Effetto dell' asbesto sulle cellule in vitro.' *Medna Lav.* **62**, 120–129

— and Paronetto, F. (1962). Adjuvant effect of silica (tridymite) on antibody production.' *Proc. Soc. exp. Biol. Med.* **110**, 390-392

Policard, A., Gernez-Rieux, C., Taquet, A., Martin, J. C., Devalder, J. and Le Bouffant, J. (1967). 'Influence of pulmonary dust load on the development of experimental infection by *Mycobacterium kansasii*.' *Nature, Lond.* **216**, 177–178

Powell, D. E. B. and Gough, J. (1959). The effect on experimental silicosis of hypersensitivity induced by horse serum. *Br. J. exp. Path.* **40**, 40–43

Price, T. M. L. and Skelton, M. O. (1965). 'Rheumatoid arthritis with lung lesions.' *Thorax* **11**, 234–240

Sakabe, H. and Koshi, K. (1967). 'Preventative effect of polybetaine on the cell toxicity to quartz particles.' *Ind. Hlth* **5**, 181–182

— — and Hayashi, H. (1971). 'On the cell toxicity of mineral dusts.' In *Inhaled Particles 3*, pp. 423–434. Ed. by W. H. Walton. Woking; Unwin

Scadding, J. G. (1964), 'Fibrosing alveolitis.' *Br. med. J.* **2**, 686–941

— and Hinson, K. F. W. (1967). 'Diffuse fibrosing alveolitis (diffuse interstitial fibrosis of the lungs). Correlation of histology at biopsy with prognosis.' *Thorax* **22**, 291–304

Scheel, L. D., Smith, B., Van Riper, J. and Fleischer, E. (1954). 'Toxicity of silica.' *A.M.A. Archs ind. Hyg.* **9**, 29–36

Schultz, R. T., Calkins, E., Milgrom, F. and Witebsky, E. (1966). 'Association of gamma globulin with amyloid.' *Am. J. Path.* **48**, 1–17

Siegfried, M. (1893). 'Über die chemischen Eigenshaften des reticulirten Gewebes.' *Fortschr. Med.* **11**, 185

Stalder, K. and Stöber, W. (1965). 'Haemolytic activity of suspensions of different modifications and inert dusts.' *Nature, Lond.* **207**, 874–875

Stöber, W. (1968). 'On the theory of silicosis. IV.' *Archs envir. Hlth* **16**, 706–707

Thiart, B. F. and Engelbrecht, F. M. (1967). 'Globulins in silicotic lungs.' *S. Afr. med.* **41**, 731–733.

Tomasi, T. B. Jr., Tan, E. M., Solomon, A. and Prendergast, R. A. (1965). 'Characteristics of an immune system common to external secretions.' *J. exp. Med.* **121**, 101–124

Torrigiani, G., Roitt, I. M., Lloyd, K. N. and Corbett, M. (1970). 'Elevated IgG antiglobulins in patients with seronegative rheumatoid arthritis.' *Lancet* **1**, 14–16

Turner Warwick, M. and Haslam, P. (1971). 'Antibodies in some chronic fibrosing lung diseases. 1. Non-organ-specific auto-antibodies,' *Clin. Allergy* **1**, 83–95

Vigliani, E. C. and Pernis, B. (1959). 'An immunological approach to silicosis.' *J. occup. Med.* **1**, 319–328

— — (1963). 'Advances in tuberculosis research.' In *Fortschritte der Tuberkuloseforschung*, Vol. 12, pp. 230–279. Ed. by H. Birkhauser, H. Bloch, and G. Canetti. Basel and New York; Karger

Voisin, G. A., Collet, A., Martin, J. C., Daniel-Moussard, H. and Toulet, F. (1964). 'Propertés immunologiques de la silice et des composés du beryllium: les formes soluble comparées aux formes insoluble.' *Revue fr. Étud. clin. biol.* **9**, 819–828

Ward, D. J., Johnson, G. D. and Holborrow, E. J. (1964). 'Antinuclear factor in rheumatoid arthritis; its incidence and clinical significance.' *Ann. rheum. Dis.* **23**, 306–310

Williams, R. C., and Kunkel, H. G. (1962). 'Rheumatoid factor, complement, and conglutin aberrations in patients with subacute bacterial endocarditis.' *J. clin. Invest.* **41**, 666–675

World Health Organization (1964). 'A nomenclature for human immunoglobulins.' *Bull. Wld Hlth Org.* **30**, 447–450

5—The Chest Radiograph

More faithful witness are eyes than ears
Heraclitus: Fragment XV

Although the diagnosis of a pneumoconiosis necessarily involves an analysis of occupational history, physical examination and lung function tests, the chest radiograph is without doubt the most informative single investigation available.

The general principles of chest radiography and radiology are admirably discussed, respectively, by Clarke (1964) and Simon (1968) among others. But when the pneumoconioses are under consideration it is particularly important that certain principles which determine the appearance of the chest radiograph should be understood if errors of interpretation are to be avoided.

Chest radiography is employed both for clinical and epidemiological purposes: the first to establish diagnosis, prognosis and guidance of treatment; the second to estimate prevalence and behaviour of disease in different communities. Our concern here is mainly with the first. Whichever the purpose, however, the highest possible standard of radiographic technique must always be sought.

RELEVANT X-RAY PHYSICS

X-rays used for diagnostic purposes are electromagnetic radiations normally within the 0·1 Å to 1 Å wavelength range (1 Å or Ångstrom unit = 10^{-10} metre) which travel in straight lines but, on encountering matter, may be absorbed or scattered in various amounts and directions by its atoms.

The *atomic number* (that is, the number of electrons around the nucleus in an uncharged atom) of an element decides its character. It is the average atomic number of a body tissue—not its atomic weight—which is responsible for the extent to which incident x-rays of given energy will be absorbed or scattered by different tissues and, hence, for the appearance of the radiographic image.

100

Absorption and scatter

The amount of absorption and scatter is also determined by the number of atoms per unit volume and consequently by the density or specific gravity of the material. Therefore, both x-ray absorption and scatter are significantly less in air than in fluids such as blood or pleural effusion.

Some x-rays pass through matter without interacting with its atoms but those which do interact are subject to a range of increasing effects. These are as follows: slight change in their direction with some loss of energy; inter-action with electrons in their orbital shells; and complete absorption by atoms resulting in the emission of electrons and secondary radiation.

Detailed consideration of these processes is inappropriate here but the enunciation of two fundamental principles is important:

(1) Some radiation is totally or partly absorbed in the material while the remainder either has its direction changed or is degraded to lower energy radiation which is scattered in all directions.

(2) The amount of scatter is dependent upon the number of electrons per gramme of irradiated material and, allowing for density, this is much the same for most elements in biological materials with the exception of hydrogen which has about twice the number (Osborn, 1969).

Production of the x-ray image

The effect of x-rays upon the conventional x-ray film is to produce blackening when it is developed. Conversely, unexposed film is transparent and appears white when viewed against white light. Materials or tissues which absorb x-rays completely and prevent them reaching the film emulsion cast 'shadows' which appear white and these are conventionally regarded as of high density. Consequently the various tissues of the body, which have different absorptive capacities for x-rays, produce a range of effects from black (for example, air) when absorption is least, through tones of grey (for example, fat and muscle), to white (for example, bone) when absorption is greatest.

Hence, it is convenient to conceive of four basic degrees of radiographic densities: 'air', 'fat', 'water' (equivalent to blood and soft tissues), and 'bone'. With the exception of air the radio-opacity of different tissues is dependent more upon their effective atomic number than upon their specific gravity (Spiers, 1946) or chemical composition. The *effective atomic number* is an expression of the resultant total absorption of x-rays by atoms of the different elements in a material and it is dependent upon the percentage by weight, the atomic number and atomic weight of each element. In the low-voltage region where photoelectric absorption is important, the contribution made by any one element to the effective atomic number of the material as a whole depends on its atomic number raised to about the third power (Johns and Cunningham, 1969). The effective atomic number for fat is given as 5·9, for muscle and water as 7·4, for air as 7·6, and for bone as about 14; the atomic numbers of phosphorus and calcium are 15 and 20, respectively. Air, in spite of the value of its effective atomic number and for reasons given in the next section, is virtually radiolucent; fat (which contains less hydrogen than water) produces a grey effect; all body fluids, muscle and solid viscera have a similar radiographic density which is equivalent to that of water

('Water Equivalent') and this produces a lighter grey effect than fat; and bone gives the densest, that is, the whitest, 'shadows' of all tissues. A radiograph of a normal shoulder (*Figure 5.1*) demonstrates these degrees of radioopacity. The contrast between the various radiodensities makes the total image.

Within the diagnostic range of x-ray energy, the absorption of rays is apparently proportional to the second or third power of the effective atomic number (Osborn, 1969) which explains not only why bone stands out so clearly, but also why extraneous materials with higher atomic numbers than

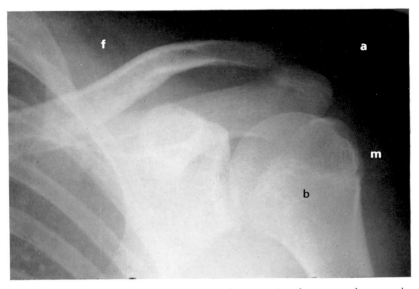

Figure 5.1. Radiograph of a normal shoulder demonstrating the contrast between the radio-opacities due to air (a), bone (b), fat (f) and muscle (m), best seen above the clavicle and flanking the humerus

the tissues cast denser 'shadows'. It is on this account that some of these materials, notably iodine and barium, are introduced into the body as contrast media, but the importance of this principle in the present context is that heavy metals such as iron, tin, antimony and barium when retained in the lungs cast particularly dense shadows which contrast sharply with the surrounding lung (*see Figure 6.4*). Table 5.1 sets out the atomic numbers of the major elements of the body and of some relevant extraneous elements.

However, it must be remembered that the image of the lung fields on the film is caused by the *sum* of superimposed radiodensities of structures and lesions throughout the thickness of the chest.

The effect of the air content of the lungs

As the values of the effective atomic numbers given in the last section suggest, air, if compressed to unit density, would in fact absorb more x-rays than unit density muscle or unit density fat. But air in the lungs is not in this state and its volume in normal lungs causes their density to be nearer that of air than that of the surrounding soft tissues—or 'water equivalent'—by a factor of about 800 (Osborn, 1969). This is due to the fact that air contains practically no hydrogen unless, as is virtually the case in the lungs, it is saturated with water vapour when it contains only about 0·8 per cent hydrogen by weight in contrast to some 10 per cent in soft tissues (Osborn, 1969). Hence, because the ratio of air density to tissue density is normally 1:800 the absorption of x-rays by air and the lungs as a whole is very substantially less than by other tissues. Furthermore, the lungs cause negligible scatter of radiation because the number of electrons per cm³ in their air is very small by comparison with the number of electrons per cm³ of the surrounding tissues. Indeed, it is calculated that the scattering effect (Scatter Attenuation Coefficient) of air is almost one thousand times less than that of soft tissues whether these be fat, muscle, blood vessels or fibrous tissue (Osborn, 1969).

Therefore, lung tissue has negligible radiodensity in contrast to that of its pulmonary blood vessels and their blood, mediastinal and other soft tissues,

TABLE 5.1

ATOMIC NUMBERS OF SOME RELEVANT ELEMENTS

Chief atomic constituents of body tissues and fluids		Elements of exogenous origin			
Hydrogen	1	Beryllium	4	Tin	50
Carbon	6	Carbon	6	Antimony	51
Nitrogen	7	Aluminium	13	Iodine	53
Oxygen	8	Silicon	14	Barium	56
Sodium	11	Vanadium	23	Cerium	58
Phosphorus	15	Chromium	24	Rare earth	
Calcium	20	Manganese	25	elements	58 to 71
		Iron	26	Tungsten	74
		Zirconium	40	Lead	82
		Silver	47	Thorium	90

and bone; an increase of soft tissue density within the lungs or the presence of radiodense dusts therefore produces additional contrasting opacities on the film. This has a direct and important bearing on an alleged obscuring effect which emphysema is wrongly, but often, supposed to have on the x-ray images of pneumoconiotic lesions (see this Chapter, page 127).

Sharpness of the radiographic image on the film
Sharpness in radiographs is limited by three factors:

(1) The penumbra around the image which is related to the size of the x-ray source and the distance of the subject from the film (*Figure 5.2*). This is reduced by increasing the distance between the x-ray source and the film, and by decreasing the size of the 'focal spot' in the x-ray tube.

(2) Movement of the subject. For example, slight body movement, failure to hold the breath, and normal movement of the heart and great vessels.

(3) Limitations imposed by film grain size and intensifying screens.

X-ray scatter within the lungs does not diminish sharpness of the image but excessive superficial fat and well-developed muscles may be responsible for sufficient absorption and scatter to cause reduction of contrast due to more or less uniform greyness of the total image. A much greater effect, of course, is produced by fluid—such as pleural effusion.

Appreciation of these points is of particular importance for the production of radiographs with the sharp definition required for investigation of all forms of pneumoconiosis, especially as these are sometimes represented by small or tenuous opacities.

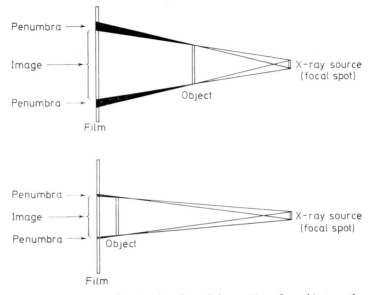

Figure 5.2. Diagram showing the effect of the position of an object on the size of the penumbra around its image on the film. The closer the object to the focal spot from which the x-rays emanate the larger the image produced. But, since the focal spot has a finite size, the penumbra is also larger, and this has the effect of blurring the edges of the image. This blurring effect can be decreased by reducing the object-film distance in relation to the focus-film distance or by reducing the size of the 'focal spot'. It is for this reason that chest films are customarily taken at 6 feet using a fine focal spot—preferably under 1 mm diameter

THE STANDARD CHEST RADIOGRAPH

Conventionally, the routine chest film is a postero-anterior (PA) view and is usually 17 × 14 inches (42·5 × 35·0 cm). During x-ray exposure the subject's breath must be held in the deepest possible inspiration; the mid-expiratory position suggested by the International Labour Office (1959) is not desirable as it is not capable of accurate control and prevents full expansion and, hence, optimal visualization of the lung fields—a matter of importance in the examination of asbestosis subjects. The technique for taking good quality films is summarized in *International Classification of Radiographs of Pneumoconioses* (ILO, 1970). Too white (under-exposed) or too dark (over-exposed) films are to be avoided, and the quality of serial films should, as far as possible, be kept comparable.

Films must be of adequate size to include the whole of the thorax from the lung apices to just below the costophrenic angles. In subjects with unduly large chests the lung bases may be incompletely visualized, in which case a wide basal view should be taken to include both costophrenic angles especially when asbestosis is suspected.

The subjects should be unclothed above the waist, and corsets and lumbar belts removed because, in addition to obscuring the lower lung fields, these

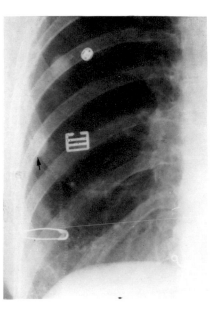

Figure 5.3. Clothing artefacts due to brassiere and blouse. Note the opacities in the right mid-zone (arrowed). A repeat film, taken after removal of clothing, was clear

limit maximal inspiratory descent of the diaphragm. Failure to remove clothing may lead to confusing artefacts. *Figure 5.3* shows the gross effect that clothing may have, but artefacts from this cause are commonly subtle so vigilance is required if they are not to be interpreted as evidence of pathology—especially if the obvious clue of pins and buttons is absent and it is taken for granted that the subject was stripped to the waist when the film was taken. This problem is more likely to be encountered in periodic radiographic examinations of workers in industry than in clinical practice.

PROCEDURE FOR INSPECTION OF THE CHEST RADIOGRAPH

Unless a systematic and consistent discipline for examining the film is followed, abnormalities may be overlooked or misinterpreted. It is also important to acquire the imaginative power of 'looking into' the two-dimensional film as if it were three-dimensional. If the quality and technique of the film is acceptable it can then be inspected by orderly stages.

Stage 1. Peripheral region
The soft tissues of the root of the neck, axillae, chest wall and diaphragm on both sides are studied and compared. The intense radio-opacity of the

diaphragm must be carefully 'looked into' to detect abnormal opacities (such as localized pleural thickening) which are only slightly different in contrast.

Next, the skeleton is inspected; clavicles, ribs (posterior, lateral and anterior aspects), scapulae, spine and sternum. In this way the occasional clues which bone lesions may give to lung disease are not missed.

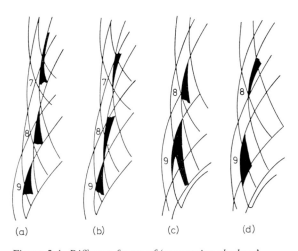

(a)   (b)   (c)   (d)

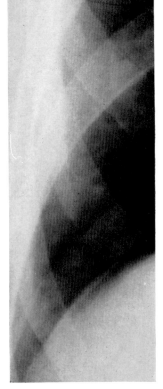

Figure 5.4. Different forms of 'companion shadows'— normal muscle shadows—of the lateral chest wall is shown in diagrams (a) to (d). (By courtesy of Drs Fletcher and Edge and the Honorary Editor of Clinical Radiology). An example in the radiograph of a 50-year-old man is seen on the right. These shadows may be mistaken for pleural lesions, a mistake which may be of importance in asbestos workers

The costal margins of the lung fields should be followed from the lung apices to the costophrenic angles and then along the diaphragm to the cardiophrenic angles. In this respect one should be familiar with the lower 'companion shadows' of the lateral chest wall which may be seen for a few rib spaces above the costophrenic angles in a proportion of normal PA films. These are triangular opacities whose lateral aspects are continuous with the rib shadows and their medial aspects usually well defined and vertical, while their lower parts lack definition. They are bilateral although not necessarily symmetrically equal and are caused by the interdigitations of the serratus anterior and external abdominal oblique muscles (*Figure 5.4*). Slight rotation of the chest during exposure of the film makes these shadows more prominent on one side than the other, when they may be misinterpreted as pleural lesions, a mistake which may occur anyway if their true nature is not recognized.

106

Stage 2. Central region

The position, size and shape of the trachea, great vessels and heart are noted. The heart shadow, especially on the left, must be 'looked through' for any abnormal opacity which may be superimposed upon it.

Stage 3. Hilar region

The position, size and shape of the hilar shadows are examined and the size and distribution of the pulmonary arteries passing to the lung fields noted.

Stage 4. Lung fields

These should be examined in two stages. First, the pulmonary arteries ('lung markings') should be followed until they are no longer visible which is usually in the outer third of the lung fields, and their branching and size (whether unduly thick or narrow) noted. These appearances are produced by vessels which run roughly parallel to the plane of the film, but those running in the anterior-posterior plane, and at right angles to that of the film, appear as oval or round opacities. If this is not understood they are sometimes wrongly interpreted as round lesions of silicosis (or some other discrete pneumoconiosis) when there is a relevant occupational history.

Second, the vessels must, as far as possible, be ignored and the lung fields 'looked into' for opacities indicating lesions in the parenchyma, and their size, shape and distribution assessed. Corresponding regions in both fields must be compared throughout.

Each lung field is arbitrarily, but conveniently, subdivided into three zones by two horizontal lines, drawn respectively through the anterior ends of the second and fourth ribs. These demarcate upper, middle and lower zones to which the distribution of abnormal shadows can be referred.

SOME COMMON CAUSES OF ERROR IN INTERPRETATION

Rotation of the subject

This causes unequal radiotranslucency of the two lung fields. If, for example, rotation is to the right a PA view will show the right field to be more translucent than the left and the right hilar region more prominent than the left.

Film taken in expiration

The lower zones of a film taken at the end of expiration have a different appearance from those of a film taken in full inspiration due to condensation of tissue radiodensities, the reduced volume of air and elevation of the diaphragm (*Figure 5.5*a and b). If the technical error of such a film, or one taken in incomplete inspiration, is not identified, misinterpretation is likely to occur. An early stage of diffuse interstitial fibrosis may be diagnosed or, if this is already present (in the form of asbestosis, for example), it may be regarded as being more advanced than it really is and the elevated diaphragm construed as evidence of contraction of the lungs.

Soft tissue shadows

Prominence of both pectoral muscle shadows, or of one more than the other on the dominant side of a muscular man, can be recognized for what they are if the discipline of inspection may be wrongly suspected. The effect of the interdigitations of serratus anteria and the external oblique muscle of the abdomen has been referred to already.

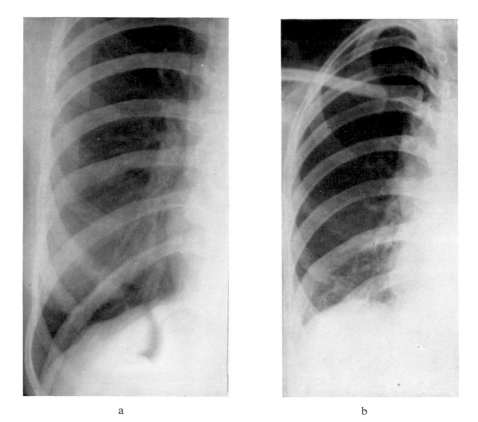

a   b

Figure 5.5. Difference in the appearances of the lower zones of normal lung fields in (a) inspiration compared with (b) expiration. The latter may be interpreted as mild diffuse interstitial fibrosis (for example, in asbestos workers)

Large breasts tend to obscure the lower lung fields and when good visualization of these zones is important this can usually be achieved by lightly binding the breasts and taking another PA film using a Potter-Bucky diaphragm.

Bronchographic contrast media

The scattered, rather dense, opacities of variable size which sometimes persist for a period of time after bronchography are sometimes a source of confusion if their cause is not recognized. However, bronchography is less often used today than it was a few years ago and many clinics use water-soluble media which disperse quickly. Bronchography has no particular value in the diagnosis of any form of pneumoconiosis.

OTHER RADIOLOGICAL TECHNIQUES

Lateral view

A lateral view should always be taken when the individual is seen for the first time, not only to define the spatial relationship of abnormal shadows seen in the PA view, but also to show the configuration of the chest, the shape and level of the diaphragm and the dimensions of the retrosternal translucence (*see* pages 129 and 130).

Anteroposterior view (AP view)

An AP view is invaluable for the clarification of uncertain or small and indistinct opacities seen in PA film because lesions which cause these may be situated rather more posteriorly than anteriorly in the lungs and are therefore more clearly defined.

Right and left anterior (first and second) oblique views

These are particularly helpful in demonstrating pleural thickening, hyaline plaque formation, and the lung fibrosis of asbestosis at an early stage. By this means the majority of pleural lesions are viewed tangentially and, thus, at their maximum radiodensity. It has been found that for this purpose more informative films are produced if the subject's chest is positioned at 45 degrees to the casette rather than at the 60 degree angle of the conventional technique (Mackenzie and Harries, 1970). (*See* Chapter 9.)

Macroradiography (magnification technique)

This employs a finer focus x-ray source—0·1 mm to 0·3 mm—than is used for the standard PA view, and the subject is placed midway between the source and the cassette (Bracken, 1964). It produces larger, but less distinct images than the standard film. It is sometimes used in the hope of detecting small discrete lesions of a pneumoconiosis before they give evidence of their presence in standard films. This is not borne out by general experience, and surveys have shown that macroradiographs of normal persons who have never been exposed to dust hazards may be interpreted as showing discrete pneumoconiotic lesions while those of persons who have been so exposed, may be regarded as normal. In practice, macroradiography offers no advantage over good quality PA and AP films examined first by naked eye and subsequently with a hand lens of ×2 or ×3 magnification. And this conclusion is corroborated by the good correlation which exists between appearances of standard PA view and post-mortem examination of the lungs (*see* later, this Chapter, page 126).

Apical view

The apical view, also known as an apicogram or lordotic view, is often of value in clarifying poorly defined and partly obscured shadows in the regions of the upper lobe apices, and may be helpful in distinguishing pneumoconiotic masses from other lesions in this region.

Tomography

Recourse to this technique is rarely required in the diagnosis of any type of pneumoconiosis. It is sometimes helpful in differentiating a confluent pneumoconiotic mass from other lesions which may resemble it, and of identifying such a mass when partly obscured by heart or mediastinal shadows; lateral tomography may then be of value.

Mass miniature radiography (MMR)

It is unnecessary to emphasize in general what a valuable technique this is, but the use of 35 mm or 70 mm films is not satisfactory for the detection of the early stages of a discrete pneumoconiosis (for example, silicosis or coal pneumoconiosis) or of a diffuse interstitial fibrosis (such as asbestosis) as they are not easily discerned on such films. Full size, standard PA films are always to be recommended. Recent technological advances with 100 mm films, however, may make these acceptable in the future.

A disadvantage of all MMR techniques is that the dose of radiation to the subject is greater by a factor of three or four than with the standard PA view.

USE OF THE CHEST RADIOGRAPH IN INDUSTRY

As an essential part of pre-employment examination the chest radiograph serves the dual purpose of identifying existing chest disease and establishing an initial point of reference by which later radiographs may be compared.

(1) It enables the majority of industrial lung diseases to be identified at an early stage.

(2) It is an invaluable epidemiological tool for defining the incidence ('attack rate') and progression of a particular lung disease in a given industrial population. This technique has been applied extensively to the identification of new cases of coal pneumoconiosis and the detection of progression of existing cases in individual collieries in Britain (Liddell and May, 1966). It is similarly used in industries in which there is a risk of other forms of pneumoconiosis, although in some (especially those involving asbestos exposure), physiological tests are needed to augment the radiographic examination.

INTERPRETATION OF THE PA RADIOGRAPH IN INDUSTRIAL LUNG DISEASE

The brightness of viewing boxes should not be less than that given by two 15-watt white fluorescent tubes.

As in the diagnosis of any lung disease, it is necessary first to establish *where* the lesions are (that is, their anatomical site) and then to deduce *what* they are (that is, their pathology). The anatomical placing of lesions demands a careful routine of inspection of the PA and lateral films such as has been described.

It must be emphasized that, in general, there is no radiographic appearance unique to any one type of pneumoconiosis. Radiographic diagnosis must be deductive in the light of all other relevant data, and the habit of 'spot' diagnosis in this branch of chest medicine is particularly apt to cause unfortunate mistakes.

Fundamentally, appearances in the lung fields due to a pneumoconiosis

TABLE 5.2

SOME CAUSES OF DISCRETE AND LINEAR LUNG OPACITIES

Discrete	Linear with or without 'honeycomb'
Infections	
Chicken pox (healed calcified lesions) in adults	
Tuberculosis; miliary, acino-nodular (*)	
Blastomycosis (*)	
Coccidioidomycosis (*)	
Histoplasmosis (*)	
Torulosis (*)	
Schistosomiasis	
Inhalation	
Dusts	
Iron	
Silver	
Barium	
Tin	
Antimony	
Cerium Oxide	
Coal and Carbon	
Free silica	Free silica (occasional)
China clay	
Asbestos	Asbestos
'Talc'	'Talc'
Beryllium (*)	Beryllium
Actinomycetes, fungi and other organic materials (extrinsic allergic 'alveolitis') (*)	Actinomycetes, fungi and other organic materials (diffuse interstitial fibrosis)
Fumes and gases	
Oxides of nitrogen (*)	
Ozone (*)	
Phosgene (*)	
Aspiration	
Dysphagia pneumonitis (*)	
Lipoid granuloma	
Diagnostic contrast	
media (bronchography) (*)	
Associated with cardiovascular disease	
Oedema (*)	
Mitral stenosis	
Haemosiderosis	
Miliary ossification	
Right-sided infective	
endocarditis (*)	
Of uncertain cause	
Sarcoidosis (*)	Sarcoidosis
Associated with erythema nodosa	Cryptogenic diffuse interstitial fibrosis ('fibrosing alveolitis')
Idiopathic haemosiderosis	
Alveolar proteinosis (*)	
Microlithiasis	

TABLE 5.2—*Continued*

Discrete	*Linear with or without 'honeycomb'*
Associated with general constitutional diseases	
'Rheumatoid' pneumoconiosis	'Honeycomb lung' and diffuse interstitial fibrosis, fibrosing 'alveolitis'
	Developmental
	Xanthomatosis
	Tuberose sclerosis
	'Rheumatoid lung'
	Sjögren's syndrome
	Scleroderma (progressive systemic sclerosis)
	Generalized lupus erythematosus
	Cystic disease of the pancreas
Reticulosis and blood disease	
Leukaemia	
Hodgkin's Disease	
Lymphosarcoma	Lymphosarcoma
Neoplastic	
Primary and secondary carcinoma	Lymphangitis carcinomatosa
Bronchiolar carcinoma	
Allergic	
Eosinophilic infiltration (*)	
Infiltration during asthma (*)	
Polyarteritis nodosa (*)	
Associated with healed inflammatory disease	
	Fibrosis
	Bronchiectasis

* Opacities which may be transient
(Modified from J. G. Scadding (1952) with the permission of Emeritus Professor Scadding and the Editor of *Tubercle*)

are of two main types: discrete, roughly round opacities of small or large size (often referred to as 'nodular')—such as occur in siderosis, silicosis and coal pneumoconiosis; and fine to coarse linear, curvilinear, and irregular opacities which are sometimes accompanied by small ring shadows with central translucencies ('honeycomb' pattern)—such as occur in asbestosis, the fibrotic stage of extrinsic allergic 'alveolitis', chronic beryllium disease and cryptogenic diffuse interstitial fibrosis. When discrete, round opacities are very small and numerous they may present an ill-defined 'ground glass' appearance but, when viewed through a ×2 or ×3 hand lens are seen never quite to lose their identity. Indefinite, fine, net-like, irregular opacities are sometimes associated with retention of dusts of low atomic number—carbon, for example—and are caused mainly by superimposition of different radio-densities and not by the pathological process alone. The term 'reticulation' is often applied to this appearance but if it is used it should be made clear that radiographic appearances are referred to and not the proliferation of reticulin fibres for which, unfortunately, the same term is sometimes used by patho-logists, especially in Britain. This derives from the confusing statement of Belt and Ferris (1942): 'Dust reticulation may be defined as a dust-ridden state of the lungs corresponding to x-ray reticulation'. Such confusion of identity must be avoided for there is no correlation between the net-like opacities and reticulin proliferation in the lungs. It is, perhaps, preferable not to use the term in either sense. 'Mottling' is frequently employed—usually as a vague and ill-understood term—to describe appearances in the lung fields but it is uninformative unless used in the sense defined by the Ministry of Health (1952), that is, 'mottling' consists of 'multiple discrete or semi-confluent shadows generally less than 5 mm in diameter; 'miliary mottling' consists of 'numerous discrete, well-defined shadows not exceeding 2 mm in diameter'.

Discrete or linear opacities are transient or permanent according to the nature of the underlying disease process and are due, therefore, to a large number of causes. A list of these—it makes no claim to be comprehensive—is given in Table 5.2.

It is clear, therefore, that failure to elicit a satisfactory occupational history and relate it to the radiographic and other features may result in non-occupational disease being wrongly interpreted as a pneumoconiosis so that appropriate treatment is delayed or not given, or in a pneumoconiosis being mistaken for non-occupational disease with the consequence of irrelevant treatment.

CLASSIFICATION OF PNEUMOCONIOSIS RADIOGRAPHS

Various systems of classification have been proposed in order to attempt standardization of description of opacities but that of the International Labour Office (ILO, 1959) has, until recently, been the most widely used. This has been modified and extended to include irregular (or 'linear') opacities (such as occur in asbestosis) and other abnormalities (ILO, 1970), and subjected to further minor revision in 1971 (Table 5.3) (Jacobson and Gilson, 1973; Liddell, 1973). This system, designed to apply to 'persistent radiological opacities in the lung fields provoked by mineral dust', seeks, in the main, to do two things: to categorize *the size or form* of opacities and to indicate their *profusion or extent* in the lung fields.

The symbol 'p' stands for 'pinpoint' opacities, 'm' for 'micronodular' and 'n' for 'nodular'; 'm' and 'n' have been renamed 'q' and 'r' in the 1971 ILO/UC Classification of Pneumoconioses to avoid phonetic confusion, but their meaning is unchanged. A transparent rule marked in millimetres will assist the inexperienced observer to assign the proper size category to these opacities. In the 1971 Classification (in contrast to that of 1959) profusion of small round opacities is expressed by reference to the zones of the lung fields: Category 1 consists of relatively few small round opacities occupying no more than two zones of both lung fields; Category 2, more numerous opacities and Category 3, very numerous opacities which may partly or wholly obscure 'normal lung markings'.

The specifications of large opacities, Categories A, B and C, are the same in the 1971 system as in the old, and the method of distinguishing between Categories B and C is shown in *Figure 5.6*; category A is readily defined with a rule.

A set of standard films illustrating all categories is issued by the ILO.

TABLE 5.3

ILO U/C International Classification of Radiographs of Pneumoconioses 1971

I. OUTLINE OF CLASSIFICATION

Feature	Short classification	Extended classification
No pneumoconiosis	0	Rounded, Irregular 0/–, 0/0, 0/1
PNEUMOCONIOSIS		
SMALL OPACITIES		
Rounded		
Profusion*	1, 2, 3	1/0, 1/1, 1/2; 2/1, 2/2, 2/3; 3/2, 3/3, 3/4
Type	p, q(m), r(n)	p, q(m), r(n)
Extent	—	zones: right, left; upper, middle, lower
Irregular		
Profusion*	1, 2, 3	1/0, 1/1, 1/2; 2/1, 2/2, 2/3; 3/2, 3/3, 3/4
Type	s, t, u	s, t, u
Extent	—	zones: right, left; upper, middle, lower
LARGE OPACITIES		
Size	A, B, C	A, B, C
Type	—	wd (well defined), id (ill defined)
PLEURAL THICKENING		
Costophrenic angle	—	Right, left
Walls and Diaphragm		
Site	pl	Right, left
Width		a, b, c
Extent		1, 2
DIAPHRAGM OUTLINE	—	Ill defined: right, left
CARDIAC OUTLINE	—	Ill defined: 1, 2, 3

PLEURAL CALCIFICATION
Site
Extent

plc

Walls, diaphragm, other; right, left
Length: 1, 2, 3

II. DETAILS OF CLASSIFICATION

		Codes	Definitions
Small opacities	**Rounded** Profusion*	0/– 0/0 0/1 1/0 1/1 1/2 2/1 2/2 2/3	The category of profusion is based on assessment of the concentration (profusion) of opacities in the affected zones. The standard films define the mid-categories (1/1, 2/2, 3/3). Category 0—small rounded opacities absent or less profuse than in Category 1 Category 1—small rounded opacities definitely present but few in number. Category 2—small rounded opacities numerous. The normal lung markings are usually still visible.
		3/2 3/3 3/4	Category 3—small rounded opacities very numerous. The normal lung markings are partly or totally obscured.
	Type	p, q(m), r(n)	The nodules are classified according to the approximate diameter of the predominant opacities. p —rounded opacities up to about 1·5 mm diameter. q(m) —rounded opacities exceeding about 1·5 mm and up to about 3 mm diameter. r(n) —rounded opacities exceeding about 3 mm and up to about 10 mm diameter.
	Extent	RU RM RL LU LM LL	The zones in which the opacities are seen are recorded. Each lung is divided into three zones—upper, middle and lower.
	Irregular Profusion*	0/– 0/0 0/1 1/0 1/1 1/2	The category of profusion is based on the assessment of the concentration (profusion) of opacities in the affected zones. The standard films define the mid-categories. Category 0—small irregular opacities absent or less profuse than in Category 1. Category 1—small irregular opacities definitely present but few in number. The normal lung markings are usually visible.
		2/1 2/2 2/3	Category 2—small irregular opacities numerous. The normal lung markings are usually partly obscured.

		Codes	Definitions
	Type	3/2 3/3 3/4 s t u	Category 3—small irregular opacities very numerous. The normal lung markings are usually totally obscured. As the opacities are irregular, the dimensions used for rounded opacities cannot be used, but they can be roughly divided into three types. s—fine irregular or linear opacities. t—medium irregular opacities. u—coarse (blotchy) irregular opacities.
	Extent	RU RM RL LU LM LL	The zones in which the opacities are seen are recorded. Each lung is divided into three zones—upper, middle and lower—as for rounded opacities.
	Combined Profusion*		When both rounded and irregular small opacities are present, record the profusion of each separately and then record the combined profusion as though all the opacities were of one type. This is an optional feature of the classification.
Large opacities	Size	A B C	Category A—an opacity with greatest diameter between 1 cm and 5 cm, or several such opacities the sum of whose greatest diameters does not exceed 5 cm. Category B—one or more opacities larger or more numerous than those in category A, whose combined area does not exceed the equivalent of the right upper zone.
	Type	wd id	As well as the letter 'A', 'B' or 'C', the abbreviation 'wd' or 'id' should be used to indicate whether the opacities are well defined or ill defined.
Other features	**Pleural thickening** Costophrenic angle	Right left	Obliteration of the costophrenic angle is recorded separately from thickening over other sites. A lower limit standard film is provided.
	Walls and diaphragm Site Width	Right left a b c	Grade a—up to about 5 mm thick at the widest part of any shadow. Grade b—over about 5 mm and up to about 10 mm thick at the widest part of any shadow. Grade c—over about 10 mm thick at the widest part of any shadow.
	Extent	0 1 2	Grade 0—not present or less than Grade 1. Grade 1—definite pleural thickening in one or more places such that the total length does not exceed one-half of the projection of one lateral chest wall. The standard film defines the lower limit of Grade 1.

Grade 2—definite pleural thickening in one or more places such that the total length exceeds one-half of the projection of one lateral chest wall.

The lower limit is one-third of the affected hemidiaphragm. A lower limit standard film is provided.

Grade 0—not present or up to one-third of the length of the left cardiac border or equivalent.
Grade 1—above one-third and up to two-thirds of the length of the left cardiac border or equivalent.
Grade 2—above two-thirds and up to the whole length of the left cardiac border or equivalent.
Grade 3—more than the whole length of the left cardiac border or equivalent.

Grade 0—no pleural calcification seen.
Grade 1—one or more areas of pleural calcification, the sum of whose greatest diameters does not exceed about 2 cm.
Grade 2—one or more areas of pleural calcification, the sum of whose greatest diameters exceeds about 2 cm, but not about 10 cm.
Grade 3—one or more areas of pleural calcification, the sum of whose greatest diameters exceeds about 10 cm.

Diaphragm
Ill defined   Right left

Cardiac outline
Ill defined (shagginess)   0 1 2 3

Pleural calcification
Site
Diaphragm
Walls   Right left
Other

Extent   0 1 2 3

Symbols

ax —coalescence of small rounded pneumoconiotic opacities
bu —bullae
ca —cancer of lung or pleura
cn —calcification in small pneumoconiotic opacities
co —abnormality of cardiac size or shape
cp —cor pulmonale
cv —cavity

di —marked distortion of the intra-thoracic organs
ef —effusion
em —marked emphysema
es —eggshell calcification of hilar or mediastinal lymph nodes
hi —enlargement of hilar or mediastinal lymph nodes
ho —honeycomb lung
k —septal (Kerley) lines

od —other significant disease. This includes disease not related to dust exposure, e.g. surgical or traumatic damage to chest walls, bronchiectasis, etc.
pq —pleural plaque (uncalcified)
px —pneumothorax
rl —rheumatoid pneumoconiosis (Caplan's syndrome
tba —tuberculosis, probably active
tbu —tuberculosis, activity uncertain

* Use of 12-point scale for small opacities. The instructions are to classify the film in the usual way into one of the four categories, 0 to 3, and if, during the process, a neighbouring category is considered as a serious alternative, record this after the formal category. Thus category 2/1 is a film which is category 2, but category 1 was seriously considered as an alternative. The film which is without doubt a category 2, i.e. a mid-category closely similar in profusion to the standard film, would be classified as 2/2. In films within category 0, a subdivision is also possible. Thus category 0/1 is a film which is category 0, but category 1 was seriously considered. Category 0/0 is a normal film without small opacities. Occasionally films look exceptionally "normal" i.e., there is exceptional clarity of the normal architecture. Provision for these is made by the category 0/−. (Reproduced by permission of ILO)

Examples of Categories 1r(n), 2q(m), 3p, A, B and C are illustrated in *Figures 5.7* to *5.11*. These are not ILO standard films, however.

When small 'round' opacities coexist with large opacities the category of the small opacities should be given first (for example, 2q) and that of the large opacity (or opacities) next (for example, B) so that the category denomination is then written 2qB. Categories A, B, and C may be observed in the absence of accompanying small, round ('background') opacities, but this is not common.

Categories 's', 't' and 'u' refer to linear and irregular opacities such as are

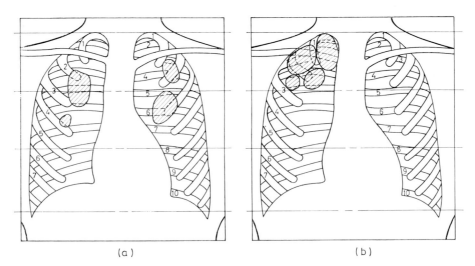

(a)   (b)

Figure 5.6. Method of categorizing large opacities. (a) represents opacities of massive pneumo-coniotic lesions; (b) shows how these are regrouped in the mind's eye, or with the aid of a transparent ruler, into the right lung field. This is Category B as the combined area lies within the confines of one-third of the field. An area extending beyond this classed as Category C

seen in asbestosis and other forms of diffuse interstitial fibrosis (fibrosing 'alveolitis'): 's' = fine, irregular or linear opacities: 't' = medium, irregular opacities; 'u' = coarse (blotchy) irregular opacities (*Figure 5.12*). The profusion (or extent) of these opacities is expressed according to the number of conventional zones (upper, middle and lower) of the lung fields which they occupy.

There are numerous additional symbols which are shown in Table 5.3.

This method of classification, it should be noted, does not specify any particular disease process nor imply degree of impairment of lung function or of respiratory disability.

Progression from lower to higher categories of profusion

Because this sort of classification of radiographs is arbitrary, it gives only a semi-quantitative scale of increasing radiographic abnormality, whereas in reality there is a continuum from normality along an abnormality scale; although, of course, a disease process may accelerate rapidly at one time, lag at another or remain permanently at a standstill at any one point. Because there

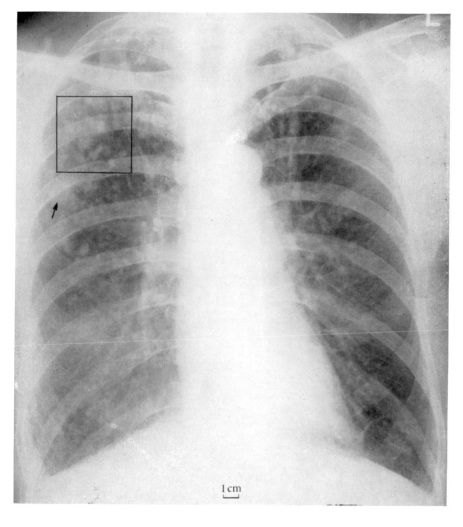

1 cm

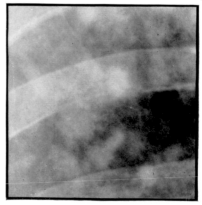

Figure 5.7. Category 1r(n)A. Opacities greater than 3 mm but less than 10 mm in diameter. The A opacity (arrowed) measures 2·5 × 1·5 cm. (Right, selected area, natural size)

119

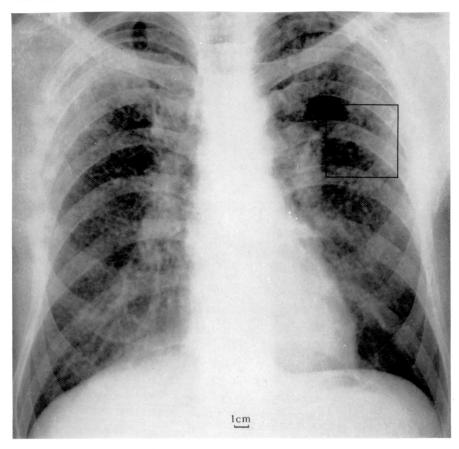

1cm

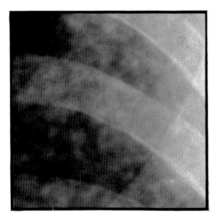

Figure 5.8. Category 2q(m). Opacities greater than 1·5 mm but less than 3 mm in diameter (Left, selected area, natural size)

120

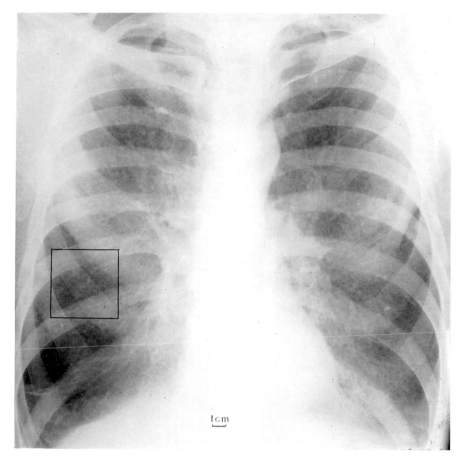

1cm

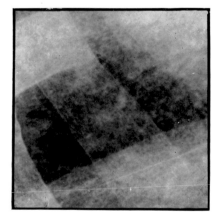

Figure 5.9. Category 3p. Opacities not exceeding 1·5 mm in diameter. (Right, selected area, natural size)

121

is a tendency to underestimate progression when the short ILO classification is used, it was suggested (Liddell, 1963) that a half category for each of the existing profusion categories should be added thus converting the four-point (Category 0 to 3) scale into a twelve-point scale (*Figure 5.13*). This modification is employed by the British National Coal Board and is adopted by the ILO (1971) classification (Table 5.3).

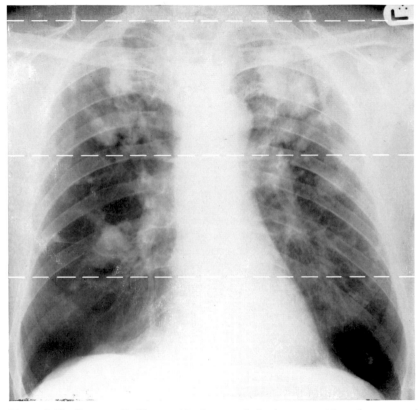

Figure 5.10. Category B. The combined area of the large opacities when grouped together (see Figure 5.6) does not exceed one-third of the right lung field

Variation of interpretation by one observer or between different observers can be reduced by this method, but its undoubted value to the epidemiologist and statistician has little application in the clinical field where analysis of this sort is not necessary.

To return to the 1971 ILO system: this is presented in 'short' and 'extended' forms: the short form closely resembles the old 1958 system; but the extended form incorporates the NCB elaboration of profusion for both 'round' and 'irregular' opacities (Table 5.3). The 'short' form is appropriate to clinical practice if the 's', 't' and 'u' categories are included, and the 'extended' form to epidemiological and other research studies.

An initial trial of the new ILO (UICC/Cincinnati) classification in use suggests that it is practical and the repeatability of film readings good (Rossiter, 1972a).

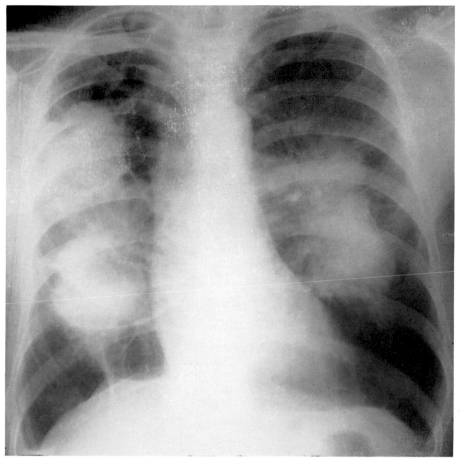

Figure 5.11. Category C. Area of large opacities exceeds one-third of the right lung field

RELEVANT ASPECTS OF PRODUCTION AND INTERPRETATION OF THE CHEST RADIOGRAPH

Effects of technical quality of radiographs on category

The technical quality of radiographs has an important effect upon their interpretation. In particular, there is a tendency when examining films which are too 'black' or too 'white' to relegate small discrete opacities to too low a category (Wise and Oldham, 1963; Pearson *et al.*, 1965), and the proportion of unsatisfactory films is greater as chest thickness (Liddell, 1961) or the ratio of body weight to sitting (stem) height (Pearson *et al.*, 1965) increases. Three points to follow from this.

(1) If normal (Category 0) radiographs are excluded, observer error tends

123

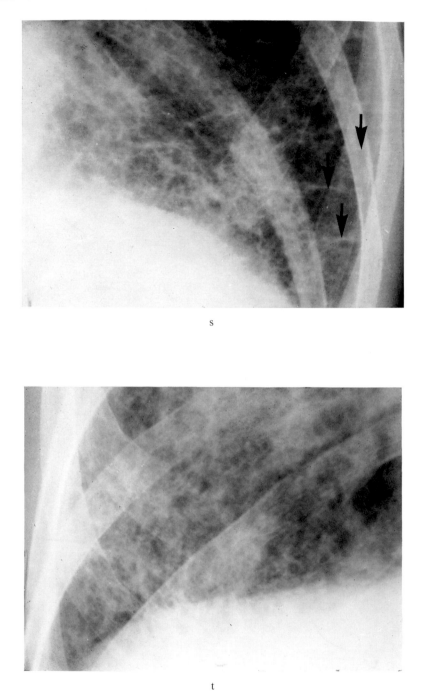

s

t

Figure 5.12. Example of ILO classification of opacities: Category s: fine, irregular or linear opacities. Arrows indicate Kerley B lines. Category t: medium, irregular opacities. Category u: (opposite page) coarse, irregular opacities. Natural size

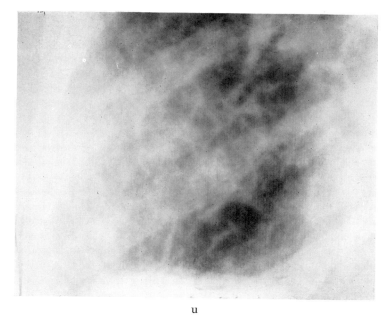

u

to be greater the lower the category. Category 1 is most likely to be obscured or lost by poor radiological technique. But, for clinical purposes, the general level of agreement becomes progressively better as the category increases.

Small round opacities, unless caused by substances of high atomic number, do not represent individual lesions, but the summation of normal and abnormal structures in the lungs. Their appearance is altered, therefore, by variation in the degree of inflation of the lungs, by slight degree of rotation of the chest, and by excess of soft tissue shadow. If the soft tissue background is much increased it becomes difficult to interpret the significance of such opacities. Furthermore, nodular pulmonary lesions may appear to be 'cystic' on the film, and linear structures, 'nodular' (Carstairs, 1961).

(2) From the epidemiological standpoint, differences in the interpretation of normal radiographs and those showing discrete small round opacities, may influence significantly the reported prevalence of a pneumoconiosis from different areas of the same country and from different countries.

(3) There is need for rigorous international standardization of radiographic technique. This has not yet been achieved and the technical difficulties involved are great.

It should be noted that most of the features of a dark (too 'black') film can be discerned if it is viewed against a very bright white light rather than on a standard viewing box. An over-'white' film is valueless.

CORRELATION OF RADIOGRAPHIC APPEARANCES WITH PNEUMOCONIOTIC LESIONS

Correlation between the number and distribution of discrete opacities on chest radiographs and the number and distribution of small pneumoconiotic

125

lesions observed *post mortem* is fairly good, in spite of the fact that the appearance of the radiograph is determined not only by the number and composition of the lesions but also by the superimposition of their own radiodensities and those of lung and chest wall structures.

Various factors operate to absorb x-rays in different types of lesion. The profusion and distribution of silicotic nodules (*see* Chapter 7) observed *post mortem* show close agreement with radiographic appearances and category; these appearances are due to the combined effect of the concentration of iron within the nodules (Otto and Maron, 1959) (referred to in Chapter 1), to collagen fibrosis, possibly to the content of free silica, and, in some cases, to deposition of calcium salts. In the case of coal pneumoconiosis,

ILO Category 0			ILO Category 1			ILO Category 2			ILO Category 3		
0/-	0/0	0/1	1/0	1/1	1/2	2/1	2/2	2/3	3/2	3/3	3/4

Figure 5.13. The NCB elaboration of the ILO classification. (By courtesy of Professor F. D. K. Liddell (Quebec) and Dr John Rogan, National Coal Board (Medical Research Memorandum, 4. 1966)

the higher the ILO category of small 'round' opacities the greater the number of foci of retained dust and the higher the proportion of fibrotic (collagen) nodules found in the lungs (Caplan, 1962). Rossiter (1972b) has shown that the radiographic appearances in coal workers are most highly correlated with the mineral content of the lungs, although iron also makes a significant contribution. Due to their different x-ray mass absorption coefficients 1·5 grammes of iron in the lungs has an equal effect in increasing the category by one unit as 16 grammes of coal (Gilson, 1968); the category of discrete ('simple') coal pneumoconiosis correlates better with the non-haem endogenous iron content (which may accumulate during phagocytosis of dust particles) (*see* Chapter 8) than with the total iron content of the lungs (Bergman, 1970). It is probable, therefore, that the effect of iron upon category reflects variation in the amounts of coal and mineral present (Rossiter, 1972b). Coal itself contributes very little to the appearances.

As might be expected, correlation of radiographic abnormality with large conglomerate or pneumoconiotic masses of whatever cause is usually good.

Correlation of radiographic appearances and diffuse interstitial fibrosis is not as good as that for discrete round pneumoconiotic lesions, but the correlation improves as the severity of the lesions increases from partial loss of alveolar wall architecture to its complete replacement by fibrous tissue with multiple cystic spaces (Livingstone *et al.*, 1964). It is difficult to detect the very early stages radiographically. These considerations apply not only to cryptogenic diffuse interstitial fibrosis but also to such diseases as chronic extrinsic allergic 'alveolitis', asbestosis and chronic beryllium disease. The correlation of radiographic appearances with a section of the corresponding lung in a case of cryptogenic diffuse interstitial fibrosis with 'honeycombing' is shown in *Figure 5.14*.

Experimental work designed to simulate linear opacities by radiographing increasing numbers of layers of plastic lattices placed at right angles to the x-ray beam has shown that, as the number of layers is increased, an appearance of discrete ('nodular' or 'mottled') opacities and ill-defined areas of relative translucency is produced—not more emphatic linear opacities (Carstairs, 1961) (*Figure 5.15*). This observation probably explains some of the discrete opacities and relative translucencies which are to be seen in many cases of diffuse interstitial fibrosis, and possibly also the small 'p' type opacities sometimes observed on the films of coal workers (*Figure 5.9*) who are subsequently found to have uniformly distributed emphysema and dust without fibrosis (*see Figure 8.20*). These appearances may be due in some cases to the effective contrast between the increased volume of air in the numerous dilated air spaces on the one hand, and the surrounding lung tissue which possesses greater radiodensity than normal owing to the combined effect of mineral dusts, endogenous iron and coal, on the other (*see also* page 103). In the case of inert dusts of high atomic number the opacities are denser and more clearly demarcated (*see* Chapter 6).

It is important to note that, in general, respiratory symptoms and patterns of impaired lung function correlate very poorly with the radiographic appearances of pneumoconiosis.

Alleged obscuring effect of emphysema
There is a fairly common belief, which has been current for more than thirty years (Rappaport, 1936, 1967; Ogilvie, 1970) that emphysema may obscure opacities which, in its absence, would have been caused by discrete (round) pneumoconiotic lesions with the result that an expected Category 2 or 3 would be converted to 0 or 1; or, contrariwise, that Category 0 could be produced in the presence of significant pneumoconiosis. This effect, it has been claimed, is produced by attenuation of x-rays due to their scatter by excess air in the lungs (Rappaport, 1936). From the physical principles already described on page 103 it is evident that this cannot be true and that both absorption and scatter of x-rays by air are very substantially less than by the tissues or by minerals, so that an increased volume of air in the lungs will tend to increase the 'visibility' of the pneumoconiotic lesions. Confirmation of this is furnished by two observations: (1) when moderate or severe emphysema is present, Categories 0 to 1 are not correlated, *post mortem*, with an unexpectedly large number of pneumoconiotic lesions (Caplan, 1962); (2) the presence of 'focal' emphysema (which cannot be identified as such radiographically) is associated with over-assessment and not under-assessment of category (Rossiter *et al.*, 1967) due, probably, to the contrast effect referred to in the last section.

Of course, displacement of lung in which there are pneumoconiotic lesions by distension of large emphysematous bullae is a different matter and is obvious radiographically.

Kerley 'A' and 'B' lines
The radiographs of some persons with a pneumoconiosis—especially if due to dusts of higher atomic number—may show the 'A' and 'B' lines first described by Kerley (1950).

'A' lines
'A' lines are fine, not more than 1 mm thick, do not branch, are usually between

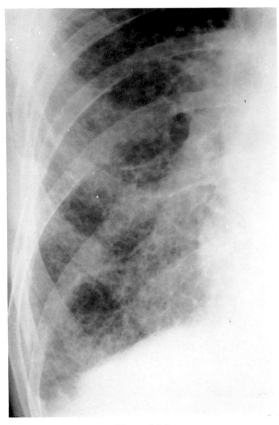

Figure 5.14a

Radiographic appearances produced by cryptogenic diffuse interstitial fibrosis (fibrosing 'alveolitis'), with cyst formation, of typical distribution. The patient was never exposed to an occupational dust hazard

2 and 4 cm long and do not pass into the periphery of the lung to reach the pleural margin.

'B' lines

'B' lines are similarly fine, short (usually less than 2 cm), are almost perpendicular to the pleural margin with which their outer end is always in contact, and can occur anywhere in the lung fields but are usually in the lower zones. 'A' lines may be due to dust surrounding or within anastomotic lymphatics; and 'B' lines, to dust in interlobular septa but not in pleural lymphatics (Trapnell, 1963) (*Figure 5.12*). Neither represent a fibrotic pneumoconiotic process.

Both lines are found more frequently in the higher categories of discrete pneumoconiosis (ILO Categories 3, A, B and C), 'B' lines being more common than 'A' (Trapnell, 1964), and both tend to be seen rather more often in the right lung than in the left (Rivers *et al.*, 1960). In my experience,

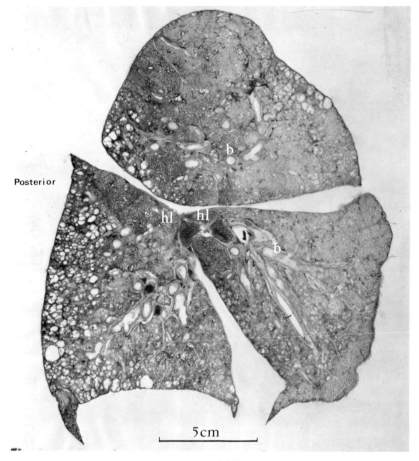

Figure 5.14b

Sagittal section of right lung. Note variable size of the ('honeycomb') cysts. The fibrosis is free of pigment; minimal carbon pigmentation in upper lobe. (b, bronchi; hl, hilar lymph nodes)

however, they are present in less than half the cases of coal pneumoconiosis in these categories—a finding confirmed by Trapnell (1964).

'A' and 'B' lines are, of course, also found in some cases of increased pulmonary venous pressure due to mitral stenosis and chronic left ventricular failure, in lymphangitis carcinomatosa and in some cases of pulmonary sarcoidosis.

RADIOGRAPHIC APPEARANCES OF EMPHYSEMA

Due to its air trapping effect panlobular emphysema when widespread and severe is readily identified by the criteria of a low, flat diaphragm, increase in size and downwards extension of the retrosternal translucent area seen in the lateral film, a narrow, vertical heart shadow, prominent hilar vessels and unduly small arterial shadows in the mid and peripheral lung fields in the PA view (Simon, 1964). Although severe panlobular emphysema is virtually excluded by a normal radiograph, lesser degrees may fail to produce these characteristic signs or give rise to only some of them (Reid and Millard, 1964; Thurlbeck *et al.*, 1970).

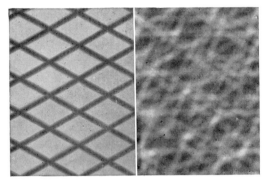

1 layer   *7 layers*

Figure 5.15

The effect produced by super-imposing an increasing number of plastic lattices lying at right angles to the x-ray beam

40 layers   *80 layers*

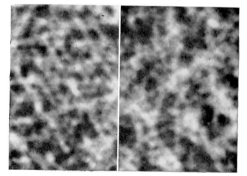

The simple pattern produced by one layer becomes progressively 'nodular' in appearance with ill-defined areas of relative translucency. (By courtesy of Dr L. S. Carstairs and the Hon. Editors of Proceedings of the Royal Society of Medicine)

On the other hand, centrilobular emphysema—whether or not associated with dust retention or pneumoconiosis—cannot be detected on standard radiographs even when it is widespread (Snider, Brody and Doctor, 1962), although it is claimed that severe grades accompanied by panlobular emphysema may sometimes be recognized (Laws and Heard, 1962).

Once established, bullae associated with local panlobular or paraseptal emphysema are usually readily recognized.

Chronic obstructive bronchitis or severe widespread panlobular emphysema may sometimes cause secondary polycythaemia in which case the pulmonary artery opacities in the middle of the lungs as well as at the hila become unduly large and prominent. Because of the 'end-on' appearance of such arteries on a PA radiograph a discrete pneumoconiosis (such as silicosis or coal pneumoconiosis) is sometimes incorrectly diagnosed; this may also occur with pulmonary artery plethora from other causes (for example, atrial septal defect).

CALCIFICATION OF THE PLEURA

Nowadays, pleural fibrosis and calcification (pleural 'plaques') are looked for in the radiographs of people who have been, or are thought to have been, exposed to an asbestos hazard (Chapter 9). When it is fairly widespread, pleural calcification is readily identified by virtue of a bizarre and irregular configuration (the so-called holly-leaf pattern) which does not correspond with any lobar or segmental distribution and which has an intensity of opacity contrasting strongly with the surrounding lung. But sometimes it is represented only by tiny opaque flecks, or short thin lines of opacity along the diaphragmatic and cardiac outlines or along the costal margin, or by small irregular areas in the lung fields. These are readily overlooked if a systematic search is not made. As described on page 109, 45-degree anterior oblique views are helpful in defining these lesions.

Anterior oblique views incidentally may also be of assistance in the investigation of malignant pleural mesothelioma (*see* Chapter 9).

It should not be forgotten, however, that calcification of the pleura, whether widespread or localized, may be due to past empyema, tuberculous pleurisy, haemothorax (as may follow chest injury), or may occur spontaneously in normal aged persons. Even when an individual has been exposed to asbestos, one or other of these may, in fact, be the true cause of the calcification. Calcification due to the first three of these causes is usually wholly or predominantly unilateral.

Calcification of costal cartilages will not be mistaken for pleural calcification if the routine for inspection is followed but the possibility of making this error must always be kept in mind; even the elect are sometimes deceived by it especially where the abnormal opacities are superimposed on the diaphragmatic shadow.

A DIRECT QUANTITATIVE RADIOLOGICAL TECHNIQUE

Direct detection of the nature and amount of an exogenous dust retained in the lungs of the living person is possible using the principle that every element has a definite 'absorption edge' which abruptly changes the transmission of x-rays through it. When radiation with energies ranging above and below the energy of the 'absorption edge' of a given element is passed through the lungs, alteration in its penetration due to the differential absorption effect of the element should be demonstrated (McCallum and Day, 1965). Theoretically, this offers a new dimension in radiographic identification of certain types of pneumoconiosis, but, in practice, it is in an experimental stage. It is limited to elements with atomic numbers greater than about 40 and, so far, has been applied only to antimony and tin (McCallum *et al.*, 1971).

PERFUSION SCINTIGRAPHY

Colour scintigraphy using 131I-labelled human albumin particles injected intravenously has demonstrated that irregular distribution of blood flow may exist in the vicinity of massive lesions of silicosis and coal pneumoconiosis (Schröder *et al.*, 1969), but this is not likely to be of practical use for purposes of routine investigation.

REFERENCES

Belt, T. H. and Ferris, A. A. (1942). 'Histology of coal miner's pneumoconiosis.' In *Chronic Pulmonary Disease in South Wales Coal Miners*, pp. 203–222. (Medical Research Council.) London; H.M.S.O.

Bergman, I. (1970). 'The relation of endogenous non-haem iron in formalin-fixed lungs to radiological grade of pneumoconiosis.' *Ann. occup. Hyg.* **13**, 163–169

Bracken, T. J. (1964). 'The technique of macroradiography in the diagnosis of industrial disease of the chest.' *Radiography* **30**, 291–298

Caplan, A. (1962). 'Correlation of radiological category with lung pathology in coal worker's pneumoconiosis.' *Br. J. ind. Med.* **19**, 171–179

Carstairs, L. S. (1961). 'The interpretation of shadows in a restricted area of lung field in the chest radiograph.' *Proc. R. Soc. Med.* **54**, 978–980

Clarke, K. C. (1964). *Positioning in Radiography*. (Ilford Publication.) London; Heinemann

Gilson, J. C. (1968). *Classification of Chest Radiographs and its Application to the Epidemiology of Pneumoconiosis*. (Report on a Symposium at Katowice, 1967.) Copenhagen; W.H.O.

International Labour Office (1959). 'Meetings of Experts on the International Classification of Radiographs of the Pneumoconioses.' *Occup. Saf. Hlth* **9**, No. 2

International Labour Office (1970). *International Classification of Radiographs of Pneumoconioses. (Revised 1968.)* Occup. Saf. Hlth Series No. 22. Geneva; I.L.O.

Jacobson G. and Gilson, J. C. (1972). 'Present status of the U.I.C.C./Cincinnati Classification of Radiographic Appearances: report of a meeting held at the Pneumoconiosis Research Unit, Cardiff, Wales, 13–15 April, 1971.' *Ann. N.Y. Acad. Sci.* **200**, 552–569

Johns, H. E. and Cunningham, J. R. (1969). *The Physics of Radiology*, 3rd Edition, pp. 210–211. Springfield; Thomas

Kerley, P. (1950). In *A Textbook of X-ray Diagnosis*, Vol. 2, pp. 404–405. Ed. by S. C. Shanks and P. Kerley. London; Lewis

Laws, J. W. and Heard, B. E. (1962). 'Emphysema and the chest film: a retrospective radiological and pathological study.' *Br. J. Radiol.* **35**, 750–761

Liddell, F. D. K. (1961). 'The effect of film quality on reading radiographs of simple pneumoconiosis in a trial of X-ray sets.' *Br. J. ind. Med.* **18**, 165–174

— (1963). 'An experiment in film reading.' *Br. J. ind. Med.* **20**, 300–312

— and May, J. D. (1966). *Assessing the Radiological Progression of Simple Pneumoconiosis*. Medical Research Memorandum 4. National Coal Board Medical Service

Liddell, F. D. K. (1972). 'Validation of classifications of pneumoconiosis.' *Ann. N.Y. Acad. Sci.* **200**, 527–551

Livingstone, J. L., Lewis, J. G., Reid, L. and Jefferson, E. E. (1964). 'Diffuse interstitial pulmonary fibrosis.' *Q. Jl Med.* **23**, 71–103

McCallum, R. I. and Day, M. J. (1965). '*In vivo* method of detecting antimony deposits in the lung by differential absorption of X-radiation.' *Lancet* **2**, 882–883

— — Underhill, J. and Aird, E. G. A. (1971). 'Measurement of antimony oxide dust in human lungs *in vivo* by X-ray spectrophotometry.' In *Inhaled Particles 3*, pp. 611–618. Ed. by W. H. Walton. Woking; Unwin

MacKenzie, F. A. F. and Harries, P. G. (1970). 'Changing attitude to the diagnosis of asbestos disease.' *Jl R. nav. med. Serv.* **56**, 116–123

Ministry of Health (1952). *Standardization of Terminology of Pulmonary Disease and Standardization of Technique of Chest Radiography*. London; H.M.S.O.

Ogilvie, C. M. (1970). 'Emphysema and coal worker's pneumoconiosis.' *Br. med. J.* **3**, 769

Osborn, S. B. (1969). Personal communication

Otto, H. and Maron, R. (1959). 'Zur Histologie der Eisenablagerungen bei Porzeillinersilikosen.' *Arch. Gewerbepath. Gewerbehyg.* **17**, 117–126

Pearson, N. G., Ashford, J. R., Morgan, D. C., Pasqual, R. S. H. and Rae, S. (1965). 'Effect of quality of chest radiographs on the categorization of coal worker's pneumoconiosis.' *Br. J. ind. Med.* **22**, 81–92

Rappaport, I. (1936). 'The phenomena of shadow attenuation and summation in roentgenography of the lungs.' *Am. J. Roentg.* **35**, 772–776

— (1967). 'Overinflation of the lungs of coal miners.' *Br. med. J.* **3**, 493–494

Reid, L. and Millard, F. J. C. (1964). 'Correlation between radiological diagnosis and structural lung changes in emphysema.' *Clin. Radiol.* **15**, 307–311

Rivers, D., Wise, M. E., King, E. J. and Nagelschmidt, G. (1960). 'Dust content, radiology, and pathology in simple pneumoconiosis of coal workers.' *Br. J. Med.* **17**, 87–108

Rossiter, C. E. (1972a). 'Initial repeatability trials of the UICC/Cincinnati classification of the radiographic appearance of pneumoconioses.' *Br. ind. Med.* **29**, 407–419

— (1972b). 'Relation between content and composition of coal worker's lungs and radiological appearances.' *Br. J. ind. Med.* **29**, 31–44

— Rivers, D., Bergman, I., Casswell, C. and Nagelschmidt, G. (1967). 'Dust content, radiology and pathology in simple pneumoconiosis of coal workers. (Further Report.)' In *Inhaled Particles and Vapours*, 2, pp. 419–434. Ed. by C. N. Davies. London; Pergamon

Scadding, J. G. (1952). 'Chronic lung disease with diffuse nodular or reticular radiographic shadows.' *Tubercle, Lond.* **33**, 352–355

Schröder, H., Magdeburg, W., Tewes, E. and Rockelsberg, I. (1969). 'Perfusion scintigraphy of the lungs in patients with silicosis and silicotuberculosis.' *Germ. med. Mon.* **14**, 551–552

Simon, G. (1964). 'Radiology and emphysema.' *Clin. Radiol.* **15**, 293–306

— (1968). *Principles of Chest X-ray Diagnosis.* 2nd Ed. London; Butterworths

Snider, G. L., Brody, J. S. and Doctor, L. (1962). 'Subclinical pulmonary emphysema. Incidence and anatomic patterns.' *Am. Rev. resp. Dis.* **85**, 666–683

Spiers, F. W. (1946). 'Effective atomic number and energy absorption in tissues.' *Br. J. Radiol.* **19**, 52–63

Thurlbeck, W. M., Henderson, J. A., Fraser, R. G. and Bates, D. V. (1970). 'Chronic obstructive lung disease. A comparison between clinical roentgenologic, functional and morphologic criteria in chronic bronchitis, emphysema, asthma and bronchiectasis.' *Medicine, Baltimore* **49**, 81–145

Trapnell, D. H. (1963). 'The peripheral lymphatics of the lung.' *Br. J. Radiol.* **36**, 660–672

— (1964). 'Septal lines in pneumoconiosis.' *Br. J. Radiol.* **37**, 805–810

Wise, M. E. and Oldham, P. O. (1963). 'Effect of radiographic technique on readings of categories of simple pneumoconiosis.' *Br. J. ind. Med.* **10**, 145–153

6—Inert Dusts

Definition

Inert dusts are inorganic (mineral) dusts which, if insoluble, cause neither substantial proliferation of reticulin fibres nor give rise to collagenous fibrosis when retained in the lungs; and, if soluble, are not toxic locally or systemically. They are classed as 'inert dusts' or 'nuisance particulates' by the ACGIH (1971) provided that they are free of toxic impurities and that their quartz content is less than 1 per cent.

Importance of inert dusts

The radiodensity of these dusts ranges from high to low (*see* Chapter 5). They may be inhaled in almost pure form or in association with fibrogenic dusts (usually free silica in the form of quartz) either as an intimate mixture produced simultaneously by one industrial process, or separately and at different times by different occupations. Dusts of low radiodensity give no evidence of their presence on a chest radiograph whereas those of high radiodensity cast small, round, well-defined and contrasted opacities throughout the lung fields and often cause pronounced opacity of hilar lymph nodes (due to their concentration in these sites) which may be interpreted as calcification by the inexperienced observer.

It is, therefore, possible to consider inert dusts according to whether they are of high or low radiodensity and whether or not their presence is associated with that of a fibrotic pneumoconiosis (such as silicosis or asbestosis), in which case the lesions due to the inert dusts are morphologically distinct from the others. But inert dusts (most notably iron oxides) may modify the fibrogenic effect of quartz, and other forms of free silica, and cause 'mixed dust fibrosis' (*see* Chapter 7) which lacks the characteristic morphology of the silicotic nodule. As noted in Chapter 3, the presence of quartz in the lungs increases the retention and interstitial and lymphatic penetration of inert dusts, but reduces their elimination by the airways. When low radiodensity dusts are contaminated by quartz as an accessory mineral of parent rock, both types of dust may be inhaled when such rocks are mined, quarried, crushed or used in particular industrial processes. It is necessary to be aware of this in order that an inert dust is not, on the one hand, wrongly considered to be

134

fibrogenic or that, on the other, the presence of a free silica risk does not go unsuspected.

DUSTS OF HIGH RADIODENSITY
BENIGN PNEUMOCONIOSIS

Iron (Atomic Number, 26): Siderosis
(σίδηρος IRON)

Sources of exposure

Dust or fume of metallic iron and iron oxide may be encountered in the following processes, although their concentrations in many industries are limited by dust control measures.

(1) *Iron and steel rolling mills* in which metal strips are subjected to much agitation with the consequent production of rust and iron scale dust.

(2) *Steel grinding* produces metallic dust.

(3) *Electric arc and oxyacetylene welding.*—The high temperature of these types of welding when applied to iron gives rise to iron oxide fume and other fumes and gases (*see* Chapter 12). The concentration of fumes in the breathing zone is often high if welders work in confined and ill-ventilated places such as tanks, boilers, and the holds of ships. Siderosis of arc welders was first described by Doig and McLaughlin (1936).

For an excellent summary of modern welding methods and their possible hazards to health the reader is referred to Challen (1965).

(4) *Polishing of silver and steel with iron oxide powder.*—The powder is usually an especially pure form of ferric oxide in a finely divided state and is often referred to as 'rouge' or 'crocus'. Polishing is done by means of power-operated buffing wheels of wool or cotton. Silver polishing is also likely to produce minute particles of metallic silver.

Ferric oxide is further used to polish plate glass, stone and cutlery.

(5) *Fettling (that is, scouring), chipping and dressing castings in iron foundries.* —Until recently this process was a common source of quartz as well as iron dust from attrition of burnt-on moulding sands adhering to the castings (*see* Chapter 8) and, therefore, liable to cause 'mixed dust fibrosis' or typical silicosis. Nevertheless, siderosis may occur alone when it may be wrongly diagnosed as silicosis.

A survey in a Sheffield steel foundry between 1955 and 1960 revealed that the average prevalence of siderosis among welders and burners in the fettling and grinding shops was 17·6 per cent (Gregory, 1970).

(6) *Boiler scaling* involves the cleaning of fireboxes, flues and water-tubes in enclosed spaces in the boilers of ships, factories, power stations and the like. A high concentration of dust is produced which contains iron and carbon, and, in coal-fired—but not oil fired—boilers, silicates and small quantities of quartz derived from the coal. Although siderosis alone may be produced, mixed dust fibrosis may also occur.

(7) *Mining and crushing iron ores.*—The important ores are magnetite, hematite and limonite.

Magnetite occurs in several geological environments and ores of the mineral are frequently associated with quartz-bearing rock and contain quartz gangue (as in Northern Sweden, where the richest deposits are found). It is

135

also found in beach sands. Therefore, quartz may sometimes be a substantial contaminant of the ore resulting in mixed dust fibrosis or silicosis in addition to siderosis in miners and crusher operators; but, again, siderosis may be observed alone.

Hematite, known also as 'specularite' and 'kidney ore', is mined chiefly in Cumberland and, until recently, in the Furness district of Lancashire where it occurs in limestone beds; but some deposits are associated with red ferruginous sandstone and are, therefore, liable to contamination by quartz. One of the largest sources in the world, near Lake Superior in Canada, is also partly contaminated by free silica because it contains interbedded layers of chert, but quartz is virtually absent from deposits at Bilbao and on the Quebec-Labrador border.

Limonite, including 'bog iron ore', is, for practical purposes, free from contaminating free silica.

It will be seen, therefore, that the likelihood of siderosis occurring alone, or accompanied by pure silicosis or mixed dust fibrosis will depend to a large extent upon the geographical origin of the ore or the site from which it comes in any one deposit. Dust is produced during mining, loading, crushing and milling of the ores.

Hematite and limonite are used as pigments in paint manufacture and, together with magnetite, are added in finely divided form to certain fertilizers. It is possible, therefore, for workers in those industries to be exposed to iron oxide dusts.

(8) *Mining, milling and mixing emery and its use as an abrasive.*—Emery is an intimate mixture of hematite, magnetite and *corundum* (aluminium oxide, Al_2O_3) which, next to diamond, is the hardest natural mineral known. At one time emery came mainly from the Grecian Island of Naxos but today Turkey is the largest producer, and smaller quantities come from the United States. It is found most commonly in pockets or lenses in crystalline limestone, gneisses and schists, or as a deposit derived from these rocks by weathering. It contains insignificant quantities of quartz, and its abrasive quality is due mainly to the aluminium oxide present.

Because emery is apt to contain variable amounts of impurities (such as plagioclase feldspar) and a constant composition cannot, therefore, be relied upon, it has been very largely replaced by artificial abrasives—principally Carborundum and synthetic corundum (*see* pp. 159, 482). On account of its particular hardness, purity and resistance to heat, Naxos emery was used for grindstones, but Turkish emery, which is softer, is still employed in the making of emery cloths and papers, in the setting up of polishing wheels and mops, in abrasive pastes and as a non-slip, wear-resisting component of concrete floors. High concentrations of emery dust have been, and occasionally still are, produced during the manufacture of most of these materials and the use of the different abrasive preparations for various polishing procedures (Bech, Kipling and Zundel, 1965; Foá, 1967).

Pneumoconiosis in emery workers, therefore, will almost certainly be siderosis unless there has also been exposure to some other dust hazard (for example, the coal-mining, pottery or asbestos industries).

(9) *Mining, pulverizing and mixing natural mineral pigments.*—Hematite and limonite have already been referred to as a source of pigments but

others are the ferruginous earths—ochre, sienna and umber clays—which consist of iron and aluminium oxides with a variable amount of siliceous impurity. These clays are mined in the United States, the Persian Gulf, Turkey, Cyprus, France, Italy and Andalusia but pulverizing and mixing are usually done by the firm which imports them. Synthetic iron pigments prepared from iron oxides, however, are now much more important than the natural products.

Siderosis may occur alone in workers who pulverize and mix natural pigments which, at this stage, have been purified by washing and dehydration; also in those who prepare synthetic pigments. Particle sizes of powdered natural pigments range from about 0·8 to 2 μm. But silicosis may also be found among miners when the quartz content of the clays is substantial, as is the case in France (Vernhes and Roche, 1955) and Italy where it varies from 2 to 35 per cent (Champeix and Moreau, 1958).

Pathology

The features of siderosis only are considered here.

Macroscopic appearances

The pulmonary pleura is marbled a rust-brown colour but, in the case of hematite, the colour may be a deep brick-red. This is due to the deposition of iron oxide in the pleural lymphatics similarly to the black pigmentation seen in the pleura of coal-miners and city dwellers.

The cut surface of the lungs reveals grey to rust-brown coloured macules (*macula*, a stain or mark) from 1 to 4 mm in diameter which are impalpable and do not stand up from the surface in contrast to silicotic nodules. They are evenly distributed but may be difficult to distinguish as individual lesions if the lungs are generally dust stained. The appearance of the lungs and lesions where hematite is involved is particularly striking due to the brick-red coloration. Some hematite lungs may also exhibit discrete nodular fibrosis or massive fibrosis when quartz is associated with the iron oxide, but this is described in Chapter 7. Typical silicotic lesions are readily distinguishable by the naked eye.

Microscopic appearances

Particles of iron fume or dust, unlike endogenous iron, do not give a Prussian blue reaction. They are present both in macrophages and are free in alveolar spaces and walls where they are mostly perivascular. Although there may be reticulin proliferation there is no collagenous fibrosis. A typical siderotic macule is shown in *Figure 6.1*. It is worth noting that natural emery when introduced into the lungs or peritoneum of rats causes neither reticulin proliferation nor collagenous fibrosis (Mellissonos, Collet and Daniel-Moussard, 1966).

Metallic silver, as well as iron, is present in the lungs of silver polishers and is taken up as a vital stain by the elastic tissue which appears grey-black in colour, in the walls of airways and arteries. This has been referred to as 'argyro-siderosis' (McLaughlin *et al.*, 1945). The silver (atomic number, 47) contributes to the effective atomic number of the mixture and, therefore, to the summation of opacities on the radiograph.

It has been suggested that the retention of iron dust may cause emphysema but there is no evidence to support this. The question of a possible relationship between iron oxides and bronchial carcinoma is referred to later.

Symptoms and physical signs

Apart from the production of reddish coloured sputum following exposure to these dusts, there are no symptoms or abnormal physical signs caused by siderosis, and if any are present they are due to some other cause.

Lung function

There is no impairment of any parameter of lung function (Enzer, Simonson and Evans, 1945; Kleinfeld *et al.*, 1969) and, although a greater prevalence of airways obstruction has been reported among electric arc welders compared

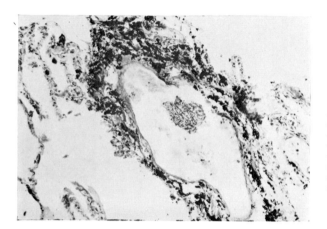

Figure 6.1. Siderosis. There is a perivascular 'cuff' of iron particles and dust-laden macrophages but no fibrosis. The alveolar walls and spaces are normal. (Original magnification × 225 reproduced at half-scale; H and E stain)

with non-welders (Hunnicutt, Cracovaner and Myles, 1964), this was related mainly to cigarette smoking. Impaired lung function in a subject with lone siderosis is due either to the effects of cigarette smoking or to non-industrial lung disease, or a combination of both.

Radiographic appearances

The standard chest radiograph shows a variable number—usually very many—of small opacities varying from 0·5 mm to about 2 mm in diameter, of striking density and associated with fewer, fine, rather less dense, linear opacities (*Figure 6.2*). Large, confluent opacities do not occur. In some cases Kerley B lines due to iron oxide dust in interlobular lymphatics are prominent. The hilar lymph nodes may appear unusually radio-opaque, due to their concentrated iron content, but are not enlarged.

Prolonged exposure to iron dust or fume is usually required to give these radiographic appearances, but in the event of exposure to high dust concentration they have been observed after as short a period as three years (Kleinfeld *et al.*, 1969).

Diagnosis

This rests upon a history of work in processes known to give rise to iron dust or fume coupled with the radiographic appearances. Siderosis can be easily overlooked if the details of the work are not known as, for example, when it occurs in woodworkers who have used emery abrasives. Biopsy of lung tissue is rarely justifiable.

It is to be borne in mind that welders may have been exposed intermittently to free silica dust if, for example, they worked in the neighbourhood of fettling or sandblasting operations in foundries (*see* Chapter 7), or to asbestos dust when working in the vicinity of insulation workers lagging boilers, pipes or other apparatus. Hence, nodular silicosis mixed dust fibrosis or asbestosis may be present together with siderosis in welders.

Differential diagnosis

Other inert dusts of high radiodensity (antimony, tin and barium, for example) may produce almost identical appearances. As a rule, the size and

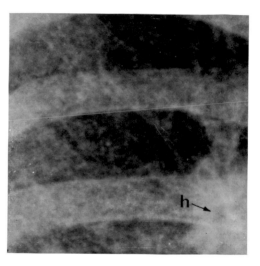

Figure 6.2. Siderosis. Numerous small (Category p) fairly radio-opaque areas. These are usually distributed uniformly in the lung fields. Film of a man who had worked 22 years crushing hematite. The category was 3p. (Natural size; h, hilar shadow)

density of the opacities of siderosis distinguish them from those of silicosis and coal pneumoconiosis, which are larger, less dense, and usually less well defined. Occasionally, tiny 'pin-head' opacities are observed in the radiographs of coal-miners (*see* Chapter 8) but their density is generally less than those of siderosis.

Miliary tuberculosis is readily distinguishable because of the lack of industrial exposure, the illness of the patient and the fact that the opacities tend to be less dense, less well defined and often most profuse in the mid-zones of the lung fields.

Some cases of 'idiopathic' sarcoidosis present a similar appearance but the lack of an industrial history, evidence of enlarged hilar lymph nodes and other clinical and investigatory features of this disorder readily establish the diagnosis. When, however, there is a history of relevant industrial exposure the differentiation may occasionally be sufficiently difficult to indicate lung biopsy.

Cryptogenic pulmonary haemosiderosis, which is commoner in men than women and in which opacities resembling those of siderosis follow repeated capillary haemorrhages (Wynn-Williams and Young, 1956; Karlish, 1962), is distinguished by recurrent haemoptysis, hypochromic anaemia and, in some cases, finger clubbing and enlargement of liver and spleen. Haemosiderosis due to mitral stenosis is readily identified in most cases if the presence of the valve disease is recognized and, though differentiation is impossible in the occasional case of a worker with mitral stenosis who has been exposed to iron oxide dusts or fumes, this is of no practical importance.

Prognosis
After the worker leaves exposure, the iron dust is slowly eliminated from the lungs over a period of years. This is reflected in the partial or complete disappearance of radiographic opacities (Doig and McLaughlin, 1948); but the greater the quantity of dust the longer the period for its elimination.

The benign nature of siderosis has been clearly demonstrated in arc welders (Doig and McLaughlin, 1936; Morgan and Kerr, 1963).

Prevention
This depends upon effective suppression of dust or fume, and exhaust ventilation methods. In many of the processes already listed concentrations have been either eliminated or greatly reduced in recent years. Nevertheless, persons who have inhaled large quantities of iron dusts in the past will continue to have abnormal chest radiographs for many years or permanently.

The TLV for iron oxide fume is 10 mg/m^3. Emery and 'rouge' are classed as 'inert' or 'nuisance particulates' by the ACGIH.

Bronchial carcinoma and iron-dust inhalation
It has been suggested that inhaled iron dust may act as a carcinogen mainly on the grounds that a higher incidence of bronchial carcinoma has been calculated to be present in hematite-miners than in the general population (Faulds and Stewart, 1956), but the methods of reaching this conclusion were criticized by Doll (1959). However, other substances (such as mineral oils and tars) with known carcinogenic potential were present in some of the work processes and the smoking habits of the workers were not analysed. Nevertheless, recent work has confirmed that West Cumberland iron-ore miners have a lung cancer mortality about 70 per cent higher than 'normal' (Boyd et al., 1970) and there is evidence of a similar lung cancer risk among iron-ore miners in Lorraine, France (Roussel et al., 1964). This might seem to increase the suspicion that iron oxides are lung carcinogens. However, it has been shown that radon concentrations are unusually high in the Cumberland hematite mines (Duggan et al., 1970) and may be the carcinogenic agency, although the identity of this is still regarded as obscure by Boyd et al. (1970) (see Chapter 12.)

In short, there is no convincing evidence to incriminate exogenous iron as a pulmonary carcinogen, although it cannot be confidently absolved.

TIN (ATOMIC NUMBER, 50): STANNOSIS
(STANNUM, TIN)

Because the atomic number of tin is almost double that of iron its radio-density is substantially greater.

Stannosis was first recognized in Germany during World War II. Shortly afterwards it was reported in Czechoslovakia (Barták and Tomečka, 1949), in the United States of America (Pendergrass and Pryde, 1948; Cutter et al., 1949; Dundon and Hughes, 1950) and, in particular detail, in the United Kingdom (Robertson and Whittaker, 1955; Robertson et al., 1961). Unlike siderosis it is very uncommon because the possibilities of industrial exposure are limited; only about 140 cases are recorded in the world literature. However, the radiographic appearance is striking.

Origins of tin ore

The chief tin ore is *cassiterite*, tin oxide, from which the tin must be recovered by smelting. The world's main tinfields are in Malaysia, Burma, Indonesia, Bolivia, China and Nigeria. The metalliferous region of South-West England is the only indigenous source in the United Kingdom from which production has been increasing in recent years after a long period of decline. The ore is found in association with acidic igneous rocks which thus contain substantial quantities of quartz.

The United Kingdom is the world's second largest importer of tin in various forms after the U.S.A.

Sources of exposure

Because the amount of tin in the crude ore is extremely small, mining procedures (drilling and loading of ore) are unlikely to cause stannosis, but the highly siliceous dust produced is a source of silicosis. Concentrates of cassiterite received by the smelters are largely freed of associated rock and the content of quartz, therefore, almost eliminated.

Processes likely to produce tin dust or fume are as follows: the emptying of bags of crude ore into skips; milling and grinding of ore (Oyanguren et al., 1957); shovelling up of spilt ore; tipping of crushed ore into the calcination furnace; charging smelting furnaces with calcined ore (molten tin issuing from these furnaces gives off tin oxide fume (Spencer and Wycoff, 1954); raking out of refinery furnaces which contain a high percentage of tin oxide and melting down tin scrap to recover tin oxide (Dundon and Hughes, 1950).

Tin dust produced by grinding, briquet making, smelting and casting contains 58 to 65 per cent tin and only 0·2 to 1 per cent quartz (Oyanguren et al., 1957). High concentration of tin dust and fume are also produced by hearth tinning where the articles to be plated are dipped by hand into molten tin (Cole et al., 1964). Tin plating is now done mainly by electrodeposition methods.

The greatest smelter tin production in 1969 was by West Malaysia and then, in order, the United Kingdom, the Netherlands, the U.S.A. and Australia (Natural Environmental Research Council, 1971).

In the float glass process (*see* page 170) glass is floated on molten tin in an

141

enclosed bath, but there is no exposure to tin fume or dust at any stage (Cameron, 1970).

Tin oxide is used as an opacifying agent for white glazes of ceramics and enamels, and has been used for polishing granite.

Pathology

Pneumoconiosis in tin-miners occurs in the form of nodular silicosis; stannosis is not seen.

Macroscopic appearances

In stannosis, naked-eye inspection of the cut surface of the lungs reveals numerous tiny (1 to 3 mm), grey-black dust macules, soft to the touch and

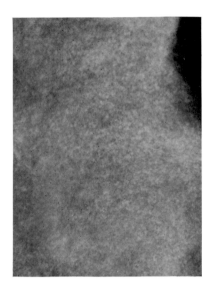

Figure 6.3. Stannosis. Postmortem radiograph of unperfused lung. Note smallness of the size and intense radio-opacity of the lesions. (Natural size)

not raised above the cut surface of the lung. Some indication of the size and profusion of these lesions, as well as their radiodensity, is given in *Figure 6.3*, a radiograph of an unexpanded lung from a tin refinery worker.

Microscopical appearances

Macrophages containing tin oxide dust particles are present in alveolar walls and spaces, perivascular lymphatics, and interlobular septa. The macules, like those of siderosis, consist of dense perivascular and peribronchiolar aggregations of dust-laden macrophages (*see Figure 6.1*). By light microscopy the intracellular particles are indistinguishable from carbon but they remain after micro-incineration (Robertson *et al.*, 1961) whereas carbon disappears; x-ray diffraction gives definitive identification. The tetragonal crystals of tin oxide exhibit strong birefringence but, as seen by the 'medical' microscope, this has no diagnostic significance (*see* Appendix) and it is important that it should not be taken to imply the presence of crystals of quartz which in any case, is poorly birefringent. There is no excess of reticulin or collagen fibres even after 50 years' exposure to tin oxide (Robertson *et al.*, 1961).

142

The quartz content of the lungs is negligible and has been estimated as substantially less than 0·2 g per lung (Robertson *et al.*, 1961) and in the same cases the amount of tin was estimated as ranging from 0·5 to 3·3 g per lung—the former value related to a man with an 11-year exposure and the latter, one with 50 years. Dust particles, single or aggregated, recovered from the lungs are from 0·1 to 0·5 μm in diameter and closely resemble furnace fume particles in size and appearance (Robertson *et al.*, 1961).

The hilar lymph nodes appear black but are not fibrotic.

Although small quantities of tin oxide have been found in the spleen and liver of a man who had stannosis (Barták and Tomečka, 1949) there is no evidence that it has any systemic toxic effect.

Tin oxide does not cause fibrosis in the lungs (Robertson 1960; Fischer and Zinnerman, 1969), liver or spleen (Fischer and Zinnerman, 1969) of experimental animals.

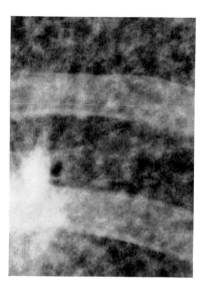

Figure 6.4. Radiographic appearances of stannosis. The opacities are denser and somewhat larger than those of siderosis. Note the density of the hilar region. Occupation, 10 years in tin ore crushing and mixing. (Natural size; by courtesy of Dr Percy H. Whitaker)

Symptoms and physical signs

There are no symptoms or abnormal physical signs due to the inhalation and retention of tin oxide dust.

Lung function

Lung function is unaffected (Robertson, 1960) and if there is any associated abnormality it is due to some other cause.

Radiographic appearances

When exposure to tin oxide dust has been heavy or prolonged numerous small, very dense opacities are scattered evenly throughout the lung fields; they may be somewhat larger (2 to 4 mm diameter) and more 'fluffy' or irregular in outline than those of siderosis—possibly due to the combined effect of superimposition and their greater radiodensity (*Figure 6.4*). Kerley

B lines are often clearly defined, and thin dense linear opacities may be seen in the upper lung zones. With lesser degrees of exposure, opacities are fewer, less dense and somewhat larger (Robertson, 1960).

Large confluent opacities do not occur and the hilar shadows, although unduly radio-opaque, are of normal size.

Diagnosis

The occupational history, lack of symptoms and physical signs and the striking density of the opacities on the radiograph are diagnostic. In the absence of a history and when opacities are fairly few they might be mistaken for silicosis, possibly for baritosis (q.v.) or for other causes of discrete bilateral lung lesions already referred to in Table 5.2.

Prognosis

Stannosis has no known effect upon health or life span. It is possible, if sufficient time were to elapse after last exposure to the dust, that the opacities would gradually disappear but this has not been reported.

Prevention

This depends upon efficient dust suppression, exhaust ventilation and good factory 'housekeeping'.

Tin oxide is classed among the 'inert' or 'nuisance particulates' by the ACGIH (1971).

BARIUM (ATOMIC NUMBER, 56): BARITOSIS

The most important compound is barytes ($BaSO_4$) known as *barite* in the U.S.A. *Witherite* ($BaCO_3$) is less important.

Baritosis ('barium lung') was first observed in Italy (Fiori, 1926) and later by other Italian workers (for example, Preti and Talini, 1939) then in Germany (Wende, 1956). A survey of a barium plant (related to duration of exposure) revealed the presence of baritosis in 48 per cent of 118 workers (Lévi-Vallensi et al., 1966).

Barytes is widely distributed throughout the world together with other minerals and is often associated with igneous, sedimentary and metamorphic rocks. Therefore, such minerals as fluorite, calcite, limestone, witherite, quartz and chert may be intermixed according to the type of deposit in which the barytes is found. In the United Kingdom deposits are almost wholly of hydrothermal origin and may thus contain varying amounts of quartz derived from the hydrothermal fluids and not from the surrounding rocks in which they lie. It is evident then that barytes from some areas will contain variable and often significant quantities of free silica.

In 1969 the world's greatest producer of barytes was the U.S.A. (mainly from Nevada, Missouri, Arkansas and Georgia), followed in magnitude by Federal Germany, the U.S.S.R., Greece, Mexico, the Irish Republic and Canada. It is of particular interest that production by the Irish Republic (County Sligo) has increased almost fortyfold since 1961. The total output by the United Kingdom (chiefly as barytes recovered as a by-product of fluoro-spar production in Derbyshire) is now very small. (National Environmental Research Council, 1971.)

Until recently, the United Kingdom was the sole world supplier of *witherite* which was mined in Northumberland and Durham, but production has now (1971) virtually ceased.

Sources of exposure and uses

During mining of the crude ore high concentrations of dust may be produced and, as indicated, in some areas this may contain either quartz in hydrothermal deposits or chert from neighbouring rocks. When mining is done by the opencast method the concentration of airborne dust is greatly reduced.

Barytes is supplied to various industries in crude form, as flotation concentrates from which contaminants have been removed, or in ground and purified form. With the exception of the crude form it is washed, leached out and then crushed or ground in the wet state. The chance of dust inhalation in these circumstances, therefore, is low, but during the drying and bagging of ground barytes, high concentrations of dust may be produced.

Ground barytes is used mainly in the oil industry as a weighting agent for drilling mud (when it is in the form of a slurry and not a dust); as a filler with weight-increasing properties in some types of paper, in linoleum, textiles, rubber, brake linings and gramophone records (until the introduction of microgroove records about 1948); in enamel paints, and in the glass industry to increase the fluidity of molten glass.

Lithopone was widely used as a pigment and filler until recent years. It is made by roasting crude, 'silica free' barytes with carbon in a rotary kiln, leaching out the product and adding zinc sulphate; the precipitate is washed, filtered dried and again calcined. At some stages of this process a mixture of barytes and carbon dusts may be present; coal was often used in the past as a source of carbon, and grinding this was a dusty process. Thus, there was the possibility of coal or carbon pneumoconiosis co-existing with baritosis. The production of lithopone (which is now mainly used in paints) has, however, decreased notably in the last decade but the results of exposure to these dusts may still be found in ex-workers. Barium, chiefly in the form of barytes but also witherite, is used in large quantities by the chemical industry. As a general rule, free silica is absent, or present in only minute amount in barytes used in industrial processes.

Accidental inhalation of barium sulphate during radiography of the alimentary tract may sometimes occur but is not likely to be confused with baritosis of industrial origin.

In recent years barium titanate has been used for many types of electronic and ultrasonic devices (such as transducers and digital computers) because of its mineral electromagnetic properties.

Pathology

Although this section is concerned with baritosis, it should be noted that if exposure has occurred to both barytes and 'free silica' dusts (as may be the case in some barytes mines) then both baritosis and silicosis may be present. But there is no evidence that the pathogenesis of the silicotic lesions is modified by barytes.

Macroscopic appearances

Many discrete grey macules are present in the pulmonary pleura and the cut surface of the lungs shows numerous discrete, impalpable macules which resemble those of stannosis. There is no confluent massing or evidence of fibrosis. Hilar lymph nodes are not enlarged.

Microscopic appearances

The appearances of the lesions are similar to those of stannosis and siderosis. The initial reaction is an insignificant mobilization of polymorphonuclear leucocytes but a brisk macrophage response together with a little intra-alveolar exudate. There is little increase of reticulin and no fibrosis. The lack of fibrotic reaction is confirmed in experimental animals (Huston, Wallach and Cunningham, 1952). Following accidental inhalation of barium meal, barium-containing macrophages fill the alveoli and small airways and some are present in alveolar walls.

It is claimed that barium can be identified by a special staining technique (Waterhouse, 1951) in which lung tissue is fixed with carefully neutralized 10 per cent formalin in 70 per cent alcohol and immersed in a 1 or 2 per cent solution of sodium rhodizonate in distilled water when an intense red colour is produced by barium compounds. As calcium reacts with this reagent under alkaline, but not neutral conditions the test may not always be successful. If positive identification is important, x-ray diffraction or spectrographic methods are advisable. Barytes particles are moderately birefringent.

Symptoms and signs

Baritosis is symptomless and causes no abnormal physical signs. There are no systemic toxic effects due to absorption of barytes from the lungs as it is poorly soluble and chemically inert.

Lung function

No abnormality of lung function has been recorded.

Radiographic appearances

Particularly dense, discrete, small opacities (usually about 2 to 4 mm in diameter) are distributed throughout the lung fields and may develop after only a few months' exposure to the dust (Pancheri, 1950). When the amount of retained barium dust is large (as may be the case after long periods of exposure) the opacities may be bigger and, indeed, large, irregular and densely opaque areas, which may give the impression of confluent lesions, may be seen (Preti and Talini, 1939); this is due to the superimposition effect of very many highly radiodense deposits. Kerley B lines are often prominent and the hilar lymph nodes may be remarkably opaque, but not enlarged (*Figure 6.5*).

As in the case of siderosis, very gradual clearing of the opacities, due to elimination of the dust, occurs after industrial exposure has ceased (Spedini and Valdini, 1939; Lévi-Valensi *et al.*, 1966).

Diagnosis

The work history presents the necessary clue and the density of the opacities should suggest the possibility of baritosis. But if exposure to the dust has been slight, or if opacities are few, confusion with other causes of discrete opacities may well occur.

It is important to remember that pneumoconiosis in barytes-miners is likely to be predominantly silicosis. For example, in the case of one such miner, many characteristic silicotic nodules were found and analysis of the lung ash revealed about 15 per cent SiO_2 by weight but only 4 per cent $BaSO_4$.

Baritosis is rare and many men in whom it is found are either elderly or have left the responsible industry some years before it is recognized. But sporadic 'new' cases continue to be observed especially when men who were exposed to the dust more than a decade previously have a chest radiograph taken for the first time.

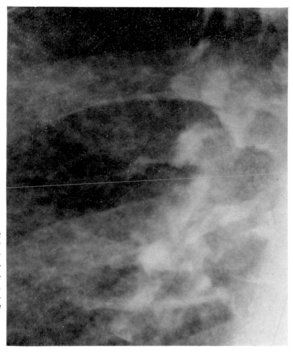

Figure 6.5. Baritosis. This is a mild case, the amount of dust in the lungs being slight, but note the degree of opacity of the hilar lymph nodes. When the dust content is high the appearances are those of a dense 'snowstorm' pattern. (Natural size)

Prognosis

The presence of barytes or witherite in the lungs is not known to have any adverse effect upon health or life expectancy. Gradual clearance of opacities can be expected over the years after the worker has left exposure.

Prevention

The same conditions as those already mentioned for iron and tin apply.

There is no TLV for barytes or witherite and they are not classed among 'inert' or 'nuisance particulates' by the ACGIH.

ANTIMONY (ATOMIC NUMBER, 51)

Antimony occurs in metamorphic deposits in quartz veins of deep-seated origin which lie in or near intrusive rocks such as the granites and as deposits

147

in limestone and shales. It is mined in South Africa, China, Bolivia, Algeria, Mexico and parts of Europe.

It is imported into other countries as *stibnite* (Sb_2S_3) ore or powder. Antimony metal, trioxide, pentoxide, trisulphate and pentasulphide are produced from the ore.

Sources of exposure and uses

Exposure to antimony dust may occur during mining, crushing the ore, and cleaning of extraction chambers which collect the oxide dust from roasting chambers (Renes, 1953). Exposure to fume may occur among antimony alloy workers and Linotype setters, but is most important among men who smelt and refine the ore.

In the United Kingdom antimony is smelted near Newcastle upon Tyne in the largest smelting plant in Europe and the chief centres in the U.S.A. are in Pennsylvania and Texas (Cooper *et al.*, 1968). The metal and white antimony trioxide are produced.

Antimony dust apparently remains suspended in the air longer than might be expected of a heavy metal (Fairhall and Hyslop, 1947) which suggests that the particle size is small; and the fine white fume of antimony oxide which is produced during smelting in the manufacture consists of particles which, on average, are less than 1 μm diameter (McCallum *et al.*, 1971). Work in the baghouse or at the furnaces is associated with most dust or fume exposure.

The metal is used chiefly as a component of lead alloys for battery plates, electrodes, pewter and printing type. Antimony oxides are employed as pigments for paints, glass and fusable enamels; in the colouring and vulcanizing of rubber, in plastics and the red tips of matches.

Pathology

Histological examination of the lungs of antimony workers has shown an accumulation of dust particles and dust-laden macrophages in alveolar walls and perivascular regions, but no fibrosis or inflammatory reaction (McCallum, 1967); the dust of antimony ore or the trioxide does not cause fibrosis in the lungs of experimental animals (Cooper *et al.*, 1968).

Small amounts of antimony have been detected in the urine of a worker some four years after he left the industry, suggesting that antimony is not fixed in the lungs and may be absorbed into the circulation in small quantities and excreted (McCallum, 1963).

Symptoms and Physical signs

There are no symptoms or abnormal physical signs.

Some workers develop skin irritation with a papular and pustular rash in the vicinity of sebaceous and sweat glands of the forearms and the thighs— especially in the flexures.

Lung function

There is no abnormality of lung function.

Radiographic appearances

There are many small, dense opacities similar to those of siderosis which vary from ILO Categories 1p to 3p (McCallum, 1963; Cooper *et al.*, 1968). Larger, confluent shadows are not seen but the hilar regions may be denser than normal (*Figure 6.6*).

A radiographic survey of 262 men in an antimony works between 1965 and 1966 revealed the presence of 44 cases (16·8 per cent) of antimony pneumoconiosis (McCallum *et al.*, 1971).

Using the differential x-ray absorption technique referred to in Chapter 5 in some of these workers McCallum *et al.* (1971) observed antimony values ranging from nil to just over 11 mg/cm² and these tended to rise the longer the period of employment in the industry and the higher the ILO Category recorded.

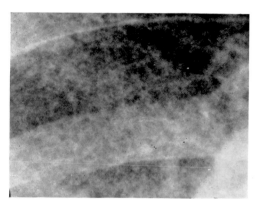

Figure 6.6. Antimony pneumo-coniosis in an antimony smelter. Category p size opacities are distributed throughout both lung fields. (Natural size; by courtesy of Dr R. I. McCallum)

Abnormal chest radiographs have been reported in men mining and smelting antimony ore in Yugoslavia (Karajovic, 1958) but those of the miners appear to have been due to silicosis.

Diagnosis

Benign antimony pneumoconiosis is rare but if the clinician is not aware that antimony in the lungs causes radiographic abnormality, or if a history of industrial exposure to antimony is not obtained in the first place, errors in diagnosis (mainly in the direction of non-industrial disease) will probably occur.

The differential diagnosis is generally similar to that of siderosis (page 139).

Prognosis

There is no known detrimental effect upon health or life expectancy.

Unlike siderosis and baritosis no evident diminution of radiographic appearance has yet been recorded.

Prevention

The principles are the same as those for tin oxide.

The TLV for antimony and antimony compounds is 0·5 mg/m³.

ZIRCONIUM (ATOMIC NUMBER, 40)

Zirconium (Zr) occurs most commonly as *zircon* (ZrO_2SiO_2) and *baddeleyite* (ZrO_2). Zircon, which is widely distributed in some igneous and sedimentary rocks, is recovered commercially from beach sands and river gravels and is concentrated by magnetic and electrostatic separation techniques to remove accessory minerals such as ilmenite, rutile, magnetite and monazite, and quartz is removed by gravitation.

Zircon is very heavy, has a low solubility and remarkable refractory properties.

Uses and sources of exposure

Zircon dust or fume may be produced when zircon concentrate is dried and calcined to remove organic material; subsequent treatment with magnetic and roll separators to remove quartz and other impurities may also give rise to dust. Dust of zirconium compounds may be produced during many of the processes in which it is used. Quartz dust may be a hazard during the milling of the raw material and in the separation processes, but is otherwise absent.

Probably the largest use of zirconium is in alloy manufacture; with silicon and manganese in steel, and in nickel–cobalt and niobium–tantulum alloys which resist neutron bombardment.

Zircon is of particular importance in the manufacture of technical refractory ceramics in the form of crucibles, tubes and boats and for high-temperature work in chemistry and metallurgy. It is increasingly, though not universally, used in foundry work in the form of oil-bonded 'sand', and for mould paints and parting powder in place of quartz sands and 'silica flour' (*see* Chapter 7). Not only does it eliminate or reduce the 'silica' risk but it possesses the additional advantage of high resistance to thermal shock. Zircon and various zirconium compounds are employed as opacifiers in ceramic enamels and in glasses and glazes because of their resistance to acid and thermal shock; and to impart high dielectric strength to electrical porcelain such as sparking plugs. Zircon is also employed as a polishing agent for glass and television tubes and in the form of 'pebbles' as a grinding medium in rotary mills.

Stabilized zirconium dioxide which can withstand temperatures higher than 1,900°C plays an important role in turbojet and rocket manufacture; and zirconium is used in the manufacture of photographic flash bulbs and in the surface reflecting material of 'space' satellites.

Pathology

The possible biological effect of zircon was investigated in experimental animals by Harding (1948) and Harding and Davies (1952) and was found to be remarkably inert in the lungs. Normal phagocytosis of dust particles and a slight accumulation of small cells occurred but there was no fibrosis or increase of reticulin. These observations were confirmed by Reed (1956). Numerous small dense opacities were revealed throughout radiographs of the animals' lungs due to the atomic number of the retained dust (Harding and Davies 1952).

There appears to be no record of pathological studies on human lungs.

Zirconium compounds have, however, the unique effect of causing sarcoid-like granulomas in the skin when applied in deodorants (Rubin *et al.*, 1956), or under experimental conditions (Shelley and Hurley, 1958) but there appears to be no radiographic evidence that they produce pulmonary granulomas when inhaled by man (Reed, 1956). However, peribronchial granulomas have been produced in rabbits by the inhalation of sodium zirconium lactate (Prior, Crouk and Ziegler, 1960) and diffuse interstitial fibrosis has occurred in a variety of experimental animals after prolonged inhalation of zirconium lactate (Brown, Mastromatteo and Horwood, 1963). The possibility that these and other zirconium compounds might produce similar effects in human lungs should be borne in mind and requires further investigation.

Symptoms and physical signs
On present evidence inhalation of zirconium and zirconium compounds apparently causes no clinical effects in man.

Lung function
No case studies are on record.

Radiographic appearances
The presence of small dense opacities (ILO Category 1 to 3p) similar to those just described in experimental animals was observed by McCallum (1967) in the chest radiographs of 8 men working in a zirconium process adjacent to antimony smelting. But no radiographic changes 'reasonably attributable to radio-opaque dusts' were found by Reed (1956) in 22 workers exposed from 1 to 5 years in a zirconium plant.

Diagnosis
The possibility of a symptomless and benign pneumoconiosis being caused by zirconium dusts should be borne in mind in view of the now widespread use of these compounds in industry. It is possible that the small opacities seen in chest radiographs of some moulders and 'knock-out' men in foundries where moulding sands and parting powders have been replaced by zircon may be caused by zirconium rather than by iron (siderosis).

Conclusion
Zirconium compounds may sometimes cause radio-opacities of a benign pneumoconiosis, and the production of lung granulomas and, possibly, diffuse interstitial fibrosis appears theoretically possible.

Threshold limit value
The TLV for zirconium compounds as zirconium is 5 mg/m³.

THE LANTHANONS OR RARE-EARTH ELEMENTS

The rare-earth elements (the lanthanons), with atomic numbers ranging from 57 to 71, occur in a variety of minerals, the most important commercially being *monazite*, a rare-earth phosphate, and *bastnaesite*, a rare-earth fluorocarbonate. Cerium (Atomic Number, 58) is the most abundant rare-earth metal but thorium oxide is also present in small amounts in monazite and yttrium which are included with the rare-earths.

Uses and sources of exposure
Cerium (usually in the form of dioxide) has been used for years in the

151

manufacture of gas mantles to provide luminosity. It is now chiefly employed as a mild abrasive for polishing lenses, mirrors and prisms; in the manufacture of fireworks, cigarette lighter 'flints'; for high temperature ceramics (such as crucibles); in light metal alloys; and, to increase light brilliance, as the nitrate, fluoride and oxide in the core of carbon arc rods. The heat of the arc evaporates the salts which accumulate as fine dust on apparatus on ledges and other objects in the work room. Benign pneumoconiosis attributed to cerium and other rare-earth elements has been reported in men who have worked in frequent contact with carbon arc lamps (Heuck and Hoschek, 1968) and in the preparation of cerium oxide (Napée, Bobrie and Lambard, 1972). Unseparated rare-earth elements are also used for various 'misch-metall' alloys some of which, like lighter 'flints', are pyrophoric; the iron alloy, for example, is employed in the manufacture of luminous projectiles and tracer bullets. Latterly small amounts of europium and yttrium oxides of high purity are being employed as phosphors in colour television tubes and mercury vapour and fluorescent lamps.

Pathology

No pathological studies of human lungs appear to be on record. However, when rare-earth dusts are inhaled or injected by the intratracheal route into experimental animals no fibrosis or other evident reaction occurs (Heuck and Hoschek, 1968). When their fluoride content is relatively high they cause acute transient pneumonitis, bronchitis and bronchiolitis, but no fibrosis (Schepers, 1955).

Symptoms, signs and lung function

No symptoms, abnormal physical signs or alteration in lung physiology are attributable to these inhaled dusts.

Radiographic appearances

Three persons (among some 67) who worked in the photographic department of an offset printers are the source of this description (Heuck and Hoschek, 1968). Chest radiographs showed small, discrete opacities of a density similar to those of baritosis throughout the lung fields (ILO Category being from 2q to 3q) (*Figure 6.7*). The presence of significant amounts of thoron as [228]Th in the expired air of two of them with a high concentration in the lungs of one demonstrated by the whole body counter was taken as proof that the opacities were caused by rare-earth elements.

There appear to be no other cases on record but the author has observed the case of a man with similar radiographic appearances who worked with cerium dioxide for six years.

Differential diagnosis

This is similar in all respects to that of other high-density dusts. The demonstration of thorium, predominantly in the lungs, by the whole body counter and the detection of radioactive elements of the thorium decay chain in expired air should, in association with the industrial history, establish the diagnosis of 'cerium pneumoconiosis'.

Prognosis

No injurious effects of cerium and the related lanthanide salts are known but the co-existence of thorium (an α-particle emitter) and its decay chain products may be harmful (*see* Chapter 12). This risk may be encountered during extraction of the rare-earths. Nothing appears to be known about possible clearance of radio-opacities after exposure has ceased, but none was evident in the case I observed years after exposure had ceased.

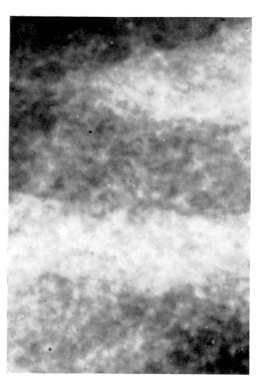

Figure 6.7. Small (Category q) opacities due to cerium dioxide. (By courtesy of Dr F. Heuck and Georg Thieme, Stuttgart)

Prevention

This depends on satisfactory dust control. No TLV for the rare-earth elements is given. The question of thorium is referred to in Chapter 12.

Awareness of the fact that a benign pneumoconiosis may result from exposure to the salts of cerium and other members of the lanthanon group is of some importance in view of their increasing use in industry which may give rise to further cases in the future. In addition, thorium decay chain products may present a hazard during the extraction process of monazite.

CHROMITE

Chromite is the mineral ore of chromium, and it consists of chromium and iron oxides (Cr_2O_3FeO). The atomic numbers of chromium and iron are 26 and 24 respectively but the effective atomic number of chromite is 22.

The world's largest producers of chromite are Rhodesia, South Africa, Turkey and the U.S.S.R. In the Transvaal it occurs in association with

153

pyroxenite, anorthosite and norite rocks and although there are occasional pegmatite veins which contain some quartz and alkaline feldspar these are few, and the amount of quartz in the mine dust is generally less than 1 per cent (Sluis-Cremer and du Toit, 1968).

The chest radiographs of miners who have been exposed to chromite mine dust for eight or more years may show small, discrete opacities similar to those of siderosis and increased opacity, but no enlargement, of the hilar shadows. There are no accompanying respiratory symptoms or signs (Sluis-Cremer and du Toit, 1968). No histological studies are available in these cases, but in view of the fact that chromite dust appears to cause only a minor cellular reaction and no fibrosis in the lungs of experimental animals (Goldstein, 1955; Worth and Schiller, 1955), Sluis-Cremer and du Toit (1968) consider the human lesions are benign and are not associated with fibrosis. However, histological examination of the lungs of three men who had worked in a chromate plant in which chromite was one of the three chromium compounds used, revealed large quantities of black pigment (identified as chromite) in the alveolar walls which were thickened, fibrotic and hyalinized (Mancuso and Hueper, 1951). Whether these changes were due to chromium, to some past inflammatory process or to some other inhaled aerosol is uncertain.

On present evidence, therefore, it appears that chromite dust is non-fibrogenic. The increased incidence of carcinoma of the lung in chromate workers is, of course, another matter, but no cases of carcinoma were observed in chromite miners (Sluis-Cremer and du Toit, 1968).

VANADIUM (ATOMIC NUMBER, 23)

Vanadium is considered here in order to point out that there is no evidence—as has been, and still is, sometimes suggested—that it or its compounds cause pneumoconiosis of inert or fibrotic type.

Vanadium is found in combination with other elements in igneous and sedimentary rocks and in some petroleum deposits because of the fossilized remains of sea squirts of the tunicate family and sea cucumbers whose normal blood consists, in part, of vanadium.

Sources of exposure and uses

Vanadium ore is first crushed and dried ('inactive ore'), finely ground in a ball mill ('active ore') and roasted; it is then mixed with sulphuric acid and the resulting precipitate, which is dried, is vanadium pentoxide. This is packed in bags. The roasting and bagging processes tend to produce most dust, grinding and crushing, rather less.

Vanadium-bearing slags, produced on a large scale during the manufacture of steel from titaniferous magnetite, are becoming an increasingly important source of vanadium in some countries (for example, South Africa and the U.S.S.R.). Other important sources of vanadium-containing dusts are furnace residues from oil refineries, soot from oil-fired boilers (Williams, 1952) and slags from the production of ferrovanadium. The soot is ground and treated with sodium hydroxide and slag is crushed, extracted with water, neutralized with sulphuric acid and filtered. In addition to vanadium,

154

carbon dust is also produced by these processes. Deposit formed on heat-exchanger tubes of gas turbines contains some 11 to 20 per cent of vanadium (Browne, 1955); its removal gives rise to much dust.

Carnotite ($K_2O.2UO_3.V_2O_5.3H_2O$), a uranium-containing vanadium mineral found in South Australia and Colorado and Utah in the USA, forms the cementing material of sandstones and, being disseminated through them, must be mined with them. After mining it is milled and processed on a large scale as a uranium source. Mining and milling may thus carry a quartz risk, but the chief potential hazard to health lies in the production of radon decay products (Archer *et al.*, 1962).

Vanadium metal is used extensively for metal alloys; ferrovanadium and molybdenum-vanadium steels, and vanadium bronze and brass. Vanadium pentoxide is a catalyst in the manufacture of sulphuric acid and phthalic anhydride. Vanadium salts are also employed in inks, dyeing processes, paints, insecticides, printing fabrics and glass production.

Pathology

Acute bronchitis and pneumonitis has been ascribed to exposure to vanadium pentoxide. This is referred to in Chapter 12.

Wyers (1946) suggested on the grounds of alleged abnormalities in chest radiographs of vanadium-exposed workers (but without the benefit of pathological examination of lungs) that permanent lung changes—interpreted as fibrosis—were caused by vanadium pentoxide. In fact, no pathological studies appear to be on record which demonstrate fibrosis in human lungs due to vanadium. However, mild cases of silicosis due to the presence of small quantities of quartz in the dust of dry sedimented dross seem to have occurred.

Rabbits exposed to low concentrations of vanadium pentoxide for more than eight months showed no evidence of lung fibrosis, and no fibrosis resulted after its injection into the peritoneum of guinea-pigs (Sjöberg, 1950).

The lack of retention of vanadium in the lungs is probably explained by its rapid absorption into the blood whence it is deposited in other organs (Hudson, 1964).

Symptoms and physical signs

Symptoms and signs of acute bronchitis with bronchospasm may apparently result from exposure to high concentrations of vanadium pentoxide dust from the soot of oil-fired boilers of ships, from furnace residues of oil refineries and from slags resulting from the production of ferrovanadium. However, although chronic cough (Dutton, 1911) and dyspnoea (Wyers, 1946) have been attributed to vanadium exposure, there is no satisfactory evidence of a causative relationship. In Dutton's cases pulmonary tuberculosis appears to have been responsible. Prospective studies of vanadium workers (Sjöberg, 1950; Vintinner *et al.*, 1955) have not shown the presence of cough, breathlessness and abnormal physical signs which can be ascribed to this cause, although 'bronchitis with broncho-spasm' appears to be enhanced by repeated exposure to europium-activated yttrium orthovanadate (Tebrock and Machle, 1968).

Tiredness and lassitude due to anaemia was at one time thought to occur

155

in vanadium workers but this has not been confirmed (Hudson, 1964); on the contrary, it appears rather to stimulate haemopoiesis. Dyspnoea from this cause, therefore, can be discounted.

Some workers exposed to vanadium dusts for long periods or in high concentration develop a greenish-black furring of the tongue. The fur contains vanadium (Hudson, 1964).

Lung function
No difference in VC between exposed subjects and controls was found by Sjöberg (1950) and Vintinner et al. (1955) did not observe any significant impairment of other spirometric values.

Radiographic appearances
Wyers (1946) reported fine linear markings ('x-ray reticulation') in three cases, but the validity of this observation—which has never been confirmed (Williams, 1952; Tebrock and Machle, 1968)—is most doubtful; discrete opacities have not been described.

Although the radiodensity of vanadium is little less than that of iron there is no evidence that it causes a benign pneumoconiosis. This may be due to its rapid absorption from the lungs.

Diagnosis
As vanadium does not cause any radiographic abnormality there can be no confusion with pneumoconiosis or other forms of lung disease. If this is not understood abnormal radiographic shadows in a worker known to have been exposed to vanadium dust or fume in the past may be wrongly attributed to this cause and the responsible disease thus overlooked.

Prevention
Measures required apply to the prevention of acute disease. TLV for vanadium pentoxide dust is 0.5 mg/m^3 and for fume, 0.1 mg/m^3.

CONCLUSION

The importance of inert dusts of high radiodensity is that they are not responsible for any symptoms, physiological impairment or progressive disease yet they produce abnormal radiographic appearances (vanadium apparently excepted) which persist either permanently or for many years after the worker has left the relevant industry. It follows whenever small discrete opacities of emphatic density are observed in the radiographs of a person with no other evidence of pulmonary disease that industrial exposure to an inert radiodense dust should always be remembered and enquired into.

In some cases the work processes in which these materials were used have been discontinued in recent years or are now carried out only on a small scale. Nevertheless, the chest radiograph may give clear evidence of past exposure years after it has ceased. Failure to recognize present or past exposure to one of these dusts as the cause of an abnormal chest radiograph will inevitably cause misdiagnosis and the likelihood of anxiety for the worker and his family.

INERT DUSTS OF LOW RADIODENSITY

Due to their low atomic numbers such dusts cause no evident radiographic abnormality but, when accompanied by free silica in the form of quartz, flint or chert, silicosis may result, in which case the appearances may be interpreted as due to the inert dust which is wrongly thought to be fibrogenic, or, if the work history is inadequate, to some unconnected disease process.

These dusts are included by the ACGIH among the 'inert' or 'nuisance particulates' which are not known to cause lung damage. Their TLV for a normal working day is given as 10 mg/m³ or 30 mppcf of total dust less than 1 per cent SiO_2, whichever is smaller (ACGIH, 1971). Five examples will be briefly considered so that their negative place in the pathogenesis of pneumoconiosis may be recognized by contrast with the siliceous dusts with which they may be contaminated at some stage or another. They are: *limestone, marble, Portland cement, gypsum* and *silicon carbide*.

Carbon, which in general behaves as an inert dust of low radiodensity, is a special case and is discussed in Chapter 9.

Limestone

Limestones (*see* Chapter 2) generally contain small—usually minute— percentages of quartz and those containing more than about 15 to 20 per cent free quartz are rare.

Industrial exposure to 'pure' limestone (that is, of less than 1 per cent quartz content) does not cause a fibrotic pneumoconiosis or abnormality of the chest radiograph even after many years' exposure (Collis, 1931; Davis and Nagelschmidt, 1956), and it has no systemic effect.

Marble and chalk are similarly harmless.

However, when limestone contains flint or chert nodules or significant quantities of quartz grains there is a risk of silicosis. This may occur when siliceous limestone is quarried, crushed, milled, cut or polished (Doig, 1955).

Cement

Portland cement is manufactured on an enormous scale in large plants throughout the industrialized world, and production has been steadily increasing since 1961. The processes involved are often very dusty and, because they are sometimes wrongly regarded as causing fibrotic pneumoconiosis, must be briefly outlined.

There are three main groups of raw materials:

(1) *Calcareous*: limestone, marl and chalk.

(2) *Argillaceous*: shale, clay, marl, mudstone and, in some countries, volcanic rocks and schists.

(3) Gypsum.

Minor components are sand, quartzite and iron dusts.

The limestone must not contain too high a proportion of quartz but should this be deficient in the total mix, it is added in the form of sand, quartzite or sandstone.

The process most commonly used involves four stages:

(1) Raw materials are crushed in roll, jaw or gyratory crushers and then ground down to optimal size for chemical reaction. Grinding is done either dry in ball or roll mills, or wet in ball mills fed with water.

(2) The raw mix is blended to the required composition.

(3) It is then calcined at a temperature of about 1,430°C to 1,650°C, usually in rotary kilns, and appears at the far end of the kiln as clinker and is cooled. Calcination drives off moisture, breaks down carbonates to oxides and forms calcium silicates and aluminates so that negligible quantities of quartz remain.

(4) Clinker, to which about 5 per cent gypsum has been added, is then ground to a fine powder in ball or race mills. The gypsum controls the setting of the finished product.

Dust collected from grinding mills, crushers and conveyers is returned to the process. Although dust from the kiln stacks may contain some silicon dioxide in addition to other oxides, this is usually collected in electrostatic or mechanical precipitators and likewise returned to the process.

Certain types of blast furnace slag may be ground to produce Portland cement directly.

Clearly then, the chance of workers being exposed to significant quantities of free silica is small but, when such exposure does occur, it is in the preparatory stages of the process in those plants where quartz is added or siliceous clays or limestones are used.

The inhalation of cement dust by experimental animals causes neither acute nor chronic pathological changes (Baetjer, 1947). However, Einbrodt and Hentschel (1966) observed an uncommon situation in which dust recovered at the end of the process (in the packaging department) contained 5 per cent quartz and gave rise to atypical collagenous nodules when injected into the peritoneum of rats.

Surveys of large numbers of cement workers in many countries have revealed either no radiographic abnormalities or only an extremely low incidence of discrete opacities (Sayers, Dallavalle and Bloomfield, 1937; Gardner et al., 1939; Sander, 1958; Jenny et al., 1960). In a study of 2,557 workers in Argentina, Vaccarezza (1950) did not find a single case of pneumoconiosis. But Hublet (1968) observed discrete opacities—mostly category 1q but also a few 2q (ILO, 1958)—in just over half of 478 men who had worked in a Belgian cement plant from five to twenty years. It is not clear what these appearances represented. However, silicotic-type nodules and conglomerate masses have been reported in men who worked at those stages in manufacture where quartz contamination was fairly high (Doerr, 1952; Prosperi and Barsi, 1957).

Conclusion

Cement dust does not cause a pneumoconiosis, but if more than 2 per cent 'free silica' is present as a contaminant, silicosis may occur after some years' exposure. This is most likely to apply in quarrying and milling of raw materials. Nevertheless, the practical fact is that pneumoconiosis among cement workers is remarkably rare.

The lack of pathogenic effects of cement dust may be contributed in some degree to its actively hygroscopic nature favouring flocculation of its particles so that the resulting aggregates are deposited very largely in the upper respiratory tract and mouth. Certainly rhinolithiasis has been a common annoyance to many workers in the industry.

Portland cement is classed among the 'inert' and 'nuisance particulates' (ACGIH, 1971).

Gypsum

Gypsum ($CaSO_4 . 2H_2O$: *see* Chapter 2) has been used for some thousands of years as a building material, for example, as mortar between the blocks of the great pyramids and in Roman buildings, and this remains its major use today.

It occurs as a sedimentary deposit which originated as a saline residue precipitated during the evaporation of enclosed basins of sea water, and is commonly associated with shale, marl and limestone. Contamination by quartz is absent or very slight—rarely more than 1 to 2 per cent (Schepers and Durkan, 1955). However, contiguous beds of shale or siliceous limestone may contribute a variable quantity of quartz which may be encountered by gypsum miners when extending underground passages or sinking shafts, and by those engaged in crushing and calcining the raw material.

It is mined by opencast and underground methods, and is also quarried, the largest of the worlds' producers being the USA, Canada, France, the USSR, Spain, Italy and the United Kingdom.

First-stage crushing of the rock is usually done at the main processing plant by ball and hammer mills. Most of the gypsum produced is calcined and used in the preparation of various plasters and plaster boards for building purposes. Quartz is either absent or present in negligible amounts in the dust produced. Milled gypsum is extensively used as a retarder in Portland cement manufacture and also in agriculture as a soil conditioner. Calcined gypsum is employed for dental moulds and orthopaedic plasters; and there is a variety of other uses.

Gypsum does not cause lung fibrosis in experimental animals (Schepers, Durkan and Dellahant, 1955) but appears, rather, to inhibit the fibrogenic effects of quartz. Neither is pneumoconiosis or any other harmful effect caused in human lungs (Riddell, 1934), although cellular infiltration may be observed around the walls of some bronchioles (Schepers and Durkan, 1955).

In short, gypsum dust does not cause a pneumoconiosis. However, small discrete radiographic opacities, consistent with mild *silicosis* or '*mixed dust fibrosis*' (*see* Chapter 7) may be observed in men who have mined or crushed quartz-contaminated gypsum rock for many years (*Figure 6.8*). It is of interest that the lesions are of limited extent and show little tendency to progress.

Silicon carbide

Silicon carbide (SiC) is a universally used artificial abrasive of a hardness only slightly less than that of diamond. It is usually known by the trade name Carborundum, but sometimes by other names such as Crystolen and Carbolon. It is impervious to the action of acids, including hydrofluoric.

To produce silicon carbide, high-grade silica, sand and finely ground carbon (preferably in the form of petroleum coke), common salt and sawdust are fused in an electric furnace at a temperature of about 2,200°C. If the temperature is too high, silicon carbide decomposes, silica is volatilized and the

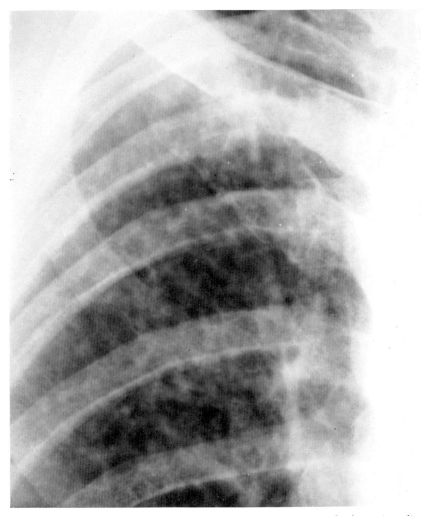

Figure 6.8. Gypsum-miner for 17 years. No other dust exposure. Little change in radiographic appearances over 10 years. (FEV₁, 3·8 l; FVC, 5·1 l; age 52 years; height, 6 ft 1 in)

carbon converted into graphite (Ladoo, 1960). At the end of the process silicon carbide crystals are surrounded by a variable amount of unreacted raw material. Fully-formed silicon carbide is then ground in crushers and mills, and impurities are removed.

It has long been used for abrasive wheels in place of the earlier, highly dangerous, sandstone wheels and is also employed as a refractory in the manufacture of boilers, forging and annealing furnaces and ceramic setter tiles.

Experimental animals exposed to high concentrations of silicon carbide dust do not develop lung fibrosis (Gardner, 1935; Holt, 1957) and, in general, it is remarkably inert. Neither is there any satisfactory evidence that it causes a pneumoconiosis in human lungs (Clark and Simmons, 1925; Miller and Sayers, 1934). Nonetheless, pneumoconiosis has been reported in workers engaged in the manufacture of Carborundum (Smith and Perina, 1948; Bruusgaard, 1949). But Bruusgaard's workers had been exposed to quartz dust from the raw material crushers, furnace residue and milling and sieving processes; those of Smith and Perina (who had significant radiographic evidence of a pneumoconiosis) had been previously exposed to other dust hazards.

There is no evidence to support the suggestion sometimes made that silicon carbide may liberate free silica or silicic acid in the lungs due to the action of tissue fluids.

Hence, although silicosis has occurred—and may still be observed—in men who have been exposed to quartz dust during the preparatory stages of the process or from furnace residue, silicon carbide dust does not cause pneumoconiosis. But the materials used to bond silicon carbide grains together contained, until recent years, variable quantities of flint, quartz, feldspar and ball and china clay, and silicosis has been recorded in men working in the bonding process (Posner, 1960). Latterly, bonding material has to a large extent been replaced by a flux (often called 'frit') which consists of silicates, borates and oxides and is almost free of quartz or flint; or substituted by rubber, synthetic resins and organic materials.

It has been suggested (Posner, 1960) that particles of quartz and flint, or tridymite and cristobalite formed by the conversion effect of furnace temperatures of 2,200°C (see Chapter 2) may be released when grinding wheels are in use, but there does not seem to be any proof of this in fact.

Very recently the U.K. Atomic Energy Authority has developed self-bonded silicon carbide in which the grains themselves are bonded together by silicon carbide during manufacture. No additional substances are used and this new ceramic material is tougher and more resistant than the previous forms. It should find a wide application in industry and its dust will almost certainly have no fibrogenic potential.

It can be concluded that there is no evidence that exposure to silicon carbide dust gives rise to a pneumoconiosis, although pneumoconiosis, due to significant exposure to quartz or carbon dusts in the course of manufacture of silicon carbide grinding wheels may occur (see Chapter 7). And it must be remembered that the use of these grinding wheels on cast iron or steel (turning or grinding) may ultimately cause *siderosis* from attrition of the metal (Buckell *et al.*, 1946); or when employed for fettling metal castings moulded in siliceous sand, may give rise to silicosis or 'mixed dust fibrosis' (see Chapter 7).

REFERENCES

Archer, V. E., Magnuson, H. H., Holaday, D. A. and Lawrence, P. A. (1962). 'Hazards to health in uranium mining and milling.' *J. occup. Med.* **4**, 55–60

Baetjer, A. M. (1947). 'The effect of Portland cement dust on the lungs with special references to lobar pneumonia.' *J. ind. Hyg. Toxicol.* **29**, 250–258

Barták, F. and Tomečka, M. (1949). 'Stannosis (coniosis due to tin).' *Proceedings of the Ninth International Congress of Industrial Medicine, London*, pp. 742–754. Bristol; Wright

Bech, A. O., Kipling, M. D. and Zundel, W. E. (1965). 'Emery pneumoconiosis.' *Trans. Ass. ind. med. Offrs* **15**, 110–115

Boyd, J. T., Doll, R., Faulds, J. S. and Leiper, J. (1970). 'Cancer of the lung in iron ore (haematite) miners.' *Br. J. ind. Med.* **27**, 97–105

Brown, J. R., Mastromatteo, E. and Horwood, J. (1963). 'Zirconium lactate and barium zirconate.' *Am. ind. Hyg. Ass. J.* **24**, 131–136

Browne, R. C. (1955). 'Vanadium poisoning from gas turbine.' *Br. J. ind. Med.* **12**, 57–59

Bruusgaard, A. (1949). 'Pneumoconiosis in silicon carbide workers.' *Proceedings of the Ninth International Congress of Industrial Medicine, London*, pp. 676–680. Bristol; Wright

Buckell, M., Garrard, J., Jupe, M. H., McLaughlin, A. I. G. and Perry, K. M. A. (1946). 'The incidence of siderosis in iron turners and grinders.' *Br. J. ind. Med.* **3**, 78–82

Cameron, J. D. (1970). (Group Medical Officer, Pilkington Bros Ltd.) Personal communication

Challen, P. J. R. (Ed.) (1965). *Health and Safety in Welding and Allied Processes.* (Institute of Welding) 2nd edition. London and Woking; Unwin

Champeix, J. and Moreau, H. L. (1958). 'Observations récentes sur les pneumoconioses par terre d'ocre.' *Archs Mal. prof. Méd. trav.* **19**, 564–573

Clarke, W. I. and Simmons, E. B. (1925). 'The dust hazard in the abrasive industry.' *J. Ind. Hyg.* **7**, 345–351

Cole, C. W. A., Davies, J. V. S. A., Kipling, M. D. and Ritchie, G. L. (1964). 'Stannosis in hearth tinners.' *Br. J. ind. Med.* **21**, 235–241

Collis, E. L. (1931). 'Occupational dust disease.' *Bull. Hyg.* **6**, 663–670

Cooper, D., Pendergrass, E. P., Vorwald, A. J., Maycok, R. L. and Brieger, M. (1968). 'Pneumoconiosis among workers in an antimony industry.' *Am. J. Roentg.* **103**, 495–508

Cutter, H. C., Faller, W. W., Stocklen, J. B. and Wilson, W. L. (1949). 'Benign pneumoconiosis in a tin oxide recovery plant.' *J. ind. Hyg. Toxicol.* **31**, 139–141

Davis, S. B. and Nagelschmidt, G. (1956). 'A report on the absence of pneumoconiosis among workers in pure limestone.' *Br. J. ind. Med.* **13**, 6–8

Doerr, W. (1952). 'Pneumokoniose durch Zementstaub.' *Virchows Arch. path. Anat. Physiol.* **322**, 397–427

Doig, A. T. (1955). 'Disabling pneumoconiosis from limestone dust.' *Br. J. ind. Med.* **12**, 206–216

— and McLaughlin, A. I. G. (1936). 'X-ray appearances of lungs of electric arc welders.' *Lancet* **1**, 771–775

— — (1948). 'Clearing of X-ray shadows in welder's siderosis.' *Lancet* **1**, 789–791

Doll, R. (1959). 'Occupational lung cancer, a review.' *Br. J. ind. Med.* **16**, 181–190

Duggan, M. J., Soilleux, P. J., Strong, J. C. and Howell, D. M. (1970). 'The exposure of United Kingdom miners to radon.' *Br. J. ind. Med.* **27**, 106–109

Dundon, C. C. and Hughes, J. P. (1950). 'Stannic oxide pneumoconiosis.' *Am. J. Roentg.* **63**, 797–812

Dutton, W. F. (1911). 'Vanadiumism.' *J. Am. med. Ass.* **56**, 1648

Einbrodt, H. J. and Hentschel, D. (1966). 'Tierexperimentelle Untersuchungen mit Arbeitsplatzstäuben ans einem Hüttenzememtwerk. *Int. Arch. Gewerbepath. Gewerbehyg.* **22**, 354–366

Enzer, N. E., Simonson, E. and Evans, A. M. (1945). 'Clinical, physiological observations on welders with pulmonary siderosis and foundry men with uncomplicated silicosis.' *J. ind. Hyg. Toxicol.* **27**, 147-158

Fairhall, L. T. and Hyslop, F. (1947). *The Toxicology of Antimony.* Suppl. to Publ. Hlth Rep. No. 195. U.S. Treasury Dept.

Faulds, J. S. and Stewart, M. J. (1956). 'Carcinoma of the lung in haematite miners.' *J. Path. Bact.* **72**, 353–366.

Fiori, E. (1926). 'Contributo alla clinica e alla radiologia delle pneumoconiosi rare.' *Osp. magg.* **3**, 78-84

Fischer, H. W. and Zinnerman, G. R. (1969). 'Lung retention of stannic oxide.' *Archs Path.* **88**, 259–264

Foá, V. (1967). 'La pneumoconiosi dei pulitori di oggetti metallici.' *Medna Lav.* **58**, 588–602

Gardner, L. U. (1935). *Experimental production of Silicosis.* U.S. Publ. Hlth Rep. 50, pp. 695–702

— Durkan, T. M., Brumfield, D. M. and Sampson, H. L. (1939). 'Survey in seventeen cement plants of atmosphere dusts and their effects upon the lungs of twenty-two hundred employees.' *J. ind. Hyg. Toxicol.* **21**, 279–318

Goldstein, B. (1965). Quoted by Sluis-Cremer, G. K. and du Toit, R. S. F. (1968) q.v.

Gregory, J. (1970). 'A survey of pneumoconiosis at a Sheffield steel factory.' *Archs envir. Hlth* **20**, 385–399

Harding, H. E. (1948). 'The toxicology of zircon: preliminary report.' *Br. J. ind. Med.* **5**, 75–76

— and Davies, T. A. L. (1952). 'The experimental production of radiographic shadows by the inhalation of industrial dusts. Part II. Zircon.' *Br. J. ind. Med.* **9**, 70–73

Heuck, F. and Hoschek, R. (1968). 'Cer-pneumoconiosis.' *Am. J. Roentg.* **104**, 777–783

Holt, P. F. (1967). *Pneumoconiosis*, p. 177. London; Edward Arnold

Hublet, P. (1968). 'Enquête relative au risque de pneumoconiose dans la fabrication des ciments de construction.' *Arch. belg. Méd. soc.* **26**, 417–430

Hudson, T. G. F. (1964). *Vanadium. Toxicology and Biological Significance.* Ed. by E. Browning. Amsterdam, London and New York; Elsevier

Hunnicutt, T. N., Cracovaner, D. J. and Myles, J. T. (1964). 'Spirometric measurements in welders.' *Archs envir. Hlth* **8**, 661–669

Huston, J., Wallach, D. P. and Cunningham, G. J. (1952). 'Pulmonary reaction to barium sulphate in rats.' *Archs Path.* **54**, 430–438

Jenny, M., Battig, K., Horisberger, B., Havas, L. and Grandjean, E. (1960). 'Arbeitsmedizinische Intersuchung im Zementfabriken.' *Schweiz. med. Wschr.* **90**, 705–709

Karajovic, D. (1957). 'Pneumoconiosis in workers of an antimony smelting plant.' *Proceedings of the 12th International Congress on Occupational Health, Helsinki*, Vol. 3, pp. 370–374

Karlish, A. J. (1962). 'Idiopathic pulmonary haemosiderosis with unusual features.' *Proc. R. Soc. Med.* **55**, 223–225

Kleinfeld, M., Messite, J., Keoyman, O. and Shapiro, J. (1969). 'Welder's siderosis.' *Archs envir. Hlth* **19**, 70–73

Ladoo, R. B. (1960). 'Abrasives.' In *Industrial Minerals and Rocks*, p. 18. Ed. in Chief, J. L. Gillson. New York; Am. Inst. Mining, Metal and Petrol Engineers

Lévi-Valensi, P., Drif, M., Dat, A. and Hadjadj, G. (1966). 'Á propos de 57 observations de barrytose pulmonaire.' *J. fr. Méd. Chir. thorac.* **20**, 443–454

McCallum, R. I. (1963). 'The work of an occupational hygiene service in environmental control.' *Ann. occup. Hyg.* **6**, 55–63

— (1967). 'Detection of antimony in process workers' lungs by X-radiation.' *Trans. Soc. occup. Med.* **17**, 134–138

— Day, M. J., Underhill, J. and Aird, E. G. A. (1971). 'Measurement of antimony oxide dust in human lungs *in vivo* by X-ray spectrophotometry.' In *Inhaled Particles 3*, pp. 611–618. Ed. by W. H. Walton. London and Woking; Unwin

McLaughlin, A. I. G., Grout, J. L. A., Barrie, H. J. and Harding, H. E. (1945). 'Iron oxide dust and lungs of silver finishers.' *Lancet* **1**, 337–341

Mancuso, T. F. and Hueper, W. C. (1951). 'Occupational cancer and other health hazards in a chromatic plant: a medical appraisal. I. Lung cancer in chromatic workers.' *Ind. Med. Surg.* **20**, 358–363.

Mellissonos, J. C., Collet, A. and Daniel-Moussard, H. (1966). 'Étude expérimentale d'un émeri naturel des cyclades.' *Int. Arch. Gewerbepath. Gewerbehyg.* **22**, 185

Miller, J. W. and Sayers, R. R. (1934). 'Physiological response of peritoneal tissue to dusts introduced as foreign bodies.' *Publ. Hlth Rep., Wash.* **49**, 80–89

Morgan, W. K. C. and Kerr, H. D. (1963). 'Pathologic and physiologic studies of welder's siderosis.' *Ann. int. Med.* **58**, 293–304

Nappée, J., Bobrie, J. and Lambard, D. (1972). 'Pneumoconiose au cérium.' *Archs Mal. prof. Méd. trav.* **33**, 13–18

Natural Environmental Research Council (1971). *Statistical Summary of the Mineral Industry.* 1964–1969. London; H.M.S.O.

Oyanguren, H., Schüler, P., Cruz, E., Guijon, C., Maturana, V. and Valenzuela, A. (1957). 'Estañosis: neumoconiosis benigna debida a inhalacion de polvo y humo de estaño.' *Revta méd. Chile* **85**, 687–695

Pancheri, G. (1950). 'Su alcune forme di pneumoconiosi particolarmente studiate in Italia.' *Medna lav.* **41**, 73–77

Pendergrass, E. P. and Pryde, A. W. (1948). 'Benign pneumoconiosis due to tin oxide. A case report with experimental investigation of the radiographic density of tin oxide dust.' *J. ind. Hyg.* **30**, 119–123

Posner, E. (1960). 'Pneumoconiosis in makers of artificial grinding wheels, including a case of Caplan's syndrome.' *Br. J. ind. Med.* **17**, 109–113

Preti, L. and Talini, P. C. (1939). 'La pneumoconiosi da bario nel quandro radiologica.' In *Bericht u. den VIII Internat. Kongr. fur Unfallund. und Berufskrankheiten. Leipzig.* pp. 963–965

Prior, J. T., Crouk, G. A. and Ziegler, D. D. (1960). 'Pathological changes with the inhalation of sodium zirconium lactate.' *Archs envir. Hlth* **1**, 297–300

Prosperi, G. and Barsi, C. (1957). 'Sulle pneumoconiosi dei lavatori del cemanto.' *Rass. Med. Ind.* **26**, 16–24

Reed, C. E. (1956). 'Effects on the lung of industrial exposure to zirconium dust.' *A.M.A. Archs ind. Hlth* **13**, 578–580

Renes, L. E. (1953). 'Antimony poisoning in industry.' *Archs ind. Hyg.* **7**, 99–108

Riddell, A. R. (1934). 'Clinical investigation into the effects of gypsum dust.' *Can. Publ. Hlth J.* **25**, 147–150

Robertson, A. J. (1960). 'Pneumoconiosis due to tin oxide.' In *Industrial Pulmonary Diseases*, pp. 168–184. Ed. by E. J. King and C. M. Fletcher. London; Churchill

— and Whittaker, P. H. (1955), 'Radiological changes in pneumoconiosis due to tin oxide.' *J. Fac. Radiol.* **6**, 224–233

— Rivers, D., Nagelschmidt, G. and Duncomb, P. (1961). 'Stannosis: Pneumoconiosis due to tin oxide.' *Lancet* **1**, 1089–1095

Roussel, J., Pernot, C., Schoumacher, P., Pernot, M. and Kessler, Y. (1964). 'Considérations statistiques sur le cancer bronchique du mineur de fer du bassin de Lorraine.' *J. Radiol. Électrol.* **45**, 541–546

Rubin, L., Slepyan, A. H., Weber, L. F., Neuheuser, I. (1956). 'Granulomas of the axillas caused by deodorants.' *J. Am. med. Ass.* **162**, 953–955

Sander, O. A. (1958). 'Roentgen re-survey of cement workers.' *A.M.A. Archs ind. Hlth* **17**, 96–103

Sayers, R. R., Dallavalle, J. M. and Bloomfield, S. G. (1937). *Occupational and Environmental Analysis of the Cement, Clay and Pottery Industries.* Public Hlth Rep. U.S. No. 238, pp. 1–50.

Schepers, G. W. H. (1955). 'The biological action of rare earths. II.' *A.M.A. Archs ind. Hlth* **12**, 306–316

— and Durkan, T. M. (1955). 'Pathological study of the effects of inhaled gypsum dust on human beings.' *A.M.A. Archs ind. Hlth* **12**, 209–217

— — and Delahant, A. B. (1955). 'The biological effects of calcined gypsum dust. An experimental study on animal lungs.' *A.M.A. Archs. ind. Hlth* **12**, 329–347

Shelley, W. B. and Hurley, H. J. (1958). 'The allergic origin of zirconium deodorant granulomas.' *Br. J. Derm.* **70**, 75–99

Sjöberg, S. (1950). 'Vanadium pentoxide dust.' *Acta med. scand.* Suppl. 238

Sluis-Cremer, G. K. and du Toit, R. S. F. (1968). 'Pneumoconiosis in chromite miners in South Africa.' *Br. J. ind. Med.* **25**, 63–67

Smith, A. R. and Perina, A. E. (1948). 'Pneumoconiosis from synthetic abrasive materials.' *Occup. Med.* **5**, 396–402

Spedini, F. and Valdini, P. L. (1939). 'Contributo allo studio della pneumoconiosi da barite.' *Radiologia med.* **26**, 1–31

Spencer, G. E. and Wycoff, W. C. (1954). 'Benign tin oxide pneumoconiosis.' *Archs ind. Hyg.* **10**, 295–297

Tebrock, H. E. and Mackle, W. (1968). 'Exposure to europium-activated yttrium orthovanadate. *J. occup. Med.* **10**, 692–696

Vaccarezza, R. A. (1950). *Higiene y Salubridad en la Industria del Cemento Portland. Su investigación en las Fábricas Argentinas.* Buenos Aires; Guillermo

Vernhes, A. and Roche, S. H. R. (1955). 'Quelques considérations sur la silicose des travailleurs de l'ocre.' *Presse méd.* **63**, 975–978

Vintinner, F. J., Vallenas, R., Carlin, C. E., Weiss, R., Macher, C. and Ochoa, R. (1955). 'Study of the health of workers employed in mining and processing vanadium ore.' *Arch. ind. Hlth* **12**, 635–642

Waterhouse, D. F. (1951). 'Histochemical detection of barium and strontium.' *Nature, Lond.* **167**, 358–359

Wende, E. (1956). 'Pneumokoniose bei Baryt und Lithoponcarberten.' *Arch. Gewerbepath. Gewerbehyg.* **15**, 171–185

Williams, N. (1952). 'Vanadium poisoning from cleaning oil fired boilers.' *Br. J. ind. Med.* **9**, 50–55

Worth, G. and Schiller, E. (1955). 'Gesundheitsschädigungen durch Chrom und seine Verbindungen. *Arch. Gewerbepath. Gewerbehyg.* **13**, 673–686

Wyers, H. (1946). 'Some toxic effects of vanadium pentoxide.' *Br. J. ind. Med.* **3**, 177–182

Wynn-Williams, N. and Young, R. D. (1956). Idiopathic pulmonary haemosiderosis in an adult.' *Thorax* **11**, 101–104

7—Diseases due to Free Silica

It is sometimes suggested that lung disease due to various forms of free silica is now so uncommon as to be of little significance as an occupational hazard. And, although it is true that, numerically, there has been a pronounced over-all reduction in both the risk and prevalence of silicosis in Britain and most major industrial countries by comparison with the 1940s and earlier, it remains important for the following reasons:

(1) In a few industries the risk and prevalence of silicosis has fallen very little, or even increased as, for example, among granite workers in Austria, Sweden and Singapore (*see* Prevalence).

(2) As siliceous minerals are ubiquitous they may be encountered at any time in a multitude of work processes. A serious risk may exist if their presence is not recognized or if the fact that exposure to large concentrations of siliceous dust for a short period of time can cause rapid onset of disease is not understood. There is a particular possibility of this occurring in newly developing countries where there are areas of intensive industrial expansion.

(3) There is—and will be for some years to come—a 'survivor population' of unknown size with silicosis.

(4) The fact that silicosis is now comparatively uncommon increases the necessity for clinical vigilance to differentiate it promptly from other lung disorders.

(5) Silicosis, unlike other forms of pneumoconiosis, predisposes significantly to the development of pulmonary tuberculosis.

Lung disease caused by free silica is of four different types which are best treated separately:

(a) Characteristic hyaline and collagenous nodular lesions due to dusts having a substantial content of quartz or flint. That is, the 'classical' or 'pure' form of *nodular silicosis*.

(b) Ill-defined, irregular, stellate fibrotic lesions due to the combined effect of dusts consisting of a mixture of free silica and an inert mineral—most commonly, iron oxide. This is referred to as *mixed dust fibrosis* (*Mischstaubpneumokoniosen*).

(c) Predominantly diffuse interstitial fibrosis (fibrosing 'alveolitis') often with a fairly well developed cellular component, caused by calcined diatomaceous earth—*diatomite pneumoconiosis*. Some cases in this group may exhibit similar microscopic features to those which characterize the last group.

(d) Alveolar lipoproteinosis-like lesions and diffuse interstitial fibrosis (fibrosing 'alveolitis'). Unlike the other three, disease in this group develops rapidly in weeks or months and can, therefore, reasonably be called '*acute silicosis*', although this term has sometimes been used to denote nodular silicosis of unusually quick development following heavy dust exposure.

I. 'PURE' OR NODULAR SILICOSIS

The term 'silicosis' should be limited to the characteristic nodular, hyaline fibrosis caused by free silica and not be used in a more general way.

SOURCES OF EXPOSURE

'Free silica' dusts consist of quartz or flint, sometimes tridymite or cristobalite (or mixtures of any of these) and, rarely, of chert.

In Britain, flint is obtained mainly as a by-product of the quarrying of chalk for the cement industry (*see* Chapter 6). Flint nodules are separated, washed and then graded by hand; no risk is attached to this process. The best grade goes to the pottery industry for which the nodules are calcined at about 600 to 1,100°C and ground, usually in a ball-mill, during which a dust hazard may exist. Ground calcined flint is also used in mastic asphalt for roofing, making a finishing surface for timber and brickwork, and occasionally in the manufacture of refractory bricks. A silicosis risk may exist in these processes. *Flint clay* is not related to flint in any way and is a kaolinitic, non-plastic refractory clay.

Chert has a very limited use, chiefly for lining ball-mills and as a raw material in certain refractories (the second may offer some dust risk), but until recent years it was employed as an abrasive 'sand'-blasting agent for cleaning the stonework of buildings—potentially a most hazardous occupation.

The dust risk is usually evident (as in quarrying, drilling and tunnelling quartz-containing rocks) but may be unsuspected by those not conversant with the details of an industrial process. For example, quartz may be encountered during mining and crushing the harmless rock, gypsum (*see* Chapter 6) or during processing the montmorrilonite clay, bentonite (Phibbs, Sundin and Mitchell, 1971).

Although the 'free silica' hazard has, in recent years, been greatly reduced or eliminated in major industrial countries, nevertheless, in some work places (often small) it still remains or has increased. As silicon dioxide is ubiquitous in Nature it is evident that it will always be available as a potential risk wherever there is an unsatisfactory standard of dust control and industrial hygiene, or where the risk is not recognized.

Only crystalline and cryptocrystalline (or microcrystalline) forms of silica are considered in this section, quartz and cristobalite being the most important members of the crystalline group, and flint, chert and chalecedony, the most important of the cryptocrystalline group.

(1) Mining, quarrying and tunnelling of siliceous rocks

Mining

During the mining of gold, tin, copper and mica, drilling, hewing, shovelling, crushing and the use of explosive charges are all productive of much dust. Wet rock drilling, introduced in 1897 but not widely used until about 1920 (Holman, 1947), is only partly successful in suppressing dust even when wetting agents are employed.

The major goldfields are in the Transvaal, the U.S.S.R., Canada, the U.S.A. and Australia. The ore usually occurs in quartz veins associated with granite masses.

Tin mining is carried on mainly in West Malaysia, Bolivia, Thailand and China. The Cornish tin-mines have produced little ore for many years past but are at present being redeveloped. Tin ore lies in relation to rocks of the granite family.

Mica, which is found in rocks of high quartz content (such as pegmatite veins), is a rich source of quartz dust during mining, crushing and milling, hence silicosis may occur (Government of India Ministry of Labour, 1953; Thiruvengadam et al., 1968). The United States of America and India are the largest mica-producing countries.

Sandstone or other siliceous sedimentary rocks may be encountered in some coal-mines during shaft sinking and the development of tunnels and roadways.

Quarrying

Granite quarrying.—The quartz content of granite varies from 10 to about 30 per cent. Quarrying is done with powered drills, wire belt saws fed with an abrasive slurry (usually aluminium oxide) and, in some quarries since the early 1950s, by a flame cutter in which the combustion of oxygen and fuel oil fed through a nozzle produces a flame with a temperature of over 2,800°C; a stream of water accompanies the flame and when they are directed against the rock it disintegrates into fragments. The flame cutter produces a dust consisting of crystalline quartz particles, the concentration of which appears to be low (that is, less than 10 ppcf), and other particles less than 0·1 μm diameter which are apparently formed by vaporization of the granite (Burgess and Reist, 1969). The significance and possible effects of these submicron particles upon the lungs requires further study, but as they undoubtedly consist of 'fused silica' (quartz glass) owing to the high temperature (*see* Table 2.1) they may be expected, like Aerosil particles, to have little fibrogenic potential (*see* page 205).

Small quarries still rely on simple methods with little mechanization. Change to elaborate mechanization in large quarries has increased the concentration of dusts.

Sandstone quarrying.—This is carried on in many countries. In the United Kingdom quarries are worked in Cornwall, the Forest of Dean, Lancashire, Cumberland, Yorkshire and Scotland. The quartz content of the stone is always high. It is obtained by drilling and 'channelling' and, if hard, by the use of light blasting charges. It may be cut further and rough hewn in the quarry.

Slate quarrying.—Sericite (white mica) is the most abundant constituent of slates but the quartz content of some may be as high as 20 to 30 per cent.

The chief slate-producing countries are the U.S.A. (Maine, Pennsylvania, Vermont and Virginia), the British Isles (North Wales—until recently the largest slate-producing area in the world—Cornwall, and Tipperary and Cork in Southern Ireland), France and Germany. Welsh slate has a particularly high quartz content, especially that from Blaenau Ffestiniog.

The fact that the quartz content of slates is variable, and is low in some, probably explains the widely different prevalence of silicosis observed in this industry in different regions.

Exposure to dust occurs during quarrying, in the sawmills where the slate is cut into blocks, and during the splitting of blocks to specified thickness and size by hand or machine. Sawing and splitting are usually done at the quarry site. Slate is still used for the manufacture of electric panels and switchboards, billiard and other table tops, and fireplaces. It is cut, trimmed and polished in the factory—activities which are also dusty.

Tunnelling.—In civil engineering, cutting tunnels and excavation for a variety of purposes may be serious and often unsuspected hazards, especially as ventilation is usually poor. Driving sewer tunnels (which may be called 'construction work') and digging graves in sandstone, both of which have caused silicosis, are the sort of examples which can be easily overlooked.

(2) Stone cutting, dressing, polishing, cleaning and monumental masonry

These stones (known as 'dimension stone' in the U.S.A.) include rough building stone, cut stone, ashlar, pavement flags, curbing and monumental stone. The most important materials for these, from the standpoint of silicosis, are sandstone and granite.

Quarried sandstone is cut by hand or machine, dressed, shaped and drilled for building and ornamental purposes, often in closed sheds, and until some 20 years ago (and rarely still) was fashioned into grindstones. Masons and their helpers who work the stone on benches (known as bankers) are likely to be exposed to high concentrations of dust when hygiene measures are inadequate. In some quarries the stone is crushed and sieved on site for road materials. This is a very dusty process although in the open air.

Men restoring or cleaning sandstone buildings with powered tools may be exposed to high local concentrations of dust.

Quarried granite is cut to specified sizes by wire or gang saws (a gang saw employs steel shot and water), ground to a desired contour or profile, and polished. In large factories these procedures are highly mechanized and subjected to local and background exhaust ventilation, but in small firms mechanical methods may be limited. Fine cutting and finishing work is done with pneumatic hand tools. Designs and inscriptions are cut through stencils by abrasive blasting.

Where standards of local and general exhaust ventilation and enclosure are high—as in the Vermont granite industry (Hosey, Trasko and Ashe, 1957)—the prevalence of silicosis has greatly decreased, but where these are lacking or deficient, it tends to be higher than in non-mechanized factories.

Monumental masons and curbstone dressers were, and occasionally still are, liable to be exposed to dust without protection.

169

(3) Abrasives

Sandstone is now rarely used for the manufacture of grindstones, but such grindstones may still be found in use. Crushed sand, sandstone and quartzite have been used for metal polishes and scouring powders, and flint or quartz are crushed and graded to make sandpaper. Tripoli (*see* Chapter 2) is crushed and made into compositions for finishing and buffing metals, and ground rottenstone is used as a base for polishes.

Crushing and pulverizing these materials and mixing and sieving them during manufacture may give rise to a substantial dust hazard, but today the machinery is usually enclosed.

Although for thirty years or more it has been known that high dust concentrations of powdered quartz and flint used in the manufacture of abrasive soaps and scouring powders may cause rapidly progressive silicosis, their use in domestic scouring powders in the United Kingdom has only recently been discontinued. Feldspar is often employed as a substitute.

(4) Glass manufacture

Pure beach and river sands are employed to produce glass and, until the mid-1960s, sand of graded particle size was used in the form of a slurry to grind and polish plate glass. Subsequently the 'float glass process' (Pilkington, 1969) has largely replaced the previous techniques for manufacturing plate glass in most major glass industries in the United Kingdom and other countries. The earlier grinding and polishing methods, therefore, have now been abandoned by large companies but may still survive in small firms.

(5) Fillers

Finely ground quartz-containing rock is used for some paints and as a filler in the rubber industry; Neuburg chalk (Neuburger Kieselkreide), which contains a high percentage of quartz (Schneider, 1966), is commonly used in Germany. Fillers employed in the manufacture of gramophone records from about 1908 to 1948 (when microgroove records were introduced) included powdered slate and rottenstone of about 10 μm or less particle size. This practice was discontinued in 1948 because of the need to reduce the signal–noise ratio in the new records (E.M.I., 1970).

Exposure is most likely to occur during the production of fillers but may exist to a variable degree during their use.

(6) Abrasive blasting

The principle of this technique consists of propelling abrasive grains at high velocity at a target by means of compressed air, water under pressure, or a controlled centrifugal force. The grains may be quartzose sands, flint or chert (sandblasting); but corundum, iron garnet [usually almadine, $Fe_3Al_2(SiO_4)_3$] and silicon carbide, which do not cause pneumoconiosis, are also used. All are previously ground to specified grain size. Steel shot (shot blasting) has commonly replaced the siliceous grains for some years past, but is more costly, tends to be less hard and deteriorates when stored. Hence, sandblasting has by no means been eliminated from industry and is apparently still extensively employed in the United States of America.

Sandblasting is used to clean metal castings and to remove 'burnt-on' moulding sand, in the preparation of metal surfaces for painting or enamelling, for cleaning building stone and concrete, and renovating stone veneer; for making inscriptions on memorial stones, and to etch glass and plastics.

If the size of the articles to be blasted is suitable, the process can be enclosed and operated by remote control and, although this does not expose the operator to dust, significant concentrations of dust may be encountered when he enters the cabinet or cleans out detritus from the floor or trap beneath. When enclosure is not possible (for example, sandblasting ships or buildings) the operator must wear a special helmet supplied with uncontaminated air—preferably compressed air to prevent the entry of dust particles.

It should be remembered that even when non-siliceous abrasives are used to clean metal castings the dust produced from 'burnt-on' moulding sand may contain large amounts of quartz. Until recent times this was a notorious hazard and dangerous exposure may still be encountered.

(7) Foundry work

Free silica dust is produced in iron and steel foundries in the following ways:

(a) Moulding
(b) Application of parting powders
(c) 'Knocking out' or 'shaking out' of castings
(d) Dressing, fettling and abrasive blasting of castings
(e) Contamination of foundry floors
(f) Maintenance and repair of refractory materials.

(a) A mould is normally made of highly refractory quartzose sand bonded with a clay (such as china clay or ball clay) and placed in a cast-iron or wooden box which splits into two or more parts. The sand is sufficiently plastic to take the 'pattern', or shape, of the casting to be made. If the casting is to be hollow a core of the desired shape is constructed from oil-bonded sand or plastic, and baked to impart strength.

When molten metal is poured in, the sand is subjected to a high temperature (about 1600°C in the case of steel) and this is sufficient to convert some of the quartz to cristobalite, which is strongly fibrogenic (see Chapter 4). It may be re-used many times over for other moulds.

For a number of years some foundries have used zircon sands as a substitute for quartzose sands, but these have the disadvantage of being costly. Olivine sands are also used; olivine consists of magnesium and ferrous orthosilicate and is non-fibrogenic in animals (King et al., 1945).

(b) Some moulds require dusting with a 'parting powder' which gives increased resistance to thermal shock when the molten metal is run in. Powders of high free-silica content have been generally used for this purpose. Inevitably this was a dusty process and, in the United Kingdom, has been controlled since 1950 by the Foundries (Parting Materials) Special Regulations which forbid the use of materials having more than 3 per cent of silicon dioxide by weight of dry material. Replacement with zircon powders is now common.

(c) After the metal has cooled, the mould and core are separated—that is, 'knocked out' or 'shaken out'—from the casting. This is also a very dusty job and a most important potential source of exposure. If the size of the cast is small enough it can be enclosed with the vibrating table which performs the task automatically, but large casts must be done by hand.

(*d*) Sand which is adherent, or burnt on to the casting, must be removed— a process known as 'fettling', 'roughing-off' or 'stripping'. Larger areas are chipped off by hammer and chisel; smaller areas are smoothed down with portable grinding wheels of carborundum or emery which is another source of iron oxide dust. Some castings are finished by abrasive blasting (*see* previous section). Small castings are cleaned in a revolving cylindrical mill which may contain steel balls (ball-mill) as an additional abrasive agency.

All fettling operations are potentially very dusty and various methods of enclosure and exhaust ventilation are applied to eliminate or reduce the dust. In the United Kingdom both the 'knock out' and fettling processes are controlled by the Iron and Steel Foundries Regulations, 1953, and abrasive blasting specifically regulated by the Blasting (Casting and other Articles) Special Regulations, 1949.

Iron foundry fettling tends to produce a mixed dust consisting of different proportions of iron oxide and quartz which is an important cause of 'mixed dust fibrosis' described later in this chapter.

(*e*) At one time all foundries had earth floors and such floors are still occasionally to be found because they have the advantage that they can be dug up to make large moulds; their disadvantage, however, is that they become highly contaminated with siliceous dust which it is impossible to eradicate.

Conditions similar to those in iron and steel foundries may be met in some non-ferrous foundries, especially brass foundries, and in the United Kingdom are controlled by the precepts of the Joint Standard Committee in Safety Health and Welfare Conditions in Non-Ferrous Foundries (1957).

(8) Ceramics

Ceramics may be defined as 'man-made articles which have been first shaped or moulded from a wide range of natural earths, minerals and rocks, and then permanently hardened by heat' (Adams, 1961).

The three main ceramic groups are defined and the essential features of Technical Ceramics and Structural Clay Products summarized in Chapter 2. Only *Pottery* and *Whiteware*—that is, bone china, porcelain and earthenware —and *Refractory Ceramics* are considered here. The manufacture of *Structural Clay Products*, the raw materials of which consist of argillaceous clays, does not normally present a 'silica risk'. But an exception to this exists in the case of some types of wall and fireplace tiles in which flint and ball clay are used and have caused, and may still cause, silicosis in men who manufacture and cut ('tile slabbers') the tiles.

(*a*) *Chinaware, porcelain, stoneware and earthenware*

The raw materials for china ware ('bone china') are china clay, china stone (that is a granitic rock containing quartz and feldspar of which a high-quality form called 'Cornish Stone' is found in the United Kingdom near St Austell), and calcined animal bone; those for stoneware are similar apart from the bone, and some fireclay (a fine-grained equivalent of ganister) may be added. The ingredients for porcelain and vitreous china are china

172

and ball clays, feldspar and quartz or flint; those for earthenware are china and ball clays, feldspar and flint but fireclay is added for some products such as sinks. The free silica content of china clay in the refined state necessary for the ceramic industry is 2 to 3 per cent; of ball clay, 5 to 25 per cent; and of natural red clay, about 30 per cent (H.M. Factory Inspectorate, 1959).

Briefly, the manufacturing processes are as follows. Non-plastic raw materials such as china stone, feldspar, fireclay, quartz and calcined flint are crushed and milled, and converted into a 'slip' by the addition of water. The plastic clay materials are also converted into a 'slip'. After the removal of contaminants the 'slips' are mixed, the mixture pumped through a press where most of the water is extruded and, if required in a plastic state for shaping, the contained air is expelled in a 'pug mill'. The final mixture is known as 'body'.

Crushing and milling calcined flint and quartz produces 'free silica' dust but the wet process does not. However, spillage and subsequent drying of non-plastic 'slip' and 'body' on benches, equipment, the floor and operatives' clothes can be a serious source of siliceous dust if the environmental conditions are not vigorously controlled by satisfactory standards of monitoring of airborne dust, local and general exhaust ventilation and special protective clothing worn by the operatives (see Health Conditions in the Ceramics Industry, 1969). Even so, the risk may not be wholly eliminated (see Prevention).

Next, 'body' is shaped on a revolving wheel (this is known as 'jollying' or 'jiggering') or pressed into the shapes desired by machine presses. If the shapes are complex, 'body' is liquefied and poured into a plaster-of-Paris (gypsum) mould ('slip-casting'), the mould allowed to dry before opening. Obviously, dried 'body' is a source of dust.

As china ware 'body' contains no flint it might be thought to offer no silicosis risk. However, silicosis has been observed in exposed workers (Posner, 1961) due, undoubtedly, to the high quartz content (about 30 per cent) of 'Cornish Stone'.

The rough surfaces and edges of the ware produced is fettled, usually by women, by applying small knives, abrasive rags and tow to the ware as it stands on a revolving wheel. This operation (known as 'towing') produces much dust and requires to be strictly controlled.

All shaped ware is then kiln fired between 900° and 1,200°C according to the type of ware (Adams, 1961). When removed from the kiln the ware is known as 'biscuit'. In the British pottery industry before about 1937 ware to be fired was placed in powdered flint for support in fireclay 'saggars'. This exposed kiln workers to high concentrations of 'free silica' dust and, consequently, there was a high prevalence of silicosis. Since that date, flint has been replaced by calcined alumina with the result that silicosis among these workers has been virtually eradicated (Posner and Kennedy, 1967).

Finally, 'biscuit' ware is glazed with liquid glaze and refired at from 1,050 to 1,400°C. The glaze usually consists of feldspar, quartz, borax, sodium carbonate and zinc oxide; except for the pulverization of quartz during preparation and the drying of glaze spillage, it does not appear to offer any risk. When ware is decorated a third 'on glaze' firing at lower temperatures

173

is required. Certain types of ceramics are fired at 1,200°C or more in order to produce in the ware a large concentration of cristobalite because this possesses a very high thermal expansion.

It should be noted that large numbers of women are employed in the pottery industry.

In the United Kingdom pottery manufacture is regulated by the Pottery (Health) Special Regulations, 1947, and the Pottery (Health and Welfare) Special Regulations, 1950.

In the United States of America, Finland and Denmark, wollastonite (see Chapter 2) is used as a substitute for flint, quartz sand, feldspar and china clay in 'body' and in 'glazes' with a consequent reduction in the potential silicosis hazard. For economic reasons of import costs and plant design it is little used in the United Kingdom other than in certain glazes and fluxes. Investigations into the possibility of synthesizing anhydrous calcium metasilicate are being conducted by the British Ceramic Research Association (Andrews, 1970).

(b) Refractory ceramics

The most important group in the present context are referred to as *acid refractories*. These include lining bricks of various sorts, cements and different types of shaped ware. Bricks and cements are used in kilns, steel furnaces, ovens in gas-making plants, boiler houses and domestic hearths.

The raw materials—ganister or 'silica rock' (that is, quartzite sandstones, sands or grits) which have a very high quartz content—are crushed (usually in dry pans), milled, screened to desired size and mixed with a controlled quantity of water and, in some cases, with small amounts of paper-mill waste and 'milk of lime'. Power presses shaped the resulting material into bricks, or it is made into shapes by hand or by the 'slip casting' method. The bricks and shapes are dried in ovens or on heated floors and then fired in a tunnel kiln at about 1,450°C. Before the bricks are fired they may be dusted with quartzite sand to prevent adherence, and this is afterwards retrieved, sieved and used again. With recurring exposure to high temperature a significant proportion of the quartz is transmuted into tridymite and cristobalite.

The end-product is referred to as 'fireclay brick' when the raw material is ganister, and as 'silica brick' when it is 'silica rock'.

Obviously this process is capable of producing large concentrations of siliceous dust.

Kiln bricklayers and others who maintain and dismantle the refractory bricks of ovens, furnaces, kilns and retorts ('retort setting') are exposed to dust from disintegrating bricks, and, in repair work, there may be an additional hazard in that the interstices of the bricks are often grouted with asbestos fibre mixed with water at the site, or with dry fibre or asbestos rope. This source of asbestos exposure is referred to in context in Chapter 9.

A coarse-grained quartzose sand with natural clay bonding is used to line the dams and runners of blast furnaces. These 'cast house' or 'runner' sands may be a source of dust.

Because, in the presence of small amounts of alkali, quartz converts to cristobalite at temperatures of about 1,200°C instead of about 1,400°C (*see*

Chapter 2) cristobalite is the principal constituent of 'silica' refractories and may also be present in many pottery bodies. Moreover, in the temperature range 1,150 to 1,250°C flint converts to cristobalite more readily than quartz and, in the presence of alkali (for example, chalk), cristobalite may be formed at a temperature as low as 950°C. In view of the fact that cristobalite is apparently more fibrogenic than quartz (Chapter 4) it may enhance the severity of the resulting lung fibrosis.

Neutral refractories are made from chrome ore, aluminium oxides or sillimanite mixed with a small quantity of plastic clay and fired at temperatures of 1,450 to 1,650°C. Under these circumstances aluminium oxides do not appear to offer any pneumoconiosis risk. Sillimanite is referred to in Chapter 9.

'*Basic*' *refractories.*—Refractory bricks and other materials are made from magnesium, chert-free dolomite and olivine rock, and they do not present any 'free silica' risk.

(9) Boiler scaling

The tubes, flues and fireboxes of boilers require cleaning and scaling at regular intervals. Coal-fired boilers collect ash and concretions which consist of quartz (derived from roof and floor rock seams of coal-mines), carbon, iron, silicates and carbonates from coal combustion. The composition is variable but the relative amounts of quartz, iron and carbon in the dust influences the type of lung lesion which may be produced. This is referred to in the next section.

Cleaning is done with brushes, hammer and chisel, and compressed air jets in enclosed and restricted spaces so that dust concentrations are high.

Ash deposited in the gas passages, flues and smoke stacks of oil-fired boilers contains no quartz but occasionally has a high content of vanadium which is naturally present in large quantity in some oils—particularly Venezuelan oil (McTurk, Huis and Eckhardt, 1956) (*See* Chapter 6).

It is worth noting that boiler scalers have often worked in close proximity to bricklayers dismantling and replacing refractory brick linings and may, therefore, have been exposed to quartz dust from this source. Furthermore, they may have been present during periodic relagging of boiler and neighbouring installations with asbestos insulating materials and even assisted the laggers.

(10) Vitreous enamelling

Enamel consists of quartz, feldspar, metal oxides and carbonates in variable quantities. These ingredients are pulverized, mixed and then fused at temperatures up to 900°C. Although the heat converts much of the quartz to silicates some remains unchanged. The resulting sinter (referred to as 'frit') is ground with water in a ball-mill and further quantities of the ingredients may be added. The mix is enamel. The process may be dusty. Enamel spraying in particular may present a hazard, especially when the inner surfaces of vessels are sprayed (Friberg and Öhman, 1957). Nowadays spraying is done in booths with special exhaust ventilation and the sprayer wears a respirator; nevertheless, the potential danger remains.

An additional risk is encountered when some enamelled objects are 'finished off' by sandblasting.

INCIDENCE AND PREVALENCE

Until World War II, silicosis was the most important and widespread form of pneumoconiosis. But since then, due mainly to substitution by other materials and hygienic measures, the incidence of new cases appears to have declined dramatically in the majority of industrial countries. But accurate statistics are rarely available as they are often based on compensation figures and, therefore, on selected cases; diagnostic criteria vary and, in some countries, coal pneumoconiosis is bracketed with 'silicosis'.

Furthermore, reliable information about the size of populations at risk is lacking.

As Table 1.2 shows, the incidence of 'new' cases in the United Kingdom is low. In the United States of America, although the disease has been virtually eliminated from the Vermont granite (Hosey, Trasko and Ashe, 1957) and metal mining industries (Flinn *et al.*, 1963), there is reason to believe that the prevalence is not otherwise decreasing (Ayer, 1969). Some increase (often due to single industrial processes) has been reported in Bulgaria, Spain (WHO, 1968), Sweden (Ahlmark and Bruce, 1967) and Singapore (Khoo and Toh, 1968). In Finland there has been no change over a thirty-year period ending in 1964, and it is anticipated that the annual number of new cases will rise in the next few years (Ahlman, 1968).

It is of interest that surveys of the granite industry in Cornwall and Devon in 1951 and 1961 (Hale and Sheers, 1963) showed little reduction in the silicosis risk and that Grundorfer and Raber (1970) found an increase among granite workers of lower Austria since 1958 due mainly to granite crushing for gravel production. Granite crushing is particularly hazardous when, as in Austria, it is a skilled and continuous occupation, but it is unlikely to be so when workers are casual and unskilled as, for example, they usually are in Sweden (Ahlmark, Bruce and Nyström, 1960) and the United Kingdom (Hale and Sheers, 1963).

A survey in an English steel foundry between 1955 and 1960 showed an average prevalence rate of silicosis (diagnosed radiographically) of 6·4 per hundred—the rate in the fettling shop being seven times higher than in the foundry itself—and 2·8 per hundred among furnace liners (Gregory, 1970).

In short, nodular silicosis is still to be reckoned with as a cause of respiratory disability and in differential diagnosis.

Pathogenesis

The evolution of silicotic nodules consists first of the formation of collagen as a result of the cytological events referred to in Chapter 4, followed later by hyalinization of the fibrous tissue as the nodules mature. Although IgG and IgM have been recorded as occurring among, and bound to, the collagen fibres and fibrohyalin of human silicotic nodules (Pernis, 1968), there is no evidence to show that a specific antigen-antibody reaction is involved in pathogenesis (*see* Chapter 4). But circulating rheumatoid factor may be found in high titre in some cases of silicosis with enhanced activity in the absence of tuberculosis and irrespective of whether rheumatoid arthritis is present or not. Thus, it is possible that some form of immunological activity, as yet unexplained in detail, may enhance local tissue damage. And though this is

176

still to be proved, the fact remains that the naked-eye and histological appearances differ from those of typical silicotic nodules and resemble Caplan-type coal nodules (*see* Chapter 8), although the pigment content is less. Unfortunately, no epidemiological studies of circulating antibodies in silicosis appear to have been done and, hence, their prevalence in this disease is unknown.

The possible operation of a genetic influence has been little explored, but a survey of a large number of fluorspar miners and their families in Sardinia appears to have uncovered evidence that a predisposition for some persons to develop silicosis and for others to resist it may be genetically determined (Gedda *et al.*, 1964).

Pathology

Macroscopic appearances

The pulmonary pleura is usually thickened due to fibrosis and is often adherent to the parietal pleura especially over the upper lobes and in the vicinity of

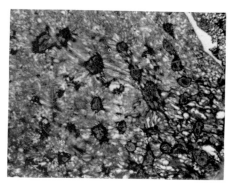

Figure 7.1. Natural size photo-graph of part of an upper lobe containing discrete silicotic nodules. Note their whorled pattern and that dust pigmenta-tion is generally slight

underlying conglomerate lesions. Thickening and symphysis may be extensive but only slight when there are no subpleural nodules.

Nodules are readily felt in the unopened lung and when it is cut are seen to vary from 2 to 6 mm in diameter, to have a whorled pattern (*Figure 7.1*) and to be grey-green to dark grey in colour. Similar lesions may be seen in the hilar nodes.

Both discrete nodules and conglomerations of nodules tend to be distributed more in the upper halves of the lungs than in the lower, and more in their posterior than anterior parts; but exceptions to this are seen. When conglomerations of nodules (which may sometimes be large enough to occupy an upper lobe) are examined by reflected light, or in whole-lung section against transmitted light, they are clearly seen to consist of closely fused individual nodules (*Figure 7.2*). Unlike confluent coal pneumoconiosis (progressive massive fibrosis) conglomerate lesions rarely develop cavities in the absence of tuberculosis. In some cases discrete nodules and conglomerations are found subpleurally and when the conglomerate lesions are calcified and fused to dense pleural fibrosis, the lung is locally encased; this is sometimes referred to as 'cuirasse' (armour plate). Occasionally, a large unilateral conglomerate nodular mass occurs with little other evidence of silicosis (Fiumicelli, Fiumicelli and Pagni, 1964).

The gross appearances of nodular silicosis are quite distinct from those of coal pneumoconiosis but silicotic lesions are sometimes found in the lungs of coal-miners who have done much drilling of siliceous rock seams (*see* Chapter 8).

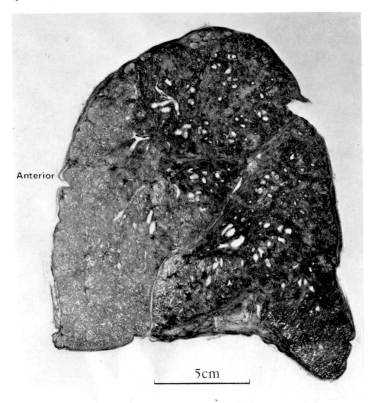

Figure 7.2. Conglomeration or matting together of silicotic nodules. Individual nodules can still be identified. Note the typical predominance of the lesions in the upper parts of the upper and lower lobes. (Paper-mounted whole sagittal section of left lung; by courtesy of Professor J. Gough)

Enlarged and fixed hilar and paratracheal lymph nodes occasionally cause distortion of the trachea, the main bronchi and branches of the pulmonary arteries near the hila (Pump, 1968), and similar pulmonary lymph nodes may restrict bronchial movements.

There appears to be a clear correlation between the amount of quartz per 100 g of lymph node tissue and the degree of calcification, and the possibility of endocrine disturbances playing some part in pathogenesis has been raised (Einbrodt and Burilkov, 1972).

Microscopic appearances

Dust particles are found either in macrophages or in the naked state in the walls of alveoli—chiefly those of respiratory bronchioles—and collected in perivascular areas. Cell death, fibroblast proliferation and reticulin formation occurs. The walls of affected alveoli are thereby thickened, in some places sufficiently to obliterate neighbouring alveolar spaces. Collagenous fibrosis follows in a concentric arrangement. Subsequently, much of the collagen becomes 'hyalinized' and the resulting near-spherical nodules consist of concentrically arranged, or whorled zones of acellular hyaline which are enclosed by a moderately cellular collagenous capsule; the cells are macrophages (which often contain carbon particles) and plasma cells (*Figure 7.3*). Giant cells are not seen. Silicotic hyaline resembles amyloid in having a higher content of carbohydrate and phospholipids than other forms of hyaline.

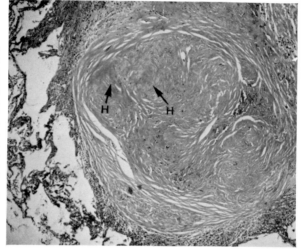

Figure 7.3. Photomicrograph of a typical silicotic nodule showing the concentric ('onion skin') arrangement of collagen fibres, some of which are hyalinized (arrowed), the cellular capsule and lack of dust pigmentation. The lesion is clearly demarcated from adjacent lung tissue which is normal. The appearances are those of a proliferative process. Compare with coal lesions (Figure 8.6) and asbestosis (Figure 9.4). (Original magnification ×55, reproduced at ×33; H and E stain

Silicotic nodules, by contrast with the lesions of coal pneumoconiosis (*see* Chapter 8), are 'proliferative' in that they contain an excess of collagen but little dust; indeed, the higher the quartz content of a dust the smaller the amount of dust required to produce a given severity of fibrosis (*see Figure 4.4*) (Nagelschmidt, 1965), and the longer quartz particles are retained in the lungs, the greater the fibrosis and the smaller the quantity necessary to cause fibrosis (Einbrodt, 1965). Continuous exposure to dust causes existing nodules to increase in size and new ones to form. But this progression may occur long after exposure has ceased and may be due either to a self-perpetuating tendency for quartz-containing macrophages to migrate and die in and around existing lesions (Heppleston, 1962) or, possibly, to the intervention of a secondary immunological reaction. The distinguishing features between typical and 'rheumatoid' silicotic nodules are referred to in a later section in this chapter and between silicotic nodules, 'rheumatoid' coal nodules and tuberculous lesions in Chapter 8.

The amount of quartz found in normal lungs exposed to industrial dusts has been estimated to be from 0·18 to 1·5 per cent of dried lung tissue and in normal hilar lymph nodes to be from 0·23 to 0·6 per cent of dried tissue (Sweany, Porsche and Douglass, 1936). In silicotic lungs the quartz content is in excess of 0·2 per cent of dried weight, commonly about 2 to 3 per cent, but may be as high as 20 per cent of the dried weight.

Alveoli in proximity to silicotic nodules are usually of normal size; occasionally scar (irregular) emphysema is seen, but is exceptional and of slight order as the nodules are proliferative and expanding. Associated centrilobular emphysema is not seen.

Nodules tend to occur in clusters and may subsequently fuse into conglomerations of varying size. These conglomerations are not amorphous masses, for individual nodules do not wholly lose their identity. It is to be noted that calcification (which is sometimes pronounced) may occur in some nodules in the absence of tuberculosis or histoplasmosis, the insoluble calcium salts being deposited mainly in the central hyaline (Moreschi, Farina and Chiappino, 1968). Central necrosis of nodules rarely occurs in the absence of complicating tuberculosis but occasionally results from ischaemic changes.

Quartz particles can be demonstrated in variable amount in the central zone of the nodules and as a halo round their periphery by accurately orientated polarized light (see Appendix) or by dark ground microscopy after microincineration of the lesions, but they are absent from the collagenous capsule.

The growth of peribronchiolar silicotic nodules may narrow or obliterate these airways, and perivascular nodules may cause obstruction of lymphatics and arteritis with eventual obliteration of some vessels and destruction of their walls. Larger elastic arteries are rarely obstructed but may be compressed.

In the rare case in which silicosis develops rapidly from the start and in which some additional unidentified determining factor (probably immunological) may play a part, the nodules are very numerous, small and lack the ordered pattern of typical nodules (*Figure 7.4*).

Much of the dust reaching the lymphatics passes to the hilar lymph nodes, but some travels to the internal mammary nodes and to more distant extrathoracic nodes, notably the supraclavicular, cervical and abdominal aortic groups. Particles gaining entry to the systemic blood stream may give rise to isolated nodules in the spleen (Belt, 1939) and liver (Lynch, 1942), but are too few to cause any functional damage.

Affected lymph nodes contain dense fibrosis or typical nodules with quartz particles. The capsular and peripheral regions of these nodes may calcify and resemble the shell of an egg. This change may appear early or late in relation to the evolution of the lung lesions, and may be present when silicotic lung disease is negligible. It has been suggested that this is due to an unusual propensity to deposit calcium salts (Chiesura, Terribile and Bardellini, 1968). There is no evidence that tuberculous infection is involved.

Tuberculosis

That silicosis predisposes to pulmonary tuberculosis has been established since the beginning of the century and in those days the majority of silicotics succumbed to it. In 1937 Gardner found evidence of co-existent tuberculosis in 65 to 75 per cent of silicotics from various industries. In recent years the rate has fallen dramatically in parallel with the general decline of tuberculosis but, nevertheless, it is still in excess of that in the general population. The more advanced the silicosis the greater the incidence of active tuberculosis is likely to be (Chatgidakis, 1963).

The enhancing effect of 'free silica' upon tuberculosis was demonstrated experimentally by Gardner (1929) by the reactivation of previously induced and healing tuberculous lesions in guinea-pig lungs after inhalation of a

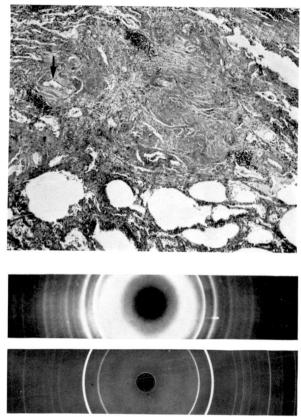

Figure 7.4

Microsection of lung from a case of rapidly
loping atypical silicosis in a man exposed to
concentrations of uncalcined quartzite sands.
e is only a suggestion of the ordered pattern
h characterizes the typical silicotic nodule;
sis, which is hyalinized in places, extends into
lar walls. Numerous plasma cells were
nt round these lesions. Occasional typical
les were also found (↓, artery). The radio-
hic features are shown in Figure 7.10. Cases
his sort are rare. (Original magnification
55, reproduced at ×33; H and E stain)

X-ray diffraction of the lung dust shows a
ong quartz pattern (by Dr F. D. Pooley)

Standard quartz pattern

quartz aerosol, and by the production of tuberculous lesions in guinea-pigs by a normally non-pathogenic strain of tubercle bacillus (RI) in the presence of quartz (Gardner, 1934). More recent experiments have confirmed the potentiating effect of quartz upon tuberculosis in guinea-pigs (Policard *et al.*, 1967) and the demonstration that this occurs at macrophage level has been referred to already in Chapter 4.

'Rheumatoid' silicotic nodules

Nodules of larger than average size (that is, 3 to 5 mm diameter), frequently with light grey necrotic centres, may be found in the presence of rheumatoid

181

arthritis or circulating rheumatoid factor without arthritis. The association was first described by Colinet (1953) in a woman who had been exposed to high concentrations of 'free silica' and has subsequently been observed by Hayes and Posner (1960) and others. To the naked eye they look like active tuberculous nodules and are easily misinterpreted as such, but acid-fast bacilli cannot be identified microscopically, nor can *M. tuberculosis* be isolated by culture or guinea-pig inoculation. In geographical areas where histoplasmosis is endemic this may be diagnosed in error but histoplasma cannot be identified in the nodules (Gough, 1959). Unlike the nodules of 'rheumatoid' coal pneumoconiosis, concentric black rings of deposited coal particles are not seen. (*See* Chapter 8.)

Microscopically, the lesions consist of an acidophilic, acellular necrotic centre in which there are the remains of collagen fibres, and at the periphery of the necrosis, fibroblasts are arranged in palisade form, although less prominently than in rheumatoid subcutaneous nodules. External to these is a zone of polymorphonuclear leucocytes and macrophages and there may be clefts containing cholesterol crystals. These are not seen in non-rheumatoid silicotic nodules. Outside this active zone are arranged normal reticulin and collagen fibres in various stages of maturation and numerous plasma cells, lymphocytes and fibroblasts. Endarteritis, consisting mainly of plasma cells and lymphocytes, is found in close proximity to the lesions. When activity in the nodules has ceased they may, like 'pure' silicotic nodules, become calcified.

Clinical features

Symptoms

It is important to emphasize that there may be no symptoms even though the radiographic appearances may be surprisingly advanced.

Cough may develop as the disease advances and is of variable severity, mainly in the mornings but sometimes intermittently throughout the day and night. In the later stages there may be prolonged and distressing paroxysms due, possibly, to irritation of nerve receptors in the trachea and bronchi by silicotic lymph node masses.

Often there is no sputum or only a small quantity of mucoid appearance raised from time to time during the day. However, in advanced disease recurrent bronchial infections tend to occur and produce quite a large volume of purulent sputum. There is no haemoptysis in the absence of complicating active tuberculosis.

Unless there is accompanying chronic obstructive bronchitis or allergic asthma there is no wheeze, although some patients who have narrowing, distortion and fixity of the trachea and main bronchi caused by contiguous silicotic nodes may complain of stridor (*see* next section), especially during effort when there is increased velocity of air flow. This is an uncommon symptom.

Breathlessness occurs as the disease advances, first during pronounced effort and later with lesser degrees of effort; it is rarely complained of at rest unless other lung disease is present. The presence and severity of dyspnoea and impairment of lung function correlates poorly with radiographic appearances.

Chest pain is not a feature of silicosis.

General health is unimpaired unless tuberculosis or congestive heart failure supervenes. Haemoptysis and loss of weight may signal the presence of tuberculosis.

Physical signs

The general physical condition is good but deteriorates with the onset of congestive heart failure and in the presence of tuberculosis. Central cyanosis is absent unless there is complicating heart or lung disease, and dyspnoea at rest suggests disease other than silicosis.

Finger clubbing is not caused by silicosis and when observed is either of congenital type or evidence of other pathology.

The chest contour is usually normal but in advanced disease there may be localized flattening of one upper zone possibly with some degree of dorsal scoliosis. Expansion remains good and equal until a late stage of the disease when it may be somewhat diminished often on one side (where underlying fibrosis is greater) more than the other.

The trachea is sometimes displaced to one side either by silicotic hilar node masses or a large distorted conglomerate mass in an upper lobe. Occasionally, hard, non-tender, silicotic lymph nodes are palpable in the neck and supraclavicular fossae.

Percussion note is unaffected unless there are areas of unusually dense pleural fibrosis—chiefly in the upper zones.

Breath sounds are normal or reduced by pleural thickening, and inspiratory and expiratory stridor (of greater or lesser intensity) may be heard over the trachea and at the open mouth when there is excessive distortion of trachea or main bronchi; when this sign is present it is persistent.

Adventitious sounds are not heard in disease uncomplicated by chronic obstructive bronchitis or tuberculosis.

In the advanced stage of silicosis the signs of right ventricular hypertrophy may eventually develop with or without those of congestive heart failure.

Investigations

Lung function

In the early radiographic stages of typical silicosis (ILO Category 2) impairment of any parameter of lung function is generally absent but in some cases slight reduction in VC and of arterial oxygen tension (on effort) may be observed. With more advanced disease, impairment is commonly present but often of a much less degree than the radiographic category might suggest. There is a decrease of TLC, VC, RV and FRC without evidence of airways obstruction and, in some cases, a slight reduction in gas transfer, although this is often remarkably little affected even in the presence of advanced disease. Oxygen desaturation is not present at rest or on moderate effort (300 kg.m/min) in the non-conglomerate stage of disease (Becklake, du Preez and Lutz, 1958), but may be observed on greater effort in some cases. As the disease progresses, inequality of gas distribution and of ventilation-perfusion ratio occurs resulting in some impairment of gas transfer in addition to the volume changes mentioned. Ventilation–perfusion imbalance and

183

arterial oxygen desaturation on effort are determined by the extent of arteritis as well as by silicotic fibrosis.

The best over-all guide to the degree of respiratory disability in conglomerate disease is the ventilatory capacity.

There is nothing characteristic in the patterns of impaired function in silicosis.

Radiographic appearances

The earliest radiographic evidence of nodular silicosis consists of small discrete opacities of moderate radiodensity which appear in the upper halves of the lung fields and vary from 1 to 3 mm diameter (ILO Category 'p' and 'q') (*Figure 7.5*). It has been claimed, however, that linear opacities accompanying

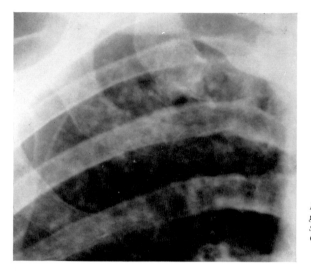

Figure 7.5. Discrete radiographic opacities of typical silicosis at an early stage. Category 'q'. (Natural size)

the normal vascular markings are the earliest evidence of silicosis but this is not generally accepted (Ashford and Enterline, 1966), and these appearances (of which it is difficult to be convinced) do not correlate with morbid anatomical evidence of silicosis.

There appears to be a clear relationship between total dust exposure and radiographic evidence of silicosis (Beadle, Sluis-Cremer and Harris, 1970).

As the disease advances, discrete opacities increase in number and size (ILO Category 'r') and occupy the lower as well as the other zones of the lung fields (*Figure 7.6*). In general they are roughly symmetrical in the two lung fields but are sometimes of disparate size and distribution. Small conglomerations (ILO Category A) may then appear—usually, but not always, in the upper zones—and subsequently develop into large and irregular opacities which may occupy the greater part of both lung fields. Bullae may be seen in the vicinity of conglomerations and there may be significant distortion of the trachea (*Figure 7.7*).

Progression may be slow and gradual over many years, may occur rapidly within a year or two, having been unchanged for years (*Figure 7.8*), or may not occur at all. These different patterns of behaviour appear to be determined mainly by the amount of siliceous dust inhaled but idiosyncratic reaction also appears to be involved. Sudden extension of abnormal opacities is most likely to be due to supervening tuberculosis but, where there is no evidence of this, it may be associated with circulating rheumatoid factor with or

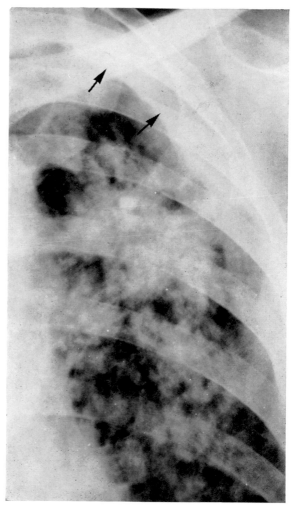

Figure 7.6. Moderately advanced silicosis with a conglomerative mass and discrete nodules in a foundry worker for 30 years. Note pleural thickening at apex of the lung (arrowed)

without the onset of rheumatoid arthritis; under these latter circumstances, signs of pleural effusion—usually unilateral—may also be present in some cases, and may recur on the opposite side.

Sometimes both discrete and conglomerate opacities are very dense due to the presence of calcification (*Figure 7.7*). These appearances are sometimes identical with those of calcified nodules in some cases of 'rheumatoid' coal pneumoconiosis. Cavitation is rarely seen in the absence of complicating tuberculosis. A unilateral conglomeration is occasionally seen without other evidence of silicosis.

Lymph node calcification is characterized by thin, very dense ring shadows around the nodes ('egg shell' calcification) and groups of nodes are involved, usually the hilar and pulmonary nodes (*Figure 7.9*), but sometimes extra-thoracic nodes are affected (Polacheck and Pijanowski, 1960). There is no correlation between the degree of hilar (and other) node calcification and the amount of silicosis or the presence of pulmonary tuberculosis (Chiesura,

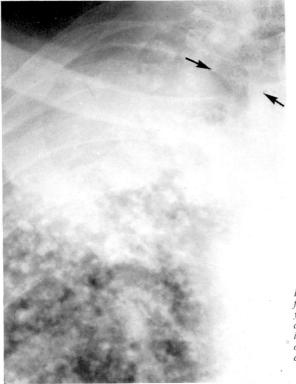

Figure 7.7. Radiograph of a fettler in an iron foundry for 26 years. Most of the small opacities represent calcified lesions. Note distortion and bowing of the trachea (arrowed) and apical thickening of the pleura

Terribile and Bardellini, 1968): it may be absent in the presence of advanced silicosis or prominent when there is little evident silicosis. Although not a pathognomonic sign—as it is occasionally seen in cases of sarcoidosis, tuber-culosis and histoplasmosis—it is highly suggestive of silicosis or exposure to free silica dust.

Evidence of pleural fibrosis is present in many cases and may be pro-nounced in advanced disease.

In those rare cases where there is rapid development of silicosis (*see* Microscopic Appearances) the radiographic appearances bear little resem-blance to those of typical silicosis and spontaneous pneumothorax may occur (*Figure 7.10*).

It is rarely necessary to employ other radiographic techniques than PA,

AP and lateral views for diagnosis, although tomography may be required to demonstrate a cavitated silicotuberculous lesion. Bronchography may demonstrate bronchial distortion, filling defects and localized bronchiectasis in cases with conglomerate masses.

Other investigations

Biopsy of lung tissue should not be required for diagnosis, although examination of a scalene lymph node may resolve occasional problematical cases by demonstrating silicotic nodules.

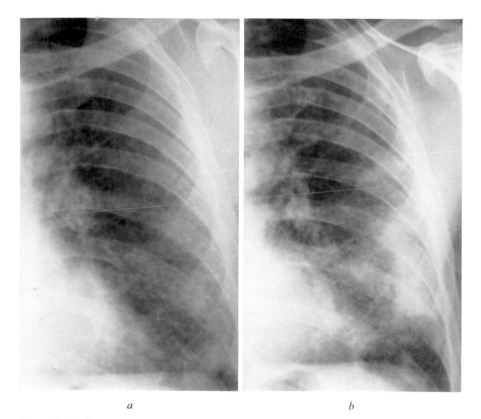

a   b

Figure 7.8. Silicosis in a man who worked 30 years as a tunneller in regions of siliceous rocks. Appearances in (a) had remained unchanged for years but progressed to those shown in (b) within 3 years. Unusual features of this case are that the lesions are predominant in the lower half of the lung field and that rheumatoid arthritis developed about 18 months before film (b); DAT, 1 : 128, ANF negative at the time of this film. No evidence of tuberculosis

It is advisable to obtain samples of sputum for culture of *M. tuberculosis* periodically, for life, as tuberculosis may develop at any time.

Tests for rheumatoid and antinuclear factors, when positive, point to the likely cause of suddenly advancing tuberculosis-negative silicosis.

Electrocardiography may be required in advanced cases to establish or refute the presence of cor pulmonale.

Investigations for sarcoidosis may be indicated on rare occasions to distinguish the two diseases (*see* next section).

The erythrocyte sedimentation rate is not raised in the absence of complicating tuberculosis or other disease.

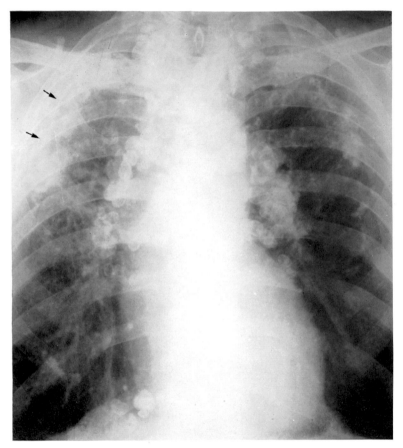

Figure 7.9. This radiograph of a man who worked 55 years in various processes in the manufacture of siliceous refractory bricks shows egg-shell calcification of many lymph nodes. Not only are hilar nodes involved but nodes of the paratracheal and mediastinal groups, the internal mammary chains and the cervical groups are similarly affected. (Egg-shell calcification of cervical nodes can also be seen in Figure 7.7.) Localized 'cuirasse' of the pleura is present in the right upper zone (arrowed) and the trachea is bowed. Egg-shell calcification of this extent is uncommon, the appearances being usually limited to the hilar nodes. Another notable feature of this case is the paucity of the pulmonary lesions of silicosis

Diagnosis

When a satisfactory occupational history is combined with good-quality radiographs, nodular silicosis should rarely be mistaken for other diseases. The chief cause of misdiagnosis is failure to recognize the 'silica' hazard of a past occupation, and the fact that the prevalence of silicosis is now low increases the possibility of this error.

An isolated conglomerate lesion (so-called 'silicoma') may be confused with bronchial carcinoma, especially in a first radiograph. Tomography may help in the distinction by revealing multiple small densities within a silicotic mass.

When silicotic lung lesions and hilar and pulmonary lymph nodes are calcified it is necessary to exclude:

(*a*) Tuberculosis

(*b*) Histoplasmosis

(*c*) Sarcoidosis. Confusion should rarely arise here but it has to be remembered that pulmonary and hilar node sarcoid lesions may calcify (Israel *et al.*, 1961; Scadding, 1967) and present a similar radiographic appearance, and non-calcified silicotic lesions in women (from past work in the pottery industry, for example) might initially be confused with sarcoid.

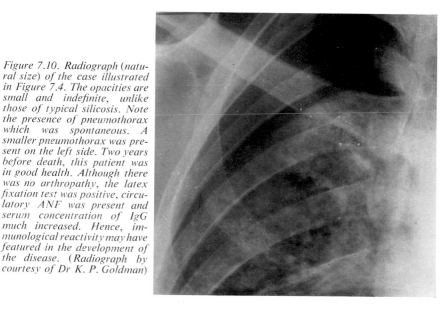

Figure 7.10. Radiograph (natural size) of the case illustrated in Figure 7.4. The opacities are small and indefinite, unlike those of typical silicosis. Note the presence of pneumothorax which was spontaneous. A smaller pneumothorax was present on the left side. Two years before death, this patient was in good health. Although there was no arthropathy, the latex fixation test was positive, circulatory ANF was present and serum concentration of IgG much increased. Hence, immunological reactivity may have featured in the development of the disease. (Radiograph by courtesy of Dr K. P. Goldman)

(*d*) Pulmonary alveolar microlithiasis. This rare disorder may occasionally be simulated radiographically by silicosis when the lesions are very small and calcified (*Figure 7.11*).

(*e*) Calcified lung lesions as a sequela of chicken pox are usually few in number, small (about 2 to 3 mm diameter) and are not accompanied by the egg-shell sign of hilar node calcification.

Complications

(1) Tuberculosis

Silicosis is the only pneumoconiosis which predisposes to the development of tuberculosis. Although the incidence of tuberculosis in silicosis has fallen dramatically since the 1950s it is still the most common complication. It may occur at any stage in the evolution of silicosis, but is most likely in the fifth and later decades in association with a moderate to severe degree of silicosis (Chatgidakis, 1963; Jones, Owen and Corrado, 1967).

In the early stage of the tuberculous disease it is difficult or impossible to recognize any change in the established radiographic appearance of silicosis, and there may be no symptoms; a recently developed cough with scanty greenish sputum may, however, give a warning signal. Subsequently the characteristic symptoms develop, sometimes with haemoptysis. Rapid radiographic changes consistent with tuberculosis are then seen, possibly with evidence of cavitation. When the disease is of indolent nature, or after healing, scar emphysema with bullae may be detected radiographically in the areas of fibrosis.

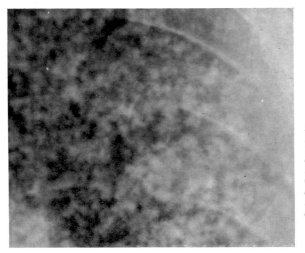

Figure 7.11. Radiograph of a North Wales slate quarry worker for 7 years. These opacities were widespread throughout both lung fields (Category 3q) and, although a little larger, resemble pulmonary alveolar microlithiasis. The lesions were probably calcified. (Natural size)

It must be remembered, however, that photochromogenic and non-photochromogenic mycobacteria are sometimes isolated from the sputum of silicotic subjects (Schepers *et al.*, 1958). These organisms may occasionally be found in association with *M. tuberculosis* (Palmhert, Webster and Lens, 1968) and, in general, are probably not pathogenic, but *M. avium* (*see* Chapter 4) is a serious, if rare, complication and is poorly sensitive to anti-tuberculous therapy; *M. kansasii* is also pathogenic. The pathogenicity of these organisms is probably potentiated by quartz and other forms of free silica and the importance of distinguishing these organisms from *M. tuberculosis* is evident.

(2) Cor pulmonale

This may develop in some cases of advanced conglomerate silicosis but right ventricular failure due to this cause (contrary to popular belief and many textbook descriptions) supervenes in only a small proportion, in whom, however, death is likely to occur in congestive heart failure. Co-existent chronic obstructive lung disease may be an important contributory factor in some of these cases, and the likelihood of cor pulmonale causing death is significantly increased when there is complicating tuberculosis by contrast with silicosis alone (Becker and Chatgidakis, 1960).

(3) Bronchitis

Episodes of acute and subacute bronchitis due to infection in deformed and rigid bronchi may occur in advanced stages of silicosis, but there is no correlation between chronic obstructive bronchitis, which is very largely associated with cigarette smoking, and silicosis (*see* Chapter 1).

(4) Emphysema

Although small areas of scar ('irregular') emphysema are sometimes observed around nodules and larger bullous areas of the same type of emphysema may be related to conglomerate lesions, emphysema is not a feature of silicosis. Centrilobular and panlobular types of emphysema may be present but are not pathogenically related to silicosis.

(5) Spontaneous pneumothorax

Spontaneous pneumothorax is an uncommon complication caused by the rupture of a bleb or bulla and the resulting pneumothorax is usually localized due to the limitations imposed by pleural symphysis. For this reason it may be unsuspected unless detected fortuitously by radiography. Rarely it may be bilateral and fatal (*Figure 7.10*).

(6) Segmental and middle lobe collapse

On rare occasions compression or occlusion of smaller bronchi by enlarged silicotic lymph nodes causes an area of lung collapse.

(7) Rheumatoid syndrome

The progression of silicosis and the appearance of the lesions in the presence of rheumatoid arthritis or rheumatoid factor without rheumatoid arthritis has already been alluded to and are important in that they are likely to be mistaken for active tuberculous disease. Eleven cases (2 per cent) of 'rheumatoid modified' silicotic nodules were found in 576 autopsies on European gold-miners studied at the Johannesburg Pneumoconiosis Research Unit (Chatgidakis and Theron, 1961), and cases have been recorded during life in women in the German pottery industry (Otto, 1969).

(8) Scleroderma (progressive systemic sclerosis)

An unusually high incidence of scleroderma has been reported among gold-miners (Erasmus, 1960), coal-miners, stone-masons and pottery and foundry workers with pneumoconiosis (Rodnan *et al.*, 1966), although not a single case seems to have been observed in British coal-miners (Rogan, 1960). Byrom Bramwell, in 1914, first drew attention to the association of silicosis and scleroderma (which he attributed to the holding of cold chisels) in stone-masons.

This would seem to be a chance association but Rodnan *et al.* (1966) have advanced evidence suggesting that the prevalence of scleroderma is higher in workers with silicosis (or coal pneumoconiosis) than in the general population. Further investigation in which the standards of diagnosis are

191

clearly defined is necessary. Immunological factors which influence the lungs and other organs may play a part in pathogenesis, but there is no suggestion that silicosis (or any other pneumoconiosis) causes scleroderma via immunological or other agencies. Diffuse interstitial fibrosis (fibrosing 'alveolitis'), by contrast, is a well recognized manifestation of progressive systemic sclerosis (Hayman and Hunt, 1952).

(9) Carcinoma of the lung
Bronchial carcinoma occasionally occurs in silicotic lungs but there is no evidence of a causal relationship between it and silicosis; indeed, the incidence of lung cancer in miners with silicosis is significantly lower than in non-silicotic males (Miners Phthisis Medical Bureau, 1944; Rüttner and Heer, 1969).

The relationship of mine radioactivity to lung carcinoma is referred to in Chapter 12.

(10) Neurological
Irreversible abductor paralysis of the left vocal cord is a rare sequel of involvement of the left recurrent laryngeal nerve in a mass of silicotic lymph nodes (Arnstein, 1941). Obviously, all other possible causes of paralysis must be excluded before this diagnosis is accepted.

(11) Oesophageal compression
Oesophageal compression with dysphagia is another rare effect of large masses of silicotic lymph nodes (Longley, 1970).

Prognosis
In general, it is unusual for normal life span to be shortened or for invalidism to be produced by uncomplicated silicosis although respiratory symptoms may be present. However, in a proportion of cases, the disease progresses remorselessly to severe respiratory disability and death often many years after the responsible industry has been left. The likelihood of invalidism and death from cor pulmonale is increased by tuberculosis if not treated promptly and successfully, which, in the majority of cases, can be achieved today (see next section).

The finding of rheumatoid arthritis or rheumatoid factor alone may signal impending progression of the disease. When chronic obstructive bronchitis or emphysema, or both, are present with large conglomerate silicotic masses or silicotuberculosis, serious invalidism and death from this cause are virtually inevitable.

Treatment

(1) Prophylactic
Because it was shown that metallic aluminium dust is capable of preventing silicosis in experimental animals (Denny, 1939), inhalation of aluminium aerosols by men with silicosis and those exposed to quartz dusts was advocated and widely employed from the early 1940s to the mid-1950s. Although it was claimed that development of silicosis and progression of existing silicosis

was prevented this has not been substantiated, and there appears to be no difference in the behaviour of the disease in treated and untreated groups (Kennedy, 1956). Experimental work in monkeys indicates that inhaled aluminium powder delays, but does not prevent, the appearance of silicotic lesions (Webster, 1968). There is the important additional feature that aluminium dust is itself capable of causing diffuse interstitial fibrosis (*see* Chapter 12).

(2) Therapeutic

There is at present no specific treatment available to halt the progress or cause resolution of human silicosis. As described in Chapter 4, PVPNO and related substances and polybetaine effectively prevent silicosis in experimental animals, but they are not suitable for use in man; for example, PVPNO is carcinogenic in animals and extremely slowly eliminated. However, a related compound, poly-2-vinylpyridine-1-oxide, is apparently neither toxic nor carcinogenic, and is at present undergoing clinical trial (Schlipköter, 1970).

Corticosteroids do not influence or halt the progress of the disease and are obviously dangerous in the presence of unrecognized tuberculous disease. They may cause resolution of a complicating 'rheumatoid' pleural effusion but, again, a tuberculous cause must be excluded.

Appropriate treatment may be required for congestive heart failure or for co-existent acute or chronic obstructive bronchitis. Unproductive paroxysmal cough requires the use of an appropriate cough suppressant drug.

Treatment of silicotuberculosis

Treatment of complicating tuberculosis demands a triple drug regime—streptomycin, PAS and isoniazid: streptomycin 1 g daily for not less than two months and PAS 10 g daily with isoniazid 200 to 300 mg daily for not less than two years in most cases (Keers, 1969). Quiescence of disease is thereby achieved in the great majority of cases; the poor results reported in the 1950s appear to have been due to inadequate regimens. However, a few individuals with advanced, cavitated silicotuberculosis may respond poorly and the development of drug resistance greatly increases the likelihood of failure and a fatal outcome.

Prevention

This depends upon the recognition of a 'free silica' hazard and upon a high standard of dust control and disposal which must be monitored by continual and random analysis of atmospheric dust in the work and 'background' areas. Whenever possible, a harmless material should be substituted.

The principles and methods of dust control are described in *The Prevention and Suppression of Dust in Mining, Tunnelling and Quarrying* by the ILO (1966) and, as they apply to the pottery industry, in *Health Conditions in the Ceramic Industry* (Davies, 1969).

The proposed TLV for 'respirable' quartz dust is given by the ACGIH (1971) in the following formulas:

$$\text{TLV in mppcf} = \frac{300}{\% \text{ quartz} + 10}$$

(*mppcf—million particles per cubic foot*)

$$\text{TLV for respirable dust in mg/m}^3 = \frac{10 \text{ mg/m}^3}{\% \text{ respirable quartz} + 2}$$

$$\text{TLV for total dust, 'respirable' and 'non-respirable'} = \frac{30 \text{ mg/m}^3}{\% \text{ quartz} + 3}$$

The TLV for tridymite and cristobalite is one-half the value calculated from the formulas for quartz.

II. MIXED DUST FIBROSIS

The term 'mixed dust fibrosis', coined by Uehlinger (1946) and adopted by Harding, Gloyne and McLaughlin (1950), applies to lesions caused by quartz and other dusts inhaled simultaneously at the one process and not to those due to dusts from different processes at different times.

When the proportion of free silica to non-fibrogenic dust in the total dust inhaled is low, the typical nodular lesion of silicosis either does not occur or is infrequent, and irregular fibrotic lesions are produced. The commonest non-fibrogenic dusts are iron oxides.

Sources of exposure

Occupations in which 'mixed dust fibrosis' have occurred most commonly are casting, fettling and sand or shot-blasting in iron, steel and non-ferrous foundries; hematite mining, although in the United Kingdom this has caused a negligible amount of fibrotic pneumoconiosis since the 1930s owing to dust suppression measures (Bradshaw, Critchlow and Nagelschmidt, 1962); cleaning and scaling boilers; and electric arc welding and oxyacetylene cutting in foundries where there has also been some exposure to siliceous dusts from neighbouring operations in addition to iron oxide fumes from the welding or cutting.

'Mixed dust fibrosis' has been well documented as occurring in iron and steel foundry workers (Uehlinger, 1946; Harding, Gloyne and McLaughlin, 1950; Ruttner, 1954; McLaughlin and Harding, 1956), non-ferrous foundry workers (Harding and McLaughlin, 1955), boiler scalers (Harding and Massie, 1951) and hematite-miners in some regions (Stewart and Faulds, 1934), and it may be found in potters. These lesions are also sometimes observed in welders who have worked in a foundry atmosphere.

Pathology

Macroscopic appearances

As in the case of nodular silicosis, the pulmonary pleura is often thickened to a variable degree and may be puckered where it overlies an intrapulmonary fibrotic mass. Distended bullae are sometimes present in these areas.

The cut surfaces of the lungs reveal irregular or stellate fibrous lesions which may vary in size from about 3 or 4 mm to confluent masses which may occupy the greater part of a lobe or lung. Characteristic, whorled, silicotic nodules are uncommonly seen either alone or within areas of fibrosis. Confluent lesions ('progressive massive fibrosis'—P.M.F.) may be present, irregular in form, and often not limited by the anatomical boundaries of lobes or segments. In some cases of hematite-miners they appear similar to the P.M.F. lesions of coal pneumoconiosis (*see* Chapter 8), though of reddish colour, and do not resemble the conglomerate masses of silicotic nodules. Cavitation is rarely found unless due to complicating tuberculous disease.

Both small and large lesions occur mainly in the upper halves and posterior zones of the lungs (but there are exceptions to this), and are rarely of similar size and distribution in the two lungs. Occasionally, only a few isolated lesions are present.

Grey-black pigment is intimately distributed through the lesions and in hematite lungs the fibrotic areas are, like the rest of the lungs, brick red in colour.

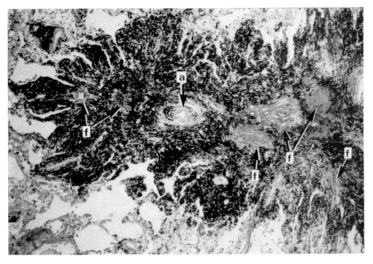

Figure 7.12. 'Mixed dust fibrosis' in an iron foundry worker. 'Medusa head' formation with much dust and randomly arranged collagenous fibrosis (f). Adjacent lung is normal (a indicates artery). (Original magnification, × 55, reproduced at × 33; H and E stain). Compare with Figure 7.3

Microscopic appearances

Iron and quartz particles accumulate in alveolar walls adjacent to respiratory bronchioles and small arteries. In lesions in which there is no quartz there is no reaction other than a slight increase of reticulin fibres (siderosis) but when small quantities of quartz are present there is fibroblastic activity leading to peribronchiolar and perivascular collagen fibrosis which obliterates neighbouring alveoli and spreads, to a greater or lesser degree, farther into the lung. Reticulin and collagen fibres are arranged in both linear and radial fashion so that individual lesions are of irregular or stellate ('Medusa head') form and not concentrically nodular (*Figure 7.12*). Separate silicotic nodules may occur, however, in some cases and occasionally both types of lesion are seen together, but the nodular component is usually immature and hyaline changes are absent. P.M.F. lesions consist of much dust which is mostly

195

extracellular, and randomly arranged, often hyalinized, collagenous fibrosis; but in other cases the fibrosis has the whorled appearance of nodular silicosis.

Scar (irregular) emphysema may be present around some 'mixed' lesions due to their concentration, and bullae with air-trapping may be found in relation to larger confluent masses. But scar emphysema is not a constant feature and in many cases it is absent or of very slight degree. Other types of emphysema which may be present are coincidental and not pathogenically related.

By contrast with nodular silicosis calcification does not occur in the 'mixed' lesions other than from healing of complicating tuberculosis.

Carbon, iron and other metallic dust particles are present in large quantity, and white doubly refractile particles may indicate quartz.

Pathogenesis
Lung dust in hematite-miners consists of hematite, quartz and mica, the quartz contributing 4 to 6 per cent of the total dust. This proportion of quartz resembles, but is rather more than, that in coal pneumoconiosis (Nagelschmidt, 1965), and, similarly to that pneumoconiosis, is not selectively concentrated in the P.M.F. lesions. The more advanced the fibrosis the higher the quartz content (Faulds and Nagelschmidt, 1962). Hematite does not give a Prussian blue reaction but intracellular haemosiderin at the periphery of the lesions does.

'Mixed dust fibrosis' appears to be due to modification of the effects of small quantities of 'free silica' (usually quartz) by the accompanying non-fibrogenic dusts. Iron oxide was early shown to inhibit the fibrogenic activity of quartz (Kettle, 1932) and, as hematite, it causes no fibrosis in experimental animals (Byers and King, 1961). According to McLaughlin (1957) the quartz content of the dust responsible for these lesions is under 10 per cent, but recent experimental work suggests that it may be appreciably higher than this (Goldstein and Rendall, 1970). If other factors play a part in pathogenesis they have not been identified. The incidence of complicating tuberculosis approaches that observed in nodular silicosis (Goldstein and Rendall, 1970) but there does not appear to be any evidence that it is involved in pathogenesis of the pneumoconiotic lesions.

Coal pneumoconiosis in some respects resembles 'mixed dust fibrosis' but there are reasons for regarding it as a distinct entity (*see* Chapter 8).

Clinical features

Symptoms, physical signs and lung function
The same considerations apply as in the case of nodular silicosis.

Radiographic appearances
When lesions in the lungs are small, the opacities they produce on the film may resemble those of discrete 'nodular' silicosis or coal pneumoconiosis; when larger, there are irregular opacities (usually in the upper and mid zones) which may be indistinguishable from those produced by fibrocaseous tuberculosis. As a rule, the well-demarcated opacities of discrete or conglomerate nodular silicosis are not observed. Calcification of lesions is not

seen unless caused by quiescent tuberculosis, and 'egg-shell' calcification of hilar lymph nodes does not seem to occur.

In iron-foundry workers, hematite-miners and boiler-scalers numerous small radiodense opacities due to siderosis may also be present throughout the lung fields.

Diagnosis

The most difficult task is to distinguish radiographically between 'mixed dust fibrosis' and healed or active tuberculosis, but the presence of cavities favours active tuberculosis. However, when there is an appropriate occupational history and sputum cultures are positive for tubercle bacilli, it is virtually impossible to exclude the presence of co-existent 'mixed dust fibrosis'.

Occasionally, isolated lesions when seen radiographically for the first time may suggest collapse-consolidation or bronchial carcinoma.

Complications

These are similar to those already described for nodular silicosis in regard to tuberculosis, cor pulmonale, chronic bronchitis, emphysema and the 'rheumatoid' changes. Circumscribed 'rheumatoid-modified' nodules with naked-eye appearances of alternating concentric rings of black pigment and yellow-grey tissue, and the microscopic features already described, have been observed in a foundry worker (Campbell, 1958) and a boiler scaler (Caplan, Cowen and Gough, 1958).

Tuberculosis complicates 'mixed dust fibrosis' less often than it does in nodular silicosis, but is substantially more frequent than in the general population.

Prognosis

This is much the same as in nodular silicosis but life expectancy is rarely shortened.

Treatment and prevention

The principles are exactly similar to those applying to nodular silicosis.

III. DIATOMITE PNEUMOCONIOSIS

Diatomite—known also as diatomaceous earth and kieselguhr—has already been referred to in Chapter 2. It is an amorphous form of silicon dioxide.

Origins

Commercially, the most important deposits occur in the United States of America (mainly in California, Nevada, Oregon and Washington), Denmark and Federal Germany. Although small quantities are produced in Scotland, Cumberland and Eire the United Kingdom relies upon imported diatomite mainly in the calcined form.

Mining and processing

Mining is done almost entirely by the open-cast method and crude diatomite is transferred to the processing plant where it is crushed, screened, re-crushed and put into storage bins for blending into qualities appropriate to various uses. Natural moisture is removed by hot-air heaters at about 260°C. It is then passed through a series of cyclones and separators to eliminate clays and other contaminants. Further processing may be done in the natural state but the greater part of the material is calcined. Calcination is done in a rotary kiln similar to that used in the manufacture of Portland cement at approximately 816 to 1,100°C; it removes organic matter and alters the structure and porosity, hence the filtration properties of the diatomite. This is referred to as *straight calcination* to distinguish it from *flux calcination* in which caustic soda or sodium carbonate is added to the diatomite as a flux before it enters the kiln and is subjected to about 1,100°C. Calcination has important implications in the pathogenesis of diatomite-induced lung disease. (*See* Pathogenesis and Pathology, this section.)

Both natural and calcined forms are next milled, passed again through separators to remove grit and coarse kiln material, then to a cyclone 'classifier' where they are divided into fine (particles less than 10 μm size, mainly 0·5 to 2·2 μm) and coarse products which are stored in baghouse hoppers and finally bagged. Straight calcined diatomite is tan coloured and flux calcined, white.

All these processes are potentially dusty but milling and bagging of calcined diatomite are the chief sources of a pneumoconiosis risk.

Processing diatomite is more advanced in the United States of America than elsewhere and world industrial demand, mainly of the calcined product, has greatly increased since World War II. A detailed description of the industry is given by Hull *et al.* (1953).

Uses of diatomite

(1) Filtration is the most important. It is used in calcined form as a filter aid in liquid form, and in the manufacture of filters for inorganic and organic liquids; especially in wine, beer and fruit juice production, the manufacture of pharmaceutical liquids and antibiotics (such as penicillin and streptomycin), and in sugar refining. It has to a large extent replaced asbestos filters which were widely used for this purpose until recently. Berkfeld filters are made from diatomite.

(2) Heat and sound insulation. It is made into refractory bricks, moulded blocks, or used as a binder for pipe covering and insulating cement, for boilers, pipes, stills, furnaces and kilns, and was (and still is) frequently mixed with asbestos fibre for insulation cements.

(3) As a filler for plastics, rubber, paper, insecticides, paints, varnishes, linoleums, floor coverings, fertilizers and in special types of paper.

(4) As an adsorbent for industrial floor sweeping powders and chemical disinfectants.

(5) As a mild abrasive in silver, metal and motor car polishes, dental pastes and hand soaps.

(6) Other uses are as a carrier for catalysts, a pozzolanic component of certain cements and concrete, for various types of building materials (board, sheets, tiles, blocks and plasters), and in electrode coatings for welding. In the United Kingdom, English and Irish diatomite is used especially in cement manufacture for which purpose it is calcined at a low temperature

to remove organic matter such as peat and, hence, is unlikely to contain a significant amount of crystalline 'silica'.

Apart from processing, therefore, exposure to diatomite (usually in calcined form) may occur to a varying degree in the manufacture of these products and when mixed by hand for insulation. Maintenance work on processing plant is also a potential source of exposure.

Prevalence

A survey in the diatomite processing industry in 1953–54 (Cooper and Cralley, 1958) showed that 25 per cent of 251 workers with more than 5 years' dust exposure and nearly 50 per cent of 101 workers exposed to high concentrations of calcined dust had radiographic evidence of pneumoconiosis which, in the main, indicated nodular and confluent lesions. The majority of these employees had been mill hands handling calcined material; there were no cases among the quarry workers.

Another radiographic survey of 869 diatomite workers revealed that of those who had been mill hands for more than five years 17 per cent had 'linear-nodular' ('simple') pneumoconiosis and 23·2 per cent confluent opacities of the ILO classification (Oechsli, Jacobson and Brodeur, 1961).

It is an uncommon pneumoconiosis. Its severity appears to correlate with the cristobalite content of the dust and duration of exposure.

Calcination was introduced into the industry in the early 1920s. Rigorous dust controls applied to one plant in the United States of America in the mid-1950s resulted in no new cases of pneumoconiosis occurring in workers recruited after that period (Cralley, Cooper and Caplan, 1966).

There appears to be no information on the prevalence among workers using calcined diatomite in the various manufacturing processes. The risk of developing pneumoconiosis is probably low but some cases may have passed unrecognized, being most likely to be interpreted as 'sputum-negative' fibrotic tuberculosis (*see Figure 7.15*).

Pathogenesis

The structural forms of silicon dioxide which may be found in diatomite has a crucial influence on its fibrogenic potential. Natural diatomite is non-crystalline (amorphous) and is associated with only minute quantities of quartz—less than 2 per cent in California, Nevada and Oregon (Cooper and Cralley, 1958)—and trace amounts of tridymite and cristobalite. When it is subjected to high temperature calcination, tridymite and cristobalite are formed at a rate directly related to the degree and duration of the applied heat (*see* Chapter 2); the cristobalite content may be about 21 per cent of the bag-house product (Cooper and Cralley, 1958). Flux calcination greatly facilitates the speed with which cristobalite is produced in the same temperature range as straight calcination (Bailey, 1947) in which case some 60 per cent cristobalite may be present in the bag-house product (Cooper and Cralley, 1958). *Figure 7.13* shows x-ray diffraction patterns of diatomite subjected to the different forms of calcination. The amount of cristobalite evolved is similar whether diatomite is of salt or fresh water origin (Cooper and Crally, 1958).

In experimental animals, natural diatomite causes infiltration of alveolar walls by macrophages, many of which contain dust particles, but no proliferation of connective tissue fibres (Tebbens and Beard, 1957); and in man there is no evidence that it causes lung fibrosis (Vigliani and Mottura, 1948; Luton *et al.*, 1956; Cooper and Cralley, 1958). By contrast, and as noted in Chapter 4, cristobalite is more fibrogenic than quartz in experimental animals (King *et al.*, 1953) and calcined diatomite has been shown to be fibrogenic in human lungs (Vorwald *et al.*, 1949). Uncalcined amorphous silicon dioxide is eliminated from the lungs more rapidly than either quartz or cristobalite (Klosterkötter and Einbrodt, 1965)—an indication of its lack of cytotoxicity.

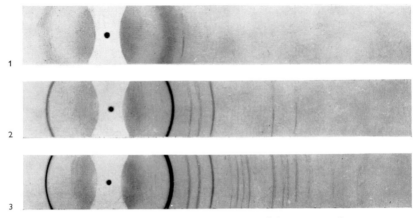

Figure 7.13. X-ray diffraction patterns of diatomite products.

(1) Crude diatomite. The presence of the diffuse band and the absence of lines indicates that this is non-crystalline or amorphous. (2) Straight calcined diatomite. The distinct lines are characteristic of cristobalite. (3) Flux calcined diatomite. Lines are further increased in intensity. Disappearance of the diffuse bands indicates conversion of amorphous silicon dioxide to cristobalite. (Reproduced by courtesy of Dr W. D. Wagner *et al.* (1968) and the Editor of the American Industrial Hygiene Association Journal)

The mean particle size of the final calcined product may be about 0·7 μm (Wagner *et al.*, 1968) which ensures penetration to the alveolar region.

Macroscopic appearances
The pulmonary pleura is often thickened.

Areas of fine and coarse, grey coloured, diffuse interstitial fibrosis of both linear and stellate form are seen in lung slices, usually in the upper halves of the lungs, although the lower halves may be involved; and the subpleural region is a common site of selection. It may be of slight or extensive order. Confluent masses of fibrosis may also be present, again chiefly in the upper zones, and may contain ischaemic cavities. Characteristic whorled silicotic nodules and conglomerations are absent.

There may be scar emphysema sometimes with bullae (especially in relation to areas of subpleural fibrosis), but often there is no emphysema.

Microscopic appearances
Early lesions consist of collections of dust-containing macrophages in alveoli,

alveolar walls and hilar lymph nodes with either no connective tissue reaction or with only a delicate reticulin proliferation (Carnes, 1954). As the lesions progress, diffuse collagen fibrosis occurs in the peribronchiolar and perivascular regions with much fibroblast activity and this extends into surrounding lung tissue as diffuse interstitial fibrosis producing thickening of alveolar walls and obliteration of adjacent alveolar spaces (*Figure 7.14*). The cellular

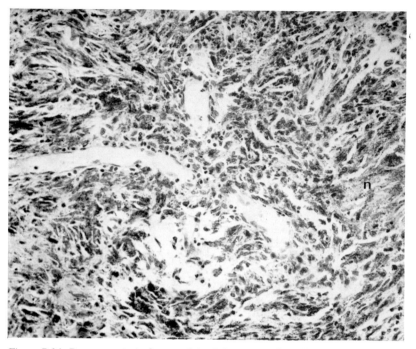

Figure 7.14. Pneumoconiosis due to calcined diatomite. The collagenous fibrosis lacks the arrangement of the typical silicotic nodule and the lesion is much more cellular. Areas of necrosis (n) are present. (Original magnification, × 225, reproduced at × 180; H and E stain. Section kindly supplied by Dr F. R. Dutra, California)

element is often prominent and the lesions, which show some predilection for the subpleural zone, may in places resemble the more cellular forms of asbestosis (Spain, 1965).

Many dust particles which can be identified as fragmented diatoms may be seen in macrophages and fibrous tissue and rather stubby, pseudoasbestos bodies with rudimentary segmentation are sometimes observed (Nordmann, 1943). The birefringence of cristobalite is low. Characteristic silicotic lesions do not occur, but 'hyalinization' may be seen in some areas of fibrosis (Vorwald *et al.*, 1949; Dutra, 1965).

The confluent masses consist of collagenous fibrosis—often unusually cellular—arranged in random fashion and showing little or no tendency to whorling. Necrosis may occur in them, sometimes with areas of calcification, due to ischaemic changes and in the absence of tuberculosis. Neighbouring blood vessels may be surrounded, and some obliterated by fibrosis.

Scar emphysema may be related to the lesions but this is not a constant finding and it appears to occur chiefly in the form of small localized bullae in the vicinity of the subpleural fibrosis.

Fibrotic lesions are also seen in the hilar lymph nodes. The quartz content of the lungs is low. In one study it was less than 2 per cent of the lungs by weight (Vorwald et al., 1949).

Clinical features

Symptoms

In general, respiratory symptoms are uncommon. When they occur they consist of morning cough, which may be non-productive, and a mild to moderate degree of breathlessness on effort; rarely, in advanced cases, there is disabling dyspnoea. Haemoptysis does not seem to occur.

Physical signs

Finger clubbing is not a feature of the disease (Cooper and Cralley, 1958).

There may be no abnormal signs but in some cases breath sounds in the upper halves of the lungs may be of bronchial type accompanied by inspiratory crepitations which may also be heard over the lower lobe regions in some cases. Signs of spontaneous pneumothorax can sometimes be elicited. In advanced cases the signs of upper zone fibrosis with tracheal displacement may be present.

Evidence of congestive heart failure due to cor pulmonale appears to be rare.

Investigations

Lung function

Comprehensive studies have been done by Motley, Smart and Valero (1956) and Motley (1960). As in the case of other types of pneumoconiosis, abnormal values correlate poorly with radiographic appearances and good pulmonary function may be associated with fairly extensive radiographic changes, but large confluent lesions are usually associated with abnormal function.

Maximum breathing capacity, timed FEV and FVC, may be slightly to moderately impaired, and arterial oxygen saturation often reduced in slight to moderate degree; RV is significantly increased and there may be some reduction in TLC and gas transfer (T_L). Uneven ventilation is present in some cases and, occasionally, there is pronounced airways obstruction.

Radiographic appearances

The earliest abnormality consists of linear or round ('nodular') opacities, or both ('linear-nodular'), in the upper and mid-zones of the lung fields and extending to their periphery. These appearances are sometimes fine and 'lace-like'. It is unusual for the discrete round opacities to exceed about 2 mm in diameter and they have low contrast with the surrounding tissues (Oechsli, Jacobson and Brodeur, 1961), rarely possessing the radiodensity of those due to nodular silicosis.

The opacities become more prominent as they coalesce and coalescent

202

lesions, which are at first indistinct, later appear as well-circumscribed homogeneous densities (ILO Category B or C). These are mainly in the upper zones and usually bilateral and may exhibit evidence of contraction,

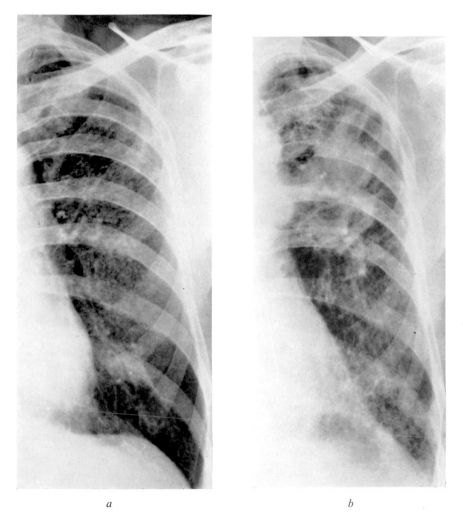

a   *b*

Figure 7.15. Diatomite pneumoconiosis in a man who spent 25 years in a processing mill with intermittent heavy exposure to flux calcined diatomite. He was removed from risk after the first film (a). The second film (b) was taken 10 years later. Tuberculin tests negative in 1953. Note the appearances of diffuse interstitial fibrosis in the lower zone. Right lung field similar.
(By courtesy of Dr W. Clark Cooper, Berkeley, Calif.)

distortion or cavitation, but rarely calcification. Appearances consistent with diffuse interstitial fibrosis may be seen in the lower zones, but have rarely been reported (*Figure 7.15*).

Enlargement or egg-shell calcification of hilar lymph nodes is not seen.

Other investigations

Apart from obtaining lung tissue for biopsy (which should rarely be necessary) there are none likely to give further assistance in establishing the diagnosis.

Diagnosis

This depends upon a history of an exposure of five or more years to calcined diatomite in processing or manufacture, and upon radiographic appearances.

Tuberculosis—active or quiescent—is the most important differential diagnosis.

Complications

There is an unusual tendency to spontaneous pneumothorax (Vigliani and Mottura, 1948; Smart and Anderson, 1952) although there is apparently no increased likelihood of tuberculosis. But when tuberculosis complicates diatomite pneumoconiosis it tends to pursue an indolent course (Smart and Anderson, 1952), and if cavitation is present, antituberculous treatment may fail to prevent relentless progression of the disease (Spain, 1965).

Prognosis

Progression to the stage of advanced confluent masses may occur years after the worker has left the industry with the disease in an early stage.

Life expectancy appears rarely to be shortened and cor pulmonale is probably exceptional. Occasionally, however, rapidly progressive disease may occur and end in fatal cor pulmonale (Luton *et al.*, 1956); this has chiefly been associated with disease due to flux calcined diatomite.

Treatment

There is no treatment to prevent or reverse the course of the disease.

Prevention

A rigid programme of dust control (monitoring of local and atmospheric dust, enclosure systems where possible, exhaust ventilation, good house-keeping and use of respirators) is necessary in diatomite processing and the use of the calcined form in manufacture. These measures, as noted already, have been applied in the major processing plants in the United States of America since the mid-1950s with excellent results.

The current Threshold Limit Value for natural diatomite is 20 mpccf, but for calcined diatomite (cristobalite) it is suggested that this should be 'one half the value calculated from the count or mass formulas for quartz'.

Submicron Amorphous Silicon Dioxide

Before concluding this section, brief reference must be made to the submicron forms of amorphous silicon dioxide which are now extensively used in industry: for example, as fillers for rubber, paints and paper; in cosmetics, inks, motor car polishes and electric light bulbs; as a diluent for insecticides and a carrying agent for catalysts. They are prepared by precipitation at high temperatures of sodium silicates (trade name Hi-Sil), hydrated calcium silicate (trade name Silene), or pure silicon tetrachloride (trade name Aerosil, Degussa or Dow Corning 'silica'). The content of non-crystalline silicon dioxide is about 99·8 per cent, and the crystalline and cryptocrystalline forms are absent. Particles are of uniform size and range from 5 to 40 nm (Volk, 1960). Neosyl, another hydrated silica precipitate, has a particles size of 100 to 200 μm but forms loose agglomerates of 1 to 10 μm diameter.

Experimental work has shown that rats exposed to these dusts exhibit no permanent lung damage, and guinea-pigs and rabbits have only a mild residual peribronchiolar and mural fibrosis (Schepers et al., 1957a, b). They appear, however, to exert an enhancing effect upon tuberculosis in guinea-pigs (Schepers et al., 1957c).

Surveys of workers to Hi-Sil and Silene (Plunkett and De Witt, 1962) and Aerosil (Volk, 1960), in which men were observed over periods of from 8 to 12 years, revealed no evidence of a pneumoconiosis or harmful effects.

Potentially, the most dusty areas in the production of these 'silicas' are the furnace room, and the bagging and loading departments but in recent years these have been controlled by dust-suppression measures.

It can be concluded that these materials are not likely to cause human pneumoconiosis.

IV. ACUTE SILICOSIS

By 'acute silicosis' is meant fibrosis of the lungs, or lesions similar to alveolar lipoproteinosis with a variable amount of interstitial fibrosis, of rapid development following intense exposure of short duration to dusts of high quartz content. Formed silicotic nodules are either not seen or are few in number in contrast with nodular silicosis of fairly rapid onset which is characterized by small immature nodules.

Sources of exposure

Attention was first drawn to this illness in workers in abrasive soap factories by Middleton in 1929 and subsequently by other authors (for example, McDonald, 1930; Chapman, 1932; Adler-Herzmark and Kapstein, 1937; Ritterhoff, 1941). Quartzite sand or sandstone were finely ground and mixed with anhydrous sodium carbonate and soap resulting in exposure to both siliceous and alkaline dusts; workers in the packing department were exposed to the mixed dusts. Today quartz is not considered a suitable abrasive for household soap powders as its hardness damages enamels and glass, nevertheless, as already stated, its use in domestic scouring powders has only recently ceased in the United Kingdom, and it is still used in non-domestic abrasive soaps.

However, exposure to high concentrations of quartz in the absence of alkalis occurs in various other ways and more important, notably, when tunnelling through rock of high quartz content (Gardner, 1933; Ashworth, 1970); when shovelling, loading and handling similar rock dusts in the holds of ships and other confined spaces, and when sandblasting with quartzite sands (Gardner, 1933; Buechner and Ansari, 1969). Indeed, any industrial process which produces very high concentrations of quartz or cristobalite of small particle size—especially if in a confined space—appears to be capable of causing this disease. Apparently sand is still frequently used in many countries for sand-blasting in spite of recommendations that it should be substituted by non-siliceous abrasives.

Incidence

The disease is undoubtedly rare. Conditions which cause it have been uncommon and its incidence may have been underestimated because the clinical, radiographic and pathological characteristics which are so different from those of 'nodular silicosis' may have not been attributed to an occupational hazard. Moreover, it has probably been diagnosed simply as tuberculosis which has, in fact, complicated some of the recorded cases.

Pathology

Macroscopic appearances

The pleura is usually much thickened and adherent and the lungs are voluminous, heavy and mostly airless.

When cut, there is grey-white consolidation interspersed by pink-red areas and widespread diffuse interstitial fibrosis which may be prominent in the upper halves of the lungs. A frothy or gelatinous fluid exudes from the cut surfaces. Silicotic nodules are either few and small or altogether absent.

Microscopic appearances

These are very variable but as Gilder pointed out some 30 years ago (McDonald, Piggott and Gilder, 1930; Chapman, 1932) they may consist of areas of acellular fibrosis, sometimes with hyaline centres, around which there is an intense small-cell infiltration; alveolar walls are thickened by fibrous tissue and, in many places, alveolar spaces are filled by an 'albuminous', acidophilic fluid containing fine granules and many cells. In 1934 Mallory drew attention particularly to the large quantity of pink staining, high-protein alveolar fluid and the presence of cuboidal cells lining, and sometimes detached from, the alveolar walls.

Recent observations (Buechner and Ansari, 1969) have shown that prominent diffuse interstitial fibrosis accompanied by infiltration of mononuclear and plasma cells occurs, together with an abundant acidophilic proteinaceous material which gives a strongly positive reaction to periodic acid-Schiff (PAS) in the alveolar apaces (*Figure 7.16*). The relative amounts of cellular infiltration, intra-alveolar material and diffuse interstitial fibrosis varies from case to case. Silicotic nodules are usually absent but, if present, are few in number and much smaller than typical nodules. Hilar lymph nodes may be enlarged and contain microscopic fibrosis and quartz crystals.

These features are closely similar to those of alveolar-lipoproteinosis (Rosen, Castleman and Liebow, 1958) in which the alveolar walls are usually (although not always) thickened by cellular infiltration, and alveolar spaces filled with a granular strongly PAS-positive proteinaceous and lipid material. The dominant cells in this material are desquamated Type II pneumocytes (Liebow, 1968) and the material itself first appears in these cells and when they disrupt it is released, together with laminated bodies, into the alveolar spaces (Spencer, 1968). Although these lesions resolve in the majority of cases, in some they leave a minor degree of diffuse interstitial fibrosis (Spencer, 1968). Of 110 cases reviewed by Davidson and McLeod (1969) at least 10 had been exposed to a free silica risk.

Pathogenesis

Because 'acute silicosis' was first identified in the abrasive soap industry, alkali (sodium carbonate) was considered to be a decisive pathogenic agent, and ingenious chemical theories suggesting that it exerted an enhancing effect on the fibrogenic potential of quartz were advanced, but these are invalidated by the fact that the same disease process occurs in the absence of exogenous alkali.

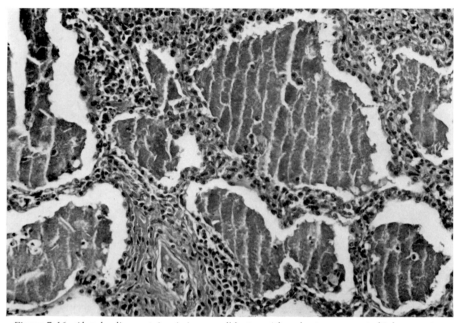

Figure 7.16. Alveolar lipoproteinosis in a sandblaster with a short exposure to high concentrations of quartzite sands (see Figure 7.17). Note cellular infiltration of alveolar walls and acidophilic proteinaceous material, which was PAS-positive, in the alveolar spaces. A few small immature silicotic nodules were present elsewhere in the lungs. (Original magnification, × 235, reproduced at × 175; H and E stain; microsection kindly supplied by Dr H. A. Buechner, New Orleans)

At least two conditions are thought to be necessary for the production of the disease:

(1) Free silica of predominantly small particle size. This is supported by experimental work in rats. Fibrogenic activity of flint administered by the intratracheal route increased significantly with decreasing particle size, and the 'optimum fibrogenic size' appeared to be between 1 and 2 μm diameter (King *et al.*, 1953). Surface area of particles, however, does not seem to be critical (Goldstein and Webster, 1966).

Furthermore, workers with this disease have often been recorded to have been exposed to the dust of finely ground quartz.

(2) High concentrations of quartz—or cristobalite—dust over a short time-period.

Rats which have inhaled particles of pure quartz, quartz and 60 per cent cristobalite, and quartz and 5 per cent cristobalite (all less than 7 μm diameter) develop lesions which are identical with those of human alveolar lipoproteinosis (Corrin and King, 1969, 1970). Commencing with a great increase in alveolar macrophages whose cytoplasm becomes swollen and vacuolated the appearances of endogenous lipid pneumonia are soon established. The macrophages break down releasing a slightly eosinophilic (acidophilic), weakly PAS-positive, floccular material into the alveolar spaces; later this becomes condensed, strongly eosinophilic and PAS-positive, and contains cholesterol crystals. Electron microscopy indicates that the lipid pneumonia causes overactivity of Type II pneumocytes which extrude large numbers of lamellar cytosomes, thought to represent pulmonary surfactant into the alveolar spaces (Klaus et al., 1962).

The production of alveolar lipoproteinosis in rats by inhalation of high concentrations of fine quartz particles has been confirmed by Gross and de Treville (1968) and by Heppleston, Wright and Stewart (1970) who showed that the alveolar material consists predominantly of lipids but also contains protein in the form of albumin and IgG derived, probably as a transudate, from serum proteins (hence the term lipoproteinosis). Serum proteins have been identified in the pulmonary washings of human alveolar lipoproteinosis (Hawkins, Savard and Ramirez-Rivera, 1967).

It is not known why these elements accumulate in the alveoli. And although quartz ingested by macrophages apparently activates the production of phospholipases (Munder et al., 1966), Heppleston, Wright and Stewart (1970) have suggested that there may be insufficient of these enzymes to lyse an excess of phospholipids produced by Type II pneumocytes. Accumulation of lipoproteinaceous material and cell debris may overwhelm normal pulmonary clearance mechanisms and isolate quartz particles from macrophages thus preventing the formation of characteristic silicotic nodules. Nor is it understood why lipoproteinosis, rather than nodular silicosis, develops following quartz inhalation as either type of lesion alone has occurred in rats which have been subjected to identical dust conditions (Heppleston, Wright and Stewart, 1970). An additional, and as yet unidentified, factor, therefore, would seem to be involved in the production of silicotic lipoproteinosis. Powell and Gough (1959) found that rabbits in which hypersensitivity was induced with horse serum developed alveolar lipoproteinosis when exposed to pure quartz dust.

To summarize: high concentrations of quartz dust of small particle size associated with an unknown factor may cause alveolar lipoproteinosis with a variable degree of diffuse interstitial fibrosis (fibrosing 'alveolitis') in man. Gough's (1967) suggestion that this factor may be immunological is at present purely speculative. There do not appear to be any reports of this disorder following exposure to calcined diatomite (cristobalite).

Clinical features

Symptoms

These develop quickly over a period of a few weeks and usually within a year or two of first exposure to the responsible siliceous dust. Malaise, fatigue, loss of weight, cough and mucoid sputum, often with pleuritic type of chest pain, are complained of; but the chief symptom is rapidly progressive dyspnoea of sudden onset.

Physical signs

The patient is usually dyspnoeic at rest and, in the later stages of the illness, orthopnoeic. The reason for this is that a large proportion of the lungs is involved by the disease process and it is possible, too, that reflex mechanisms (*see* Chapter 1) also play a part. Central cyanosis may be present together with fever ranging from 37·2°C (99°F) to 40°C (105°F).

There may be finger clubbing, impaired percussion note, and pleural rub. Breath sounds are either diminished or of bronchial type depending upon the degree of pleural thickening. Crepitations are usually heard over the greater part of the lung fields.

Investigations

Lung function

Tests have shown a restrictive defect (Buechner and Ansari, 1969) but severe reduction of TLC and gas transfer with consequent arterial oxygen desaturation can also be expected.

Radiographic appearances

Early changes consist of a diffuse haze in the lower zones of the lung fields (Pendergrass, 1958); thereafter opacities ranging from 'ground glass' type to a mixture of coarse linear and rounded opacities scattered throughout the lung fields rapidly develop but, in other cases, there is a pattern of small round opacities of alveolar consolidation which resemble miliary tuberculosis in the lower half of the lung fields. Haziness in both lung fields due to diffuse pleural thickening may also be seen (*Figure 7.17*).

Other investigations

Sputum may contain amorphous material with a strongly positive PAS reaction, and in some cases tubercle bacilli may be isolated. It may be necessary to obtain lung tissue for biopsy to establish the diagnosis.

Diagnosis

If a detailed occupational history is not elicited, the diagnosis will in all probability be missed. Confusion may occur with miliary tuberculosis, sarcoidosis, pneumonia of various types and collagen diseases which involve the lungs.

Complications

Tuberculosis may develop and infection by atypical mycobacteria has also been reported (Buechner and Ansari, 1969).

Prognosis

Spontaneously occurring alveolar lipoproteinosis apparently resolves completely in the majority of cases but 'silica'-induced disease appears to be

P   209

uniformly fatal within about one year of development of the first symptoms.

Treatment

There appears to be no effective treatment, corticosteroids being of little avail. However, if the diagnosis is made early, massive bronchopulmonary lavage to remove the alveolar material and intermixed 'silica' may offer hope of recovery (Hawkins, Savard and Ramirez-Rivera, 1967). Complicating tuberculosis must be treated vigorously.

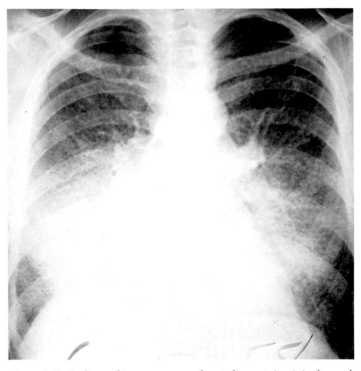

Figure 7.17. Radiographic appearances of acute lipoproteinosis in the sand-blaster referred to in Figure 7.16. (Reproduced by courtesy of Dr H. A. Buechner and the Editor of Diseases of the Chest)

Prevention

The same principles as outlined for 'nodular silicosis' and diatomite pneumo-coniosis apply. It is especially important that there should be an awareness of the dangers of high concentrations of quartz dust even over a short period of time.

REFERENCES

Adams, P. J. (1961). *Geology and Ceramics*. Department of Scientific and Industrial Research, Geological Survey and Museum. London; H.M.S.O.
Adler-Herzmark, J. and Kapstein, G. (1937). 'Weitere Untersuchungen über Silkos in Österreich.' *Wien. med. Wschr*, **87**, 433–441
Ahlman, K. (1968). 'Silicosis in Finland.' *Work Envir. Hlth* **4**, Suppl. 1

Ahlmark, A. and Bruce, T. (1967). 'The current pneumoconiosis situation in Sweden.' *Scand. J. Resp. Dis.* **48**, 181–188

— — and Nyström, A. (1960). *Silicosis and Other Pneumoconioses in Sweden.* Stockholm; Svenska Bokförlaget, London; Heinemann

Andrews, R. W. (1970). *Wollastonite.* Institute of Geological Sciences. London; H.M.S.O.

Arnstein, A. (1941). 'Non-industrial pneumoconiosis, pneumoconio-tuberculosis and tuberculosis of the mediastinal and bronchial lymph glands in old people.' *Tubercle, Lond.* **22**, 281–295

Ashford, J. R. and Enterline, P. E. (1966). 'Radiological classification of pneumoconiosis.' *Archs envir. Hlth* **12**, 314–330

Ashworth, T. G. (1970). 'Acute silico-proteinosis; case report in an African.' *S.Afr. med. J.* **44**, 1214–1216

Ayer, H. E. (1969). 'The proposed ACGIH mass limits for quartz; review and evaluation.' *Am. ind. Hyg. Ass. J.* **30**, 117–125

Bailey, D. A. (1947). 'Conversion of silica during ignition.' *J. ind. Hyg. Toxicol.* **29**, 242–249

Beadle, D. G., Sluis-Cremer, G. K. and Harris, E. (1970). 'The relationship between the amount of dust breathed and the incidence of silicosis.' In *International Conf. on Pneumoconiosis, Johannesburg, 1969*, pp. 250–254. Dept. of Mines, Republic of South Africa.

Becker, R. J. P. and Chatgidakis, C. B. (1960). 'The heart in silicosis.' *Proceedings of Pneumoconiosis Conference, Johannesburg, 1959*, pp. 205–216. Ed. by A. J. Orsenstein. London; Churchill

Becklake, M. R., du Preez, L. and Lutz, W. (1958). 'Lung function in the silicosis of the Witwatersrand gold mines.' *Am. Rev. Tuberc. pulm. Dis.* **77**, 400–412

Belt, T. H. (1939). 'Silicosis of the spleen: a study of the silicotic nodule.' *J. Path. Bact.* **49**, 39–44

Bradshaw, F., Critchlow, A. and Nagelschmidt, G. (1962). 'A study of airborne dust in haematite mines in Cumberland.' *Ann. occup. Hyg.* **4**, 265–273

Bramwell, B. (1914). 'Diffuse scleroderma: its frequency; its occurrence in stone-masons; its treatment by fibrinolysin-elevations of temperature due to fibrinolysin injection.' *Edinb. med. J.* **12**, 387–401

Buechner, H. A. and Ansari, A. (1969). 'Acute silico-proteinosis.' *Dis. Chest.* **55**, 174–284

Burgess, W. A. and Reist, P. C. (1969). 'An industrial hygiene study of flame cutting in a granite quarry.' *Am. ind. Hyg. Ass. J.* **30**, 107–112

Byers, P. D. and King, E. J. (1961). 'Experimental infective pneumoconiosis with *Mycobacterium tuberculosis* (var. *muris*) and haematite by inhalation and by injection.' *J. Path. Bact.* **81**, 123–134

Campbell, J. A. (1958). 'A case of Caplan's syndrome in a boiler scaler.' *Thorax* **13**, 177–180

Caplan, A., Cowen, E. D. H. and Gough, J. (1958). 'Rheumatoid pneumoconiosis in a foundry worker.' *Thorax* **13**, 181–184

Carnes, W. H. (1954). Quoted by Oechsli, Jacobson and Brodeur (1961) in 'Diatomite pneumoconiosis: roentgen characteristics and classification.' *Am. J. Roentg.* **85**, 263–270

Chapman, E. M. (1932). 'Acute silicosis.' *J. Am. med. Ass.* **98**, 1439–1441

Chatgidakis, C. F. (1963). 'Silicosis in South African white gold miners.' *Med. Proc.* **9**, 383–392

— and Theron, C. P. (1961). 'Rheumatoid pneumoconiosis (Caplan's syndrome).' *Archs envir. Hlth* **2**, 397–408

Chiesura, P., Terribile, P. M. and Bardellini, G. (1968). 'Le calcificazioni "a guscio d'uovo" nella silicosi: elementi tratti dall'' osservazioni di 52 casi.' *Minerva med., Roma* **59**, 5960–5968

Colinet, E. (1953). 'Polyarthritis chronique évolutive et silicose pulmonarie.' *Acta physiother. Rheum. belg.* **8**, 37–41

Cooper, W. C. and Cralley, L. J. (1958). *Pneumoconiosis in Diatomite Mining and Processing.* Publ. Hlth Serv. Publn No. 601. Washington; U.S. Dept. Hlth Educ. and Welf.

Corrin, B. and King, E. (1969). 'Experimental endogenous lipid pneumonia and silicosis.' *J. Path.* **97**, 325–330
— — (1970). 'Pathogenesis of experimental pulmonary alveolar proteinosis.' *Thorax* **25**, 230–236
Cralley, L. J., Cooper, W. C. and Caplan, R. E. (1966). 'A ten years' epidemiological follow-up of workers in the diatomite industry in the U.S.' In *Proc. of 15th Int. Congr. Occup. Hlth, Vienna*. Quoted by Wagner *et al.* (1968). *Am. ind. Hyg. Ass. J.* **29**, 211–221
Davidson, J. M. and MacLeod, W. M. (1969). 'Pulmonary alveolar proteinosis.' *Br. J. Dis. Chest* **63**, 13–28
Davies, C. N. (Ed.) (1969). *Health Conditions in the Ceramics Industry*, pp. 101–170. Oxford; Pergamon
Denny, J. J., Robson, W. D. and Irwin, D. A. (1939). 'Prevention of silicosis by metallic aluminium.' *Can. med. Ass. J.* **40**, 213–228
Dutra, F. R. (1965). 'Diatomaceous earth pneumoconiosis.' *Archs envir. Hlth* **11**, 613–619
Einbrodt, H. J. (1965). 'Quantitative und qualitative Untersuchungen über die Staubretention in der menschlichen Lungen.' *Beitr. Silkosforsch.* **87**, 1–105
— and Burilkov, T. (1972). 'Mineral dust content of the lung tissue and lymph nodes in egg-shell calcification.' *Int. Arch. Arbeitsmed.* **30**, 223–236
E.M.I. Records (Gramophone Co. Ltd.) (1970). Personal communication
Erasmus, L. D. (1960). 'Scleroderma in gold miners.' *Proceedings of Pneumoconiosis Conference, Johannesburg*, pp. 426–435. Ed. by A. J. Orenstein. London; Churchill
Faulds, T. S. and Nagelschmidt, G. S. (1962). 'The dust in the lungs of haematite miners from Cumberland.' *Ann. occup. Hyg.* **4**, 225–263
Fiumicelli, A., Fiumicelli, C. and Pagni, M. (1964). 'Contributo allo studio della silicosi massiva unilarale isolata.' *Medna Lav.* **5**, 516–530
Flinn, R. H., Brinton, H. P., Doyle, H. N., Cralley, L. J., Harris, R. L., Westfield, J., Bird, J. H. and Berger, L. B. (1963). *Silicosis in the Metal Mining Industry. A Revaluation. 1958–1961.* Publ. Hlth Serv. Publn No. 1076. Washington; U.S. Government Printing Office
Friberg, L. and Öhman, H. (1957). 'Silicosis hazards in enamelling. A medical technical and experimental study.' *Br. J. ind. Med.* **14**, 85–91
Gardner, L. W. (1929). 'Studies on experimental pneumonokoniosis, V.' *Am. Rev. Tuberc.* **20**, 833–875
— (1933). 'Pathology of the so-called acute silicosis.' *Am. J. Publ. Hlth* **23**, 1240–1249
— (1934). 'Pathology, human and experimental.' 1st Saranac Symposium on Silicosis. Trudeau Sch. Tuberc. Saranac Lake. N.Y. Ed. by B. E. Kuechle.
— (1937). 'The significance of the silicotic problem.' 3rd Saranac Symposium on silicosis. Trudeau Sch. Tuberc., Saranac Lake. N.Y. Ed. by B. E. Kuechle
Gedda, L., Bolognesi, M., Bandino, R. and Brenci, G. (1964). 'Ricerche di genetica sulla silicosi die minatori della Sardegna.' *Lavaro Um.* **16**, 555–562
Goldstein, B. and Rendall, R. E. G. (1970). 'The relative toxicities of the main classes of minerals.' In *Pneumoconiosis. Proceedings of the International Conference. J'burg. 1969*, pp. 429–434. Ed. by H. A. Shapiro. Capetown; Oxford University Press
— and Webster, I. (1966). 'Intratracheal injection into rats of size-graded silica particles.' *Br. J. ind. Med.* **23**, 71–74
Gough, J. (1959). 'Rheumatoid pneumoconiosis.' *Bull. post Grad. Comm. Med. Univ. Sydney* **15**, 280–284
Gough, H. (1967). 'Silicosis and alveolar proteinosis.' *Br. med. J.* **1**, 629
Government of India Ministry of Labour (1953). *Silicosis in mica mining in Bihar*. Office of the Chief Advisor Factories Report No. 3
Gregory, J. (1970). 'A survey of pneumoconiosis at a Sheffield steel foundry.' *Archs envir. Hlth* **20**, 385–399
Gross, P. and de Treville, R. T. P. (1968). 'Experimental "acute" silicosis.' *Archs envir. Hlth* **17**, 720–725
Gründorfer, W. and Raber, A. (1970). 'Progressive silicosis in granite workers.' *Br. J. ind. Med.* **27**, 110–120

H.M. Factory Inspectorate (1959). *Industrial Health. A Survey of the Pottery Industry in Stoke-on-Trent*. London; H.M.S.O.

Hale, L. W. and Sheers, G. (1963). 'Silicosis in West Country granite workers.' *Br. J. ind. Med.* **20**, 218–225

Harding, H. E. and McLaughlin, A. I. G. (1955). 'Pulmonary fibrosis in non-ferrous foundry workers.' *Br. J. ind. Med.* **12**, 92–99

— and Massie, A. P. (1951). 'Pneumoconiosis in boiler scalers.' *Br. J. ind. Med.* **8**, 256–264

— Gloyne, S. R. and McLaughlin, A. I. G. (1950). *Industrial Lung Diseases in Iron and Steel Foundry Workers*. Ed. by A. I. G. McLaughlin. London; H.M.S.O.

Hawkins, J. E., Savard, E. V. and Ramirez-Rivera, J. (1967). 'Pulmonary alveolar proteinosis. Origins of proteins in pulmonary washings.' *Am. J. clin. Path.* **48**, 14–17

Hayes, D. S. and Posner, E. (1960). 'A case of Caplan's syndrome in a roof tile maker.' *Tubercle, Lond.* **41**, 143–145

Hayman, L. D. and Hunt, R. E. (1952). 'Pulmonary fibrosis in generalised scleroderma.' *Dis. Chest.* **21**, 691–704

Heppleston, A. G. (1962). 'The disposal of dust in the lungs of silicotic rats.' *Am. J. Path.* **40**, 493–506

— Wright, N. A. and Stewart, J. A. (1970). 'Experimental alveolar lipo-proteinosis following the inhalation of silica.' *J. Path.* **101**, 293–307

Holman, A. T. (1947). 'Historical relationship of mining silicosis and rock removal.' *Br. J. ind. Med.* **4**, 1–29

Hosey, A. D., Trasko, V. M. and Ashe, H. B. (1957). *Control of Silicosis in the Vermont Granite Industry*. P.H.S. Publ. No. 557. Washington, D.C.; U.S. Dept of Hlth Educ. and Welfare

Hull, W. Q., Keel, H., Kenney, Jr., J. and Gainson, B. W. (1953). 'Diatomaceous earth.' *Ind. Engng Chem.* **45**, 256–269

International Labour Office (1966). *The Prevention and Suppression of Dust in Mining. Tunnelling and Quarrying. Third International Report 1958–1962*. Geneva; I.L.O.

Israel, H. L., Sones, M., Roy, R. L. and Stein, G. N. (1961). 'The occurrence of intrathoracic calcification in sarcoidosis.' *Am. Rev. resp. Dis.* **84**, 1–11

Joint Standing Committee on Safety Health and Welfare Conditions in Non-ferrous Foundries (1957). Ministry of Labour and National Service. First Report. London; H.M.S.O.

Jones, J. G., Owen, T. E. and Corrado, H. A. (1967). 'Respiratory tuberculosis and pneumoconiosis in slate workers.' *Br. J. Dis. Chest.* **61**, 138–143

Keers, R. Y. (1969). 'The treatment of silicotuberculosis.' In *Health Conditions in the Ceramic Industry*, pp. 63–69. Ed. by C. N. Davies. Oxford; Pergamon

Kennedy, M. C. S. (1956). 'Aluminium powder inhalations in the treatment of silicosis of pottery workers and pneumoconiosis of coal miners.' *Br. J. ind. Med.* **13**, 85–99

Kettle, E. H. (1932). 'The interstitial reactions caused by various dusts and their influence on tuberculous injections.' *J. Path. Bact.* **35**, 395–405

Khoo, O. T. and Toh, K. K. (1968). 'Morbidity of silicosis in Singapore.' *Singapore med. J.* **9**, 186–191

King, E. J., Mohanty, G. P., Harrison, C. V. and Nagelschmidt, G. (1953). 'The action of flint of variable size injected at constant weight and constant surface into the lungs of rats.' *Br. J. ind. Med.* **10**, 76–92

— Rogers, N., Gilchrist, M., Goldschmidt, V. M. and Nagelschmidt, G. (1945). 'The effect of olivine on the lungs of rats.' *J. Path. Bact.* **57**, 488–491

Klaus, M., Reiss, O. K., Tooley, W. H., Piel, C. and Clement, J. A. (1962). 'Alveolar epithelial cell mitochondria as source of the surface-active lung lining.' *Science* **137**, 750–751

Klosterkötter, W. and Einbrodt, H. J. (1965). 'Quantitative tiexperimentelle Untersuchungen über den Abtransport von Staub aus den Lugen in die regionalen Lymphknoten.' *Archs Hyg.* **149**, 367–384

Liebow, A. A. (1968). 'New concepts and entities in pulmonary disease.' In *The*

Lung, pp. 332–333. Ed. by Averill A. Liebow and David E. Smith. Baltimore; Williams and Wilkins

Longley, E. O. (1970). 'Oesophageal compression due to silicotic mediastinal lymph glands.' *Trans. Soc. occup. Med.* **20**, 69

Luton, P., Champeix, J., Ravet, M. and Vallaud, A. (1956). 'Observations récentes sur la pneumoconiose par terre a diatomées.' *Archs Mal. prof. Méd. trav.* **17**, 125–148

Lynch, K. M. (1942). 'Silicosis of systemic distribution.' *Am. J. Path.* **18**, 313–321

McDonald, G., Piggott, A. P. and Gilder, F. W. (1930). 'Two cases of acute silicosis with a suggested theory of causation.' *Lancet* **2**, 846–848

McLaughlin, A. I. G. (1957). 'Pneumoconiosis in foundry workers.' *Br. J. Tuberc.* **51**, 297–309

— and Harding, H. E. (1956). 'Pneumoconiosis and other causes of death in iron and steel foundry workers.' *Archs ind. Hlth* **14**, 350–378

McTurk, L. C., Huis, C. H. W. and Eckardt, R. E. (1956). 'Health hazards of vanadium containing residual oil ash.' *Industr. Med. Surg.* **25**, 29–36

Mallory, T. B. (1934). 'Cabot case records of the Massachusetts General Hospital, Case 20102.' *New Engl. J. Med.* **210**, 551–554

Middleton, E. L. (1929). 'The present position of silicosis in industry in Britain.' *Br. med. J.* **2**, 485–489

Miners Phthisis Medical Bureau (1944). *Report upon the work of the M.P.M.B. for three years ended 31st July 1941*. Pretoria; Union of South Africa Government Printer

Moreschi, N., Farina, G. and Chiappinio, G. (1968). 'La silicosi pulmonaire calcificata.' *Medna Lav.* **59**, 111–124

Motley, H. L. (1960). 'Pulmonary function studies in diatomaceous earth workers. 2. A cross section survey of 98 workers on the job.' *Ind. Med. Surg.* **24**, 370–378

— Smart, R. H. and Valero, A. (1956). 'Pulmonary function studies in diatomaceous earth workers. 1. Ventilatory and blood gas exchange disturbance.' *Archs ind. Hlth* **13**, 165–174

Munder, P. G., Modolell, M., Ferber, E. and Fischer, H. (1966). 'Phospholipoide in quarzgeschädigten Makrophagen.' *Biochem. Z.* **344**, 310–313

Nagelschmidt, G. (1965). 'A study of lung dust in pneumoconiosis.' *Am. ind. Hyg. Ass. J.* **26**, 1–7

Nordmann, M. (1943). Die Staublunge der Kieselgurarbelter. *Virchows Arch. path. Anat. Physiol.* **311**, 116–148

Oechsli, W. R., Jacobson, G. and Brodeur, A. E. (1961). 'Diatomite pneumoconiosis: roentgen characteristics and classification.' *Am. J. Roentgen.* **85**, 263–270

Otto, H. (1969). 'Results of latex tests in 6,000 porcelain workers.' In *Health Conditions in the Ceramic Industry*, pp. 91–98. Ed. by C. N. Davies. Oxford; Pergamon

Palmhert. H., Webster, I. and Lens, C. (1968). 'Atypical mycobacteria and infections of the lung in the South Africa mining industry.' *S. Afr. Pneumocon. Rev.* **3**, 6

Pendergrass, E. P. (1958). *The Pneumoconiosis Problem*, pp. 95–97. Springfield; Thomas

Pernis, B. (1968). 'Silicosis.' In *Textbook of Immunopathology*. Vol. 1. Ed. by P. A. Meischer and H. J. Muller-Eberhardt, pp. 293–301. New York and London; Grune and Stratton

Phibbs, B. R., Sundin, R. E. and Mitchell, R. S. (1971). 'Silicosis in Wyoming bentonite workers.' *Am. Rev. resp. Dis.* **103**, 1–17

Pilkington, L. A. B. (1969). 'The float glass process.' *Proc. R. Soc.* **314**, 1–25

Plunkett, E. R. and De Witt, B. J. (1962). 'Occupational exposure to Hi-Sil and Silene.' *Archs envir. Hlth* **5**, 469–472

Polacheck, A. A. and Pijanowski, W. J. (1960). 'Extrathoracic egg-shell calcifications in silicosis.' *Am. Rev. resp. Dis.* **82**, 714–720

Policard, A., Gernez-Rieux, C., Tacquet, A., Martin, J. C., Devulder, B. and Le Bouffant, L. (1967). 'Influence of pulmonary dust load on the development of experimental infection by *Mycobacteria kansasii*.' *Nature, Lond.* **216**, 177–178

Posner, E. (1961). 'Pneumoconiosis and tuberculosis in the North Staffordshire pottery industry.' In *Symposium on Dust Control in the Pottery Industry*. Stoke; British Ceramic Research Assoc. Spec. Publ. 27, pp. 5–18.

Powell, D. E. B. and Gough, J. (1959). 'The effect on experimental silicosis of hypersensitivity induced by horse serum.' *Br. J. exp. Path.* **40**, 40–43

Pump, K. K. (1968). 'Studies in silicosis of the human lung.' *Dis. Chest* **53**, 237–246

Ritterhoff, R. J. (1941). 'Acute silicosis occurring in employees of abrasive soap powder industries.' *Am. Rev. Tuberc.* **43**, 117–131

Rodnan, G. P., Benedek, T. G., Medsger, T. A. and Cammarata, R. J. (1967). 'The association of progressive systemic sclerosis (scleroderma) with coal miner's pneumoconiosis and other forms of silicosis.' *Ann. int. Med.* **56**, 323–334

Rogan, J. M. (1960). Discussion. *Proc. of Pneumocon. Conf., J'burg*, p. 435. Ed. by A. J. Orenstein. London; Churchill

Rosen, S. H., Castleman, B. and Liebow, A. A. (1958). 'Pulmonary alveolar proteinosis.' *New Engl. J. Med.* **258**, 1123–1142

Rüttner, J. R. (1954). 'Foundry worker's pneumoconiosis in Switzerland (anthrasilicosis).' *Archs ind. Hyg.* **9**, 297–305

— and Heer, H. R. (1969). 'Silicosis and lung cancer.' *Schweiz. med. Wschr.* **99**, 245–249

Scadding, J. G. (1967). *Sarcoidosis*, pp. 141–149. London; Eyre and Spottiswoode

Schepers, G. W. H., Durkan, T. M., Delahant, A. B., Creedon, F. T. and Redlin, A. J. (1957a). 'The biological action of Degussa submicron silica dust (Dow Corning silica), 1.' *Archs ind. Hlth* **16**, 125–146

— Delahant, A. B., Schmidt, J. G., von Wecheln, J. C., Creedon, F. T. and Clark, R. W. (1957b). 'The biological action of Degussa submicron silica dust (Dow Corning silica), 3.' *Archs ind. Hlth* **16**, 280–301

— — Fear, E. J. and Schmidt, J. G. (1957c). 'The biological action of Degussa submicron silica dust (Dow Corning silica), 4. *Archs ind. Hlth* **16**, 363–374

— Smart, R. H., Smith, C. R., Dworski, M. and Delahant, A. B. (1958). 'Fatal silicosis with complicating infection by an atypical acid fast photochromic bacillus.' *Ind. Med. Surg.* **27**, 27–36

Schlipköter, H. W. (1970). 'Ätiologie und Pathogenese der Silikose sowie ihre kausale Beeinflussung.' *Naturwissenschaften* **197**, 39–105

Schneider, H. (1966). 'Silikosegefahrrdung durch Neuburger Kieselkreide.' *Int. Arch. Gewerbepath. Gewerbehyg.* **22**, 323–341

Smart, R. H. and Anderson, W. H. (1952). 'Pneumoconiosis due to diatomaceous earth. Clinical and X-ray aspects.' *Ind. Med. Surg.* **21**, 509–518

Spain, D. M. (1965). In Editorial to 'Diatomaceous earth pneumoconiosis' by F. R. Dutra (1965). *Archs envir. Hlth* **11**, 619

Spencer, H. (1968). 'Alveolar proteinosis.' In *The Pathology of the Lung*, pp. 684–688. Oxford; Pergamon

Stewart, M. J. and Faulds, J. S. (1934). 'Pulmonary fibrosis in haematite miners.' *J. Path. Bact.* **39**, 233–253

Sweany, H. C., Porsche, J. D. and Douglass, J. R. (1936). 'Chemical and pathological study of pneumoconiosis with special emphasis on silicosis and silico-tuberculosis.' *Archs Path.* **22**, 593–633

Tebbens, B. D. and Beard, R. R. (1957). 'Experiments on diatomaceous earth pneumoconiosis. 1. Natural diatomaceous earth in guinea-pigs.' *A.M.A. Archs ind. Hlth* **16**, 55–63

Thiruvengadam, K. V., Anguli, V. C., Shetty, P., Sanibandam, S. and Kosairam, R. (1968). 'Silicosis in a mica-mine worker.' *J. Indian med. Ass.* **51**, 248–250

Uehlinger, E. (1946). 'Übermischstaubpneumo-Koniosen.' *Schweiz. Z. Path. Bakt.* **9**, 692–700

Vigliani, E. C. and Mottura, G. (1948). 'Diatomaceous earth silicosis.' *Br. J. ind. Med.* **5**, 148–160

Volk, H. (1960). 'The health of workers in plant making highly dispersed silica.' *Archs envir. Hlth* **1**, 125–128

Vorwald, A. J., Durkan, T. M., Pratt, P. C. and Delahant, A. B. (1949). 'Diatomaceous earth pneumoconiosis.' *Proc. IX Int. Congr. Ind. Med., Bristol*, pp. 726–741. Bristol; Wright

Wagner, W. D., Fraser, D. A., Wright, P. G., Dobrogorski, O. J. and Stokinger, H. E. (1968). 'Experimental evaluation of the threshold limit of cristobalite-calcined diatomaceous earth.' *Am. ind. Hyg. Ass. J.* **19**, 211–221

Webster, I. (1968). 'Prevention of silicosis.' *S. Afr. Pneumocon. Rev.* **4**, 11–12

World Health Organisation (1968). 'Pneumoconiosis.' *Report on the Katowice Symposium, 1967*, pp. 29–31. Copenhagen; Regional Office for Europe

8—Pneumoconiosis due to Coal and Carbon

The pneumoconiosis which occurs in workers in coal, graphite and other types of carbon is considered separately from silicosis because:

(1) The pathology is quite distinct from that of nodular silicosis.

(2) There is uncertainty as to what part—if any—quartz plays in pathogenesis.

(3) Coal pneumoconiosis has been more extensively studied than silicosis.

Terminology

The Committee on Industrial Pulmonary Disease (Medical Research Council, 1942) proposed the term *coal-worker's pneumoconiosis* although, perhaps, 'coal pneumoconiosis' is adequate to the purpose. *Anthraco-silicosis* takes for granted that this pneumoconiosis is a form of silicosis but as this is doubtful it is best avoided. The recently current term, *black lung*, is uninformative and capable of including any of the 'pulmonary conditions which may be present in a coal-miner's chest' (Gross and de Treville, 1970); it should have no place in medical terminology.

The pathological appearances and behaviour of this pneumoconiosis are closely similar, if not identical, irrespective of whether it is due to exposure to coal, graphite or synthetic carbons. Since about 1948 in the United Kingdom the terms *simple pneumoconiosis, infective nodule, complicated or infective pneumoconiosis* and *progressive massive fibrosis* have been used to describe the various stages of the lesions. 'Simple pneumoconiosis' refers to small, discrete dust macules (*macula*, a stain or spot) or nodules not larger than about 5 mm in diameter which were believed to be uncomplicated by any other causative factor than the coal- or carbon-dust (Gough and Heppleston, 1960) in contrast to somewhat larger nodules previously thought to be associated with past infection (that is, 'infective nodules'), and the massive lesions consisting of dust and fibrosis which were considered to result from the 'complication' of a modified tuberculous process. The objection to these terms is that they are not simply descriptive but assume a mode of pathogenesis which is either unproven or not universally operative. 'Progressive massive fibrosis' (P.M.F.) refers to larger confluent masses of dust and

217

collagen fibrosis and is synonymous with 'complicated pneumoconiosis'; although these lesions are not always continuously progressive it is otherwise a satisfactory and widely current term and is used throughout this chapter.

SOURCES OF EXPOSURE

COAL

The composition of coal and meaning of 'rank' of coal are briefly described in Chapter 2.

Coal-mining

The highest concentrations of dust have always occurred underground and mostly at the 'coal-face' (that is, a working place on the solid surface of a coal-seam which has separate intake and return roadways). In the United Kingdom coal was obtained by use of pick and shovel until the beginning of this century when machine-cutting methods were introduced and increasingly used over the following years. Hand-powered drills and cutters with water infusion to suppress dust also came into use during this period and in some collieries were employed until the early 1960s. In general, coal-getting has been almost completely mechanized since then. Men working at the coal-face have been known variously as coal-hewers, coal-getters and colliers.

A disadvantage of mechanical methods is that machines—unlike men— do not distinguish between rock intrusions and coal so that in some regions more quartz is contributed to the atmosphere than by hand-got methods.

Coal is loaded either manually or by mechanical means from the coal cutter on to a conveyor belt which carries it to a loading point, thence to be taken by a haulage system to the bottom of the pit shaft. From here it is lifted to the surface. As the coal-seam is developed, conveyers are dismantled and re-erected for re-positioning. Different types of haulage have been used: trucks ('tubs' or 'trams') drawn on a railway, previously by ponies, but now by diesel or electric locomotives, or by a continuous wire rope system powered by a stationary engine. Until recently the point at which the conveyor discharged the coal into the trucks was extremely dusty.

Other work on the coal-face includes 'advancing' it and shot-firing to loosen the coal; this involves boring shot holes and placing and firing an explosive charge, although some new methods do not employ explosives.

Men who make new underground roadways ('developers'), increase the height of the 'roof' and erect supports ('rippers'), increase other roadway and airway dimensions ('dinters') or keep roadways in good repair ('repairers') are exposed to variable amounts of 'stone' dust as coal-dust. The composition of this varies according to the type of rock intrusion (*see* Chapter 2) but shale is usual and sandstone common. And so, drilling, shot firing and other work in these rocks may give rise to significant quantities of quartz-dust. Men working on the sinking of coal-mine shafts are particularly likely to have been exposed to the dust of quartz-bearing rocks.

In general, concentrations of dust are very low in haulage roadways and in the vicinity of the pit shaft bottom.

Since 1910 'stone dust' has been spread periodically along roadways and elsewhere in coal-mines to prevent coal-dust explosions, and shales, limestone and gypsum have been used. As shales have a high quartz content (Nagelschmidt and Godbert, 1951) and certain limestones may contain as much as 9 per cent (Beal, Griffin and Nagelschmidt, 1953), regulations to control the type of dust employed have been applied in the United Kingdom and the United States of America. Therefore, 'stone dusting' in the coal-mines of these countries is unlikely to have been a silicosis risk in the last 15 to 20 years.

Colliery surface work

Men who work as sorters on the 'screens' (that is conveyors carrying coal) remove shale and rock, and break and grade the coal. Dust concentrations are very low and ventilation is good.

Coal-trimming

This involves loading, stowing and levelling coal in ships' holds. A mechanical loader deposits the coal into the hold, where the men shovel it into place. Dust concentrations in the holds are high. Pneumoconiosis in this occupation was first suspected by Collis and Gilchrist (1928) and later confirmed by Gough (1940).

GRAPHITE

Natural graphite, known also as plumbago, is elemental crystalline carbon mixed with a variety of mineral impurities. When the crystals are visible to the naked eye it is called 'flake' graphite; when they are small, or crypto-crystalline, it is known as 'amorphous' graphite. Amorphous graphite is the type most used in industry. Graphite is widely distributed geographically in igneous, sedimentary and metamorphic rocks; the most important commercial graphite occurs in metamorphous siliceous sediments, in veins of graphite-gneiss, quartzites, schists and marble (as in Ceylon, Madagascar, Madras and Brazil). When mined, therefore, it contains variable quantities of quartz: 3·6 to 10 per cent 'free silica' has been reported in samples from Ceylon, Korea and South-West Africa (Harding and Oliver, 1949); about 11 per cent in samples from Italy (Parmeggiani, 1950); and 5·24 per cent in samples from Pennsylvania (Ladoo and Myers, 1951). Mica, iron oxides and other minerals may also be present.

Artificial graphite is almost pure crystalline carbon, made by subjecting coal or petroleum coke to a temperature of almost 3,000°C in an electric furnace. In contrast with natural graphite it contains negligible traces of free silica (Mantell, 1968). However, significant quantities of quartz and cristo-balite are present in pyrolitic graphite (or retort carbon) because this is formed by deposition of carbon on the refractory brick surfaces of retorts, but its use is very limited. The manufacture of synthetic graphite was an extremely dusty process until after World War II.

Uses of graphite

(1) *Refractory ceramics and crucibles.*—Carbon is very resistant to thermal shock.

Natural flake graphite (usually from Ceylon and Madagascar) mixed with

219

various proportions of bond clay and sand is used to make blast furnace hearths and linings, and, with the addition of china clay, to make crucibles and ladles for the chemical and non-ferrous metallurgical industries. The preparation of these materials and subsequent trimming of the products before firing was until recently (and in some instances may still be) a very dusty process. It is evident that there was the possibility of exposure to quartz dust as well as to graphite (*see* Pathology section). These ingredients have been replaced to a large extent by artificial graphite, bitumen and certain metals.

Natural graphite has many applications in rockets, missiles, furnaces and moulds.

(2) *Foundry facings.*—Pulverized natural graphite is mixed with sand, clay or talc to give a smooth surface to the mould sand before molten metal is added. It is important in the casting of bells.

(3) *Steel and cast iron manufacture.*—Flake graphite is used to increase the hardness and strength of the metal.

(4) *Pencils.*—Amorphous graphite of high purity is finely ground and mixed in varying proportions with clay. The wet mix is extruded through dies and fired. The famous mines in Borrowdale, Cumberland, which produce graphite for this purpose were started in the middle of the sixteenth century.

(5) *Lubricants.*—Either artificial or natural graphite of high purity is used after being ground to a fine powder and mixed with oil or employed without. There must be no abrasive impurities such as quartz.

(6) *Neutron moderators in atomic reactors.*—These are manufactured from large blocks of artificial graphite.

(7) *Electrodes.*—Carbon electrodes for electrolytic processes in the chemical and metallurgical industries are made from artificial graphite.

(8) *Electrotyping.*—High-purity natural graphite is used as a parting compound dusted on to wax moulds and re-applied after the print impression is taken. This was a very dusty process which has largely been replaced by other methods since the early 1950s. However, the use of graphite for this purpose was still recorded in 1968 (Mantell).

The use of pyrolytic graphite is virtually restricted to the manufacture of carbon brushes and metal alloys.

Graphite miners (notably in Ceylon) may develop pneumoconiosis after some 15 to 20 years in the industry (Dassanayake, 1948; Ranasinha and Uragoda, 1972). Grinding, mixing and bagging graphite for any of the processes just enumerated is a potential source of high concentrations of dust and, in some, of significant quantities of quartz; but today, dust control measures are usually applied, and in most large industries are very efficient. Pneumoconiosis both in discrete and P.M.F. form is well documented among natural graphite workers (Lochtkemper and Teleky, 1932; Faulkner, 1940; Dunner and Bagnall, 1949; Gloyne, Marshall and Hoyle, 1949; Parmeggiani, 1950; Jaffé, 1951; Haferland, 1957; Gaensler *et al.*, 1966), and it has also been recorded in workers in artificial graphite (Zahorski, 1961).

LAMP BLACK

Lamp black is the smoke of an unobstructed hydrocarbon flame deposited on the floors of condensing chambers. It is an amorphous carbon used mainly as a paint pigment and an oil-absorption agent. It contains no quartz.

CARBON BLACK

Carbon is liberated from flames produced by various methods from natural gas, petroleum distillates and residues, or mixed oil and gas; or by a non-flame, 'thermal' method using natural gas in a heated air-free chamber (Mantell, 1968). As refractory chambers are employed in some of these processes it is possible that a trace quantity of quartz or cristobalite might be present in the final product.

Some stages of the manufacturing process are likely to be dusty. This was especially so during the 1930s when, for example, a carbon black plant in Texas was visible a mile or so away due to the production of black dust; since then, however, the standard of dust control in this industry in the United States of America has been very high, but it has lagged far behind in some plants in European countries, Japan, South America and India (Mantell, 1971). Collection and packaging of carbon black has always been a dusty and dirty job.

A particularly pure form of carbon black—known as acetylene black—is produced by thermal decomposition of acetylene.

Carbon black, unlike lamp black, is hard, brilliant and mainly crystalline.

Uses of carbon black

It is most extensively employed as a filler and colouring agent in rubber, plastics, gramophone records (in which it constitutes some 2 per cent of the ingredients) and printing inks; it is also used in paints and enamels, in the manufacture of carbon electrodes, and carbon paper, and as a filter aid, decolouring agent and clarifier.

Significant exposure to the dust has occurred mainly in the production of carbon black, while being emptied from bags, and weighed and mixed with other materials. Trimming and polishing carbon arc rods was also dusty. Pneumoconiosis due to carbon black has been recorded by Miller and Ramsden (1961).

Carbon electrode manufacture

The materials used are either anthracite and coke or petroleum coke. Anthracite has been mostly employed in the United Kingdom and, after purification, it is virtually pure carbon as the quartz content is then of the order of only 0·20 to 0·84 per cent (Mantell, 1968). The materials are calcined, ground to size, mixed with pitch, pressed or extruded into appropriate shapes and then baked in a furnace. The electrodes—which may be very large—are finally drilled and threaded in a machining department. The first stages of this process were very dusty until about 1950 since when grinding plants have usually been totally enclosed, and smoke and gases from the baking furnaces collected and scrubbed (Mantell, 1971). Although quartz is virtually absent (about 0·1 per cent), pneumoconiosis has been reported in workers in this industry (Watson *et al.*, 1959; Okutani, Shima and Sano, 1964). (*See* Pathogenesis.)

221

EPIDEMIOLOGY

In the late 1940s the prevalence of coal pneumoconiosis in the United Kingdom was high due to lack of adequate dust-control measures and a greatly increased production drive during the years of World War II. Dust control did not become effective till after 1950, but the incidence of new cases of both 'simple' and P.M.F. types of disease has fallen dramatically since the 1950s (*see* Table 1.2). The prevalence of all radiographic categories of pneumoconiosis in 53 collieries was 15·7 per cent in 1959 and 9·7 per cent in 1970 (National Coal Board, 1971, 1972). This result, due to dust control, is reflected in *Figure 8.1*. Somewhat similar trends seem to have occurred in other coal-producing

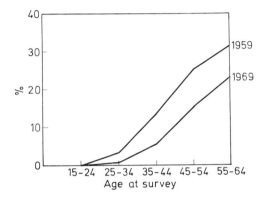

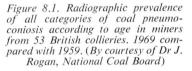

Figure 8.1. Radiographic prevalence of all categories of coal pneumoconiosis according to age in miners from 53 British collieries. 1969 compared with 1959. (By courtesy of Dr J. Rogan, National Coal Board)

countries as a result of the general adoption of dust-suppression methods in the 1950s; for example, the prevalence in working miners in the coalfields of Philadelphia and West Virginia in the period 1963 to 1964 was 9·5 per cent for all categories of pneumoconiosis and all age groups (World Health Organization, 1968). The number of men who develop pneumoconiosis per 1,000 workers per year is referred to as the *attack rate* of pneumoconiosis.

Progression of coal pneumoconiosis is related to the radiographic category when a man is first seen and, apparently, by individual susceptibility which increases as dust concentrations increase (Jacobsen *et al.*, 1971)—the 'host response' referred to in Chapter 4. In turn, category is also related to past dust exposure (Fay and Ashford, 1961) and correlates with the content of dust in the lungs (*see Figure 8.18*). The 'attack rate' of P.M.F. is substantially increased in men with Category 2 or more 'simple' pneumoconiosis but appears to have fallen in Category 3 cases in recent years (Cochrane, 1962; McLintock, Rae and Jacobsen, 1971) (*Figure 8.2*). The probability today of a man with no pneumoconiosis progressing to Category 2 or more after 35 years' exposure to different dust concentrations is small (*Figure 8.3*) (Jacobsen *et al.*, 1971). However, increased mechanization at the coal-face and longer running of the machinery which have been occurring in British coal-mines in the past ten years indicate the necessity for rigorous application of dust-suppression measures if an increase in the prevalence of 'simple' pneumoconiosis is to be prevented.

There is a geographic variation in the 'attack rate' of P.M.F. which is also related to category of 'simple' pneumoconiosis (McLintock, Rae and Jacobsen, 1971); it is highest in the South Wales and lowest in the Scottish and South Midlands coalfields (National Coal Board, 1970). The opacities of 'rheumatoid' coal pneumoconiosis are exceptional as they tend to develop in individuals with Category 0 to 1 radiographs. Expenditure of energy at

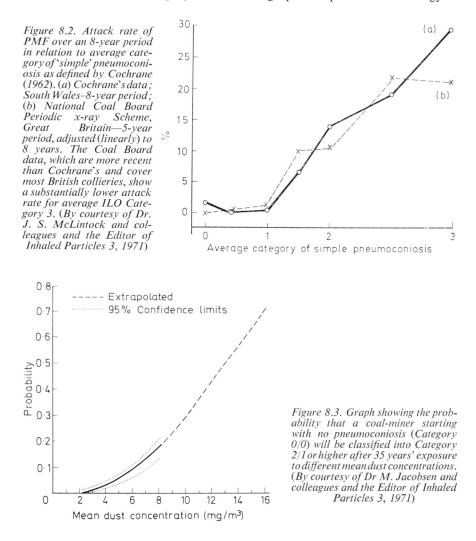

Figure 8.2. Attack rate of PMF over an 8-year period in relation to average category of 'simple' pneumoconiosis as defined by Cochrane (1962). (a) Cochrane's data; South Wales–8-year period; (b) National Coal Board Periodic x-ray Scheme, Great Britain—5-year period, adjusted (linearly) to 8 years. The Coal Board data, which are more recent than Cochrane's and cover most British collieries, show a substantially lower attack rate for average ILO Category 3. (By courtesy of Dr. J. S. McLintock and colleagues and the Editor of Inhaled Particles 3, 1971)

Figure 8.3. Graph showing the probability that a coal-miner starting with no pneumoconiosis (Category 0/0) will be classified into Category 2/1 or higher after 35 years' exposure to different mean dust concentrations. (By courtesy of Dr M. Jacobsen and colleagues and the Editor of Inhaled Particles 3, 1971)

work, smoking habits, body type, and tuberculous infection (either exogenous or endogenous) do not appear to influence the P.M.F. 'attack rate' (Cochrane, 1962), but age may (McLintock, Rae and Jacobsen, 1971). Outside the United Kingdom P.M.F. is said to be common in the coalfields of Europe and China, and less common in those of the U.S.A. and U.S.S.R. (Cochrane, 1960).

The *rate of progression* of P.M.F. is influenced chiefly by age; the younger a man with a Category A radiograph the more likely is progression to occur,

223

and this is also true if he leaves coal-mining. But progression of the 'rheumatoid' lesions is exceptional and may be rapid at any age.

The standardized mortality ratio for miners and ex-miners in a South Wales mining area has been found to be unrelated to the category of 'simple' pneumoconiosis but appears to increase when the area of P.M.F. shadows on the radiograph is substantially in excess of 20 cm^2 (Cochrane, Moore and Thomas, 1961a, b). Parkes (1971) found the average age of death from all causes in 88 miners and ex-miners with Category B or C pneumoconiosis who died in the quinquennium 1966 to 1970 was 70 years, the range being from 53 to 85 years.

The prevalence of pneumoconiosis caused by graphite and other forms of carbon is not known but must be very low because the number of men exposed in the past was small by comparison with coal-miners, and dust control has been fairly generally operative in recent years. But it is likely that some men have escaped diagnosis. Apparently there have been no new cases of pneumoconiosis in the carbon electrode industry in the United States since the mid-1940s (Mantell, 1971).

PATHOLOGY

The pulmonary pleura is marbled blue-black by subpleural deposits of dust and is not thickened unless it overlies a confluent pneumoconiosis mass (P.M.F.) in which case it is often fibrotic and puckered. Apart from this, pleural fibrosis should lead one to suspect the presence of some other disease process.

Discrete Lesions ('Simple' Pneumoconiosis)

Macroscopic appearances

When the lungs are cut through with a knife a variable number of black dust macules (ranging from few to very many) are seen and are commonly predominant in the upper halves of the lungs, but may be distributed symmetrically throughout (*Figure 8.4*). Between these lesions the lung tissue is frequently free of dust pigment. Some lungs are uniformly pigmented black so that individual macules are not discernible, but much of this pigment can usually be washed away by a stream of water to reveal the macules. Macules are not raised above or depressed below the cut surface and they yield no sense of induration to the touch. Interlobular septa and the subpleural region are commonly dust pigmented.

Black, indurated nodules, some 2 to 5 mm in diameter, which stand out from the cut surface and are readily palpable, may also be present—again in variable numbers—and are usually distributed in the upper parts of the upper and lower lobes; but in some cases nearly all the lesions are nodular and may be scattered throughout the lungs, dust macules being virtually absent (*Figure 8.5*). They may also occur in satellite groups around areas of P.M.F. Although many nodules are round (that is, of near spherical form) some are of stellate or irregularly linear shape. Nodules larger than 5 mm and less than 3 cm diameter have, as mentioned earlier, sometimes been referred to as 'infective nodules'.

224

As the nodules are uniformly black they are readily distinguishable from silicotic nodules (*see Figure 7.1*) although 'rheumatoid' Caplan-type nodules may closely resemble silicotic lesions—a mistake that has often been made.

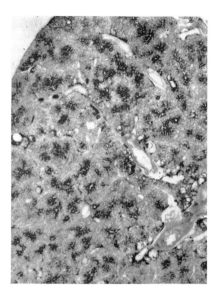

Figure 8.4. Coal-dust macules. Emphysema is absent from these lesions. (From paper lung section, natural size)

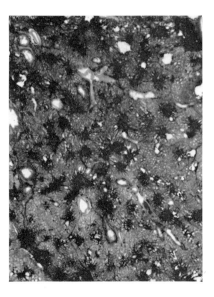

Figure 8.5. Coal nodules. They are indurated and more clearly demarcated than macules. Some nodules exhibit very slight scar (irregular) emphysema. (From paper-mounted lung section, natural size)

However, silicotic nodules or 'mixed dust fibrosis' are sometimes found together with coal or carbon nodules when there has been a significantly siliceous component in past dust exposure.

As stated in Chapter 1, in many cases, emphysema of centrilobular type with holes more than 1 mm in diameter is present in a variable proportion of dust macules—'focal emphysema' of Gough (1947). This is discussed in more detail later. Emphysema is rarely associated with nodular lesions, but when it is, it is of scar (or 'irregular') type and of mild degree.

Microscopic appearances

Dust macules consist of intra- and extracellular dust particles concentrated mainly around or near respiratory bronchioles and their vessels, and in Lambert's canals. There is some proliferation of reticulin fibres, demonstrable by silver impregnation, which loosely enmeshes particles and cells. There is

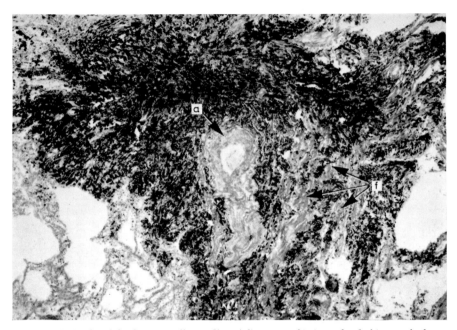

Figure 8.6. Coal nodule showing collagen fibres (f) arranged in irregular fashion, and a large quantity of coal-dust which is both intra- and extracellular. The appearances are in pronounced contrast with those of the typical silicotic nodule (see Figure 7.3). (a, artery; original magnification, × 55, reproduced at × 44; H and E stain)

no collagenous fibrosis. Dust-containing macrophages are present in great numbers in some alveolar spaces some of which may become completely filled and consolidated. Dust accumulations may also be found in the small aggregations of lymphoid tissue at the divisions of respiratory bronchioles and in the adventitia of accompanying arterioles which, however, otherwise remain intact (Wells, 1954a); capillaries, on the other hand, are often obliterated.

Nodular lesions consist of much dust, macrophages and both collagen and reticulin fibres which run in random directions in contrast to the characteristic concentric arrangement of collagen in silicotic nodules (*Figure 8.6*). The proportion of reticulin to collagen is higher than in silicotic nodules. Scar emphysema surrounds contracted nodules of stellate form.

'Curious', or pseudo-asbestos, bodies may be found in areas of dust concentration in both coal and graphite pneumoconiosis (Tylecote and Dunn, 1931; Williams, 1934; Town, 1968). They are shorter than asbestos bodies (*see* Chapter 9) but may be similarly segmented. The refractive index is similar to asbestos bodies (Gloyne, 1932–33). Their cores consist of slender spicules of coal or carbon, and the segmented deposit is golden-yellow when unstained and gives a positive Prussian blue reaction for iron. They are not likely to be confused with asbestos bodies by the experienced observer.

Vasculitis with foci of plasma cells and lymphocytes may be present around some nodules, and rheumatoid factor (IgM) has been found in coal (nodules with no histological evidence of rheumatoid changes in 7 of 35 cases (Wagner and McCormick, 1967)). (*See* Pathogenesis.)

Centrilobular emphysema with dust ('focal emphysema')

Emphysema of 'distensive' centrilobular type is seen in some coal and carbon macules. Depending upon the level and plane of section, these lesions appear either as black cuffs of dust or pigment around dilated respiratory bronchioles or as 'rosettes' of similar proportions with small black centres surrounded by dilated, partly pigmented, alveolar walls. This has been regarded by Gough (1947) and Heppleston (1947, 1953) as a distinctive form of emphysema—'focal emphysema'—believed to result from the weakening of the muscular walls of those respiratory bronchioles in which dust has accumulated and which, in turn, causes them to dilate due to the traction effect of the negative transpulmonary pressure exerted during inspiration (Heppleston, 1968).

But the existence of 'focal emphysema' as distinct from 'distensive' centrilobular emphysema is not universally accepted (Reid, 1967; Heath, 1968). Some pathologists do not consider that these lesions are essentially different from those found in the general population apart from the presence of dust. None the less, Heppleston (1968) is confident that they are in fact distinguishable, although only by the use of three-dimensional micro-techniques; and he points to a loss of smooth muscle in the affected respiratory bronchioles as causing a reduction in their elastic recoil and, hence, dilatation. Against this, however, Macklem (1968) has argued that loss of smooth muscle is unlikely to result in diminution of elastic recoil. Although 'focal emphysema' has for years been stated to be always of 'distensive' type (Gough, 1960), Gough has recently (1968) asserted that, in time, it may become 'destructive'.

There are a number of reasons for doubting that 'focal emphysema' is a separate or exceptional form of emphysema. Coal or carbon macules are often seen without emphysema (*see Figures 8.4, 8.7*). When macules are numerous and scattered throughout the lung those with the most advanced emphysema tend—as is the case with centrilobular emphysema without dust—to be predominant in the upper parts of the upper and lower lobes. In some cases a majority of macules may be emphysematous whereas, in others, an apparently similar amount of dust is associated with negligible emphysema; and the duration of dust exposure and age of death may be the same in both. Again, under the dissecting microscope dust may be found in only one segment of a dilated respiratory bronchiole while the remainder of

227

the wall is dust free. One would not expect to see such variable features as these if 'focal emphysema' were due primarily to the result of dust accumulation. Furthermore, there is no reason to suppose that soot and pigment are more likely to be the cause of 'distensive' centrilobular ('focal') emphysema than that they have accumulated in established areas of emphysema in preference to normal lung (Heard and Izukawa, 1963). On present evidence it is justifiable to believe that the same *post hoc* or *propter hoc* question applies equally to coal and carbon dusts.

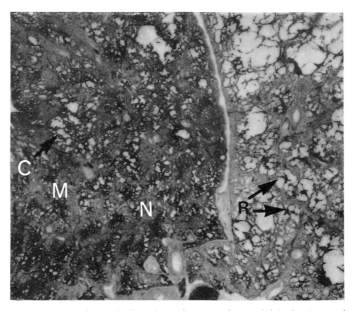

Figure 8.7. Coal-miner's lung (apical region of upper lobe) showing coal macules and nodules without associated emphysema (M, N), mild dust-pigmented centrilobular emphysema (C) and irregular emphysema around dust-pigmented scars forming 'rosette' patterns (R). By contrast, the moderately severe centrilobular emphysema in the apical region of the lower lobe (right upper corner of picture) is completely free of dust.
(Paper-mounted lung section, natural size)

Dust may also be present in the alveolar walls of panlobular (*see Figure 1.12*) and paraseptal emphysema (Heard, 1969) but there is nothing to indicate that it is causally responsible.

To summarize, although 'distensive', dust-pigmented centrilobular ('focal') emphysema is often a feature of the lungs of coal and carbon workers it is not a *sine qua non* since it is not always or uniformly present, and it is also found in the general population. Because the concept of 'focal emphysema' as a separate entity is controversial it might be preferable to replace this term by 'centrilobular emphysema with dust' as a counterpart to 'centrilobular emphysema without dust'.

However, it must be emphasized that whatever the truth of the matter may be, it is of no importance in practice because centrilobular emphysema with dust does not cause any symptoms or physical signs and, although it has been suggested that it may be responsible for a slight reduction in gas transfer and arterial oxygen found in some cases of apparent 'simple' coal pneumoconiosis, this reduction is too small to be of clinical significance (*see* Lung Function).

Emphysema in general

It has been claimed by Ryder *et al.* (1970) that there is a significant overall excess of all types of emphysema in coal miners with pneumoconiosis. But this conclusion is questionable as the miners studied were a minority of the total mining population in the United Kingdom (Rae, Muir and Jacobsen, 1970); other important sources of bias were present (Fletcher, 1970; Gilson and Oldham, 1970) and the definition of emphysema was ambiguous. Similarly, a more recent assertion by the same authors that 'simple' coal pneumoconiosis usually causes progressive impairment of ventilation which is not related to radiographic category but is due to emphysema which cannot be detected on the x-ray film (Lyons *et al.*, 1972) is also to be questioned because their conclusion that the emphysema is due to the pneumoconiosis is contrary to their own evidence (Fletcher, 1972a; Higgins, 1972; Oldham and Berry, 1972). As the data showed no quantitative relationship between the severity of emphysema and the amount of dust in the lungs as revealed by radiographic category it is difficult to conclude that the emphysema is caused by the coal dust (Fletcher, 1972b).

Finally, it is worth noting the following points: the observation by Caplan (1962) that Category 0 to 1 radiographs of coal-miners are associated with minimal 'simple' pneumoconiosis but often with a 'moderate or severe' degree of emphysema when the lungs are examined, is in agreement with the low mean dust content of the lungs in these cases (Rossiter *et al.*, 1967; Rossiter, 1972a); 'simple' pneumoconiosis in coal workers is closely related to the dust content of the lungs (Rossiter, 1972b); and no correlation between the radiographic signs of dust retention, on the one hand, and widespread emphysema, on the other, was found in coal-miners by Caplan, Simon and Reid (1966).

PROGRESSIVE MASSIVE FIBROSIS (P.M.F.)

Macroscopic appearances

These black fibrotic masses usually favour the upper halves and posterior parts of the lungs but there are many exceptions to this. They may be found in the centre of the lung, in the base of a lower lobe, or in the lingula or middle lobe (*Figure 8.8*). They may be bilateral and roughly symmetrical in size and outline or, more commonly, of disparate shape, size and distribution in the two lungs. Sometimes only a single mass occurs. When a mass is near the periphery the overlying pulmonary pleura is often puckered and fibrotic and may be adherent to the parietal layer. A remarkable feature of these lesions is their variable conformation and the fact that they are frequently not confined by the anatomical boundaries of lobes, segments or septa. Therefore, when cut across they may be round, elliptical or linear in shape and so well circumscribed that they appear almost encapsulated and as if dropped into the lung which is neither distorted nor evidently compressed adjacently;

229

but in other cases they are of irregular shape with poorly defined margins which extend in stellate fashion into the surrounding lung (*Figure 8.9*). Scar emphysema, sometimes with bullae, may surround some irregular masses, but is exceptional and does not occur in relation to circumscribed masses. Bullae may remain distended due to air-trapping after the lung has been removed from the chest.

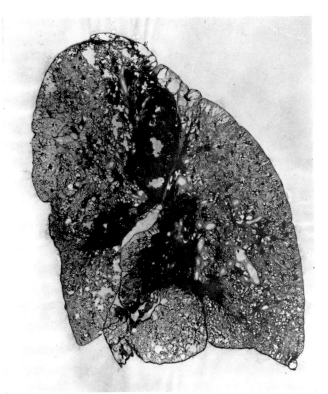

Figure 8.8. P.M.F. in a coal-miner's lung. The upper lobe lesion is irregular in outline, contains necrotic cavitated areas, is well demarcated from adjacent lung tissue and is not associated with scar emphysema. The masses in the lingula and lower lobe are less commonly seen than lesions in the upper half of the lung. (From paper-mounted lung section; approximately ×0·4 natural size)

A massive lesion or nodule is arbitrarily defined as P.M.F. when its diameter exceeds 3 cm (James, 1954). The cut surface of the mass is commonly homogeneously black—although there may be grey patches—and is uniformly hard or rubbery. Some masses, however, contain pultaceous areas of necrosis which scintillate due to the presence of cholesterol crystals, and others are black, shaggy-walled cavities caused by the previous evacuation of the necrotic contents into a connecting airway. After evacuation such cavities often refill with fluid of similar composition to blood plasma (Gernez-Rieux *et al.*, 1958). Occasionally, small caseous or calcified areas indicative of tuberculosis are seen within a mass.

Coal or carbon P.M.F. is readily distinguished from silicotic conglomeration by an excess of black dust and by the absence of matted individual silicotic nodules with a grey whorled pattern which characterize the latter. 'Simple'

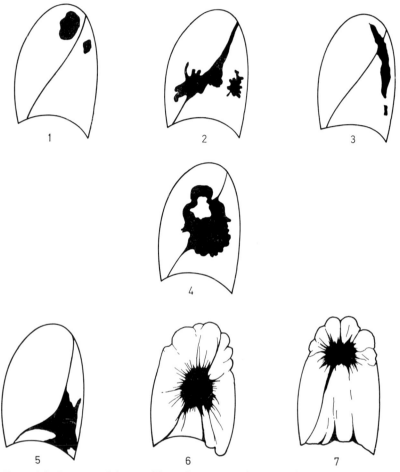

Figure 8.9. Diagram of the variable conformations of P.M.F. which may be seen when the lung is cut in the sagittal plane. (1) Solid, well circumscribed mass without scar emphysema; (2) and (3) roughly linear and irregular masses. Often these do not respect lobar boundaries; (4) large, well circumscribed, cavitated central mass without scar emphysema. When bilateral, masses of this sort usually cause obliteration of many pulmonary artery branches, leading to cor pulmonale; (5) irregular contracted mass in the uncommon location of the lower lobe; (6) contracted irregular central mass with scar emphysema; (7) contracted irregular mass in upper part of lung with severe scar and bullous emphysema

dust macules or nodules, or both, usually accompany the masses to a greater or lesser degree, but in some cases they are virtually absent. When the dust is graphite or some other form of carbon the lungs are often intensely and uniformly black.

If there has been past exposure to fairly high concentrations of quartz as well as to coal or carbon dust typical—but sometimes immature—silicotic nodules or areas of 'mixed dust fibrosis' (*see* Chapter 7) may be present in addition to the coal or carbon lesions, and there may be egg-shell calcification of the hilar lymph nodes. This is seen particularly in coal-miners who have done much rock drilling in shaft sinking or road developing or repairing, or who worked in collieries with heavily faulted ground. Indeed, in some mining areas, silicotic nodules—both discrete and conglomerate—may predominate, there being only slight characteristic coal pneumoconiosis; for example, in the United Kingdom, the Wigan area of Lancashire (Spink and Nagelschmidt, 1963) and the West Cumberland area (Faulds, King and Nagelschmidt, 1959). Silicotic nodules have also been observed with carbon pneumoconiosis in men who worked with natural graphite in the manufacture of carbon refractories (Gloyne, Marshall and Hoyle, 1949).

Hilar lymph nodes are usually black, firm and slightly enlarged.

Microscopic appearances
The structure of P.M.F. is identical to coal nodules (and 'infective nodules') and consists of a large quantity of coal (or carbon) dust, lymphocytes, dust-laden macrophages and dense bundles of reticulin and collagen fibres some of which are hyalinized. Bronchioles are usually annihilated but remnants of small pulmonary arteries and arterioles may be found in which there is progressive invasion by dust-bearing fibrous tissue from adventitia to intima to the point of obliteration; at this stage fragments of elastic lamina (revealed by elastic tissue stains) are the only evidence that these vessels existed (Wells, 1954a). At the periphery of P.M.F., arteries are partly or completely obstructed by endarteritis and the bigger the mass, the larger and more proximal are the arteries involved. Thrombosis may occur in these arteries and spread in retrograde fashion sometimes as far as the main pulmonary artery branches (Wells, 1954b), but embolism from this source is rare. Arterial obstruction may cause ischaemic colliquative necrosis within the mass and if a bronchus is eroded the necrotic material is expelled in the sputum resulting in cavitation as already described. Similar changes may be found in the small arteries around coal nodules and in pneumoconiosis due to graphite (Pendergrass *et al.*, 1968).

In some cases plasma cells are very prominent in endarteritis adjacent to P.M.F. and immunofluorescent techniques have demonstrated that rheumatoid factor (IgM) is present in these cells (Wagner and McCormick, 1967) even though the masses show none of the features of 'rheumatoid' coal nodules (*see* next section). In addition, rheumatoid factor has been found in aggregations of plasma cells and in subcapsular follicles in hilar lymph nodes in these cases (Wagner and McCormick, 1967). This suggests the possibility of immune reactivity being involved in the pathogenesis of some P.M.F. lesions. In others, caseous areas with the histological characteristics of tuberculosis are present and may yield tubercle bacilli on culture; but such cases are exceptional.

Occasionally, typical or immature silicotic lesions are found within a mass, but the amount of collagen in P.M.F. is substantially less than it is in silicotic conglomerations.

It is of interest that the collagenous tissue elaborated in P.M.F. appears to

232

be similar to that of parietal pleural plaques in asbestos workers, and to be typical of collagen produced in response to injury or irritation, and that there is a similar propensity to calcification in both processes. (Wusteman, Gold and Wagner, 1972).

'RHEUMATOID' COAL PNEUMOCONIOSIS (CAPLAN'S SYNDROME)

This is a modified form of coal pneumoconiosis, first described by Caplan in 1953, in which large nodular lesions are associated with rheumatoid

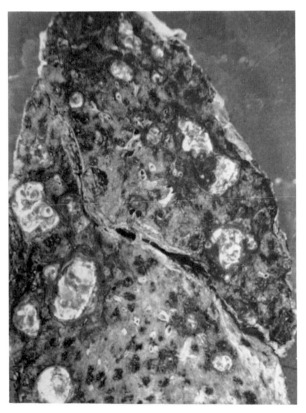

Figure 8.10. Large, well circumscribed and encapsulated necrobiotic (Caplan) nodules. Discrete, 'non-rheumatoid' coal nodules are also scattered in the lung; these are not often so numerous in 'rheumatoid' coal pneumoconiosis as in this case. (Approximately ¾ natural size; courtesy, Dr R. M. E. Seal)

arthritis. Its existence as a distinct entity has since been widely confirmed by others and the concept of the syndrome extended to include the occurrence of similar, as well as less distinctive, lesions in the absence of rheumatoid arthritis though associated with circulating rheumatoid factor (Caplan, Payne and Withey, 1962). Rheumatoid arthritis may precede or occur years after the appearance of the lung lesions, and in some cases never develops.

233

The prevalence of 'rheumatoid' pneumoconiosis among 21,000 coal-miners in the East Midlands coalfield in the United Kingdom has been reported to

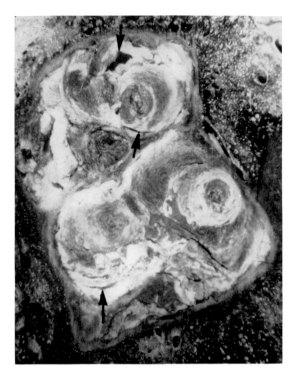

Figure 8.11. Collection of necrobiotic nodules in apex of the lower lobe in Figure 8.10. Note clefts (arrowed) and circular zones of dust. (Magnification × 2·75 approx; courtesy of Dr R. M. E. Seal)

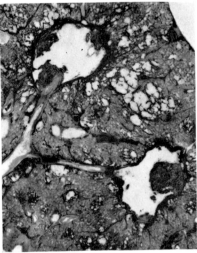

Figure 8.12. Cavitation of Caplan nodules adjacent to small bronchi. Collier with active rheumatoid arthritis, DAT 1: 128. Note scarcity of ordinary lesions of coal pneumoconiosis.(From paper-mounted lung section, natural size)

vary from 2·3 to 6·2 per cent of men with pneumoconiosis in different collieries (Lindars and Davies, 1967). This is similar to the proportion of persons with circulating rheumatoid factor in the general population (*see* page 78).

234

Macroscopic appearances

The pulmonary pleura is thickened, often more on one side than the other, in a proportion of cases. The nodules vary from about 0·3 cm to 2·0 cm diameter, but may be up to 3 cm diameter, and are scattered irregularly in any part of the lungs although they have some propensity for the upper zones. Their cut surface has a characteristic concentric arrangement of alternating black and grey-white to yellow bands due respectively to laminated collections of dust and to necrotic collagen (*Figure 8.10*). Liquefaction in the lighter areas may appear as clefts and may contain collections of cholesterol crystals (*Figure 8.11*); indeed whole nodules may become necrotic and, if they are connected with airways, discharge their contents into them leaving small cavities which subsequently close in most cases (*Figure 8.12*). These lesions are now often referred to as 'necrobiotic' nodules. If their contents are not discharged they may calcify, and in some cases many such calcified nodules are seen. Aggregation of nodules into composite groups occasionally occurs and these may closely resemble a conglomeration of typical silicotic nodules (*Figure 8.13*). Inspection of a 'rheumatoid' coal nodule with a hand-lens helps to distinguish its features from those of a silicotic nodule, but microscopy is sometimes required for confirmation.

Coal-dust macules or nodules are usually absent in the majority of these cases but, when present, they are of typical appearance indicating that the 'rheumatoid' process does not necessarily involve all the pneumoconiotic lesions (*Figure 8.10*).

Microscopic appearances (*Figure 8.14*)

The centres of most of the nodules consist of necrotic tissue in which there are no surviving cells and which stains pink with haematoxylin and eosin; its collagen content is variable. A blue-staining area of cellular infiltration surrounds this zone and in some instances forms a complete circle and in others a segment only, depending upon the plane of section; the cells are macrophages, polymorphonuclear leucocytes, fibroblasts and occasionally, multinucleated giant cells. More peripherally there are circumferentially arranged collagen fibres, fibroblasts and numerous plasma cells. Fibroblasts adjacent to the necrotic area are often grouped in palisade formation though not so strikingly as in subcutaneous rheumatoid nodules. Special stains for 'fibrinoid' are not helpful (Gough, Rivers and Seal, 1955). By contrast with silicotic nodules, clefts containing cholesterol crystals are often present. During periods of activity, dust-containing macrophages migrate into the lesions and later disrupt and discharge their dust load which remains distributed in concentric rings. Necrosis in these active zones is the cause of the segmental clefts. Numerous plasma cells and lymphocytes are an important feature in the collagenous zones.

Arteries around the nodules exhibit endarteritis in which plasma cells are significantly more predominant than in 'non-rheumatoid' pneumoconiosis; IgM is present in their walls (Wagner and McCormick, 1967) and in the cells (Wagner, 1971), and 7S γ globulin (presumably IgG) has been observed near the centres and in the outer collagenous zones of the nodules (Pernis *et al.*, 1965).

When activity in the nodule has ceased the necrotic areas tend to calcify

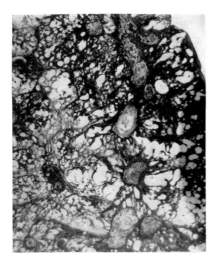

in which case the multiple concentric rings of dust are the only remaining evidence suggestive of their 'rheumatoid' origin. In those cases where the nodules are small (4–5 mm diameter) and numerous, their microscopical features are similar.

Figure 8.13. Small 'rheumatoid' coal nodules resembling silicotic nodules. (From paper-mounted lung section, natural size)

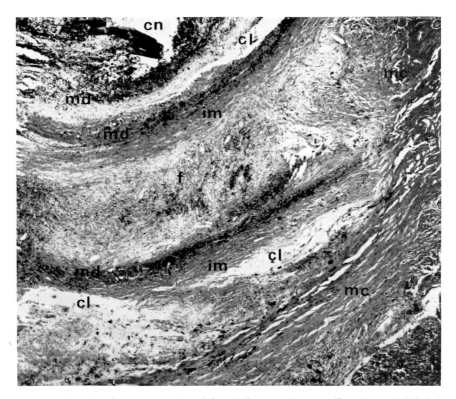

Figure 8.14. Necrobiotic (Caplan) nodule. Coal-miner 18 years. (See Figure 8.26.) (cn) central area of necrosis; (md) zones of macrophage infiltration and coal-dust; (cl) clefts; (f) zone of fibroblasts and other cells; (im) immature collagen; (mc) mature collagen. (Original magnification ×45, reproduced at ×40; Martius scarlet blue stain)

236

Bacteriology

Tubercle bacilli cannot be isolated by culture or guinea-pig inoculation from any of these lesions.

Distinguishing features

'Rheumatoid' coal nodules, clearly, are distinct from the typical nodules of coal pneumoconiosis or silicosis, and they show evidence of immunological reactivity. The features which distinguish between Caplan necrobiotic nodules, typical silicosis and tuberculosis may be summarized as follows:

Gross appearances

Caplan nodules are generally discrete, up to 3 cm diameter but may be larger, and are sometimes formed into composite groups. They are distributed at random in the lungs. There is a clear-cut concentric ring pattern of dust in nodules sectioned through or near their centres, and necrosis with cavitation is fairly common in one or more lesions.

TABLE 8.1

	Nodules of coal pneumoconiosis	Caplan nodules	Typical silicotic nodules	Tuberculosis and dust
Dust lamination	−	+ + +	−	+
Palisading of fibroblasts	−	+	−	+
Cholesterol crystal spaces	−	+ +	−	+
Central necrosis	−	+ +	+ (rare)	+ +
Calcification	+ (rare)	+ +	−	+ +
Excess of peripheral lympho- cytes and plasma cells	−	+ +	−	−
M. tuberculosis (culture or guinea-pig inoculation)	−	−	−	+ + +

Typical silicotic nodules may also be discrete but, as a rule, are smaller than Caplan nodules and tend to occupy the upper halves of the lungs. Conglomerations of nodules are usually more closely matted than composite Caplan nodules. Concentric rings of dust are either absent or very poorly defined but occasionally the gross appearances may be identical. Central necrosis is rare (*see* Chapter 7). The occupational history should point to silicosis.

Tuberculous lesions are not defined or circumscribed like Caplan nodules and tend to agglomerate in irregular form and occupy the upper parts of the lungs. Dust rings are rarely present and caseation is often evident.

Microscopical appearances

These and the bacteriological findings are shown in Table 8.1.

Differentiation on histological grounds alone may present some difficulty at times but the correct diagnosis of 'rheumatoid' pneumoconiosis can be made in almost all cases by gross inspection of the lesions—possibly with the aid of a hand-lens—by an experienced observer.

DIFFUSE INTERSTITIAL FIBROSIS

Diffuse interstitial fibrosis—sometimes with honeycombing—is occasionally found in association with coal pneumoconiosis and has also been observed

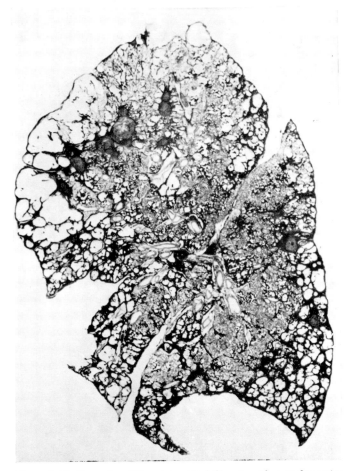

Figure 8.15. Extensive diffuse interstitial fibrosis with cyst formation ('honeycombing') with typical Caplan-type nodules. The honeycomb areas and periphery of the nodules are intensely dust pigmented. The rest of the lung is virtually free of dust pigmentation and ordinary lesions of coal pneumoconiosis. Coal-miner with rheumatoid arthritis. (From paper-mounted lung section provided by Professor J. Gough; slightly less than half natural size)

in graphite pneumoconiosis (Gaensler *et al.*, 1966; Pendergrass *et al.*, 1968). The fibrotic areas between the cysts are usually, but not invariably, heavily dust pigmented. They are predominant in the subpleural zones of the lower lobes but are occasionally widespread in all lobes. In a few cases typical Caplan nodules may be found together with honeycombing in the same lungs (*Figure 8.15*) and circulating rheumatoid factor, with or without accompanying rheumatoid arthritis, is present in such cases.

Diffuse interstitial fibrosis and coal-dust together may cause 'p' type opacities on the chest radiograph (*see* page 127).

DUST CONTENT OF THE LUNGS

The total amount of dust in lungs with coal pneumoconiosis is greatly in excess of that found in lungs with nodular silicosis and it consists mainly of coal, but non-coal dust and a small amount of quartz is also present (*see Figure 4.4*). Rivers *et al.* (1960), in the United Kingdom, found that it ranged from 5 to 88 g in lungs with 'simple' pneumoconiosis and, of this, quartz formed 2 per cent. Another British study (Nagelschmidt *et al.*, 1963), which also included lungs with P.M.F., showed considerable differences in both mean total dust and quartz content, the latter being increased in rock drillers; but, in the absence of histological evidence of silicosis, collier's lungs with P.M.F. contained only 2 to 3 per cent quartz (Nagelschmidt, 1960). Similar free silica concentrations have been found in the lungs of West Virginia bituminous-coal miners although the total dust was lower, and a higher concentration of trace elements compared with the lungs of non-miners was also present (Carlberg *et al.*, 1971).

The mean size of coal particles recovered from the lungs has been referred to in Chapter 3.

The amount of quartz expressed as a percentage of dried lung has been estimated to be 0·02 per cent or less in the pneumoconiosis of carbon electrode workers (Watson *et al.*, 1959), and similar values have been found by Otto and Einbrodt (1958). Analyses of graphite lungs have shown that free silica as a percentage of dry lung weight has varied from none (Rüttner, Bovet and Aufdermaur, 1952) to 0·12 per cent (Town, 1968), 0·35 per cent (Pendergrass *et al.*, 1967) and 0·50 per cent (Harding and Oliver, 1949).

So, the quartz content ranges from negligible in carbon pneumoconiosis to very small in coal pneumoconiosis by contrast with some 20 per cent of total dust in nodular silicosis (Nagelschmidt, 1960).

PATHOGENESIS

Only a brief review of this complex and incompletely solved problem is appropriate here.

From what has been said earlier the quartz content of coal-mine dust may range from negligible to large, depending upon the geology of the mines and the occupation of the miner but, in general, it tends to be low. Similarly, the quartz content of natural graphite varies considerably, but is less than 0·4 per cent in artificial graphite and carbon black.

Quantity and type of coal-dust

Past exposure to dust is well correlated with radiographic category (Fay and Ashford, 1961) and the amount of 'simple' coal pneumoconiosis is closely related to the dust content of the lungs (Rossiter, 1972b); the greater the exposure and, hence, the greater amount of dust in the lungs, the higher the

239

category. The probability of P.M.F. developing is related to the category of 'simple' pneumoconiosis (*see* section on Epidemiology).

The rank of coal (*see* Chapter 2) does not influence the naked eye or microscopical features of coal pneumoconiosis which are identical in the United Kingdom and the U.S.A. (Heppleston, 1951) and elsewhere. High-rank coals, such as anthracite, are associated with a greater prevalence of pneumoconiosis than low-rank coals (Hicks *et al.*, 1961; Lainhart and Morgan, 1971); and, experimentally, elimination of inhaled, high-rank coal-dust from the lungs of 'specific-pathogen-free' rats is lower than low-rank coal-dust (Heppleston, Civil and Critchlow, 1971). Furthermore, lung dust composition varies with rank; the higher the rank, the higher the coal percentage and the lower the quartz percentage (Bergman and Cassell, 1972). However, there is evidence that the effects attributed to rank are related more to the mass of dust inhaled (Jacobsen *et al.*, 1971).

Hence, the quantity of coal-dust retained in the lungs appears to be the most important factor in pathogenesis, but rank may play a subsidiary part.

Effect of quartz

Coal and carbon are not cytotoxic (Chapter 4), and in the lungs of experimental animals they behave as inert dusts causing only mild reticulin proliferation; but when large quantities of these dusts are mixed with small quantities of quartz, reticulin proliferation is significantly increased (Ray, King and Harrison, 1951). Quartz, by itself, in a concentration of 4 per cent causes fibrosis in the lungs and hilar lymph nodes of rats (Schlipköter *et al.*, 1971); but the fibrogenic effect of much larger concentrations of quartz is substantially reduced by the presence of coal-dust and with lower concentrations (3 per cent) the inhibitory effect is even more pronounced (Schlipköter *et al.*, 1971). Administration of PVPNO with quartz reduces the fibrogenic effect still further (*see* Chapter 4) suggesting that this effect is due to quartz (Schlipköter, 1970).

If these observations apply to man they would seem to imply that even a small quantity of quartz, though muted in its effect by coal- and clay-dusts, may play an important part in the pathogenesis of coal pneumoconiosis.

On the other hand, many authorities contend that quartz plays no part in the aetiology of coal or carbon pneumoconiosis. The chief reasons for this are: first, cases of 'simple' pneumoconiosis and P.M.F. have occurred in men exposed to carbon black (Miller and Ramsden, 1961; Lister and Wimborne, 1972), artificial graphite (Dunner and Bagnall, 1949; Zahorski, 1961) and coal and coke mixtures used in electrode manufacture (Otto and Einbrodt, 1958; Watson *et al.*, 1959) in which the quartz content was negligible—0·1 per cent or less (Okutani, Shima and Sano, 1964); 'simple' coal pneumoconiosis and P.M.F. ranging in size from the radiographic equivalent of Categories A to C has a similar low value in all (Nagelschmidt, 1960), and the amount of quartz in the P.M.F. lesions themselves is insignificantly higher than it is in the rest of the lung or in other lungs with 'simple' pneumoconiosis only (Nagelschmidt *et al.*, 1963). Hence selective concentration of quartz does not appear to be a factor in the development of P.M.F. Policard *et al.* (1967) found that the effect on the lungs of rats of samples of coal-dust with a quartz content varying from 0 to 4·9 per cent from thirteen French collieries was inhibited by the aluminium silicate—in the form of kaolin, illite and montmorillonite—which they also contain. These authors suggest that this observation virtually exonerates quartz from playing a significant role in the development of coal pneumoconiosis.

PROGRESSIVE MASSIVE FIBROSIS

Four theories have been advanced for the genesis of these lesions.

(1) *Local concentration of quartz.*—Higher quartz concentrations have been supposed to occur in some parts of the lungs than in others and provoke more prolific fibrogenesis—modified by coal-dust—than elsewhere. But, as just indicated, lung analysis does not support this and there is no reason to suppose that quartz concentrations might be higher in one area of a lung than another. Furthermore, an epidemiological study of chest radiographs of British coal-miners over a five-year period does not support the quartz hypothesis (McLintock, Rae and Jacobsen, 1971).

(2) *Total lung dust.*—After accumulation of a certain quantity of coal- or carbon-dust, local fibrogenesis is triggered off in some unknown way. But dust concentrations may sometimes be as high in lungs in which there are only 'simple' lesions as they are in those with P.M.F. Hence, although the quantity of total dust probably plays a dominant role it is unlikely that it can be a simple one.

(3) *Tuberculosis.*—An alleged modification of tuberculous disease by coal-dust has held a dominant place for years.

James (1954) reported that evidence of tuberculosis was present in 40 per cent of 454 cases of confluent masses at autopsy, culture or guinea-pig inoculation being positive in 36 per cent. Rivers *et al.* (1957) also cultured tubercle bacilli from 35 per cent of cases with P.M.F. However, during life, the recovery rate of tubercle bacilli from the sputum of South Wales miners with P.M.F. has usually been very low—1·1 per cent (Cochrane, Cox and Jarman, 1952) and 2·7 per cent (Marks, 1961); but Kilpatrick, Heppleston and Fletcher (1957) found a 'positive sputum' in 7·7 per cent of men with cavitated P.M.F. due, undoubtedly, to the selection of the cases. It is exceptional to find evidence of tuberculosis in these lesions today.

Concentration of soot and pigment in the area of tuberculous disease in the lungs of town dwellers has often been observed due, probably, to migration of soot-laden macrophages to the site. It is likely that a similar process occurs when tuberculosis develops in lungs containing coal-dust.

Nevertheless, there is strong evidence against the tuberculous hypothesis. It is not supported by epidemiological study (Cochrane, 1962), and no differences in tuberculin sensitivity was demonstrated in South Wales between miners and ex-miners with P.M.F. and men with either no pneumoconiosis or 'simple' pneumoconiosis only (Hart, Cochrane and Higgins, 1963). In Holland, Hendriks and Bleiker (1964) found no correlation between tuberculin sensitivity and category of pneumoconiosis. But, by contrast, Fritze *et al.* (1969) observed an above-average prevalence of positive tuberculin reactors in a survey of 1,700 coal-miners in the Federal German Republic. Prolonged treatment with antituberculous drugs in 'sputum negative' miners

R   241

does not prevent progression of P.M.F. (McCallum, 1961; Ball *et al.*, 1969), and the majority of the masses do not show any microscopical evidence of tuberculosis. Finally, it appears that although the collagen content of the lung is significantly increased in lungs with fibrocaseous and inactive fibrotic tuberculous lesions it is only slightly more in P.M.F. compared with the rest of the lung (Wagner, 1970).

Because 'opportunist' mycobacteria occur (mainly as secondary invaders) more frequently in miners with pneumoconiosis than in the general population it has been suggested that they may be important in the pathogenesis of P.M.F. (Marks, 1961). This remains to be proved. In experimental animals coal-dust and photochromogenic bacilli cause areas of confluent fibrosis (with a low proportion of collagen to reticulin) which subsequently regresses (Byers and King, 1959); and coal-dust with *M. kansasii* gives rise to cellular lesions without fibrosis which subsequently resolve completely (Gernez-Rieux *et al.*, 1965).

(4) *Immunological factors.*—As already described, both immunologically competent cells and rheumatoid factor (IgM) have been demonstrated at the periphery of some non-'rheumatoid' coal nodules and P.M.F. lesions, and in the hilar lymph nodes (Wagner and McCormick, 1967). Hence, immunological activity is not confined to typical Caplan-type nodules, and probably plays a part in some way in the genesis of some cases of P.M.F.

Patients with rheumatoid arthritis have been shown to have a defect of iron metabolism in addition to immunological hyper-reactivity; this appears to be due to iron deficiency caused either by abnormal iron-binding capacity of plasma proteins or by mobilization of tissue iron via abnormal channels which results in a low serum iron level in the presence of normal, erythropoiesis (Weinstein, 1959). It is of interest, therefore, that a similar defect in iron metabolism has been observed in seropositive coal miners with P.M.F. but without any evidence of rheumatoid arthritis (Chan, 1969a), although the significance of this remains to be elucidated.

The possibility of a genetic influence has been little studied. Hutchinson (1966) recorded that the degree and progression of coal pneumoconiosis was somewhat similar in monozygotic and dizygotic twin brothers. A survey of 1250 Welsh coal-miners and examiners (Higgins *et al.*, 1963), revealed no convincing association between ABO or rhesus blood groups, or secretor status and coal pneumoconiosis. If there is a genetic effect it is most likely to act through the medium of immune reactivity.

To summarize, it appears that the chief factor in the pathogenesis of 'simple' pneumoconiosis or P.M.F. is the mass or quantity of respirable coal- or carbon-dust; that the rank of coal may have some effect but that the part played by quartz is uncertain and, in some cases, non-existent. The development of P.M.F. is probably due to several causes in addition to the amount of dust, tuberculosis being of minor importance.

'RHEUMATOID' COAL NODULES

A significant association of circulating rheumatoid factor and radiographic evidence of rheumatoid coal pneumoconiosis, with and without arthritis, by comparison with 'simple' coal pneumoconiosis and P.M.F. without arthritis was demonstrated by Caplan, Payne and Withey (1962) (*Figure 8.16*).

The pathogenesis of the lesions is uncertain but, as the presence of immuno-logically competent cells and rheumatoid factor (IgM) in and around the nodules suggests, it is almost certainly determined by an immunological reaction in the presence of much smaller amounts of dust than are associated with conventional P.M.F. This is supported by the fact that rheumatoid pneumoconiosis usually occurs with little or no 'background' of 'simple' pneumoconiosis, and that in one epidemiological study its prevalence was similar to that of circulating rheumatoid factor in the general population (Lindars and Davies, 1967) (*see* page 234).

It has been suggested that persons with the rheumatoid diathesis are unduly

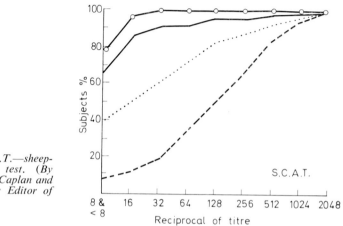

Figure 8.16. S.C.A.T.—sheep-cell agglutination test. (By courtesy of Dr A. Caplan and colleagues and the Editor of Thorax)

sensitive to small changes in autologous protein and that particles of coal-dust alter surface-absorbed serum protein so that it reacts with rheumatoid factor (Payne, 1963) and enhances antigen-antibody reaction. But this is not supported by more recent observations (Jones, Edwards and Wagner, 1972) and an alternative hypothesis proposes that non-specific lung damage or fibrosis may expose IgG-like antigens in basement membrane and give rise to rheumatoid factor (McCormick, 1972). But this does not explain the patho-genesis of the typical lesion of 'rheumatoid' coal pneumoconiosis. It may be that a cellular rather than immunological mechanism is initially involved. Investigation of the problem continues.

Miall (1955) showed that there was no increased prevalence of rheumatoid arthritis among miners and ex-miners with P.M.F. compared with an agricultural population, indicating that the pathogenesis of the arthritis is not related to dust exposure nor to the P.M.F. process in the lungs (*Figure 8.17*). This observation is in keeping with the similar prevalence of 'rheuma-toid' pneumoconiosis in colliers and that of circulating rheumatoid factor in the general population in the United Kingdom (*see* page 234).

The status of the tuberculin test in 'rheumatoid' pneumoconiosis does not appear to be known but coexistent tuberculosis is very rare.

DIFFUSE INTERSTITIAL FIBROSIS WITH COAL OR CARBON PNEUMOCONIOSIS

On present knowledge there is no clear evidence of a causal relationship between coal- (or carbon-) dust and diffuse interstitial fibrosis (fibrosing 'alveolitis'); indeed, the incidence of the cryptogenic form of the disease in

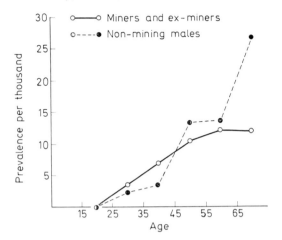

Figure 8.17. Prevalence of confirmed rheumatoid arthritis in miners and non-miners in Wales. There is no increased prevalence among the miners and ex-miners. (By courtesy of Dr W. E. Miall (1955) and the Editor of Annals of Rheumatic Diseases)

the general population is not known. It is probable that the pathogenesis of the fibrosis will prove to have an immunological basis—at least in part.

CLINICAL FEATURES

Symptoms

'Simple' pneumoconiosis is symptomless. When cough, sputum, wheeze or breathlessness are complained of they are due to coincidental lung disease—most frequently, in the United Kingdom, chronic obstructive bronchitis. Among British coal-miners smoking has been found to be the chief factor contributing to respiratory symptoms (Ashford *et al.*, 1970).

There is little correlation between radiographic category of P.M.F. and respiratory symptoms. Category A lesions cause no symptoms and larger masses may be associated with either no symptoms or with symptoms ranging from the trivial to very severe respiratory disability. The reasons for this variability are referred to in the section on Lung Function.

There is usually no sputum associated with P.M.F. if the subject is a non-smoker; when there is, it is generally of small volume but may be large if there is infection in distorted and dilated bronchi in proximity to a mass of P.M.F. It is commonly gelatinous and grey coloured (due to small quantities of coal- or carbon-dust), but may become much darker during chest infection which causes increased elimination of coal-dust even years after the man has ceased to be exposed to dust. In the absence of active tuberculosis (or other causes) haemoptysis is extremely rare in cases of P.M.F., but is not uncommon —although consisting of little more than staining of the sputum with blood— in cases of 'rheumatoid' pneumoconiosis; this, in association with the radio-graphic appearances of cavitation (*see* Radiographic Appearances), may

244

compound a mistaken diagnosis of 'sputum negative' tuberculosis. Large haemoptysis is very rare. Jet-black sputum is produced by the occasional rupture of P.M.F. with ischaemic necrosis into a bronchus; it may be large in amount, suddenly raised by distressing paroxysmal coughing and may continue in smaller amounts for some days. It consists of mucus containing large quantities of coal- (or carbon-) dust with cholesterol crystals and, occasionally, small amounts of blood.

Cough is, in general, related to cigarette smoking and the quantity or viscidity of the sputum. But in some cases of large P.M.F. lesions cough may be frequent, severe and paroxysmal although productive of a negligible amount of sputum, and is often provoked by effort. The reason for this is uncertain: it may be related to 'irritation' of the trachea and main bronchi by large adjacent masses.

Men with P.M.F. uncomplicated by severe scar emphysema or chronic airways obstruction rarely complain of breathlessness at rest but may do during or after effort.

Pain in the chest is sometimes complained of and is usually mild and transient; it appears to arise from thoracic muscular 'strains' but rarely may be due to cough fracture of the ribs.

Physical signs

There are no characteristic abnormal physical signs of coal or carbon pneumoconiosis.

Finger clubbing is not a feature of either 'simple' pneumoconiosis or P.M.F. The author found only 7 cases of undisputed clubbing in 252 men with Category B or C lesions (3 per cent). However, it is present, though rarely severe, in some men with 'p'-type category radiographs (see page 239).

Central cyanosis is not seen in the absence of airways obstruction of 'blue bloater' type or unrelated heart disease.

'Simple' pneumoconiosis and many cases of P.M.F. (even Category C) cause no abnormal signs. But impaired breath sounds and expiratory wheezes are found when massive lesions are associated with severe scar emphysema. Wheezes and rhonchi are more commonly due to coincidental chronic obstructive bronchitis. The trachea is occasionally drawn to one side on which the upper chest wall may be slightly flattened and limited in expansion due to an underlying large, contractile mass of P.M.F. Inspiratory and expiratory stridor caused by distortion of large airways may be heard at the mouth in such cases. In some men with Category 'p' radiographs, persistent inspiratory crepitations are present over the lower halves of both lungs.

Signs of pleural effusion may sometimes be present and may indicate the onset or exacerbation of rheumatoid disease. In these circumstances polyarthritis and subcutaneous rheumatoid nodules must be looked for.

Large, bilateral P.M.F. lesions may be accompanied by signs of pulmonary heart disease and, ultimately, congestive failure.

INVESTIGATIONS

Lung function

There are no abnormal physiological patterns which are characteristic of coal or carbon pneumoconiosis and so lung function tests are of no help in establishing the diagnosis.

In men with 'simple' pneumoconiosis no significant impairment of lung function is found in the absence of chronic airways obstruction, other lung

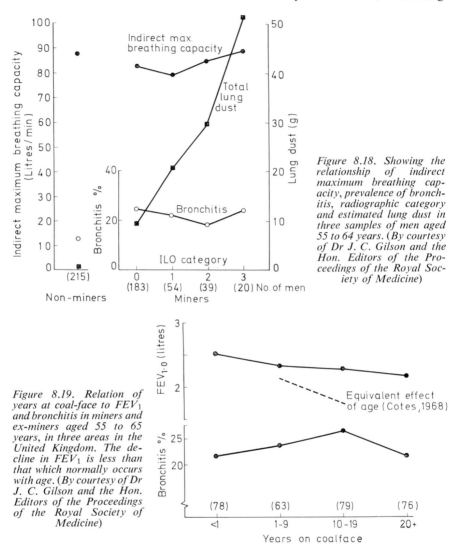

Figure 8.18. Showing the relationship of indirect maximum breathing capacity, prevalence of bronchitis, radiographic category and estimated lung dust in three samples of men aged 55 to 64 years. (By courtesy of Dr J. C. Gilson and the Hon. Editors of the Proceedings of the Royal Society of Medicine)

Figure 8.19. Relation of years at coal-face to FEV_1 and bronchitis in miners and ex-miners aged 55 to 65 years, in three areas in the United Kingdom. The decline in FEV_1 is less than that which normally occurs with age. (By courtesy of Dr J. C. Gilson and the Hon. Editors of the Proceedings of the Royal Society of Medicine)

disorders or the effects of smoking. In some mining populations, however, a slight fall of FEV_1 and FVC may be present in comparison with non-miners (Cotes, 1968; Lainhart and Morgan, 1971). Cochrane and Higgins (1961) found that ventilatory function did not decline with increasing radiographic category of 'simple' pneumoconiosis (*Figure 8.18*) and, although Rogan et al. (1961) observed a slight reduction, this was not significant when age was taken into account. Equally, the duration of exposure to coal-mine dust has no evident effect on FEV_1 (Cochrane and Higgins, 1961; Higgins *et al.*, 1968) (*Figure 8.19*). Lung volumes and mechanics are not affected and gas transfer is usually normal.

However, a proportion of men with 'p'-type category chest radiographs have a slightly reduced gas transfer factor compared with those with Category 'q' ('m') (Englebert and de Coster, 1965; Lyons *et al.*, 1967; Cotes *et al.*, 1971). This reduction does not appear to be explained on the grounds of occupational exposure, past chest illness or airways obstruction although it is significantly greater among smokers than non-smokers (Cotes *et al.*, 1971). In these cases the alveolar–arterial oxygen (A–a) gradient may be increased (Frans *et al.*, 1970) and arterial oxygen tension slightly reduced at rest, but these changes

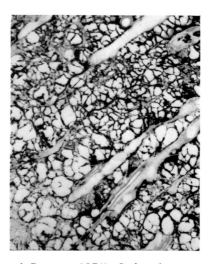

Figure 8.20. Coal-dust-pigmented panlobular emphysema which was almost uniform throughout both lungs. No fibrotic lesions of coal pneumoconiosis were found in any part of either lung. The radiographic appearances, which are shown in Figure 5·9, were ILO Category 'p'. (From paper-mounted section)

tend to correct on effort (Lapp and Seaton, 1971). It has been suggested, but not confirmed, that the underlying cause of these changes may be some diminution of the pulmonary capillary bed (Lapp and Seaton, 1971), although lung photoscanning techniques indicate that the vascular bed is normal in most cases of 'simple' coal pneumoconiosis (Seaton, Lapp and Chang, 1971). There also appears to be a larger physiological dead space relative to tidal volume than in category 'q' cases, and there may be some increase in ventilation during maximal exercise (Cotes and Field, 1972).

As these observations have attracted some attention the following points are worth noting:

(1) There is much more difficulty in relegating abnormal radiographic appearances accurately to the 'p' category than to the 'q' and 'r' categories, and this is particularly influenced by x-ray technique (*see* Chapter 5).

(2) No studies correlating the nature of the underlying lung pathology with the physiological changes appear to have been reported so that it cannot be taken for granted that they are due to coal pneumoconiosis. Indeed, both fine diffuse interstitial fibrosis and dust-pigmented panlobular emphysema (*Figure 8.20*) observed after death are not uncommonly associated with category 'p' radiographs in life (Parkes, 1972). (*See also* Chapter 5.)

(3) The physiological abnormalities are very small (Cotes *et al.*, 1971)

and are not associated with respiratory symptoms or with a reduction of capacity for heavy work (Lavenne, 1968, 1970).

Therefore, these observations, which are of considerable academic interest and require careful longitudinal investigation, have no evident practical significance in the individual case.

In P.M.F. there is a wide variation in the pattern and severity of impaired function which correlates very poorly with the radiographic appearances. It is determined variously, by the size and anatomical site of the masses, the amount of associated vasculitis and the presence or absence of scar (irregular) or panlobular emphysema and chronic obstructive bronchitis. Total lung capacity and vital capacity are usually reduced and residual volume increased, both as an absolute value and as a percentage of total lung capacity; ventilatory capacity may be reduced and, in some cases, there is irreversible airways obstruction. Compliance may be reduced but not to the extent commonly observed in asbestosis. The ventilation–perfusion ratio is impaired to a greater or lesser degree and gas transfer is reduced so that, in a proportion of cases, there is hypoxaemia on effort. The presence of a significant reduction in the vascular bed by large, central masses and associated arteritis accentuates these changes. Ventilation on effort may be normal or increased. Reduction in the ventilatory capacity is one of the best simple guides to the severity of disability in men with P.M.F.

Typical 'rheumatoid' coal pneumoconiosis of Caplan type (1953) is often accompanied by remarkably little impairment of function, presumably because only a small amount of lung tissue is involved, the remainder being normal. But atypical cases with confluent lesions exhibit, in varying degree, the changes just described.

Radiographic appearances

The earliest abnormal appearances consist of a few small, ill-defined opacities which can be distinguished peripherally from vascular shadows and are seen mainly in the upper and middle zones.

Category 'q' ('m') is the most commonly encountered size of opacity; category 'r' ('n') is relatively uncommon, and a definite Category 'p', more so. Opacities of different category may be present in the one film but one category usually predominates. The good correlation which exists between the profusion of opacities (Categories 1 to 3) and the lesions found in the lungs *post mortem* is referred to in Chapter 5 and the relationship to total lung dust is shown in *Figure 8.18*. Category correlates well with the iron content of the lungs which is itself highly correlated with the coal and mineral content (Caswell, Bergman and Rossiter, 1971; Rossiter, 1972a).

The opacities of 'simple' pneumoconiosis tend to be distributed in the upper halves of the lung fields until the Category 3 stage when the whole of the lung fields are more or less equally involved. P.M.F. opacities are also more likely to be seen in the upper halves of the lung fields than in the lower, but there are many exceptions to this. They may be unilateral or bilateral and, if the latter, roughly symmetrical or asymmetrical (*Figure 8.21*). Sometimes they are found in the middle and lower zones, in which case a single opacity may be obscured by the heart shadow and can only be made clearly visible by lateral or oblique views. There is usually a 'background' of

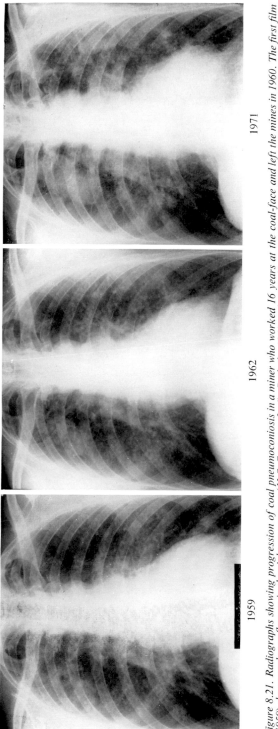

1959   1962   1971

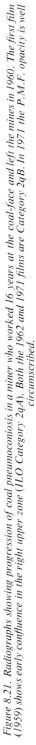

Figure 8.21. Radiographs showing progression of coal pneumoconiosis in a miner who worked 16 years at the coal-face and left the mines in 1960. The first film (1959) shows early confluence in the right upper zone (ILO Category 2qA). Both the 1962 and 1971 films are Category 2qB. In 1971 the P.M.F. opacity is well circumscribed.

Category 2 or 3 'simple' pneumoconiosis with P.M.F. but in occasional cases there is little or none; it would be interesting to know if these are associated more with evidence of immunological activity than those with Category 2 or 3.

P.M.F. opacities vary greatly in shape as well as size. They may be round, ovoid, sausage-like, or linear in outline, and, as a rule, are well demarcated from adjacent lung (*Figure 8.22*); but some have irregular projections and may be associated with Kerley B lines (Trapnell, 1964). Cavitation is indicated

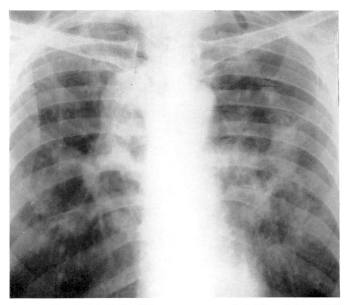

Figure 8.22. Coal P.M.F. of bizarre appearance in left lung field. P.M.F. close to mediastinum on the right. Autopsy confirmation

by a well-defined translucency in an opacity (*Figure 8.23*), and sometimes there is evidence of a fluid level. In most cases the cavity vanishes and the appearances revert wholly or partly to what they were before cavitation occurred. Areas of dense radio-opacity indicative of calcification may be present (*Figure 8.24*). P.M.F. of irregular, stellate outline is often associated with evidence of bullous emphysema, distortion of the lung and shift of trachea and mediastinum to the affected side. Occasionally, a mass may shift position over a period of years due mainly to hyperinflation of adjacent emphysematous lung.

The signs of 'egg shell' calcification of hilar lymph nodes, similar to those which may occur in silicosis (*see* Chapter 7), are present in a small proportion of cases of coal and natural graphite pneumoconiosis irrespective of the category rating. But, according to Jacobsen *et al.* (1967), they are more often found with P.M.F. than 'simple' pneumoconiosis and the author's observations have been similar (*Figure 8.24*). It is related to past exposure to dust from siliceous rock in shaft sinking or developing and maintaining colliery roads and airways; or to the quartz of natural graphite.

The opacities of 'rheumatoid' coal (or carbon) pneumoconiosis are a special case both in their appearance and behaviour. Typically they are round, fairly dense, vary from about 0·3 to 3·0 cm in diameter (occasionally up to 5 cm), are irregularly scattered in the lung fields, often in the lower zones, and are

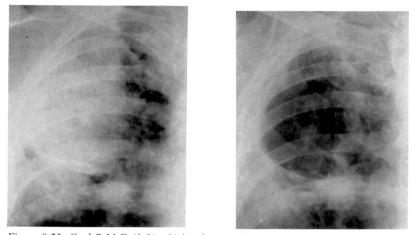

Figure 8.23. Coal P.M.F. (left) which subsequently became cavitary (right). Copious black sputum was expectorated during the development of the cavity which eventually disappeared

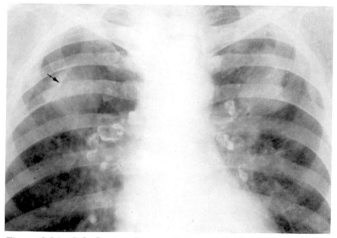

Figure 8.24. Calcification (arrowed) in coal P.M.F. This sign, which sometimes requires tomography for demonstration, is helpful in distinguishing P.M.F. from circumscribed bronchial carcinoma. Eggshell calcification of the hilar lymph nodes is also present. Case of a collier for 30 years some of which time was spent rock-drilling in drifts

usually moderate in number (Caplan, 1953) (*Figure 8.25*), but in some cases there may be only two or three or just a solitary opacity (*Figure 8.26*). Individual opacities are of variable density and are rarely completely homogeneous. The superimposition effect of a number of nodules may give the

251

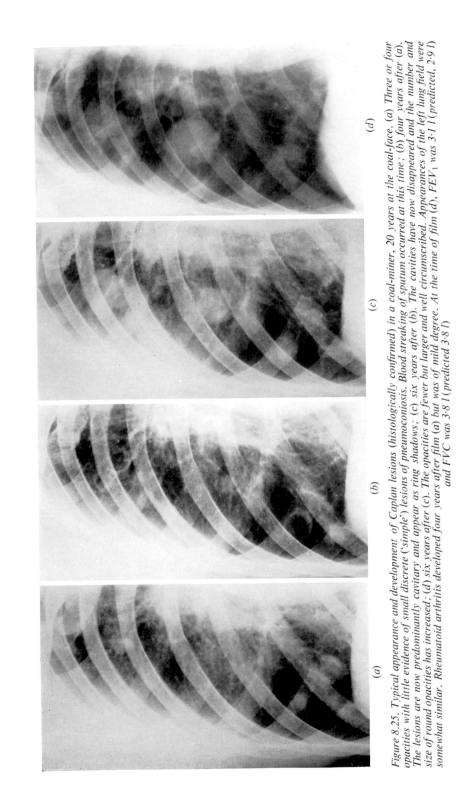

(a) (b) (c) (d)

Figure 8.25. Typical appearance and development of Caplan lesions (histologically confirmed) in a coal-miner, 20 years at the coal-face. (a) Three or four opacities with little evidence of small discrete ('simple') lesions of pneumoconiosis. Blood streaking of sputum occurred at this time; (b) four years after (a). The lesions are now predominantly cavitary and appear as ring shadows; (c) six years after (b). The cavities have now disappeared and the number and size of round opacities has increased; (d) six years after (c). The opacities are fewer but larger and well circumscribed. Appearances of the left lung field were somewhat similar. Rheumatoid arthritis developed four years after film (a) but was of mild degree. At the time of film (d), FEV_1 was 3·1 l (predicted, 2·9 l) and FVC was 3·8 l (predicted 3·8 l)

appearance of a lobulated mass. As a rule, and unlike most cases of ordinary P.M.F., there may be no 'background' of 'simple' pneumoconiosis and, when the Caplan opacities are few, there may be diagnostic difficulty if rheumatoid arthritis is absent; if a 'background' is present it is seldom more than Category 1. Evidence of calcification is a fairly common feature when the lesions are inactive. In some cases the opacities are small and numerous and many may be calcified (*Figure 8.27*); in others they are irregular and poorly defined (Caplan, Payne and Withey, 1962), and yet again are occasionally indistinguishable from ordinary P.M.F. Other radiographic appearances which may occur are a mixture of the features of diffuse interstitial fibrosis in the lower lung fields together with large or small round 'rheumatoid' opacities elsewhere; and signs of pleural effusion—a recognized complication of rheumatoid disease (Ward, 1961) first remarked upon by Fuller in 1860—which are usually unilateral but may involve both sides at different times (*Figure 8.26*). 'Rheumatoid' pneumoconiosis may be seen in more than one member of a family.

Characteristically, 'rheumatoid' lesions develop quickly and usually progress more rapidly than 'conventional' P.M.F. Progression may continue steadily or cease for a variable time—sometimes years—before proceeding. In general, the chief distinguishing radiographic features of 'rheumatoid' pneumoconiosis are its unusual appearances and erratic behaviour. Calcification of inactive, small type lesions is easily mistaken for healed tuberculosis, histoplasmosis or silicosis.

Typical Caplan nodules are prone to undergo cavitation and give rise to single or multiple ring shadows (*Figure 8.25*). These may subsequently revert to the original appearances owing to the cavity refilling, or virtually disappear due to its closure in which case only an ill-defined linear opacity remains.

In rare instances the appearances are atypical and progress with remarkable speed, usually in association with fulminating rheumatoid arthritis, to a fatal outcome (*Figure 8.28*).

The prevalence of rheumatoid arthritis in South Wales miners and ex-miners with characteristic Caplan-type chest films has been found to be over 50 per cent (Miall *et al.*, 1963). The onset of arthritis may precede, occur simultaneously with, or post date, the development of the opacities by months or years. Circulating rheumatoid factor is invariably present, and there is no correlation between the radiographic extent of 'rheumatoid' pneumoconiosis and the severity of rheumatoid arthritis; occasionally subcutaneous nodules may be the only external evidence of rheumatoid disease. In some cases either the radiographic appearances or the arthritis do not develop until late in life, years after exposure to coal-mine dust has ceased. Similar round opacities are seen rarely in persons who have never been exposed to industrial dusts (Locke, 1963; Noonan, Taylor and Engleman, 1963) in association with circulating rheumatoid factor with or without arthritis.

It should be noted, however, that a coal-miner with rheumatoid arthritis, even of severe degree, may have little or no evidence of pneumoconiosis and none of Caplan lesions. But continued observation is necessary in such cases as the chance of 'rheumatoid' pneumoconiosis ultimately developing is high. Similarly, but rarely, the appearances of uncomplicated 'simple' coal pneumoconiosis may remain unchanged over many years although associated

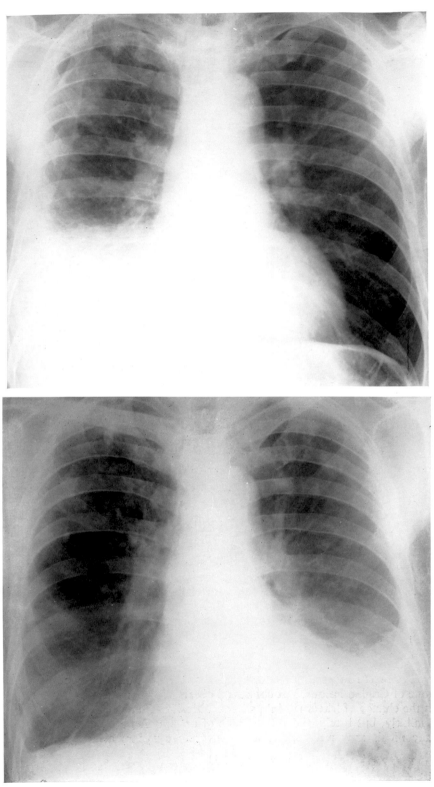

Figure 8.26

with active rheumatoid arthritis and 'rheumatoid' pneumoconiosis does not develop.

The term 'Caplan's syndrome' is legitimately applicable only to fairly large round opacities in coal-miners *with* rheumatoid arthritis, but it is evident that the concept now extends far beyond the confines of Caplan's original description (1953) and that arthropathy may be absent.

Typical appearances of diffuse interstitial fibrosis have been observed in association with graphite pneumoconiosis (Gaensler *et al.*, 1966; Pendergrass *et al.*, 1968).

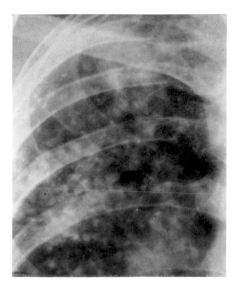

Figure 8.27. Small calcified 'rheumatoid' coal nodules. Severe arthritis with large, calcified subcutaneous nodules

Photoscanning of the lung fields after intravenous injection of albumin–131I correlates well with the vascular pathology (q.v.). The vascular bed is normal in 'simple' pneumoconiosis except in the case of larger 'nodular' opacities—which may be of 'rheumatoid' type—when small avascular areas are revealed. But avascular zones of varying extent are found in and around all P.M.F. lesions (Seaton, Lapp and Chang, 1971).

Bacteriology

When the radiograph shows a cavitated P.M.F. or opacities of recent development, sputum should be cultured for tubercle bacilli and opportunist mycobacteria. Tubercle bacilli are very rarely recovered from the 'rheumatoid' cases whether or not the lesions are cavitated.

Serology

The DAT and latex fixation tests (*see* Chapter 4) are positive in almost all

Figure 8.26. Asynchronous development of pleural effusions in a coal-miner with rheumatoid arthritis. There are only a few opacities indicative of small Caplan nodules which, with DAT 1:1024 and subcutaneous nodules, some preceded the onset of arthritis by years. Biopsy of the pleura revealed non-specific pleurisy only. This man's brother and daughter have rheumatoid arthritis. (The lower film was taken 11 months after the upper one)

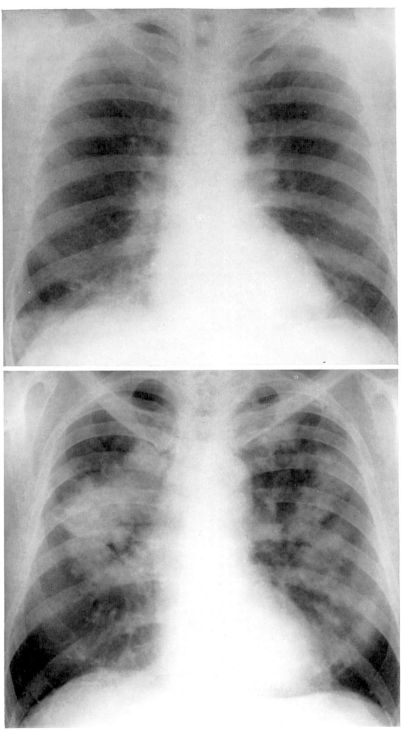

(a)

(b)

Figure 8.28

cases of 'rheumatoid' pneumoconiosis whether rheumatoid arthritis is present or not, but variation in titre may be observed over a period of time. Some cases of 'conventional' P.M.F. are also associated with circulating rheumatoid factor, but the prevalence is not yet known. In those cases where diffuse interstitial fibrosis coexists with pneumoconiosis, circulating rheumatoid factor is also often found.

The prevalence of antinuclear factor in coal pneumoconiosis is not yet known.

Haematology

Mild normochromic, a slightly hypochromic, anaemia is fairly common among coal-miners with P.M.F. in South Wales and haemodilution due to expanded plasma volume appears to be an important determining factor (Chan, 1969b) in addition to low serum iron already referred to. The cause is unknown.

Other investigations

Electrocardiography may be indicated to verify the presence of right ventricular strain and pulmonary hypertension in P.M.F. cases. But this is not normally observed until FEV_1 is reduced to about 1·0 litre or less. Cardiac catheterization is never justifiable for routine investigation.

DIAGNOSIS

Occupational and medical histories, and the radiographic appearances together provide the diagnosis. It should rarely be necessary to resort to lung biopsy.

Occasionally, the radiographic appearances of miliary tuberculosis or collagen diseases such as polyarthritis nodosa resemble 'simple' coal pneumoconiosis, although the quality of the opacities is slightly different and the patients are usually ill. Sarcoidosis is sometimes a cause of misdiagnosis in young coal-miners but if the principles of differential, and not 'spot', diagnosis are continually in mind this should not occur.

It is worth remembering that coal pneumoconiosis may co-exist with other types of pneumoconiosis (for example, asbestosis) in men who have had varied industrial exposure. P.M.F. opacities are not likely to cause diagnostic error apart from three important circumstances:

(1) *Tuberculosis.*—Large fibrocaseous tuberculous lesions and P.M.F. may be mistaken for each other especially in the presence of category 2 or 3 'simple' pneumoconiosis. In the former case, the patient is often unwell and has lost weight; tubercle bacilli can usually be cultivated from his sputum, and antituberculous treatment causes resolution of radiographic appearances in greater or lesser degree. In the latter, the man is commonly in good

---

Figure. 8.28. An example of explosive development of 'rheumatoid' coal pneumoconiosis. After 35 years as a coal-miner, the radiographic appearances were as shown in (a) (ILO Category 3p). Three years later, massive opacities had appeared and rapidly increased in size and number (b). Pain and stiffness with intermittent swelling had been present in many joints for about 10 years, but there was little clinical evidence of arthritis at the time of film (b). Latex fixation test, positive. At autopsy the lesions had the characteristic appearances of Caplan-type nodules which had become confluent with liquefactive necrosis in places

health even if complaining of some respiratory disability. P.M.F. with ischaemic cavitation is frequently mistaken for tuberculous disease but there is a history of coughing up jet-black sputum from which tubercle bacilli cannot be isolated.

The now rare 'bronchial abscess' form of tuberculosis (Clegg, 1953) produces fairly dense round radiographic opacities from 1 to 2 cm diameter which are identical to typical Caplan nodules in appearance but are usually few in number, tubercle bacilli may be cultured from the sputum, and rheumatoid arthritis and circulating rheumatoid factor are absent.

(2) *'Rheumatoid' coal pneumoconiosis.*—When these lesions are few and contain cavities they are particularly likely to be diagnosed as tuberculous even when no tubercle bacilli are cultured from the sputum; and, when calcified, they may be interpreted as healed tuberculosis or even histoplasmosis. Comparison with past radiographs and the presence of rheumatoid arthritis or circulating rheumatoid factor help to resolve the problem. If lesions are neither cavitated nor calcified they may be mistaken for secondary tumour deposits (especially those from prostatic carcinoma), although opacities due to tumour usually have a more homogeneous appearance. Large haemoptysis is strongly against a diagnosis of 'rheumatoid' pneumoconiosis.

As a general rule the diagnosis of ordinary P.M.F. is less likely and that of Caplan lesions more likely to be correct in those cases where 'simple' pneumoconiosis is either absent or is no more than category 1.

The distinguishing pathological features of Caplan's nodules are described under Pathology.

(3) *Bronchial carcinoma.*—It is obviously important to distinguish between P.M.F. and bronchial carcinoma radiographically and this is possible in most cases. But difficulty may arise if a patient is seen for the first time or after a number of years when the evolution of the opacity in question cannot be followed. Features which are helpful in distinguishing P.M.F. are variable radiodensity of the opacity, irregular linear opacities at its periphery, or evidence of calcification within the lesion (*Figure 8.24*). Tomography may clarify these features. When cavitation is present the lesions may be indistinguishable but, in the case of P.M.F., there is usually a recent history of expectoration of jet-black sputum. If an opacity is seen to develop and enlarge rapidly in a film series it is most likely to represent a carcinoma. Occasionally when P.M.F. increases rapidly in size in a man with rheumatoid arthritis, it may be mistaken for carcinoma with hypertrophic pulmonary osteoarthropathy if care is not taken to distinguish between these two arthropathies and to identify circulating rheumatoid factor.

Bronchoscopy may be unhelpful but bronchography, in the case of P.M.F., shows that bronchi adjacent to the mass, although distorted and displaced, are not occluded; whereas in the case of peripheral carcinoma of the lung they are often abruptly occluded or gradually narrowed to the point of disappearance ('rat tail' sign) (Goldman, 1965a).

Occasionally it may be impossible to make the distinction between the lesions without thoracotomy, but before this is undertaken biopsy of a scalene node may prove the presence of carcinoma deposits from an upper zone mass.

PROGNOSIS AND COMPLICATIONS

The important influence of the radiographic category of 'simple' pneumoconiosis on the development of P.M.F. is referred to on page 223. The presence of rheumatoid arthritis or circulating rheumatoid factor alone is often associated with sudden progression of pneumoconiosis lesions and dictates more frequent observation of the man than would otherwise be necessary. Although the life expectancy of younger men with large P.M.F. lesions may be shortened due either to respiratory disease or to cor pulmonale, this is exceptional and it is not uncommon to find men in their seventh or eighth decades with similar categories who die from non-respiratory causes. Prognosis is not worsened by the presence of ischaemic cavitation. Occasionally, after many years of apparent inactivity, P.M.F. may progress to considerable size in men in their seventies.

Cor pulmonale

'Simple' pneumoconiosis does not cause pulmonary heart disease or cor pulmonale. Cor pulmonale does not occur in all cases of P.M.F. but is likely to do so when the masses are large, central and bilateral, when there is concomitant chronic airways obstruction, or with the onset of acute bronchitis or bronchopneumonia.

Tuberculosis and other infections

If tuberculosis develops in the presence of P.M.F., permanent decline in ventilatory capacity may occur in some cases in spite of effective antituberculous treatment. Antituberculous treatment has been reported to be less effective in men with coal pneumoconiosis than in men with tuberculosis only (Medical Research Council/Miner's Chest Diseases Treatment Centre, 1963), but there is reason to believe that this was due to irregularity of treatment (Annotation, 1967), and at least one other study has shown satisfactory results (Ramsey and Pines, 1963).

Opportunist mycobacteria may establish themselves in lungs with P.M.F. (Kamat, Rossiter and Gilson, 1961; Marks, 1970). Of these, M. kansasii is the most common but M. peregrinum has been recorded (Ball et al., 1969), as has M. avium which, although rare, carries a very poor prognosis because of its unresponsiveness to treatment.

Infestation of ischaemic P.M.F. cavities with aspergilli—usually A. fumigatus—occasionally occurs and may cause haemoptysis.

'Rheumatoid' pneumoconiosis

As already mentioned, 'rheumatoid' pneumoconiosis behaves erratically and may progress dramatically in a very short period of time, and pleural effusion is an occasional complication.

Chronic bronchitis

The question of chronic obstructive bronchitis and dust exposure has been discussed in Chapter 1, where it was indicated that there is no convincing evidence to suggest a causal relationship between the two, or between chronic obstructive bronchitis and 'simple' pneumoconiosis in coal-miners (Gilson, 1970). A recent survey of coal-miners under 45 years of age which did reveal a significant association between 'bronchitis' (defined as persistent cough and phlegm) and exposure to coal-mine dust proved to be inconclusive because of the assumptions which were made in determining the relevant indices, but the important influence of smoking was again clear (Rae, Walker and Attfield, 1971).

There are some anomalous aspects to this problem which are highlighted by a controlled study of two West Virginia coal-mining communities (Enterline and Lainhart, 1967). Miners from both communities complained of more respiratory symptoms than non-mining controls and ventilatory capacity was lower among the miners than the non-miners in one community, but not in the other in which there was no difference; and, furthermore, the wives had similar respiratory symptoms to those of their miner husbands in the one community, but not in the other. This observation remains unexplained.

In short, it has not been established that chronic obstructive bronchitis is causally related to 'simple' pneumoconiosis or exposure to coal-dust although, of course, transient simple bronchitis is present after exposure to dust (*see* Chapter 1).

Carcinoma of the lung

There is no evidence that coal pneumoconiosis predisposes to carcinoma of the lung. The mortality rate from bronchial carcinoma among Welsh coal-miners with pneumoconiosis is substantially lower than among non-miners of comparable age, and lower among underground than surface workers (Goldman, 1965b); a similarly low rate has also been observed among English coal-miners (Kennaway and Kennaway, 1947). Furthermore, survival time is greater among men with Category 2 or 3 'simple' pneumoconiosis than those with Category 0 (Goldman, 1965c). The reason for this has not been satisfactorily explained, but it seems to be a specific effect of occupation.

Miscellaneous

P.M.F. does not cause fatal haemoptysis but intermittent blood streaking is not uncommon. Copious jet-black sputum from rupture of an ischaemic cavity, although alarming, is usually harmless, and permanent aspiration sequelae do not appear to have been reported.

It is sometimes suggested that the likelihood of death from coronary artery disease may be increased by coal pneumoconiosis in the P.M.F. stage (and, indeed, by other types of advanced fibrotic pneumoconiosis and by chronic airways obstruction) due to an additional burden of hypoxia. But the evidence points, in fact, in the opposite direction and indicates rather that P.M.F. is associated with an unduly low rate of coronary thrombosis (Sanders, 1970; Lindars *et al.*, 1972) and that chronic hypoxia tends to protect the patient from myocardial infarction (Samad and Noehren, 1965; Mitchell, Walker and Maisel, 1968; Nonkin *et al.*, 1968). This is supported by the observation that hypoxia is a common stimulus to interarterial coronary anastomoses in man (Zoll, Wessler and Schlesinger, 1951).

Retrograde spread of a pulmonary artery thrombus (*see* page 232) may occasionally lead to embolism and, consequently, pulmonary infarction but this is rarely fatal. Other complications, remarkable for their rarity, which may occur are spontaneous pneumothorax and permanent abductor paralysis of the left recurrent laryngeal nerve by P.M.F. in the upper part of the left lung adjacent to the hilum.

Finally, it should be noted that life prognosis in P.M.F. cases is, in general, much better than is commonly supposed.

The question as to whether oxides of nitrogen from shot firing, and other sources, in mines has any permanent effect on miners' lungs is discussed briefly in Chapter 12.

TREATMENT

No treatment affects the pneumoconiosis, but treatment is required for chronic obstructive bronchitis, cor pulmonale or tuberculosis. In cases where sudden expectoration of large amounts of black sputum has occurred from excavated P.M.F., reassurance and mild sedation is indicated. Reassurance is also necessary when haemoptysis occurs in cases of 'rheumatoid' pneumoconiosis or 'conventional' P.M.F.—provided that other causes have been confidently excluded.

Complicating tuberculosis is treated as outlined in Chapter 7. Although the results are as good as those in the general population in most P.M.F. cases, there are occasional exceptions in which recurrent relapse occurs due, possibly, to partial incarceration of the tuberculous process in a P.M.F. lesion.

In the event of infection by opportunist mycobacteria the organism must be carefully typed and tested against as many drugs as possible before treatment is started. Photochromogenic (Group I) organisms often respond well to a regime of at least 8 mg/kg/day of isoniazid with standard doses of PAS and streptomycin, but other drugs may be required. Non-chromogens (Group III), which include *M. avium*, respond poorly to treatment with any drug.

There is no evidence that 'rheumatoid' pneumoconiosis is influenced by corticosteroids, but they should be tried in the rare case of fulminating progressive disease.

Respiratory infections in patients with advanced P.M.F. must always be treated promptly and adequately in order to prevent the development or worsening of congestive heart failure. Oxygen is valuable in patients with a much reduced respiratory reserve, not only in relieving dyspnoea, but in promoting diuresis.

PREVENTION

In the United Kingdom prevention rests on three principles, approved dust conditions, pre-employment examination and periodic medical examination, which are employed by the National Coal Board (NCB).

Approved dust conditions
These were introduced by the NCB in 1949 and have been progressively modified since. Until 1969 concentrations of respirable dust were measured in terms of the number of 1 to 5 μm particles per cubic millimetre, but since

then the NCB (1969) has recommended their measurement in terms of mass. The reason for this is that a suitable instrument for measuring mass concentration became available in 1964 (Dunmore, Hamilton and Smith, 1964) and that gravimetric sampling has been found to be a better index of a hazard to health (Jacobsen *et al.*, 1971). This instrument—designed by the British Mining Research Establishment (MRE)—is a four-channel elutriator which selects particles in the 1 to 5 μm size range.

The standards approved by the National Joint Pneumoconiosis Committee of the Ministry of Technology and operating since April 1970 are as follows (Jacobsen *et al.*, 1970.)

(1) Dust conditions at a colliery working place are 'Approved' when the mean mass concentration of dust does not exceed:

(*a*) 3·0 mg/m³ in stone drivages.

(*b*) 8·0 mg/m³ in all other locations.

Although the concentration of airborne dust in collieries varies from place to place and from time to time, a representative average figure for the British coal-mining industry as a whole appears to be 5 to 6 mg/m³ (McKerrow, 1972).

(2) By mass concentration of dust is meant the respirable size range collected by the standard four-channel elutriator. The sampling period is the 'working shift', and sampling is continuous from the time men reach the working place to the time they leave it. (For details *see* National Coal Board, 1969; Jacobsen *et al.*, 1970.)

Pre-employment examination

Every juvenile and adult has a thorough medical examination and chest radiograph before entry, after which he is graded respectively as 'fit for any mining employment', 'fit for restricted employment' or 'unfit' and rejected for mining employment. A candidate with lung disease would not, therefore, be accepted.

Periodic medical examination

Since 1964, by legal requirement, all young miners in the United Kingdom under 18 years of age are examined annually. Older miners have chest radiographs taken every two years. Young men who develop Category 1 pneumoconiosis are removed from dust exposure; however, since 1963 there have been no cases in miners under 24 years of age (NCB 1970). Older miners with Category 2 or 3 can return to work provided they are in 'Approved Dust Conditions' (*see* next section) and are medically examined at intervals.

It is calculated that in collieries where the 8·0 mg/m³ standard is just being met, the long-term mean concentration of dust would be 4·3 mg/m³, and that if a man with no initial evidence of pneumoconiosis (ILO Category 0) were to be exposed to this concentration over a period of 35 years he would have only a 3·4 per cent chance of developing Category 2 'simple' pneumoconiosis by the end of his working life. Accordingly, it is estimated that, if this standard is effectively implemented and as older men retire from the scene, the present prevalence of pneumoconiosis in the United Kingdom should be at least halved in 35 years (Jacobsen *et al.*, 1971). (*See Figure 8.3.*)

Periodic chest radiographs are a valuable index of the effectiveness of dust control and of the 'attack rate' of pneumoconiosis.

Stone dusting to prevent coal-dust explosions

Pulverized limestone is used. It must satisfy the requirements that it shall not contain more than 5 per cent total silica of which free silica is not more than 3 per cent.

Shale dust has been discontinued since the early 1950s because of high quartz content.

Coal-mine dust standards in the U.S.A.

These are controlled by the Federal Coal Mines Health and Safety Act of 1969. The present (1971) standard is that the average concentration of respirable dust during each shift shall not exceed $3 \cdot 0$ mg/m³. By 1973 the standard is to be $2 \cdot 0$ mg/m³, although some latitude is permitted to allow time for improvement in ventilating systems until December 1975, when it will be mandatory for all coal-mines.

The standard reference sampling instrument employed is the MRE elutriator.

Anti-explosion rock dusts can be pulverized limestone, marble, anhydrite, shale and adobe, but limestone is preferred; they should not contain more than 'a total of 5 per cent free and combined silica (SiO_2)' (Bureau of Mines, 1960).

Graphite dust

Threshold Limit Values of the American College of Governmental and Industrial Hygienists (1971) are as follows:

Natural graphite. 15 million parts per cubic foot of air (mppcf).

Synthetic graphite (classed as a 'Nuisance Particulate') 30 mppcf or 10 mg/m³, whichever is the smaller.

REFERENCES

Annotation (1967). 'Tuberculosis and pneumoconiosis.' *Lancet* **2**, 410

Ashford, J. R., Morgan, D. E., Rae, S. and Sowden, R. R. (1970). 'Respiratory symptoms in British coal miners.' *Am. Rev. resp. Dis.* **102**, 370–381

Ball, J. D., Berry, G., Clarke, W. G., Gilson, J. C. and Thomas, J. (1969). 'A controlled trial of anti-tuberculosis chemotherapy in early complicated pneumoconiosis of coal workers.' *Thorax* **24**, 399–406

Beal, A. J., Griffin, O. G. and Nagelschmidt, G. (1953). *The Health Hazard of Limestone and Gypsum used for Stone Dusting in Coal Mines.* Safety in Mines Research Establishment, Ministry of Fuel and Power. Res. Rep. No. 72

Bergman, I. and Casswell, C. (1972). 'Lung dust and lung iron contents of coal workers in different coalfields in Great Britain.' *Br. J. ind. Med.* **29**, 160–168

Bureau of Mines (1960). *American Practice for Rock Dusting Underground Bituminous-coal and Lignite Mines to Prevent Coal Dust Explosions.* (ASA Standard M13. 1–1960, UDC 622. 81.) United States Department of the Interior

Byers, P. D. and King, E. J. (1959). 'Experimental and infective pneumoconiosis with coal, kaolin and mycobacteria.' *Lab. Invest.* **8**, 647–664

Caplan, A. (1953). 'Certain unusual radiological appearances in the chest of coal miners suffering rheumatoid arthritis.' *Thorax* **8**, 29–37

— (1962). 'Correlation of radiological category with lung pathology in coal-workers' pneumoconiosis.' *Br. J. ind. Med.* **19**, 171–179

— Payne, R. B. and Withey, J. L. (1962). 'A broader concept of Caplan's syndrome related to rheumatoid factors.' *Thorax* **17**, 205–212

Caplan, A., Simon, G. and Reid, L. (1966). 'The radiological diagnosis of wide-spread emphysema and categories of simple pneumoconiosis.' *Clin. Radiol.* **17**, 68–70

Carlberg, J. R., Crable, J. V., Limtiaca, L. P., Norris, H. B., Holtz, J. L., Maur, P. and Wolowicz, F. R. (1971). 'Total dust, coal, free silica and trace metal concentrations in bituminous coal miners' lungs.' *Am. ind. Hyg. Ass. J.* **32**, 432–440

Caswell, C., Bergman, I. and Rossiter, C. E. (1971). 'The relation of radiological appearance in simple pneumoconiosis of coal workers to the content and composition of the lung.' In *Inhaled Particles, 3*, pp. 713-724. Ed. by W. H. Walton. Woking; Unwin

Chan, B. W. B. (1969a). 'Serum iron and iron kinetics in coal workers with complicated pneumoconiosis.' *Br. J. ind. Med.* **26**, 65–70

— (1969b). 'Haemodilution as a cause of anaemia in coal workers.' *Br. J. ind. Med.* **26**, 237–239

Clegg, J. W. (1953). 'Ulcero-caseous tuberculous bronchitis.' *Thorax* **8**, 167–179

Cochrane, A. L. (1960). 'Epidemiology of coal workers pneumoconiosis.' In *Industrial Pulmonary Diseases*, pp. 221–231. Ed. by E. J. King and C. M. Fletcher. London; Churchill

— (1962). 'The attack rate of progressive massive fibrosis.' *Br. J. ind. Med.* **19**, 52–64

— and Higgins, I. T. T. (1961). 'Pulmonary ventilatory functions of coal miners in various areas in relation to the X-ray category of pneumoconiosis.' *Br. J. prev. soc. Med.* **15**, 1–11

— Cox, J. G. and Jarman, T. F. (1952). 'Pulmonary tuberculosis in the Rhondda Fach.' *Br. med. J.* **2**, 843–853

— Moore, F. and Thomas, J. (1961a). 'The prognosis value of radiological classi-fication in cases of progressive massive fibrosis.' *Tubercle, Lond.* **42**, 64–71

— — — (1961b). 'The radiographic progression of progressive massive fibrosis.' *Tubercle, Lond.* **42**, 72–77

Collis, E. L. and Gilchrist, J. C. (1928). 'Effects of dust on coal trimmers.' *J. ind. Hyg. Toxicol.* **10**, 101–109

Cotes, J. E. (1968). *Lung Function*. 2nd Ed. Oxford; Blackwell

— and Field, G. B. (1972). 'Lung gas exchange in simple pneumoconiosis of coal workers.' *Br. J. ind. Med.* **29**, 268–273

— Deivanayagam, C. N., Field, G. B. and Billiet, L. (1971). 'Relation between types of simple pneumoconiosis (p or m) and lung function.' In *Inhaled Particles, 3*, pp. 633–641. Ed. by W. H. Walton. Woking; Unwin

Crable, J. V., Keenan, R. G., Kinser, R. E., Smallwood, A. W. and Maner, P. A. (1968). 'Metal and mineral concentrations in lungs of bituminous coal miners.' *Am. ind. Hyg. Ass. J.* **19**, 106–110

Dassanayake, W. L. P. (1948). 'The health of plumbago workers in Ceylon.' *Br. J. ind. Med.* **5**, 141–147

Dunmore, J. H., Hamilton, R. J. and Smith, D. S. G. (1964). 'An instrument for the sampling of respirable dust for subsequent gravimetric assessment.' *J. scient. Instrum.* **41**, 669–672

Dunner, L. and Bagnall, D. J. T. (1949). 'Pneumoconiosis in graphite workers.' *Br. J. Radiol.* **22**, 573–579

Englert, M. and DeCoster, A. (1965). 'La capacité de diffusion pulmonaire dans l'anthrasilicose micronodulaire.' *J. fr. Med. Chir. thorac.* **19**, 159–173

Enterline, P. E. and Lainhart, W. S. (1967). 'The relationship between coal mining and chronic non-specific respiratory disease.' *Am. J. publ. Hlth* **57**, 484-495

Faulds, J. S., King, E. J. and Nagelschmidt, G. (1959). 'The dust content of the lungs of coal workers from Cumberland.' *Br. J. ind. Med.* **16**, 43–50

Faulkner, W. B. (1940). 'Bilateral pulmonary abscess secondary to pneumokoniosis.' *Dis. Chest.* **6**, 306–307

Fay, J. W. J. and Ashford, J. R. (1961). 'A survey of the methods developed in the National Coal Board's Pneumoconiosis Field Research for correlating environ-mental exposure with medical condition.' *Br. J. ind. Med.* **18**, 175–196

Fletcher, C. M. (1970). Correspondence. *Br. med. J.* **4**, 176

— (1972a). Correspondence. *Br. med. J.* **2**, 353

— (1972b). Correspondence. *Br. med. J.* **3**, 116

Frans, A., Portier, N., Veriter, C., Brasseur, L. and Lavenne, F. (1970). 'Lung diffusing capacity for carbon monoxide and alveolar-arterial tension differences for oxygen and carbon dioxide in coal miners still at work.' In *Pneumoconiosis.* (Proceedings of the International Conference, J'burg, 1969, pp. 514–518. Ed. by H. A. Shapiro. Cape Town; Oxford University Press)

Fritze, E., Gundel, E., Ludwig, E., Muller, G., Muller, H. O. and Petersen, B. (1969). 'Die gesundheitliche Situation van Bergar beitern einer Kohlenzeche.' *Dt. med. Wschr.* **94**, 362–367

Fuller, H. W. (1860). *On Rheumatism, Rheumatic Gout and Sciatica, their Pathology, Symptoms and Treatment.* 3rd ed. pp. 305–326. London; Churchill

Gaensler, E. A., Cadigan, J. B., Sasahara, A. A., Fox, E. O. and MacMahon, H. E. (1966). 'Graphite pneumoconiosis of electrotypers.' *Am. J. Med.* **41**, 864–882

Gernez-Rieux, C., Balgaires, E., Fournier, P. and Voisin, C. (1958). 'Une manifestation souvent méconus de la pneumoconiose des mineurs: La liquéfaction aseptique des formations pseudatumorales.' *Sem. Hôp. Paris* **34**, 1081–1089

— Tacquet, A., Voisin, C. and Devulder, B. (1965). 'Le role des infections dans la pathogenie des fibroses massives progressives des mineurs de charbon.' *Medna Lav.* **56**, 500–516

Gilson, J. C. (1968). *Pneumoconiosis. Report on a Symposium, Katowice, June, 1967,* p. 69. Copenhagen; World Health Organization

— (1970). 'Occupational bronchitis.' *Proc. R. Soc. Med.* **63**, 857–864

— and Oldham, P. D. (1970). Correspondence. *Br. med. J.* **4**, 305

Gloyne, S. R. (1932–33). 'The morbid anatomy and histology of asbestos.' *Tubercle (Edin.)* **14**, 445–451; 493–497; 550–558

— Marshall, G. and Hoyle, C. (1949). Pneumoconiosis due to graphite dust. *Thorax* **4**, 32–38

Goldman, K. P. (1965a). 'The diagnosis of lung cancer in coal miners with pneumoconiosis.' *Br. J. Dis. Chest* **59**, 141–147

— (1965b). 'Mortality of coal-miners from carcinoma of the lung.' *Br. J. ind. Med.* **22**, 72–77

— (1965c). 'Prognosis of coal miners with cancer of the lung.' *Thorax* **20**, 170–174

Gough, J. (1940). 'Pneumoconiosis in coal trimmers.' *J. Path. Bact.* **51**, 277–285

— (1947). 'Pneumoconiosis in coal workers in Wales.' *Occup. Med.* **4**, 86–97

— (1960). 'Emphysema in relation to pneumoconiosis.' In *Proceedings of the Pneumoconiosis Conference', J'burg. 1959,* pp. 200–204. Ed. by A. J. Orenstein. London; Churchill

—(1968). 'The pathogenesis of emphysema.' In *The Lung,* pp. 109–133. Ed. by A. A. Liebow and D. E. Smith. Baltimore; Williams and Wilkins

— and Heppleston, A. G. (1960). 'The pathology of the pneumoconioses.' In *Industrial Pulmonary Diseases,* pp. 23–36. Ed. by E. J. King and C. M. Fletcher. London; Churchill

— Rivers, D. and Seal, R. M. E. (1955). 'Pathological studies of modified pneumoconiosis in coal-miners with rheumatoid arthritis (Caplan's syndrome).' *Thorax* **10**, 9–18

Gross, P. and de Treville, R. T. P. (1970). 'Black lungs.' *Archs envir. Hlth* **20**, 450–451

Haferland, W. (1957). 'Graphitstaublunge und Silikose.' *Arch. Gewerbepath. Gewerbehyg.* **16**, 53–62

Harding, H. E. and Oliver, G. B. (1949). 'Changes in the lungs produced by natural graphite.' *Br. J. ind. Med.* **6**, 91–99

Hart, J. T., Cochrane, A. L. and Higgins, I. T. T. (1963). 'Tuberculin sensitivity in coal worker's pneumoconiosis.' *Tubercle, Lond.* **44**, 141–152

Heard, B. E. (1969). *Pathology of Chronic Bronchitis and Emphysema.* London; Churchill

— and Izukawa, T. (1963). 'Dust pigmentation of the lungs and emphysema in Londoners.' In *Fortschritte Staublungenforschung,* pp. 249–255. Ed. by H. Reploh and W. Klosterkötter. Dinslaken; Niederrheinische Druckerie

265

Heath, D. (1968). In *Form and Function in the Human Lung*, p. 35. Ed. by G. Cumming and L. B. Hunt. Edinburgh and London; Livingstone

Hendriks, C. A. M. and Bleiker, M. A. (1964). 'Tuberculin sensitivity in coal miners with pneumoconiosis.' *Tubercle, Lond.* **45**, 379–383

Heppleston, A. G. (1947). 'The essential lesion of pneumoconiosis in Welsh coal workers.' *J. Path. Bact.* **59**, 453–460

— (1951). 'Coal worker's pneumoconiosis.' *Archs ind. Hyg.* **4**, 270–288

— (1953). 'The pathological anatomy of simple pneumoconiosis in coal miners.' *J. Path. Bact.* **66**, 235–246.

— (1968). In *Form and Function in the Human Lung*, pp. 35–36. Ed. by G. Cumming and L. B. Hunt. Edinburgh and London; Livingstone

— Civil, G. W. and Critchlow, A. (1971). 'The effects of duration and intermittency of exposure on the elimination of high and low rank coal dusts.' In *Inhaled Particles, 3*, pp. 261-270. Ed. by W. H. Walton. Woking; Unwin

Hicks, D., Fay, J. W. J., Ashford, J. R. and Rae, S. (1961). *The Relation between Pneumoconiosis and Environmental Conditions.* London; National Coal Board

Higgins, I. T. T. (1972). Correspondence. *Br. med. J.* **2**, 713

— Higgins, M. W., Lockshin, M. D. and Canale, N. (1968). 'Chronic respiratory disease in mining communities in Marion County, West Virginia.' *Br. J. ind. Med.* **25**, 165–175

— Oldham, P. D., Kilpatrick, G. S., Drummond, R. J. and Bevan, B. (1963). 'Blood groups of miners with coal-workers' pneumoconiosis and bronchitis.' *Br. J. ind. Med.* **20**, 324-329

Hutchinson, J. E. M. (1966). 'Twins with coal-workers' pneumoconiosis.' *Br. J. ind. Med.* **23**, 240–244

Jacobsen, G., Felson, B., Pendergrass, E. P., Flinn, R. H. and Lainhart, W. S. (1967). 'Eggshell calcification in coal and metal miners.' *Semin. Roentgenol.* **2**, 276–281

Jacobsen, M., Rae, S., Walton, W. H. and Rogan, J. M. (1970). 'New dust standards in British coal mines.' *Nature, Lond.* **227**, 445–457

— — — (1971). 'The relation between pneumoconiosis and dust-exposure in British coal mines.' In *Inhaled Particles 3*, pp. 903–917. Ed. by W. H. Walton. Woking; Unwin

Jaffé, F. A. (1951). 'Graphite pneumoconiosis.' *Am. J. Path.* **17**, 909–923

James, W. R. L. (1954). 'The relationship of tuberculosis to the development of massive pneumokoniosis in coal workers.' *Br. J. Tuberc.* **48**, 89–101

Jones, B. M., Edwards, J. H. and Wagner, J. C. (1972). 'Absorption of serum proteins by inorganic dusts.' *Br. J. ind. Med.* **29**, 287–292

Kamat, S. R., Rossiter, C. E. and Gilson, J. C. (1961). 'A retrospective clinical study of pulmonary disease due to "anonymous mycobacteria" in Wales.' *Thorax* **16**, 297–308

Kennaway, E. L. and Kennaway, N. M. (1947). 'A further study of the incidence of cancer of the lung and larynx.' *Br. J. Cancer* **1**, 260–298

Kilpatrick, G. S., Heppleston, A. G. and Fletcher, C. M. (1957). 'Cavitation in the massive fibrosis of coal workers' pneumoconiosis.' *Thorax* **9**, 260–272

Ladoo, R. B. and Myers, W. M. (1951). *Non-metallic Minerals*, p. 250. New York and London; McGraw-Hill

Lainhart, W. S. and Morgan, W. K. C. (1971). 'Extent and development of respiratory effects.' In *Pulmonary Reactions to Coal Dust*, pp. 29–56. Ed. by M. M. Key, L. E. Kerr and M. Bundy. New York and London; Academic Press

Lapp, N. L. R. and Seaton, A. (1971). 'Pulmonary function.' In *Pulmonary Reactions to Coal Dust*, pp. 153–177. Ed. by M. M. Key, L. E. Kerr, and M. Bundy. New York and London; Academic Press

Lavenne, F. (1968). 'Assessment of lung function in silicosis and mixed dust pneumoconiosis.' In *Pneumoconiosis.* Report in the 1967 Katowice Symposium. EURO 0379. Copenhagen; W.H.O.

— (1970). Discussion. In *Pneumoconiosis. Proceedings of the International Conference, J'burg, 1969*, p. 521. Ed. by H. A. Shapiro. Cape Town; Oxford University Press

Lindars, D. C. and Davies, D. (1967). 'Rheumatoid pneumoconiosis. A study in colliery populations in the East Midlands coalfield.' *Thorax* **22**, 525–532

— Rooke, G. B., Dempsey, A. N. and Ward, F. G. (1972). 'Pneumoconiosis and death from coronary heart disease.' *J. Path.* **108**, 249–259

Lister, W. B. and Wimborne, D. (1972). 'Carbon pneumoconiosis in a synthetic graphite worker.' *Br. J. ind. Med.* **29**, 108–110

Lochtkemper, I. and Teleky, L. (1932). 'Studien über Staublunge; die Staublunge in einzelnen besonderin Betrieben und bei besonderen Arbeiten.' *Arch. Gewerbepath. Gewerbehyg.* **3**, 600–672

Locke, G. B. (1963). 'Rheumatoid lung.' *Clin. Radiol.* **14**, 43-53

Lyons, J. P., Clarke, W. G., Hall, A. N. and Cotes, J. E. (1967). 'Transfer factor (diffusing capacity) for the lung in simple pneumoconiosis of coal workers.' *Br. Med. J.* **4**, 772–774

— Ryder, R., Campbell, H. and Gough, J. (1972). 'Pulmonary disability in coal workers' pneumoconiosis.' *Br. Med. J.* **1**, 713–716

McCallum, R. I. (1961). Treatment of progressive massive fibrosis in coal miners. *Proceedings XIII International Congress on Occupational Health, New York*, 741–745

McCormick, J. N. (1972). Quoted by Jones, B. M., Edwards, J. H. and Wagner, J. C. (1972) q.v.

McKerrow, C. B. (1972). 'Silicosis and coalworkers' pneumoconiosis.' In *Clinical Aspects of Inhaled Particles*, pp. 130–155. Ed. by D. C. F. Muir. London; Heinemann

McLintock, J. S., Rae, S. and Jacobsen, M. (1971). 'The attack rate of progressive massive fibrosis in British coal miners.' In *Inhaled Particles, 3*, pp. 933–950. Ed. by W. H. Walton. Woking; Unwin

Macklem, P. T. (1968). Discussion of Session One. In *Form and Function in the Human Lung*, pp. 33–34. Ed. by G. Cumming and L. B. Hunt. Edinburgh and London; Livingstone

Mantell, C. L. (1968). *Carbon and Graphite Handbook*. New York and London; Wiley

— (1971). Personal communication

Marks, J. (1961). 'Infective pneumoconiosis due to anonymous mycobacteria.' *Br. med. J.* **2**, 1332

Marks, J. (1970). 'New mycobacteria.' *Hlth Trends* **3**, 68–69

Medical Research Council (1942). *Report by the Committee on Industrial Pulmonary Disease.* S.R.S. 243, p. 11. London; H.M.S.O.

—/Miners Treatment Centre (1963). 'Chemotherapy of pulmonary tuberculosis with pneumoconiosis.' *Tubercle, Lond.* **44**, 47–70

Miall, W. E. (1955). 'Rheumatoid arthritis in Wales. An epidemiological study of a Welsh mining community.' *Ann. rheum. Dis.* **14**, 150–158

— Caplan, A., Cochrane, A. L., Kilpatrick, G. S. and Oldham, P. D. (1953). 'An epidemiological study of rheumatoid arthritis associated with characteristic chest X-ray appearances in coal miners.' *Br. med. J.* **2**, 1231–1236

Miller, A. A. and Ramsden, F. (1961). 'Carbon pneumoconiosis.' *Br. J. ind. Med.* **18**, 103–113

Mitchell, R. S., Walker, S. H. and Maisel, J. C. (1968). 'The causes of death in chronic airway obstruction. II. Myocardial infarction.' *Am. Rev. resp. Dis.* **98**, 611–612

Nagelschmidt, G. (1960). 'The relation between lung dust and lung pathology in pneumoconiosis.' *Br. J. ind. Med.* **17**, 247–259

— and Godbert, A. L. (1951). *The Health Hazard of Shales used for Stone Dusting.* Safety in Mines Res. Estab., Min. of Fuel and Power., Res. Rep. No. 19

— Rivers, D., King, E. J. and Trevella, W. (1963). 'Dust and collagen content of lungs of coal workers with progressive massive fibrosis.' *Br. J. ind. Med.* **20**, 181–191

National Coal Board (1969). *Approved Conditions for Airborne Dust.* F 4040. London; N.C.B.

— (1971). Medical Service and Medical Research: Annual Report 1969–1970. London; N.C.B.

National Coal Board (1972). Medical Service and Medical Research: Annual Report 1970–1971. London; N.C.B.

Nonkin, P. M., Dick, M. M., Baum, G. L. and Gables, C. (1964). 'Myocardial infarction in respiratory insufficiency.' Archs intern. Med. 113, 42–45

Noonan, C. D., Taylor, F. B. Jr. and Engleman, E. P. (1963). 'Nodular rheumatoid disease of the lung with cavitation.' Arthritis Rheum. 6, 232–240

Okutani, H., Shima, S. and Sano, T. (1964). 'Graphite pneumoconiosis in carbon electrode makers.' In XIV International Congress of Occupational Health, 1963. Vol. 11. (Internat. Congr. Series No. 62.) Amsterdam; Excerpta Med.

Oldham, P. D. and Berry, G. (1972). Correspondence. Br. med. J. 2, 292–293

Otto, H. and Einbrodt, H. J. (1958). 'Lugenstaubanalyse bei exzessiver Anthracose und ihre versicherung-srechtliche Bedeutung.' Frankf. Z. Path. 69, 404–415

Parkes, W. R. (1972). Unpublished observations

Parmeggiani, L. (1950). 'Graphite pneumoconiosis.' Br. J. ind. Med. 7, 42–45

Payne, R. B. (1963). Rheumatoid Pneumoconiosis. Thesis for Degree of Doctor of Medicine to the University of South Wales and Monmouthshire, Cardiff

Pendergrass, E. P., Vorwald, A. J, Mishkin, M. M., Whildin, J. G. and Werley, C. W. (1967). 'Observations on workers in the graphite industry. Part 1.' Med. Radiogr Photogr. 43, 70–99

— — — — — (1968). 'Observations on workers in the graphite industry. Part 2.' Med. Radiogr Photogr. 44, 1–17

Pernis, B., Chiappino, G., Gilson, J. C., Wagner, J. C., Caplan, A. and Vigliani, E. C. (1965). 'Studies on Caplan's nodules by means of immunofluorescence.' Beitr. Silkosforsch. Bd. 6, 339–341

Policard, A., Letort, M., Charbonnier, J., Martin, J. and Daniel-Moussard, H. (1967). 'Recherches sur les interactions charbon-quartz dans le développement des pneumoconioses des houilleurs.' Archs Mal. prof. Méd. trav. 28, 589–594

Rae, S., Muir, D. C. F. and Jacobsen, M. (1970). 'Coal workers' pneumoconiosis. (Correspondence.)' Br. med. J. 3, 769

— Walker, D. D. and Attfield, M. D. (1971). 'Chronic bronchitis and dust exposure in British coal mines.' In Inhaled Particles, 3, pp. 883–894. Ed. by W. H. Walton. Woking; Unwin

Ramsey, J. H. R. and Pines, A. (1963). 'The late results of chemotherapy in pneumoconiosis complicated by tuberculosis.' Tubercle, Lond. 44, 476–479

Ranasinha, K. W. and Uragoda, C. G. (1972). 'Graphite pneumoconiosis.' Br. J. ind. Med. 29, 178–183

Ray, S. C., King, E. J. and Harrison, C. V. (1951). 'The action of small amounts of quartz and larger amounts of coal and graphite on the lungs of rats.' Br. J. ind. Med. 8, 68–73

Reid, L. (1967). The Pathology of Emphysema. London; Lloyd-Luke

Rivers, D., James, W. R. L., Davies, D. G. and Thomson, S. (1957). 'The prevalence of tuberculosis at necropsy in massive fibrosis of coal workers.' Br. J. ind. Med. 14, 39–42

— Wise, M. E., King, E. J. and Nagelschmidt, G. (1960). 'Dust content, radiology and pathology in simple pneumoconiosis of coal workers.' Br. J. ind. Med. 17, 87–108

Rogan, J. M., Ashford, J. R., Chapman, P. J., Duffield, D. P., Fay, J. W. J. and Rae, S. (1961). 'Pneumoconiosis and respiratory symptoms in miners at eight collieries.' Br. med. J. 1, 1337–1342

Rossiter, C. E. (1972a). 'Relation between content and composition of coal worker's lungs and radiological appearances.' Br. J. ind. Med. 29, 31–44

— (1972b). 'Evidence of dose-response relation in pneumoconiosis.' Trans. Soc. occup. Med. 22, 83–97

— Rivers, D., Bergman, I., Caswell, C. and Nagelschmidt, G. (1967). 'Dust content, radiology and pathology in simple pneumoconiosis of coal workers.' In Inhaled Particles and Vapours, II, pp. 419–434. Ed. by C. N. Davies. Oxford; Pergamon

Rüttner, J. R., Bovet, P. and Aufdermaur, M. (1952). 'Graphit, Caborund, Staublunge.' Dt. med. Wschr. 77, 1413–1415

Ryder, R., Lyons, J. P., Campbell, H. and Gough, J. (1970). 'Emphysema in coal workers' pneumoconiosis.' *Br. med. J.* **3**, 481–487

Samad, I. A. and Noehren, T. H. (1965). 'Myocardial infarction in pulmonary emphysema.' *Dis. Chest* **47**, 26–29

Sanders, W. L. (1970). 'Heart disease and pneumoconiosis.' *Thorax* **25**, 223–225

Schlipköter, H. W. (1970). Ätiologie und Pathogese der Silikose ihre kausale Beeinflussung. *Naturwissenschaften* **197**, 39–105

— Hilscher, W., Pott, F. and Beck, E. G. (1971). 'Investigations into the aetiology of coal workers' pneumoconiosis, with the use of PVN-oxide.' In *Inhaled Particles, 3*, pp. 379–389. Ed. by W. H. Walton. Woking; Unwin

Seaton, A., Lapp, N. L. and Chang, C. H. J. (1971). 'Lung scanning in coal workers' pneumoconiosis.' *Am. J. resp. Dis.* **103**, 338–349

Spink, R. and Nagelschmidt, G. (1963). 'Dust and fibrosis in the lungs of coal workers from the Wigan area of Lancashire.' *Br. J. ind. Med.* **20**, 118–123

Town, J. D. (1968). 'Pseudoasbestos bodies and asteroid giant cells in a patient with graphite pneumoconiosis.' *Can. med. Ass. J.* **98**, 100–104

Trapnell, D. H. (1964). 'Septal lines in pneumoconiosis.' *Br. J. Radiol.* **37**, 805–810

Tylecote, F. E. and Dunn, J. S. (1931). 'Case of asbestos-like bodies in the lungs of a coal miner who had never worked in asbestos.' *Lancet* **2**, 632–633

Wagner, J. C. (1970). 'Complicated coal workers' pneumoconiosis.' In *Pneumoconiosis. Proceedings of International Conference, Johannesburg 1969*, pp. 306–308. Ed. by H. A. Shapiro. Cape Town; Oxford University Press

— (1971). 'Immunological factors in coal workers' pneumoconiosis.' In *Inhaled Particles, 3*, pp. 573–576. Ed. by W. H. Walton. Woking; Unwin

— and McCormick, J. N. (1967). 'Immunological investigations in coal workers' disease.' *J. R. Coll. Physicians, Lond.* **2**, 49–56

Ward, R. (1961). 'Pleural effusion and rheumatoid disease.' *Lancet* **2**, 1336–1338

Watson, A. J., Black, J., Doig, A. T. and Nagelschmidt, G. (1959). 'Pneumoconiosis in carbon electrode makers.' *Br. J. ind. Med.* **16**, 274–285

Weinstein, I. M. (1959). 'A correlative study of the erythrokinetics and disturbances of iron metabolism associated with the anaemia of rheumatoid arthritis.' *Blood* **14**, 950–966

Wells, A. L. (1954a). 'Pulmonary vascular changes in coalworkers' pneumoconiosis.' *J. Path. Bact.* **68**, 573–587

— (1954b). 'Cor pulmonale in coal worker's pneumoconiosis.' *Br. Heart J.* **16**, 74–78

Williams, E. (1934). ' "Curious bodies" found in the lungs of coal workers.' *Lancet* **2**, 541–542

World Health Organization (1968). *Pneumoconiosis. Report on a Symposium, Katowice, 1967*. Annex. 1, p. 47. Copenhagen; Regional Office for Europe

Wusteman, F. S., Gold, C. and Wagner, J. C. (1972). 'Glycosaminoglycans and calcification in the lesions of progressive massive fibrosis and pleural plaques.' *Amer. Rev. Resp. Dis.* **106**, 116–120

Zahorski, W. (1961). 'Pneumoconiosis dans l'industrie du graphite artificial.' *Proceedings XIII International Congress on Occupational Health, New York*. pp. 828–832

Zoll, P. M., Wessler, S. and Schlesinger, M. J. (1951). 'Interarterial coronary anastomoses in the human heart with particular reference to anaemia and relative cardiac anoxia.' *Circulation* **4**, 797–815

9—Diseases due to Asbestos and other Silicates

Introduction

The asbestiform group of minerals are more important than any other inhaled materials—mineral or non-mineral—because their use in industry is widespread and diverse, and they are capable of causing serious disability and early death from lung fibrosis (*asbestosis*) and malignant tumours. Although asbestosis was first recognized in 1907 (Murray) and attention drawn to it again in 1924 (Cooke), it was not until 1930 (Merewether and Price) that the gravity of the problem was appreciated and an attempt made both in Britain and the United States (Sayers and Dreesen, 1939) to control the industrial hazard. The measures introduced, however, did not include the majority of industrial uses of asbestos. The potential danger of asbestiform minerals, in fact, has become generally recognized only since the latter part of the 1950s.

Although there is no doubt about the gravity of asbestos-induced disease and of the urgent need to ensure that effective preventive measures are generally applied, sensational reporting by various news media has unfortunately given an exaggerated impression of the risks of exposure of individuals to asbestos materials and of the outcome of disease, with the result that much anxiety has been caused, not only among patients who know they have asbestosis, but also among healthy past and present asbestos workers and members of the general public. Hence, it is imperative that the physician should have a balanced knowledge of the degree of risk which may exist and of the patterns of disease in order that he may bring appropriate confidence and reassurance to the patient.

Asbestos-induced disorders are:

(1) Diffuse interstitial fibrosis (fibrosing 'alveolitis') of the lungs (asbestosis).
(2) Pleural fibrosis and plaque formation.
(3) Malignant mesothelioma of pleura or peritoneum.
(4) Possibly bronchial carcinoma without asbestosis.
(5) Skin corns.

270

Other silicates may be associated with the development of pneumoconiosis; they are talc, china clay (kaolin), fuller's earth, bentonite and mica. It is appropriate, therefore, to consider them in this chapter. Sillimanite, which has been questioned as a cause of lung fibrosis, also receives brief mention.

ASBESTOS

'Asbestos' ($\dot{\alpha}+\sigma\beta\epsilon\sigma\tau os$, unquenchable) is a collective term embracing some of the metamorphic, fibrous, mineral silicates of different chemicals composition. These belong to the *serpentine* or *amphibole* groups (*see* Chapter 2):

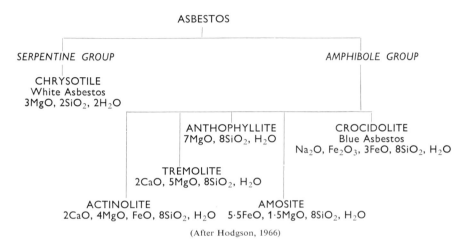

(After Hodgson, 1966)

The most important of these in industry is chrysotile which represents some 90 per cent of world asbestos production. Crocidolite and amosite are next in importance and anthophyllite, tremolite and actinolite have only a limited use.

Asbestos was first introduced into modern industry about 1878 and since 1910 the production and consumption of these minerals has grown to enormous proportions (*see* Tables 9.1 and 9.2). Because crocidolite is particularly associated with the development of malignant mesothelioma of the pleura and peritoneum its use has been greatly restricted in the United Kingdom since 1970 although in Western Europe, the United States of America and Japan imports have been continually increasing.

It is sometimes asserted that asbestos is indestructible, but this is not correct. It is true, in general, that the various asbestos types possess good resistance to weathering and to heat but at certain temperatures all decompose. Chrysotile breaks down to forsterite (an anhydrous silicate, $3\ Mg_2SiO_4$) and silicon dioxide (SiO_2) between 800° and 850°C; crocidolite breaks down between 800° and 900°C; amosite, between 600° and 900°C, and anthophyllite, between 850° and 1000°C (Hodgson, 1966). Hence, under industrial and other conditions which generate high temperatures, decomposition will occur. With the exception of chrysotile all forms of asbestos are highly resistant to acids and chemicals.

271

Exposure to an asbestos hazard can be considered from two standpoints:

(1) Industrial (including 'neighbourhood') exposure.

TABLE 9.1

WORLD PRODUCTION OF ASBESTOS—BY TYPES

By courtesy of Asbestos Research Council

Year	Anthophyllite	Amosite	Crocidolite	Chrysotile	Total
1910	–	–	1,320	84,330	86,150
1920	–	203	6,147(a)	184,100	190,450
1929(b)	–	10,664	7,331	372,865	390,860
1940	5,323	15,863	9,529	410,208	440,923
1950(c)	11,350	37,850	28,500	928,500	1,006,000
1960(d)	9,950	61,250	82,500	2,046,000	2,200,000
1965	12,400	72,800	119,000	2,628,000	2,832,000
1968	11,800	86,850	107,810	2,793,540(e)	3,000,000
1970	13,450	95,850	135,100	3,150,100	3,394,500(f)

All figures are in long tons.
Colonial Office Reports of Mineral Resources or other sources consulted give no figures for anthophyllite production before 1940.
(a) Figures reported are of all grades and may include quantities of chrysotile and amosite. Detailed figures available from another source from 1919 give the production of South African asbestos as 3,908 tons, consisting of: amosite 802 tons, crocidolite 3,088 tons, chrysotile 18 tons.
(b) Nearest year to the decadal quoted in the sources available.
(c) These figures exclude tonnages known to have been produced in Czechoslovakia, Romania, U.S.S.R., China and Korea.
(d) 1960: these figures exclude tonnages known to have been produced in Czechoslovakia, Romania and Korea.
(e) This figure does not include details for Rhodesia which were not available.
(f) The world total for 1970 excludes asbestos known to have been produced in Czechoslovakia, Romania, Eritrea and North Korea.

TABLE 9.2

CONSUMPTION OF ASBESTOS—MAIN USER COUNTRIES

By courtesy of Asbestos Research Council

Country	1910	1920	1929	1940	1950	1960	1965	1968	1970
U.K.	–	20,738	27,298	93,503	116,109	150,566	152,175	158,850	141,152
U.S.A.	–	149,925	234,942	233,315	649,669	633,266	709,679	729,806	657,572
Belgium	–	N/A	20,673	N/A	20,884	52,843	60,039	59,163	53,035
France	–	N/A	N/A	13,827	38,304	82,064	107,047	125,047	149,252
Germany	–	6,692	14,065	11,004	13,623	130,310	170,462	183,666	171,929
Italy	–	4,067	6,900*	13,258	24,420	72,389	83,464	111,098	130,238
U.S.S.R.	11,600	1,603*	27,000*	N/A	N/A	446,200	955,500	488,195	647,785
Japan	–	4,887	10,147	25,000	12,159	91,018	145,345	220,550	314,427

* These figures are based on different sources which are not entirely consistent in certain respects; and some assumptions have been made, but it is thought that they give a reasonable indication of the trend of production.
All figures are in long tons and are obtained by deducting exports from imports plus production (where applicable) of categories variously described as unmanufactured, crude, fibre, shorts and waste.
Figures for the U.K. alone do not include imports which, though described as unmanufactured, are classified as waste material. Recent figures for these additional imports are:

1960—9,870; 1965—18,149; 1968—12,178; 1970—6,377

(2) Non-industrial exposure of the general population to asbestos-containing products.

(1) Industrial

Uses of asbestos

It is impossible to enumerate all past and present uses: for chrysotile alone these were already extensive in the 1930s (Ross, 1931) and, for all forms of asbestos, are now estimated to be more than a thousand (Hendry, 1965).

The manufacture of *asbestos-cement products* consumes the greatest quantity of asbestos fibre; these products consist of tiles, corrugated roofing, gutters, drain pipes, chimneys, pressure piping and flat sheets. The fibre, which is mainly chrysotile—although up to 40 per cent crocidolite has been used (Hodgson, 1966)—acts as a reinforcing agent. Fibre is milled to appropriate size mixed with cement as a slurry and then passed on to a conveyer to make sheeting, or into moulds for making pipes and other shapes. Water is then extruded and the product air-cured for some 28 days. Sheeting and pipe sections require cutting to desired size specifications. In the United Kingdom the quartz content of the cement mixture is negligible but in the United States it may average about 18 per cent and present a silicosis risk.

The *floor tiling industry* takes the next largest quantity of chrysotile. Some 10 to 30 per cent of short fibre acts as a reinforcing agent and filler in asphalt floorings and with organic resins for vinyl tiles. In the manufacture of tiles, fibre is added to the mix in controlled amounts from a hopper, pressed into sheet form, calendered and cut to required size and shape. Asbestos–asphalt mixtures have, it seems, been suggested as road surfacing material.

Fibre is used widely for *insulation and fire-proofing.* Low-density asbestos-cement products are made in sections for pipe and boiler covering; amosite mixed with calcium silicate or light-weight magnesia has similar use as well as an important place for lining ships' bulkheads. Until the late 1960s laggers mixed chrysotile or amosite and, occasionally, crocidolite with water by hand and applied the mixture after stripping away pre-existing lagging— an unavoidably dusty job. Insulation, fireproofing and soundproofing is also done by spraying a fibre mixture (chrysotile or amosite with a bonding liquid) on to walls, ceilings, girders and spandrils of buildings, and ships' bulkheads; crocidolite has also been used for the same purpose. This technique has been extensively used in shipbuilding and repair since the middle of World War II.

Asbestos textiles for safety curtains, fireproof clothing, conveyor belts and the wicks of oil heaters incorporate chrysotile and crocidolite. Because of the high resistance of crocidolite to acids it is used for filtration cloths. Fibre (mainly chrysotile) from which grit and extraneous matter has been removed is carded on fast-moving cylinders and, for the manufacture of cloth, is incorporated with cotton, after which it is dry spun, woven or plaited. This operation is being replaced by a wet process. Graphite, incidentally, is sometimes used as a lubricant for the manufacture of rope packings.

Chrysotile is the main constituent (about 80 per cent) of *asbestos paper products* which include millboard, insulating papers, engine gaskets, roofing felts, wall coverings, soldering pads, cooking mats and flooring felt.

Another very important application of chrysotile is in *friction materials*— most notably brake linings and clutch facings—which consist of about

60 per cent of fibre mixed with phenolic resins and sometimes other minerals.

Chrysotile '*floats*' are used in plastics, paints and welding rods; and chrysotile also has an extensive application in filters for drugs, wines, beers and other fluids.

A limited use of crocidolite (but important from the point of view of disease potential) was in the manufacture of respirator filters—especially gas masks during World War II. Chrysotile has found unusual uses as 'snow' in motion picture production, for Christmas decoration, and for the manufacture of Santa Claus whiskers (Ross, 1931). It has also been incorporated into the filter tips of cigarettes in the United States but not, as far as is known, in Britain (Tobacco Research Council, 1970).

Anthophylite has a much more restricted application, being used as a filler in rubber and plastics. However, it has the oldest history having been employed in the making of cooking pottery in Finland since about 2500 B.C. (Noro, 1968). Of least importance are tremolite and actinolite, but they find some use as fillers and filter materials.

Sources of exposure

Chrysotile asbestos is mined mostly by opencast methods. The asbestos risk is low and, as the serpentine rocks in which chrysotile occurs contain no quartz, there is no risk of silicosis.

Amphibole asbestos is obtained mainly by underground methods which involve drilling, blasting and shovelling. The related rocks (banded iron-stones) contain significant amounts of quartz. Dust is controlled by 'wetting down' methods. The asbestosis risk is low but silicosis may occur. Although pure fibre was present in the final milling process in a crocidolite mine (closed in 1966) in Western Australia, quartz was also present in dust from the crushers and shakers, and in the early stages of milling. Under such conditions asbestosis and silicosis may occur together (McNulty, 1968).

Ore from the mines, in lump (or 'cob') form, is sorted by hand and then milled; 'cobbing' (that is, separating fibre from the rock) was, until very recently, done by women and children in South Africa. The crushing and milling processes were notoriously dusty until a few years ago, but enclosure and dust collection methods have improved this situation.

Extraction of fibre ('fibreizing' or disintegrating) is next done to provide fibre of a quality (or size) appropriate to the process for which it is to be used and is, therefore, often carried out in the factory. This was very dusty and dangerous until the late 1940s, since when methods of total enclosure have virtually eliminated pollution of the general factory atmosphere.

Bagging of fibre may still be a dusty operation, but during the late 1960s conditions were greatly improved by a pressure packing system which is employed both in the production of chrysotile and amphibole fibre. Bags now consist of polythene-lined hessian or woven polythene, and are 'leak proof.' Previously bags were of hessian only and were readily damaged in transit with the leakage of much dust. Dockers working in the holds of ships were especially exposed to this hazard, but truck drivers and loaders were also at some risk. Transport of bags in sealed containers has now eliminated this hazard at all stages. Regulations in the United Kingdom to enforce these measures are referred to later.

Mixing of fibre for manufacturing processes has been, and may still be, productive of much dust. The same applied to insulation or lagging materials (in which fibre was loosely bound) until the late 1960s since when little or no asbestos has been used. The dismantling of old lagging is inevitably productive of large amounts of dust which is difficult to control. Men who built and maintained steam locomotives were often exposed to asbestos lagging materials. Spraying of fibre on to walls and ceilings is perhaps the most dusty and potentially dangerous process of all. Lagging and de-lagging operations and asbestos spraying of bulkheads in the confined space of ships and submarines have produced high concentrations of dust (Harries, 1971a). Cutting, sawing and trimming asbestos-cement products, on the other hand, yields little asbestos dust as most of the fibre is captive in the cement; but some fibres may escape (Greenburg, 1970). Filing and grinding brake linings probably releases some chrysotile fibres but the 'blowing-out' of brake lining drums with compressed air during servicing produces only a very low level of contamination (Hickish and Knight, 1970).

Dust exposure was high in the asbestos textile industries some years ago and emanated from dry carding, weaving and spinning of fibre; cleaning the rollers of the carding machines was especially dusty. The majority of these processes have been enclosed since about the end of the 1950s although various methods of dust suppression have been in operation since before World War II.

Unexpected sources of past exposure, other than those already noted, included operating machines for twisting asbestos string round welding rods (a dusty job often done by women in the 1930s) and the use of asbestos rope or fibre, either dry or mixed with water, to grout the expansion gaps between refractory bricks in furnaces and kilns. Because furnace and kiln workers and some insulation workers in ships who use asbestos materials as well as refractory bricks for lining boilers are often known as 'brick-layers' their exposure to asbestos may not be suspected. It is worth noting that there is no risk to arc welders using equipment with asbestos-coated electrodes as the temperature of the arc is more than sufficient to cause complete decomposition of the asbestos.

Protective clothing made from asbestos textile may release some fibres when worn (Bamber and Butterworth, 1970), as may unlined fire-fighting asbestos helmets (Lumley, 1971); and men cleaning and maintaining exhaust ventilation ducts and dust disposal units may be exposed to high concentrations of dust. Laundry workers may have been potentially at risk from asbestos used in lining rollers and ironing machines and for insulation.

The risk of developing asbestosis is highest in the textile and insulation processes where fibre is most finely divided, and is least in mining of the ore where airborne fibres are few.

Neighbourhood ('para-occupational') sources

Workers who have never used asbestos may have been exposed to it frequently or occasionally during work done in their vicinity by others; for example, maintenance fitters and electricians in asbestos-processing factories, or stokers, fitters and others around whom de-lagging and lagging operations are frequently carried out (as in boiler houses, power stations and ships).

(2) Non-industrial

Residents in the immediate vicinity of asbestos-mines and dumps or processing factories from which exhaust effluent carrying the dust was discharged into the outside air may have been exposed to significant atmospheric contamination. In general, this latter practice is long past in Britain although it continued well into the 1950s in some European countries. Air samples taken recently from the vicinity of a textile factory in Britain and examined by a sensitive x-ray diffraction technique were not found to contain chrysotile asbestos (Rickards and Badami, 1971); but the authors do not state whether or not sampling coincided with peak production in the factory. Attention has also been drawn to a past potential hazard to the housewife who cleaned or laundered dust-contaminated overalls in the home (Newhouse and Thompson, 1965), although it has to be remembered that in the 1920s and 1930s women often worked in the asbestos industry prior to marriage.

In view of public anxiety about asbestos materials it should be noted that environmental exposure in the home and elsewhere from products in which the asbestos fibre is captive is most improbable (Walther, 1970). Such products include floor tiles, partitions, ceilings, roofs, pipes, installed thermal and acoustic insulations, and brake linings of cars and other vehicles. However, the installation and sanding of vinyl-asbestos floor tiles may be a source of exposure (Murphy et al., 1971). Dust surveys of different locations in different types of building which are known to incorporate asbestos products—including sprayed asbestos—in their construction have shown that fibre concentrations were well below that which the British Occupational Hygiene Society has recommended as a negligible hazard for a lifetime's occupational exposure, that is, 0.4 fibre/cm^3 (Byrom, Hodgson and Holmes, 1969). But if sprayed asbestos insulation is not protected from damage by efficient sealing it may become friable so that fragments fall on to the floor, ledges and elsewhere where they may collect and are thus a potential hazard to health (Lumley, Harries and O'Kelly, 1971). Fear has been expressed that the surrounding air will be contaminated by abrasion of brake shoes when in operation; however, the heat generated at the point of contact exceeds the temperature at which chrysotile is decomposed and more than 98 per cent of fibre is destroyed (Speil and Leineweber, 1969) so that danger from this source is improbable.

AERODYNAMIC BEHAVIOUR OF ASBESTOS FIBRES

The aerodynamic behaviour of fibrous particles is, as pointed out in Chapter 3, determined differently from that of compact particles. This is important not only in explaining the degree to which fibres penetrate to the depth of the lungs but also in the design of dust sampling instruments.

The 'free falling speed' (see Chapter 3) of fibres is determined by the square of their diameter and is little influenced by their length. Hence, a fibre with a length of 200 μm or more and a diameter of about 3 μm has the same 'free falling speed' as a unit density spherical particle of 10 μm diameter; that is, the fibre has an 'equivalent (aerodynamic) diameter' of 10 μm (Timbrell, 1965). Fibres with a diameter of less than 3 μm will tend to escape *sedimentation* and *inertial impaction* suffered by those with a greater 'free falling speed' and so penetrate to the level of respiratory bronchioles (Timbrell, 1970), although many very long fibres are captured by nasal hairs. The greater the

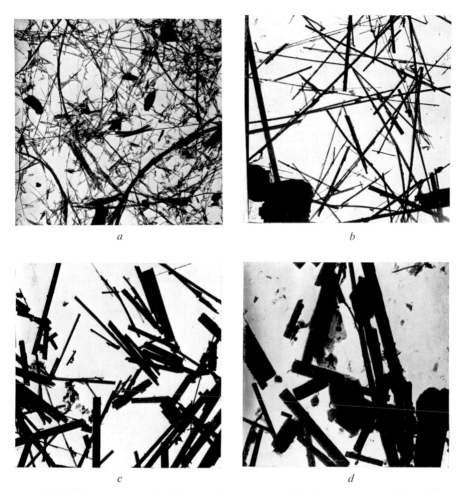

Figure 9.1. Electronmicrographs showing characteristics of the four important asbestos fibre types: (a) chrysotile; (b) crocidolite; (c) amosite; (d) anthophyllite. (Original magnification ×4,500 reproduced at quarter scale. By courtesy of Dr F. D. Pooley)

length of a fibre the more likely it is to suffer *interception* by the decreasing diameter of peripheral airways (Timbrell, Pooley and Wagner, 1970). Furthermore, the flexural modulus—or degree of *harshness*—of fibres appears to be of particular significance. Most amphiboles are harsh and stiff even when extremely fine but most chrysotile fibres are soft, or semi-harsh, and curly (*Figure 9.1*); harsh chrysotile fibres (which are relatively rigid) have little commercial use (Speil and Leineweber, 1969). The curling of long soft chrysotile fibres renders them more liable than rigid amphibole fibres to interception higher up the small airways (Timbrell, 1970). This effect may ensure that more chrysotile fibres are intercepted on the ciliary 'escalator' than pass deeply into the non-ciliated region, whereas more amphibole fibres (such as crocidolite) penetrate beyond the reach of ciliary clearance.

Fibres found in the alveolar regions of the lungs are less than 3 μm in diameter, their mean diameter being usually less than 1 μm (Timbrell, Pooley and Wagner, 1970). It appears that the longest fibres tend to be found in the respiratory bronchioles and alveolar ducts, and short fibres deeper in the acini (Timbrell, Pooley and Wagner, 1970). Some fibres—or fibrils—are beyond the resolution of the optical microscope and their diameter may be as small as 0·010 μm (Timbrell, Pooley and Wagner, 1970). The different abilities of chrysotile and other types of asbestos fibre to penetrate to the periphery of the lungs is undoubtedly important in the pathogenesis of malignant mesothelioma of the pleura (*see* later).

ASBESTOS

Definition
In this book 'asbestosis' means fibrosis of the lungs caused by asbestos dusts ('lungs' being understood in the sense defined in Chapter 1) which may or may not be as associated with fibrosis of parietal or pulmonary pleura.

Pathology

Macroscopic features
The external appearances of the lungs depend very much on the extent and severity of disease. When it is slight, the lungs are of normal size but, when severe, they are small, pale, firm and rubbery. The pulmonary pleura is usually thickened, varying from a slight loss of translucency (due to a thin layer of fibrosis) to widespread fibrosis (with fusion of both pulmonary and parietal layers) which tends to be most evident over the lower half of the lungs. Occasionally, there are localized areas of hyaline fibrosis with the hardness of cartilage. Although fibrosis of the pulmonary pleura is almost always present when lung fibrosis is advanced it does not necessarily match it in severity.

When the lungs are cut, their pleural margins usually stand out clearly due to subpleural fibrosis which extends into the intralobular septa. In the early stages a patchy, fine grey-coloured fibrosis is seen and felt in the lungs and becomes a widespread fibrotic network in advanced disease. It tends to be most evident in the lower parts of the lungs (that is, the lower lobes, lingula and middle lobe) beneath the diaphragmatic and posterolateral pulmonary pleura to a depth of about 1 to 2 cm, but it may spread into the depths of these lobes (*Figure 9.2*). As a rule the fibrosis is most prominent in the lower lobes—exceptionally in the lingula and middle lobe—and, in advanced disease, the lower parts of the upper lobes are similarly involved. Very occasionally, and atypically, this distribution is reversed, the fibrosis being predominant in the upper parts of the lungs (*see Figures 9.13, 9.14*). Whatever the distribution, however, the fibrotic areas may contain small cysts which are rarely

278

more than about 3 mm in diameter, although occasionally they may be as large as 8 mm. Rarely, large fibrotic masses ('massive fibrosis') which are not associated with tuberculosis, and in which there may be patches of necrosis, are present in the lower parts of the lungs, but are sometimes confined to the upper (*see Figure 9.15*). More rarely still there may be necrotic nodules of varying size in the presence of rheumatoid arthritis or circulating rheumatoid factor alone (Rickards and Barrett, 1958; Telleson, 1961; Morgan, 1964). In most cases there are small, discrete grey-black macules (1 to 3 mm diameter) throughout the lungs resembling those seen in 'town dwellers' lung'.

Silicotic nodules may also be found in the lungs of men who worked

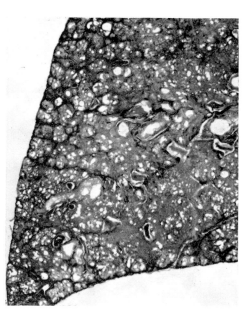

Figure 9.2. Moderately severe asbestosis. No small cysts present in this specimen. (Paper-mounted section, natural size)

crushing and milling ore at some asbestos-mines and in the United States of America in asbestos cement workers. They tend to be mainly in the upper parts of the lungs.

Textbooks sometimes state the emphysema (of unspecified type) is common and often limited to the lower parts of the lungs. This is not correct. Of course, some areas of lungs affected by asbestosis may be the seat of any type of emphysema but it is curiously uncommon. Scar emphysema does not occur as a result of asbestosis although in some cases contraction of the lower lobes may cause overinflation of the upper lobes.

Bronchiectasis is occasionally present in areas of severe fibrosis, but is infrequent.

Hilar lymph nodes are not enlarged.

Microscopic appearances

The initial site of involvement is in the alveoli of the respiratory bronchioles in which asbestos fibres and macrophages collect. A thin reticulin network

279

gradually evolves and envelops the cells and fibres. Collagenous fibrosis then replaces the reticulin fibres until these alveoli are obliterated. Hence, the primary lesion is a plastering of the alveoli from within the lumen of the respiratory bronchioles and not an interstitial fibrosis (Wagner, 1965) (*Figure 9.3*). Some degree of bronchiolitis obliterans may develop. Structures

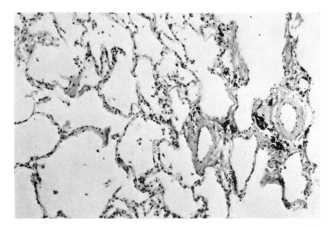

Figure 9.3. Very early stage of asbestosis showing peribronchiolar fibrosis. The alveolar walls are not yet involved. (Biopsy specimen; original magnification, × 50, reproduced at × 100; van Gieson stain; by courtesy of Dr K. F. W. Hinson)

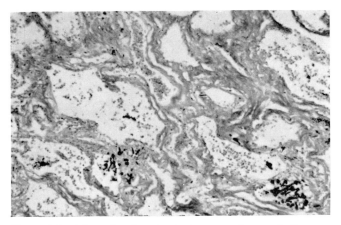

Figure 9.4. Asbestosis of moderate to severe degree. Collagenous fibrosis is widespread in the alveolar walls and alveolar spaces are partly obliterated. Whole and fragmented asbestos bodies are present. (Original magnification, × 50, reproduced at × 100; van Gieson stain; by courtesy of Dr K. F. W. Hinson)

distal to the respiratory bronchioles are not involved at this stage. Later the fibrosis spreads into the alveolar ducts, atria and alveolar walls obliterating many alveoli (Gloyne, 1932–33; Hourihane and McCaughey, 1966) but sparing the peripheral parts of the acini. It is now diffuse interstitial fibrosis ('fibrosing alveolitis') (*Figure 9.4*). In spite of this obliteration the elastic network of alveolar walls is often seen to be intact when elastic tissue stains are used indicating that much of the fibrosis is intra-alveolar (Webster, 1970a). But in areas where the fibrosis is solid, alveolar architecture is completely replaced by a mass of collagen which has a peculiarly strong affinity for haematoxylin. Numerous macrophages—some of which contain short asbestos fibres—may be present in neighbouring patent alveoli the walls of which are thickened by fibrosis and cellular infiltration.

Asbestos bodies are present in relation to the fibrosis (*see* next section).

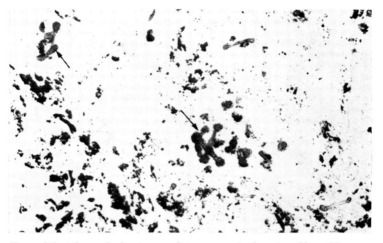

Figure 9.5. Asbestos bodies (arrowed) in an unstained section of lung. The group near the centre of the field consists of typical segmented and 'dumb-bell' forms and also fragments of bodies which have disintegrated. Most of the other particles in the photograph are carbon. (Magnification × 235)

Microscopic fibrosis may be found when on gross examination its presence is unsuspected or indefinite; the early pathological changes precede clinical, physiological and x-ray evidence of the disease process. In order that the *extent* of lung involvement can be properly assessed the International Union against Cancer (1965) has recommended that at least six blocks of tissue should be taken from specified sites as follows:

(1) Apex of right upper lobe, pleural surface.
(2) Right middle lobe, lateral pleural surface.
(3) Right lower lobe, middle of basal surface.
(4) Left upper lobe, central section.
(5) Lingula, central section.
(6) Left lower lobe, central basal section.

This can be combined with a system of grading *severity of fibrosis* to obtain a standard method for assessing the *degree of asbestosis* in the lungs as a whole. Such a method has been suggested by a Working Group on the Biological Effects of Asbestosis (Hinson *et al.*, 1972). There are four grades of *extent of lung involvement*:

281

(A) None. (B) Less than 25 per cent. (C) 25 to 50 per cent. (D) over 50 per cent.

And five grades of *severity of fibrosis*.

(1) *None*.

(2) *Minimal*. Slight proliferation of reticulin fibres around respiratory bronchioles with asbestos bodies. Usually confined to lower lobes.

(3) *Slight*. Proliferation of reticulin fibres confined to the walls of respiratory bronchioles of scattered acini. Occasional asbestos bodies and fibre fragments in their walls and lumina either free or in macrophages. More acini and alveolar ducts are involved as disease advances. This grade is classed as an 'asbestos reaction' rather than asbestosis.

(4) *Moderate*. Increased peribronchiolar reticulin fibre proliferation some of which is replaced by collagen. Bronchiolar vessels are also involved. The lesions are fairly widespread (though individual) throughout the sections and there is septal thickening. Cuboidal metaplasia of the alveolar epithelium of respiratory bronchioles and alveolar ducts is present in some cases.

(5) *Severe*. Large areas of collagenous fibrosis distorting bronchioles which may be narrowed to clefts. Some alveoli around these survive and are lined by cuboidal epithelium. The walls of distal alveoli are thickened by fibrosis and usually contain many asbestos bodies and fibres.

A proportion of asbestos fibres is visible with the optical microscope but many fibres can only be detected by the electron microscope (Timbrell, Pooley and Wagner, 1970). Fibre types may be positively identified by x-ray diffraction and by electron diffraction and microprobe techniques (Skikne, Talbot and Rendall, 1971).

Massive fibrotic lesions consist of diffuse hyaline fibrosis with areas of concentric fibrosis which are sometimes necrotic or calcified and are associated with endarteritis. The quartz content of these lesions has varied from 0·17 to 0·73 mg per 100 mg of tissue compared with 0·02 to 0·07 mg per 100 mg in control lung tissue. Whole or fragmented asbestos bodies are usually present in the lesions and diffuse interstitial fibrosis in adjacent lung tissue (Solomon *et al.*, 1971).

The 'necrobiotic' nodules of the rheumatoid variant are microscopically similar to subcutaneous rheumatoid nodules and are found in areas of asbestosis (Rickards and Barrett, 1958) and, when large, they may be more fibrotic although still exhibiting the characteristic cell reaction. Asbestosis may be minimal in the presence of large nodules (Telleson, 1961; Morgan, 1964; Mattson, 1971). Asbestos bodies have been observed in contiguous lung tissue of all the reported cases.

Centrilobular emphysema which is seen in some of the dust macules is similar to that in the lungs of town dwellers and there is no significant reticulin proliferation (Heard and Williams, 1961), but asbestos bodies are sometimes present in clusters.

There is little dust and negligible fibrosis in the hilar lymph nodes.

Asbestos bodies

First described by Fahr and Feigel in 1914, these may be found in the lungs after as little as two months exposure to asbestos (Simson, 1930). They are long structures (sometimes as much as 80 μm in length), golden yellow or brown in colour, which consist of an asbestos fibre wholly or partly coated with layers of iron-containing protein. This coat, which stains blue with Perl's reagent, is usually segmented giving a 'string of beads' appearance and both ends of the 'body' are bulbous. Some bodies, however, show little segmentation. Ultimately, they disintegrate and various stages of degeneration up to the point of beaded fragments in phagocytes and extracellular dark brown segmented granular fragments are seen (*Figure 9.5*). Uncoated fibres are also present and electron microscopy indicates that they greatly outnumber asbestos bodies and may be found in their absence (Pooley *et al.*, 1970). In advanced asbestosis several million fibres may be recovered from a gramme of lung tissue. All three major types of asbestos—chrysotile, crocidolyte and amosite—produce bodies.

Asbestos bodies and uncoated fibres may be seen singly or in groups together with carbon-laden macrophages in and adjacent to fibrosis in the walls of respiratory bronchioles (Heard and Williams, 1961). They are usually present in large numbers, but may occasionally be difficult to find in lungs with a severe degree of fibrosis.

Asbestos bodies can be simply demonstrated for routine purposes by smearing fluid from the cut surface of the lung bases on to a microscope slide and examing it unstained, first by scanning with a 16 mm objective and then using a 4 mm objective for verification. A more searching, but simple method consists in expressing lung fluid from pieces of a lower lobe into a vessel and centrifuging it; the deposit is then examined in similar fashion (Whitwell and Rawcliffe, 1971). Bodies are, however, more readily identified in lung tissue, by examining an unstained 30 μm section rather than the standard 6 to 7 μm section.

Asbestos bodies may also be present in the sputum and may be detected by dissolving the specimen with 4 per cent sodium hydroxide and examining the centrifuged deposit by phase contrast microscopy or by standard microscopy with the substage condenser lowered. Because sputum is swallowed the bodies, which are resistant to gastro-intestinal enzymes, can be found in the faeces (Gloyne, 1931).

However, asbestos bodies and fibres may be difficult to find by these methods in lung tissue or scrapings and in sputum if they are scanty or masked by the presence of other dusts. Under these circumstances the simple technique devised by Gold and Kerr (Gold, 1967) is of particular value. Many chrysotile fibres are less than 5 μm thick and so are beyond the range of the optical microscope; in fact, it appears probable that the majority of asbestos fibres in the lungs may be beyond this range.

It is important to understand that the presence of asbestos bodies in the sputum is not proof of asbestosis (or any other asbestos-induced disease) but only signifies past exposure to asbestos.

Specificity of asbestos bodies
'Curious', or pseudo-asbestos, bodies which are often found in lungs with coal or graphite pneumoconiosis have already been alluded to in Chapter 8. Although these may be segmented, are golden yellow and give a positive Prussian blue reaction they are differentiated by the fact that they have a black core and are usually shorter and thicker than asbestos bodies. However,

bodies which are indistinguishable may sometimes be found in the lungs of talc workers with or without 'talc' pneumoconiosis and are due to fibres of the amphibole tremolite and, possibly, chrysotile, which may be present in some forms of 'talc' (*see* Talc Pneumoconiosis).

Asbestos bodies, or bodies which are closely similar, have been found at autopsy in the lung fluid of 20 to 48 per cent of adults in urban areas with no known exposure to asbestos (Thomson Kaschula and McDonald, 1963; Cauna, Tolley and Gross, 1965; Anjilvel and Thurlbeck, 1966), but by contrast with asbestosis their numbers are small. Intensive searching has demonstrated 'bodies' in almost 100 per cent of such cases (Ultidjian, Gross and de Treville, 1968). Sections of lung tissue of persons who died in London between 1936 and 1966 showed that the incidence of asbestos bodies rose from zero in 1936 to 20 per cent in 1966, and that this increase correlates with the cumulative total of asbestos imported into the United Kingdom from 1910 onwards (Um, 1970). A similar study in New York showed that the incidence altered little between 1934 to 1967, being between 53 and 60 per cent (Selikoff and Hammond, 1970).

Some authorities doubt that these bodies always contain asbestos fibres (Gross, Cralley and de Treville, 1967; Wright, 1969) on the grounds that satisfactory proof of this is lacking, that many non-asbestos minerals of fibrous nature are present in the environment (Cralley *et al.*, 1968a), and that bodies similar to asbestos bodies may be produced in experimental animals by filamentous ceramic aluminium silicate fibres and fine glass fibres (Davis, Gross and de Treville, 1970). Gross, de Treville and Haller (1969) reported that although some 90 per cent of asbestos used in the United States of America is chrysotile, the electron diffraction pattern of bodies in a group of city dwellers, not exposed to asbestos occupationally, failed to demonstrate the presence of chrysotile. Accordingly, it was proposed that the non-committal term *ferruginous body* is preferable to asbestos body (Gross, Cralley and de Treville, 1967).

This is a complex problem which cannot be discussed in detail, but recent investigations indicate that 'bodies' found in the lungs of some members of the general population often do contain asbestos fibres. Electron micro-probe analysis has demonstrated amosite in the cores of bodies in the lungs of New Yorkers but identification of chrysotile was equivocal (Langer, Rubin and Selikoff, 1970). This may be explained by the fact that, unlike other forms of asbestos, chrysotile splits into submicroscopic fibrils and its magnesium is rapidly leached out under the biological conditions of the lungs (Langer, Rubin and Selikoff, 1970; Morgan and Holmes 1970). Electron microscopy has revealed that uncoated, chrysotile fibres beyond the resolution of the optical microscope are commonly found in the lungs of residents of New York City (Langer, Rubin and Selikoff, 1970; Selikoff, Nicholson and Langer, 1972) and London (Pooley *et al.*, 1970), that asbestos bodies represent only a fraction of the inorganic fibrous particles present (Langer *et al.*, 1971), and that they are rarely found on chrysotile fibres and then only on straight fibre bundles over several micrometres in length. The majority of asbestos bodies seen under the light microscope, therefore, are formed on amphibole fibres (Pooley, 1972). These observations indicate that 'asbestos bodies' detected by the optical microscope are likely to contain some form of

284

asbestos other than chrysotile. In the United States of America tremolite 'talc', which has been found in some cosmetic talcum powders (Cralley *et al.*, 1968b), may be responsible for a proportion of 'ferruginous bodies'.

In view of the relationship not only of asbestosis but also of malignant mesothelioma and, possibly, of bronchial carcinoma to past asbestos exposure

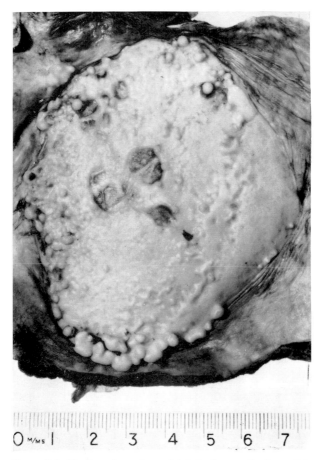

Figure 9.6. Hyaline plaque in parietal diaphragmatic pleura. It is well circumscribed, of both flat and nodular form and was partly calcified

it is obviously important that the significance and epidemiology of 'ferruginous bodies' in human lungs in relation to possible development of future disease should be established.

In experimental animals the formation of asbestos bodies involves phagocytosis of a fibre by alveolar macrophages, accumulation of endogenous iron (ferritin) in the phagosome containing the fibre and compaction of iron on to the fibres (Davis, 1965; Suzuki and Churg, 1969) which appear to be coated with a hyaline layer containing acid mucopolysaccharides (Governa and Rosanda, 1972). A similar process may occur in man.

HYALINE PLEURAL PLAQUES

These are distinct from the fibrosis of the parietal and pulmonary pleura which is an invariable accompaniment of asbestosis as they may be found both in the absence and in the presence of asbestosis. They are bilateral and consist of elevated areas of hyaline fibrosis which are usually well circumscribed, of irregular shape, and have a smooth, polished, slightly convex, ivory-coloured surface which resembles articular cartilage; some are multinodular (the nodules having a mammillated appearance), and others consist of a combination of both forms (*Figure 9.6*). They are found mainly in the parietal pleura and only exceptionally and, to a minor degree, in the pulmonary layer; and symphysis of the two layers does not occur. They tend to be distributed in the middle and lower posterolateral regions of the pleura and to favour the pleura over the ribs and the aponeurotic part of the diaphragm (although there are exceptions to this). They may also be found in the parietal pericardium. Irregular areas of calcification of greater or lesser extent are often present in the plaques.

Only a minority of plaques found *post mortem* or at thoracotomy are calcified or radio-opaque.

Microscopic appearances

The greater part of a plaque consists of avascular, acellular, laminated collagen with hyaline changes, but a few spindle-shaped fibroblasts may be found between the fibres. In some plaques the fibres stain predominantly for elastic tissue rather than collagen (Roberts, 1971) and may be 'pseudo-elastic fibres' due to changes in the composition of collagen. Dystrophic calcification is present in areas where collagen has undergone degeneration. The surface is usually acellular but, at an early stage of development, appears to be covered by a mesothelial cell lining (Thomson, 1970). The deepest (that is, external) parts show fibroblastic activity, sometimes with lymphocytes and plasma cells, and there is some vascularity. This suggests that plaques are, in fact, of extrapleural rather than pleural origin (Thomson, 1970), as *Figure 9.7* appears to confirm.

'Asbestos bodies' can be recovered from the lungs in about half the cases (Hourihane, Lessof and Richardson, 1966; Meurman, 1966) but rarely from the plaques themselves. However, asbestos fibres can be found in plaques although they are few in number and an extensive search is required (Thomson, 1970). In the majority of cases asbestosis (pulmonary fibrosis) is absent.

There appears, therefore, to be an association between past asbestos exposure and pleural plaques and, although this is not the only cause, it is said to be the most common (Hourihane, Lessof and Richardson, 1966)—at least in urban communities (see later). However, as in the case of asbestos bodies, plaques do not establish a diagnosis of asbestosis, but are a pointer to the possibility of past exposure to asbestos.

Pathogenesis

Asbestosis

The chief factors which appear to determine the onset of asbestosis are the length of time during which the worker is exposed to asbestos and that fibres are retained in his lungs (Sluis-Cremer, 1970), and, possibly, the concentrations of dust inhaled. But the severity and duration of development of disease sometimes correlates poorly with the intensity of past exposure. It is probable that fibrosis is mostly related to those fibres which, because of their curvature, are readily intercepted at bronchiolar level (*see* page 278 and Chapter 3). Chrysotile, crocidolite, amosite and anthophyllite are all capable of causing asbestosis.

Little work has been done to determine the amount of asbestos in the lungs of asbestos workers but it appears to be very small, ranging from 0·001 to 0·6 per cent of the lung weight (Sundius and Bygdén, 1938; Beattie and Know, 1961; Nagelschmidt, 1965), and to have no clear relationship

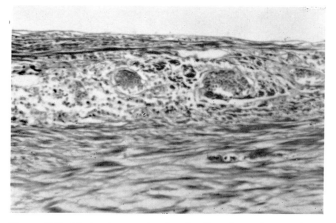

Figure 9.7. Photomicrograph of a hyaline plaque in an asbestos worker. This lies external to the parietal pleura which is seen at the outline of the section. (Original magnification, ×80, reproduced at ×160; van Gieson stain; by courtesy of Dr K. F. W. Hinson)

with the severity of fibrosis (Nagelschmidt, 1965). This implies strong biological activity and is in keeping with the fact that the relationship between radiographic changes and dust exposure is weaker and between changes in lung function and mortality stronger in asbestosis than in coal pneumoconiosis (Rossiter, 1972).

The effects of asbestos fibres upon macrophages and other aspects of pathogenesis are described in Chapter 4.

Following inhalation of chrysotile by guinea-pigs, fibres are found in alveolar macrophages and giant cells accumulate in terminal bronchioles (Davis, 1965). Giant cells appear to be formed by aggregations of dust containing macrophages. Later, collagen fibres line the respiratory bronchioles and alveolar ducts. Crocidolite, amosite and anthophyllite appear to have a similar effect (Holt, Mills and Young, 1966). Only short chrysotile fibres (that is, less than 20 μm), which are most likely to be ingested by macrophages, cause fibrosis when inhaled by the rat (Donna and Cappa,

1967). The stimulus which provokes fibroblastic activity, and hence fibrosis, is unknown but may be provided by some factor (or factors) released from dust-laden macrophages. The suggestion that these cells may be transformed into fibroblasts (Davis, 1965) is not generally accepted. That the cytopathogenic action of chrysotile is different from that of quartz is supported by the fact that polyvinyl pyridine-N-oxide (PVPNO) has no inhibitory effect upon chrysotile *in vivo* or *in vitro* by contrast with its pronounced effect on quartz (Davis, 1972).

Administration of crocidolite by inhalation to monkeys has shown that, initially, dust is found in the alveoli of respiratory bronchioles and in the alveolar ducts with an accumulation of alveolar macrophages (desquamative 'alveolitis') and the presence of bronchiolitis (Webster, 1970a). Reticulin fibres then form in alveolar spaces and are subsequently converted into collagen. There is no direct association between the resulting diffuse interstitial fibrosis and asbestos fibres or bodies. When fibres have been ground to particles about 2 μm in size, dust-containing macrophages collect in perivascular tissues but negligible reticulin and no collagen formation occurs even after five years (Webster, 1970a). Although there are species differences in response to different types of asbestos (Wagner, 1963) the crucial behaviour of alveolar macrophages is apparently common to all, and it is likely that the early events seen in the monkey reflect the development of the asbestosis man.

In the past, a theory of mechanical irritation by the fibres was proposed to explain fibrogenesis but there is no evidence to support this; and a solubility theory which postulated the production of silicic acid and its effects upon fibroblasts is equally unfounded. A recently advanced auto-immune theory (Pernis, Vigliani and Selikoff, 1965) suggests that abnormal globulin is either produced or localized by dust-containing macrophages and results in an antigen-antibody reaction which is marked by the presence of circulating rheumatoid factor; but, as yet, there is no proof to support this. However, as pointed out in Chapter 4, the prevalence of both circulating antinuclear and rheumatoid factors is unusually high in asbestosis—25 per cent and 22·6 per cent of cases respectively—but is similar (2·6 per cent) to that in the general population among asbestos workers who do not have asbestosis (Turner Warwick and Haslam, 1971). On present evidence these antibodies cannot be regarded as directly involved in the pathogenesis of asbestosis although it is possible that, in a proportion of cases, immunological activity may play an important part in some way (for example, an adjuvant effect of asbestos) in determining the course of the disease process (Turner Warwick and Parkes, 1970). It is interesting in this respect that macrophages containing IgM and complement—but no increase in numbers of plasma cells—have been found on biopsy of some lungs with asbestosis (Turner Warwick, 1972, unpublished observations), and that chrysotile and anthophyllite samples have been found to absorb rheumatoid factor (Jones, Edwards and Wagner, 1972).

The pathogenesis of massive fibrotic lesions is an enigma. It may be that quartz is involved because the lesions seem virtually to be limited to asbestos-miners (notably in South Africa where the quartz content of asbestos country rock is fairly high) in whom the quartz content of the lesions has been found to range from 0·17 to 0·73 mg per 100 mg of tissue compared with values of 0·02 and 0·07 mg per 100 mg in control lung tissue (Solomon *et al.*, 1971). An association with tuberculosis has not been established either during life or after death although, in experimental animals, asbestos dust exerts a mild, but short-lived, stimulating effect on tubercle bacilli and causes more extensive fibrosis when it is in the same region as tubercle bacilli than is produced by the bacilli alone (Vorwald, Durkan and Pratt, 1951). It is suggested that exposure to high concentrations of asbestos dust over a short period of time combined with low quartz concentrations are the determining factors (Solomon *et al.*, 1971). However, Webster (1972) has demonstrated the development of areas of fibrosis up to 1·5 cm diameter in both upper and lower lobes of Vervet monkeys exposed to long fibre asbestos in the absence of an initiating tuberculous infection.

The formation of asbestos bodies is believed to be a defence mechanism by the lungs against deposited fibres.

Hyaline pleural plaques

It is generally accepted that past asbestos exposure is related to the formation of hyaline and calcified plaques, and that all types of fibre may be responsible. However, the observation that plaques may be endemic in populations with no known exposure to asbestos or may show quite different prevalence in workers apparently similarly exposed to the same type of fibre (*see* Epidemiology section) raises the possibility that other factors may be of importance. Apatite—but not asbestos fibres—has been found by spectrographic analysis in plaques of Canadian chrysotile miners (Cartier, 1965).

Radiographically demonstrable plaques are rarely seen less than twenty years after the commencement of asbestos exposure.

It is difficult to explain satisfactorily why plaques occur predominantly in the parietal pleura and are localized rather than diffuse when asbestos fibres and bodies are found throughout the lungs. The suggestion (Thomson, 1970) that rigid fibres penetrate the pulmonary pleura and pass to the parietal pleura leaves much to be explained, and the hypothesis (Heard and Williams, 1961) that fibrin is deposited on the parietal pleura and becomes organized from beneath assumes, as Kiviluoto (1960) suggested, that trauma by fibres initiates the process.

Calcified pleural plaques are also observed after exposure to tremolite (Siegal, Smith and Greenburg, 1943; Smith, 1952) (*see* Talc Pneumoconiosis).

In short, not only is the pathogenesis of pleural plaques associated with asbestos exposure obscure, but it appears likely that they have causes other than asbestos which have not yet been identified.

Epidemiology

Asbestosis

In 1967 it was estimated that there was about 20,000 asbestos workers in the United Kingdom (Ministry of Labour, 1967); but this figure did not include the unknown, but probably large, number of persons working regularly or intermittently in the vicinity of asbestos operations.

There are few accurate statistics on the incidence and prevalence of asbestosis but it is known that the disease is most common in persons who have worked in milling and disintegrating ore, in heat and sound insulation (lagging and spraying fibre) and in dockyards. In general, figures are derived from two sources: compensation records and death certificates; undoubtedly they underestimate the true situation. The trend of new cases diagnosed for compensation in the United Kingdom is shown in Table 1.1.

It appears that an overall increase in incidence has occurred in most industrial countries in the last 30 or more years which is due mainly to heightened awareness and recognition of the disease, the cumulative effect of time lapse since the years when there was little dust control, substantial increase in the use of asbestos and expansion of the working population exposed. However, in those industries (asbestos cement and textiles in particular) in the United Kingdom which have been subject to the dust control measures imposed by the Asbestos Industry Regulations (1931) since 1933 a striking decline in new cases of asbestosis has occurred over the last 30 years (Knox, Doll and Hill, 1965; Smither, 1965), but a similar trend has not occurred in industries where these Regulations have not applied. And it must be emphasized that only a proportion of workers who have been, or who are, at risk can be identified; the total number is unknown.

There is no information as to whether asbestosis is more likely to develop as a result of exposure to one type of fibre rather than another because asbestos workers have in general been exposed to different types of fibre in one process or successively in a variety of processes over the years. An additional difficulty is that retrospective records of work details and the types of asbestos used have not been kept in the majority of industries. Accurate records of this information and of dust count data are imperative for systematic prospective knowledge of the magnitude of risk and the behaviour of asbestos-induced disease.

Until the late 1940s pulmonary tuberculosis often occurred with asbestosis but in latter years it has been no more common in workers with asbestosis than among the general population. This is exemplified by a London asbestos factory in which 31 per cent with asbestosis between 1931 and 1949 had active tuberculosis (Wyers, 1949) compared with four cases of healed tuberculosis between 1957 and 1964 (Smither, 1965). In short, the earlier high incidence of tuberculosis was similar to that existing in other populations of the same social class, and the present situation indicates that asbestosis, unlike silicosis, does not predispose to the development of tuberculosis.

Pleural plaques

For reasons given earlier, radiographic surveys underestimate the prevalence of plaques. However, pleural thickening and plaque formation has been detected fairly commonly among asbestos workers and residents (usually over 40 years of age) in the immediate neighbourhood of asbestos industries. Prevalence is related to intensity of exposure to asbestos: for example, in a naval dockyard 28 per cent of men with continuous exposure were found to have pleural thickening compared to 1·9 per cent among those slightly and intermittently exposed (Sheers and Templeton, 1968); a similar relationship was observed in 150 cases of pleural calcification among 1,117 New York insulation workers (Selikoff, 1965), and in Belfast insulation workers the frequency of both pulmonary and pleural abnormality determined by chest radiographs increased from 13 per cent of those who worked less than 10 years to 85 per cent in those who had worked 30 years or more (Langlands, Wallace and Simpson, 1971).

The occurrence of plaques appears to be world wide. Prevalence varies from about 1 per cent in a radiographic survey of neighbourhood cases (Kiviluoto, 1960) to 52 per cent of autopsies in an urban population in Finland (Meurmann, 1966). In Glasgow they have been found in 12·3 per cent of 334 hospital autopsies accompanied by asbestos bodies in the lungs in about 85 per cent (Roberts, 1971). They are also common in South Africa. Autopsy observations show that calcified plaques are less common than uncalcified.

Plaques have been observed in agricultural communities with no known exposure to asbestos (Zolov, Burilkov and Babadjov, 1967) and, in one such community in Czechoslovakia, both flat and nodular plaques were found in 6·6 per cent of 9,760 persons examined; and similar lesions were also encountered in cattle in the same area (Rous and Studený, 1970). It is of particular interest that in the Canadian chrysotile mining complex, plaques were detected in 90 per cent of a large number of employees in four mines, but in only 10 per cent of employees in four other mines, while no cases were found at all among a similarly large number of employees in the largest mine 65 miles distant from the others (Cartier, 1965). These observations give support to the view that some other agency than asbestos may be partly or wholly responsible for the production of plaques, or that fibres from different geological areas may differ in physical properties and, hence, in their ability to reach the periphery of the lungs. On the other hand, in a tobacco-growing area of Bulgaria where pleural plaques are endemic among the human population, soil samples have demonstrated the presence of small amounts of anthophyllite, tremolite and sepiolite derived from outcropping rocks (Burilkov and Michailova, 1970).

Clinical features

Symptoms

The symptoms of *asbestosis* are of insidious onset and the time lag between their being first noticed by the patient and his past asbestos exposure is very variable; in some cases (especially when exposure has been heavy) this period may only be a few years, but in others it may be so long that he may have altogether forgotten that he worked with asbestos. This emphasizes the need for direct questioning at a certain point in taking the occupational history.

As a rule, breathlessness on effort is the most important first symptom, slight at first and then increasing in severity. In most cases this increase occurs slowly over a period of years, but in some rapid worsening may occur within the space of one or two years, and in others there may be very little change over a decade. When breathlessness has become at least moderate in degree some patients complain of inability to take in a full breath which they notice at rest as well as on effort; when breathlessness is severe they may, in addition, find that they cannot yawn. These symptoms (which occur with any advanced diffuse interstitial fibrosis) are caused by the increased stiffness (reduced compliance) of the lungs imposed by fibrosis.

Breathlessness is often out of proportion to the extent of the physical signs in the lungs and of radiographic appearances.

Cough at the onset may be negligible or absent, but is later complained of in almost all cases; it is characteristically dry or productive of only a small quantity of viscid mucoid sputum which may be difficult to raise and provokes paroxysms of coughing which may be very distressing. Exercise may precipitate a coughing bout. But some patients with advanced asbestosis may have remarkably little cough.

Sputum, when present, is rarely of large volume, is usually mucoid and tends to be raised in the first few hours after getting up in the mornings; this, of course, is also influenced by smoking habits. Cough and sputum throughout the day (as noted by Elmes, 1966) appears to be the exception rather than the rule. Occasionally, however, sputum is purulent and of fairly large volume, in which case it may be due to the uncommon complication of bronchiectasis.

Haemoptysis is caused by some other disease process and not by asbestosis; bronchial carcinoma complicating asbestosis may be responsible.

Lassitude is a common complaint in advanced disease but is sometimes experienced when clinical, physiological and radiographic abnormalities are mild.

Chest pain is not a feature of asbestosis. But poorly localized aching or sudden, transient sharp pains are sometimes complained of and in some patients who are anxious about the disease appear to be of psychoneurotic origin, but in those with severe dyspnoea they may arise from intercostal and other chest wall muscles. It must be noted, however, that persistent pain may be the first evidence of malignant mesothelioma of the pleura (see later).

Pleural plaques, in the majority of cases, do not cause any symptoms but occasionally, when very extensive, they may be associated with a mild degree of dyspnoea on effort.

Physical signs

Central cyanosis may be seen in advanced asbestosis usually after effort, but is uncommon. It is rarely severe except in some cases where there is co-existent chronic airways obstruction.

Clubbing of the fingers and toes is frequently present though its severity varies from case to case. It may be slight in the presence of advanced disease or severe with apparently mild asbestosis. But some patients (possibly about a quarter of all cases of asbestosis) never develop clubbing. Occasionally, it progresses with remarkable rapidity and is then usually associated with similar progression of the lung fibrosis. It is the author's impression, even when clubbing is of mild degree, that the presence of nailbed fluctuation is associated with actively advancing lung fibrosis. Rarely, hypertrophic pulmonary osteoarthropathy occurs in the absence of bronchial carcinoma.

Warts, or corns, were common until recently in the skin of the dorsal and palmar surface of the hands and forearms of asbestos workers but, although some lesions acquired years ago are still occasionally to be seen, they have become rare in the United Kingdom since the mid-1960s. They consist of areas of advanced keratosis in which asbestos fibres are found

(Alden and Howell, 1944), and remain for long periods unless the fibres are removed (which workers quickly learn to do themselves), whereupon they disappear.

Expansion of the chest is normal when the disease process is at an early stage but becomes impaired as it advances. The impairment affects the lower part of the thorax and is usually similar on both sides; it increases as the disease advances. Measurements of basal expansion from full expiration each time the worker is examined is, therefore, a valuable index of progress of the disease. In cases of mild disease, expansion is usually normal (that is, $2\frac{1}{2}$ inches (6·3 cm) or more) but in advanced disease may be reduced to $\frac{1}{2}$ inch (1·2 cm) or less.

Crepitations are heard early in the development of the disease, patchily, in the lower lobe regions usually posteriorly but often first in the lower axilla and sometimes in the middle lobe and lingular regions. At this stage they are of fine (that is, high pitched), crisp quality and may only be heard at the end of *full* inspiration. It is important, therefore, that during auscultation the subject should breathe as deeply as possible. As fibrosis progresses, crepitations of fine to medium crackling quality are heard throughout inspiration, and later become widespread in the lower lobes, middle lobe and lingula, and may extend into the upper lobes posteriorly. They are persistent and are not dispersed or altered by coughing. Hence, persistent inspiratory crepitations of crisp quality are an important sign and may be present before respiratory symptoms or definite abnormalities of the chest radiograph or routine lung function tests at rest. Exceptionally, in advanced asbestosis they are either absent or scanty towards the end of inspiration; the explanation for this may be that restriction of chest movement is then severe enough to prevent sufficient expansion of the lungs to produce these sounds.

Rhonchi are unusual. A pleural rub can sometimes be heard at any site over the lower regions of the lungs and is often bilateral. This sign is not necessarily correlated with the location of plaques or evident pleural fibrosis.

Loss of weight is not a feature of asbestosis but occurs sometimes in advanced disease and commonly in the presence of complicating bronchial carcinoma or malignant mesothelioma.

Investigations

Sputum

Identification of asbestos bodies in the sputum of a worker with a history of asbestos exposure gives no additional information but when no such history can be obtained this may be a helpful clue to the diagnosis of asbestosis and also in the differential diagnosis of malignant mesothelioma of the pleura.

Erythrocyte sedimentation rate

This is frequently raised, especially in individuals with moderately extensive or advanced asbestosis.

Serology

It has already been noted that circulating antinuclear and rheumatoid factors

293

may be present in almost one-quarter of cases of asbestosis though the significance of this is not known. Thus identification of these antibodies in an asbestos worker with diffuse interstitial fibrosis does not help in distinguishing whether or not the fibrosis is due to asbestos or to some other cause. But the presence of rheumatoid factor with an otherwise inexplicable pleural effusion in an asbestos worker may indicate that the effusion is a manifestation of 'rheumatoid disease'.

Lung function

Lung function tests have three applications:

(1) As an important aid in establishing diagnosis
(2) To evaluate progress of established disease
(3) For periodic observation of healthy asbestos workers

(1) *Diagnostic.*—Physiological tests alone cannot prove the diagnosis of asbestosis; they reveal only the abnormal patterns of function which characterize diffuse interstitial fibrosis (fibrosing 'alveolitis') from any cause. But in combination with occupational history, abnormal physical signs and chest radiographs they give strong confirmatory evidence of the presence of the disease and indicate its severity. For this reason they are an essential part of the investigation of suspected cases of asbestosis.

The earliest detectable abnormality of lung function appears to be an increase in static elastic pressure which precedes symptoms and physical signs of lung disease, definitive changes in other parameters of lung function and radiographic abnormality (Jodoin *et al.*, 1971); but this test is not suitable for routine use as it is complex, causes some discomfort to the subject and demands a high degree of co-operation.

For practical purposes, the most important tests are those which determine the lung volumes (TLC, RV, FRC and VC), ventilatory capacity (FEV_1, FVC and FEV per cent) and gas transfer; assessment of arterial oxygen saturation is a useful additional, but not requisite, test. Determination of compliance is not essential in establishing the diagnosis.

In the early stages of the disease, hyperventilation on exercise due to hypoxaemia caused by reduction in gas transfer may be observed in the absence of any abnormality in the other parameters of lung function or of radiographic abnormality. Under these circumstances all these tests are normal at rest. When fibrosis is more advanced the changes in function are those of the 'restrictive syndrome' (*see* Chapter 1) with impaired gas transfer. TLC and FRC are diminished but RV is either little changed (so that RV/TLC is increased) or is decreased; VC, FVC and FEV_1 are reduced—and to a severe degree when disease is advanced—but the FEV_1/FVC percentage is usually normal or greater than normal. Airways obstruction is uncommon but when present is usually related to cigarette smoking and co-existing chronic obstructive bronchitis. However, it has been suggested that it may also be caused by obstruction of the smaller airways (Jodoin *et al.*, 1971; Muldoon and Turner Warwick, 1972) possibly by asbestos fibrosis of respiratory bronchioles. This requires verification by studies correlating detailed physiological data during life with the pathology of the small airways in a sufficient number of cases. A case has been observed which appears to support the contention (Heard and Turner Warwick, 1973). Compliance is also reduced and gas transfer impaired to a greater or lesser degree, due both to reduction of the membrane component and to ventilation–perfusion imbalance. Arterial oxygen desaturation occurs on exercise.

The presence of persistent basal crepitations is fairly well correlated with reduction of TLC and gas transfer, but radiographic abnormality is poorly correlated with the degree of functional impairment (Hunt, 1965; Kleinfeld et al., 1966); and, although some observers (for example, Bader et al., 1961; Kleinfeld et al., 1966) found no consistent relationship between duration of asbestos exposure and impaired lung function, there is evidence that it exists (Harries, 1971b; Becklake et al., 1972). Reduction in gas transfer may precede clinical and radiographic abnormalities (Hunt, 1965) and, apparently, occurs more rapidly than reduction in FVC in exposed workers (Murphy et al., 1972).

The tests which have proved most sensitive in the early detection of asbestosis are VC, gas transfer and compliance. Reduction of VC—in the absence of significant airways obstruction—has been found to be the best single test for discriminating workers with asbestosis from those without (Thomson, Pelzer and Smither, 1965; Becklake et al., 1970); and it may be impaired some 10 to 15 years before moderate or advanced fibrosis is apparent radiographically (Bader et al., 1970). This is a fortunate circumstance in that VC is a simple test requiring apparatus which is readily portable and inexpensive, but it must be properly maintained and the test correctly performed if the results and their interpretation over the years are to be valid.

In the absence of evidence of asbestosis, calcified pleural plaques, even when extensive, cause no abnormality of lung function (Leatheart, 1968), but diffuse pleural fibrosis (without calcification) is sometimes associated with a mild restrictive defect and impairment of gas transfer on effort. However, lung function values tend to be lower in individuals with the radiographic signs both of pleural abnormality and of asbestosis than in those with signs of asbestosis alone.

(2) *Progression of established disease.*—Once the diagnosis of asbestosis is established, progress of the disease can be adequately assessed at subsequent re-examination by VC, FVC and FEV_1; decline in VC and FVC values greater than that due to the normal ageing effect over a period with a normal FEV_1/FVC percentage indicates progress of fibrosis in the absence of other causes of the 'restrictive syndrome'. The VC is the most sensitive index of progression of asbestosis (Bader et al., 1965; Becklake et al., 1970). If there is a substantial increase of respiratory symptoms or abnormal physical signs of radiographic appearances it is desirable to repeat the more comprehensive tests.

(3) *Periodic observation of healthy asbestos workers.*—The suggestion made by Leathart (1960) that the VC of all asbestos workers 'should be measured at regular intervals and that a progressive decline should be taken as a warning of impending disease' is good practical advice. VC, FVC and FEV_1 should be recorded in every new entrant to an asbestos hazard and annually in all healthy asbestos workers (*see* also Preventive Measures).

Radiographic appearances

These can be considered under three headings according to their underlying cause:

(1) Pulmonary fibrosis (asbestosis).
(2) Pleural fibrosis and plaques.
(3) Pleural effusion.

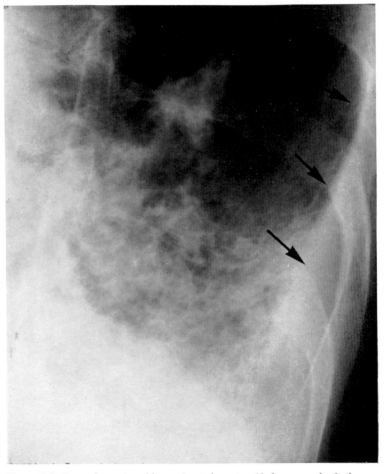

Figure 9.8. Part of anterior oblique view taken at a 45-degree angle. It demonstrates pleural thickening (arrowed) and fairly advanced asbestosis with an appearance of small cysts

Pulmonary fibrosis.—By contrast with silicosis and coal pneumoconiosis the abnormal appearances of asbestosis predominate in the lower halves of the lung fields in the great majority of cases, in common with those of cryptogenic and some other forms of diffuse interstitial fibrosis (fibrosing 'alveolitis') from which they are indistinguishable.

The earliest abnormality is to be sought in both lower zones near the costophrenic angles and is sometimes more easily identified on the 45-degree first oblique view (*Figure 9.8*) than the standard PA view (Mackenzie and Harries, 1970). The first perceptible abnormality consists of more fine vessel opacities than is normal in these regions with thickening of the vascular markings where they branch and divide. Linear opacities which look like extensions of vascular markings may reach to the periphery or cross, giving a net-like

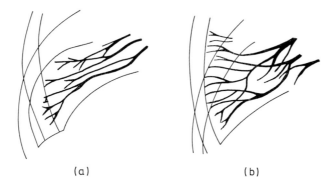

(a)   (b)

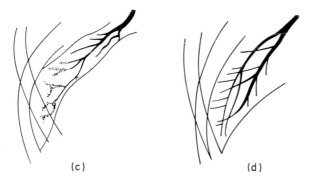

(c)   (d)

Figure 9.9. Diagram showing the various radiographic patterns of early asbestosis. (a) more small vessel markings than is normal; (b) vessel markings tend to be thickened where they branch and divide, an appearance occasionally seen in normal chests. Vessels may have the same calibre over the peripheral 2 or 3 cm and extend to the pleural margin. Branches cross giving a coarse net-like appearance; (c) fine, 'nodular' opacities 1 to 2 mm in diameter accompanying the smaller peripheral vessels; (d) horizontal linear pattern resembling Kerley B lines. Some of these lines are continuous with vessel markings and do not reach the pleural margin. (Reproduced by courtesy of Drs D. E. Fletcher and J. R. Edge and the Honorary Editor of Clinical Radiology)

appearance (*Figure 9.9*) (Fletcher and Edge, 1970). Initially these opacities are tenuous (*see Figure 5.12*) but they become progressively coarser and, when few, may resemble Kerley B lines although often they do not reach the pleura. As the disease advances, both types of appearance spread into the mid zones but only exceptionally to any degree into the upper zones (*Figure 9.10*). Another early abnormality consists of minute bead-like opacities, 1 to 2 mm in diameter, close to distal branches of the pulmonary arteries

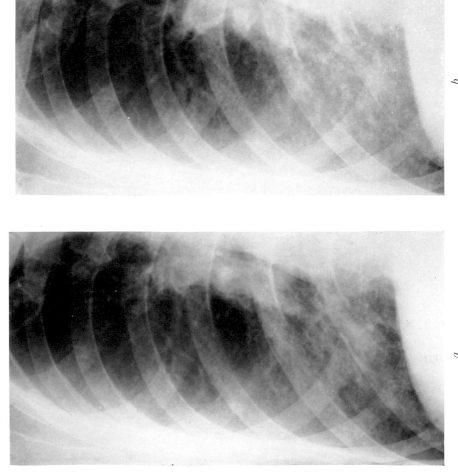

Figure 9.10. Rapid progression of asbestosis which has extended into the mid-zone of the lung field. Film (b) was taken 2 years after (a). Eighteen years' asbestos exposure. DAT, 1 : 32; ANF, negative; no evidence of rheumatoid arthritis. Lung function at time of film (a): TLC 5·0 l (7·5 l); RV/TLC% 48 (33); FRC 2·9 l; (4·3 l); FVC 2·8 l (5·0 l) FEV₁ 2·3 l (4·0 l); FEV₁/FVC% 82 (80); Tₗ CO/min. per mmHg 14·2 ml (32 ml). (Figures in parentheses are predicted normal values)

b

a

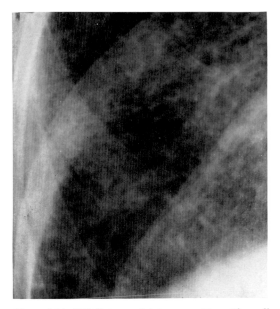

Figure 9.11. ILO Category 'p'-type opacities with small 'honeycomb' appearances in asbestosis. Man with 4 years' asbestos exposure. ANF positive; DAT negative

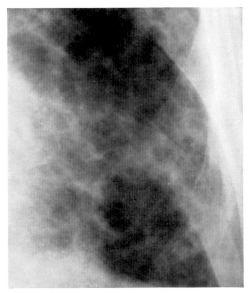

Figure 9.12. 'Honeycomb' pattern in asbestosis

in the costophrenic angles (Fletcher and Edge, 1970). Occasionally minute 'p'-type opacities persist in the lower zones as the predominant abnormality (*Figure 9.11*). A good hand lens and a bright light facilitate identification of early changes.

With progression of disease a cystic or 'honeycomb' appearance may develop in the lower halves of the lung fields, but the 'cystic spaces' rarely exceed about 5 mm diameter (*Figure 9.12*).

When linear and 'cystic' opacities are established in the lower zones the costophrenic angles are frequently obliterated, and evidence of a greater or lesser degree of pleural thickening (often more on one side than the other) is present. The heart outline may become blurred and ill-defined—an appearance commonly described as 'shaggy'; this is due to superimposition of the radiodensities of the heart and fibrosis of the lung, pleura and parietal pericardium. Examples of asbestosis of ILO categories 's', 't' and 'u' are shown in *Figure 5.12*.

In most cases, these appearances are almost symmetrically equal but sometimes they are more prominent on one side than the other; and, rarely, more in the upper and mid-zones than in the lower. It is difficult to be certain of the authenticity of dominantly upper zone cases but the case shown in *Figures 9.13* and *9.14* appears indisputable.

As the disease advances the area of the lung fields decreases due to fibrotic contraction (*Figure 9.10*), and undue translucency of both upper and mid-zones indicative of hyperinflation may be seen. In other cases there are indefinite, roughly rounded opacities in the lower and mid-zones which correspond to small masses of solid fibrosis in the lungs. Discrete 'nodular' opacities resembling those of silicotic nodules may occasionally be present in the upper zones (Nice and Ostrolenk, 1968) and have been described as common in South Africa (Solomon, 1969), although they are rarely observed in the United Kingdom. It seems probable that these opacities in fact represent silicotic lesions caused by quartz in the banded ironstone in which crocidolite and amosite are found; as much as 20 per cent quartz has been recorded in the dust of crushing-mills (Solomon, 1969). In general, these appearances tend to be confined to the films of miners and millers of amphibole asbestos and are not observed in those of asbestos workers exposed to chrysotile or amphiboles from which contaminating country rock has been removed—unless, of course, they have also worked in contact with other fibrogenic dusts in the past. Therefore, appearances of both nodular lesions and diffuse interstitial fibrosis of asbestosis may, under some circumstances, be seen on the one film.

Because crocidolite and amosite ores and their country rock may also contain the iron minerals magnetite and hematite, small discrete opacities of siderosis may be present on the films of some asbestos-miners and millers (*see* Chapter 6).

Rarely, large discrete opacities (up to about 2 cm diameter) indicative of 'rheumatoid' nodules may occur either with or without accompanying evidence of asbestosis (Rickards and Barrett, 1958; Telleson, 1961; Morgan, 1964; Mattson, 1971). When 'isolated' these opacities closely resemble those seen in the films of the typical Caplan syndrome (Morgan, 1964; Mattson, 1971) (*see Figure 8.25*).

300

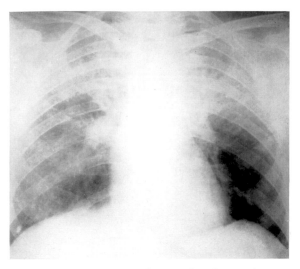

Figure 9.13. Appearances indicative of predominantly upper zone fibrosis in an asbestos insulation worker

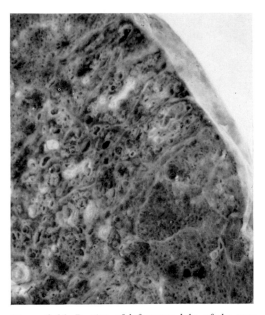

Figure 9.14. Portion of left upper lobe of the case shown in Figure 9.13. The features are those of asbestosis with very small cystic spaces. Histological appearances were those of asbestosis with numerous asbestosis bodies. No exposure to pigeons or budgerigars. Avian and other precipitins negative. (Natural size)

301

Larger opacities of confluent or massive fibrosis are also sometimes encountered and, although not seen in the United Kingdom, in South Africa they are more common in asbestos-miners than in coal- or gold-miners (Solomon, 1970). They are usually located in the lower lung field on one or both sides; less often, in one or both upper lung fields. Unilateral opacities of this type may be mistaken for bronchial carcinoma which commonly occurs in the lower parts of the lungs in asbestosis. In some cases they are

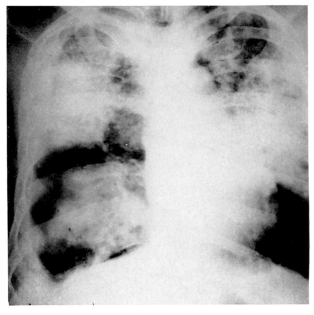

Figure 9.15. Radiograph of a young man with about 10 years' high dust exposure in a North Cape (S. Africa) crocidolite-mine. In addition to the large opacities, smaller round opacities are present as well as evidence of extensive pleural thickening over the right lung. (Reproduced by courtesy of Dr A. Solomon and colleagues and the Editor of Environmental Research)

widespread (*Figure 9.15*) (Solomon *et al.*, 1971). Their histology is described earlier.

Occasionally, bronchography demonstrates cylindrical and saccular bronchiectasis in the lower lobes, middle lobe or lingula (Leatheart, 1960).

The patterns of progression of disease are referred to under 'Prognosis'.

Pleural fibrosis and plaques.—For descriptive purposes it is convenient to distinguish the appearance of pleural thickening (fibrosis) from those of hyaline plaques by restricting the latter term to localized pleural thickening *not* involving the costophrenic angles which occupies less than four interspaces (Sheers and Templeton, 1968). A variable degree of obliteration of both costophrenic angles is a common, but not invariable, accompaniment of asbestosis from an early stage; and the combination of the signs of parenchymal fibrosis and diffuse pleural thickening is frequent.

Plaques are not visible radiographically until the thickness of their fibrous

302

tissue or the amount of calcium deposition is sufficiently radiodense, hence they are often undetected and their prevalence underestimated during life. None the less, some which are capable of being identified are overlooked. The reasons for this are: the observer's failure to inspect the costal margins and the outlines of the heart and diaphragm systemically; faintness and lack

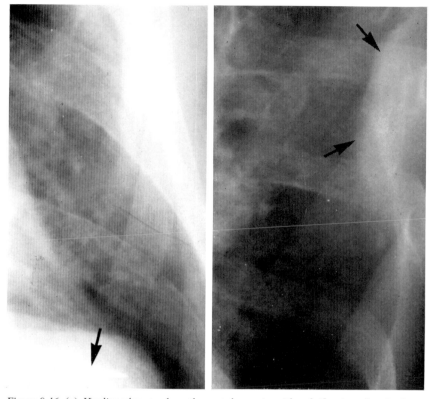

Figure 9.16. (a) Hyaline plaques along the costal margin with calcification of a diaphragmatic plaque (arrowed). (b) The 45-degree anterior oblique view clearly demonstrates the costal plaque (arrowed). (Natural size)

of definite outline of non-calcified plaques when viewed *en face* in the PA projection; failure to take an anterior oblique view—preferably at 45 degrees (Mackenzie and Harries, 1970)—to display the lesions tangentially at their maximum radiodensity (Anton, 1968).

Lower 'companion shadows' (*see* Chapter 5), although uncommon, must not be confused with plaques; they are usually bilateral but not necessarily symmetrical, although their similarity on the two sides is evident. Fibrous plaques, on the other hand, although invariably bilateral are not symmetrical. They are slightly to moderately protuberant opacities along the lateral chest wall in the middle and lower zones of the lung fields (*Figure 9.16*) and contiguous with subcostal rims for which they may be mistaken; they may also be seen along the line of the diaphragm.

303

Calcified plaques are more obvious than uncalcified plaques but may be missed when they are small or superimposed on the relative radiodensity of ribs, pulmonary arteries or diaphragm—especially if the film is underexposed. In most cases they are bilateral and when seen *en face* are irregular, or 'map-like', in outline and, owing to the fact that calcification is patchy, have a variable density (*Figure 9.17*). Calcified plaques may also be present in the diaphragm (as lateral views clearly demonstrate) or skirt the left border of the heart shadow. They are uncommon in the upper zones of the lung fields. Confusion with costal cartilages will not occur if orderly inspection of the film is carried out (*see* Chapter 5).

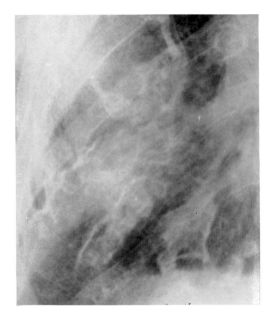

Figure 9.17. Irregular pattern presented by partly calcified plaques on the costal surface of the lung.

The location of plaques in the parietal pleura can be confirmed during life by ciné-radiography which reveals that the lung moves independently of the calcified lesions, whereas they move synchronously with the chest wall (Selikoff, 1965).

Calcified or uncalcified plaques are often observed in the absence of any evidence of asbestosis.

However, the plain fact that pleural fibrosis with or without calcification is fairly common among persons with no known exposure to asbestos should not be lost sight of. In a study of a large number of persons attending chest clinics in and around the Birmingham area in the United Kingdom, no evident association between pleural shadowing and asbestos exposure was detected (British Thoracic and Tuberculosis Association/MRC Pneumoconiosis Unit, 1972).

The prevalence of rounded opacities, irregular small opacities and pleural thickening in chrysotile miners and millers in Quebec has been found to rise considerably with increasing dust exposure. But these workers were exposed to crocidolite, amosite, diatomite, talc and quartz dusts. The prevalence of pleural changes was strikingly different in the two mines although production methods were similar; this may have been due to the fact that radiographic control was introduced ten years earlier in the mine with the lower prevalence and the consequent transfer of men with slight radiographic abnormalities to less dusty jobs. (Rossiter *et al.*, 1972.)

Pleural effusion.—A basal pleural effusion may occasionally be found at any stage of development of asbestosis and has been observed in the absence of evident lung fibrosis in some asbestos workers (Sheers and Templeton, 1968; Gaensler and Kaplan, 1971); it resolves slowly but may leave the signs of residual pleural thickening. Such effusions may be associated with circulating rheumatoid factor (Eisenstadt, 1964, 1965). It must, however, be borne in mind that pleural effusion may not only be a presenting feature of bronchial carcinoma complicating asbestosis, or of malignant pleural mesothelioma, but also of unrelated disease processes; until extensive epidemiological study has been applied to this problem a causal relation between asbestos exposure or asbestosis and pleural effusion cannot be regarded as proven. To this end a prospective survey has been in progress in the United Kingdom since about 1970 (Harries, 1971b).

The revised ILO Classification of Radiographs of the Pneumoconiosis (1971) provides category symbols for description of discrete, linear and 'honeycomb' 'parenchymal' opacities and of the various types of pleural shadow (*see* Table 5.3).

Diagnosis

Asbestosis

From what has been said already, the criteria for diagnosis can be summarized as follows:

(1) Known past exposure to the asbestos group of minerals.

(2) The presence of pleural plaques or of asbestos bodies in the sputum may support or suggest past exposure.

(3) Dyspnoea on effort.

(4) Persistent basal inspiratory crepitations with or without finger clubbing.

(5) Appearances consistent with diffuse interstitial fibrosis on the chest radiograph in the lower halves of the lung fields.

(6) Reduction of VC, TLC and gas transfer (T_L and D_m).

In the early stage of the disease, (3) and (5) may not yet be present and physiological abnormality may consist solely of hyperventilation and oxygen desaturation on exercise, and possibly slight reduction in VC. Crepitations are almost always present but are usually localized and may only be heard at the end of a full inspiratory effort. Given evidence of past asbestos exposure, the early diagnosis of asbestosis, therefore, depends first upon the presence of basal crepitations, second upon the chest radiograph and third upon abnormal lung function tests.

It must be emphasized, however, that the symptoms, physical signs, physiological abnormalities and radiographic appearances of asbestosis are no different from those of other forms of diffuse interstitial fibrosis (for example, cryptogenic, scleroderma, systemic lupus erythematosus and 'rheumatoid lung'). The absence of the diagnostic criteria of such diseases and evidence of past asbestos exposure practically establishes the diagnosis of asbestosis. Overlap occurs with 'rheumatoid lung' because circulating rheumatoid factor may be present in some 22·6 per cent of cases of asbestosis (Turner Warwick and Haslam, 1971) and it is also possible for 'rheumatoid lung' to occur in asbestos workers. There is at present no means of resolving this problem but when diffuse interstitial fibrosis is found with rheumatoid factor alone or with rheumatoid arthritis in a person with known asbestos exposure, asbestosis should be diagnosed.

It has been suggested that removal of lung tissue by thoracotomy (Gold and Cuthbert, 1966) or trephine needle (Steel and Winstanley, 1968) for biopsy should be undertaken in any case of uncertainty. But the proper application of the diagnostic criteria just enumerated enables the diagnosis to be made in the majority of cases before definitive radiographic changes occur. It is undesirable to subject people who are not patients in the accepted sense to either of these procedures unless there is a real possibility of some other treatable disease which cannot be otherwise identified. This is further emphasized by the fact that it is by no means certain that early diagnosis and removal of the worker from exposure prevents progression of disease (*see* section on Prognosis).

Microscopic diagnosis—whether by biopsy or post-mortem examination of lung tissue—rests on the features described earlier although those of the fibrosis are not pathognomonic. However, its distribution in the lower halves of the lungs and the presence of clusters of asbestos bodies and fibres establishes it as asbestosis. But when asbestos bodies are difficult to find, or are few in number, the diagnosis may be problematical; diffuse fibrosis with only an occasional asbestos body after careful searching should, as a general rule, probably not be diagnosed as asbestosis. It has been suggested (Hinson, 1971) that the presence of hypertrophic smooth muscle or lymphoid hyperplasia in the areas of fibrosis renders the diagnosis of asbestosis less likely. There are no specific cytological appearances on optical microscopy.

Cystic spaces are sometimes seen in the fibrotic zones but are usually of much smaller size than those which occur in the 'honeycomb' lung of diffuse interstitial fibrosis due to other, non-occupational causes. But 'honeycombing' may result from exposure to nickel (Jones Williams, 1958) or aluminium fumes, and its occasional occurrence in coal and graphite workers has already been alluded to (Chapter 8).

The finding of asbestos bodies in the sputum does *not* establish a diagnosis of asbestosis. The use of electron microscopy for positive identification of asbestos fibres in lung tissue is not practical for routine examination.

The clinician should remember that another form of pneumoconiosis may co-exist with asbestosis: for example, siderosis in amphibole miners and millers, and in arc welders who have worked with laggers; silicosis in amphibole miners and millers, and in refractory bricklayers who have used asbestos fibres and rope for grouting kilns or furnaces; or silicosis or coal pneumoconiosis in men who followed other occupations before or after being exposed to asbestos.

Pleural plaques

The recognition of fibrous and calcified plaques on the chest radiograph is described in Chapter 5. They appear to be a fairly reliable guide to past asbestosis provided that chest injury, haemopneumothorax (spontaneous, artificial or traumatic) or infection (mainly tuberculous pleurisy) can be excluded, although these are commonly unilateral and associated with evidence of general pleural thickening, whereas plaques are usually bilateral.

Pleural thickening or calcified plaques, however, are not an indication or proof of the coexistence of asbestosis (diffuse interstitial fibrosis).

The question of a relationship between pleural thickening, calcified plaques and asbestos exposure must be critically appraised in each case. Clinical experience in some districts indicates that pleural thickening (often of minor order) is common whereas pleural calcification is not, and that careful history taking frequently reveals evidence of past pulmonary or pleural inflammation or of chest injury; in many cases no history of past exposure to asbestos can be obtained.

Pleural effusion

Although it appears that pleural effusion in asbestos workers may sometimes be followed later by the development of asbestosis all other causes of effusion must be excluded before it is attributed to asbestos exposure; in particular, the possibility of an effusion being a presenting sign of malignant pleural mesothelioma should be kept in mind.

Prognosis

The development and severity of asbestosis is related more to continual than to intermittent asbestos exposure but there appears to be little doubt that individual susceptibility both of development and progression of the disease varies considerably; among men with similar exposure some subsequently have severe asbestosis, some mild and others apparently none. As a general rule, however, once acquired, asbestosis progresses slowly and relentlessly although, in some cases, it develops rapidly (for example, within a period of two or three years) from the start or years after being first diagnosed (*see Figure 9.10*). Either way, progression continues long after exposure to asbestos has ceased. The usual slow progress is exemplified by those patients (who may be in their sixth or seventh decades) in whom the disease proclaims itself, or first comes under medical supervision, twenty or thirty years after they have left the responsible industry. In some cases the disease is apparently arrested and no further progression occurs. The relationship between radiographic changes and exposure to dust is substantially weaker and that between mortality and alteration in lung function much stronger in asbestos workers than in coal-miners due to the biological activity of asbestos compared with coal-mine dust (Rossiter, 1972). Immunological and, possibly, other unidentified factors may also contribute to the rate of progression and severity of asbestosis.

There appears to be no certainty that removing workers with minimal asbestosis from further exposure effectively prevents progression; nor does there seem to be any means of identifying those who are likely to show serious progression in the long run and those who are not, but where the disease develops rapidly from the start the probability is that it will continue to do so. It is not yet (1973) clear whether unduly rapid progression is significantly more likely to occur in subjects with circulating antinuclear or rheumatoid factors than in those without.

In the United Kingdom severe respiratory disability occurs at a later age today than it did thirty years ago—usually after the fourth decade; this is due primarily to disease being, on the whole, less severe since the application of dust-control measures in industries subject to the 1931 Asbestos Industries Regulations which came into force in 1933. But many exceptions to this are seen in insulation and other workers who were not covered by these regulations and who have been exposed to uncontrolled concentrations of asbestos —often in confined spaces—until 1970 when the Asbestos Regulations 1969 came into operation (*see* section on Preventive Measures).

Before 1940 the average age of death in men with asbestosis in the United Kingdom was about 49 years but in the early 1960s it was about 60 (Buchanan, 1965); and in large textile and cement factories where dust-control measures have been in force since about 1933, only men with long service and severe asbestos exposure have died from respiratory disease at a younger age than men in the general population (Newhouse, 1969). Hence, today, many persons with asbestosis live a normal life span and die of unrelated causes, but the chances of dying ultimately from respiratory failure or cor pulmonale remain fairly high among workers who have been in uncontrolled dust conditions, or in whom the disease is established in the fourth decade or earlier. Because of longer survival the risk of developing the complication of bronchial carcinoma (*see* next section) is correspondingly higher.

Complications

Carcinoma of the lung
A relationship between asbestosis and carcinoma of the lung was suggested in 1935 (Lynch and Smith) and in the United Kingdom Merewether in 1949 reported that 14·7 per cent of male workers with asbestosis died of pulmonary malignancy; in 1963 this figure had risen to over 50 per cent (Buchanan, 1965). Similar trends have been observed in the United States of America and elsewhere. In part this increase is due to workers with asbestosis now living longer than they did some years ago, thereby increasing the period of time in which lung cancer can occur; and, of course, there has been a steady rise in cigarette consumption (*see* Table 1.3).

As a rule the tumour arises in the vicinity of the fibrosis and, therefore, occurs chiefly in the lower lobes (Jacob and Anspach, 1965); it may be of any cell type and, although it has been thought to be usually of squamous type, adenocarcinoma—especially of peripheral type—may predominate.

It has also been claimed that asbestos exposure in the absence of asbestosis may be associated with an excess mortality from bronchial carcinoma (Selikoff, Churg and Hammond, 1964; Enterline, 1965; Jacob and Anspach, 1965) which may be seven or eight times the expected rate (Selikoff, Hammond and Churg, 1968); but post-mortem examinations were not made in all the cases analysed. In the United Kingdom, in 1955, no such association was found by Doll in chrysotile workers without asbestosis. More recently an excess mortality from cancer of the lung and pleura, apparently related to severe asbestos exposure and cigarette smoking, has been found in male and female asbestos workers (Berry, Newhouse and Turok, 1972); however, the proportion of smokers among the women was higher than the national average (Newhouse *et al.*, 1972). Selikoff, Hammond and Churg (1968) calculated that asbestos workers ran about ninety times the risk of dying of bronchial carcinoma than non-smokers who never worked with asbestos, but, as the number of non-smokers was small it is difficult to determine the true rate among them. It is possible that there is a synergistic carcinogenic effect between cigarette smoke and asbestos dust (Meurman *et al.*, 1970) and the evidence suggests that this is more likely to be due to multiplicative than to independent action (Doll, 1971; Berry, Newhouse and Turok, 1972). Further investigation is required to establish that asbestosis is not present in such cases.

A tumour-initiating agent might be present in the natural mineral oils found in crocidolite and amosite or in contaminating oils from jute bags used to transport and store fibre (Roe, Walters and Harington, 1966); or in chromium and nickel which have a limited carcinogenic potential for man (Kazantzis, 1972) and are known to contaminate chrysotile, crocidolite and amosite (Cralley, Keenan and Lynch, 1967); or, possibly, in the iron of crocidolite and amosite (Harington and Roe, 1965). But there is no satisfactory evidence to support any of these contentions.

The occurrence of bronchial carcinoma has not been predominantly associated with any one type of fibre (Wagner, 1971).

Rigorous control of factory hygiene can reduce the mortality rate from bronchial carcinoma to the national average, as has been shown over a period of about thirty years in a textile factory using mainly chrysotile (Hill, Doll and Knox, 1966; Knox *et al.*, 1968). And there is nothing to suggest that numbers of the public who may have been exposed to low concentrations of asbestos in the general air run an increased risk of developing bronchial carcinoma.

Carcinoma of the gastro-intestinal tract

More deaths than might be expected from carcinoma of stomach and colon have been reported in asbestos workers in the United States of America (Enterline, 1965; Mancuso, 1965; Selikoff, Hammond and Churg, 1970), but the evidence is not strong enough to suggest a causal association; and, in the United Kingdom, no unexpected incidence of gastro-intestinal cancer has so far been observed (Ministry of Labour, 1967).

Carcinoma of the ovary

A causal relationship has also been suggested between asbestos exposure and ovarian carcinoma (Keal, 1960; Graham and Graham, 1967) the incidence of which has apparently been rising in industrially advanced Western countries since the turn of the century (Graham and Graham, 1967). However, the evidence is circumstantial and epidemiological investigation is required. Some of Keal's cases, in fact, proved (as he himself had suggested) to be malignant mesotheliomas of the peritoneum when re-examined by Hourihane (1964). (*See* section on Malignant Mesothelioma.)

309

Neoplasia of the haemopoieitic system

An unexpectedly large number of neoplastic haemopoietic diseases has been observed in some persons who apparently had asbestosis. These included multiple myeloma, lymphatic leukaemia, acute leukaemia, lymphoblastoma, myelo-proliferative diseases and Waldenström's macroglobulinaemia (Lieben, 1966; Gerber, 1970). This problem has not yet been analysed epidemiologically and on present evidence the association of these neoplasias with asbestosis or asbestos exposure cannot be regarded as other than chance.

Cor pulmonale and respiratory failure

Patients with advanced asbestosis may subsequently develop cor pulmonale, death ultimately occurring in congestive heart failure; but this is by no means invariable and the cause of death may be unrelated. Complicating bacterial or viral pneumonia is likely to precipitate respiratory failure with or without congestive heart failure.

Tuberculosis

A high rate of pulmonary tuberculosis was observed in persons with asbestosis in the 1930s and 1940s (Wood and Gloyne, 1934; Middleton, 1936; Smither, 1965), but in recent years the incidence is no higher than in the general population (Enterline, 1965; Smither, 1965). Undoubtedly the earlier findings were simply a reflection of the greater prevalence of tuberculosis in the working urban population of that period. There is no evidence that either asbestosis or asbestos exposure predispose to the development of tuberculosis or impair the effectiveness of antituberculous treatment.

Bronchitis and emphysema

There is no evidence to suggest that chronic obstructive bronchitis is causally related to asbestosis and, contrary to statements which have appeared in some textbooks, asbestosis does not cause emphysema.

Bronchiectasis

It has already been noted that bronchiectasis sometimes develops in areas of asbestosis due, apparently, to cicatrical traction on the walls of small bronchi, but is rarely severe enough to give rise to the typical clinical manifestations of bronchiectasis.

Psychological

The anxiety which may be caused to many patients by publicity given to the possible fatal outcome of asbestosis and the risk of bronchial carcinoma and malignant mesothelioma should be borne in mind for, although some may disguise this successfully, it is often responsible for much distress both to them and their families.

Treatment

There is no treatment at present known which will arrest or retard the progress of asbestosis and, although corticosteroids may bring about symptomatic improvement with some reduction of dyspnoea (possibly due to an effect on lung receptors), this appears to be short-lived. Equally there is no proof that removing the patient from dust exposure reduces the rate of progression, but obviously this recommendation will depend upon his age, severity of disease and, if he continues at work, whether the hygienic conditions are such that the level of airborne fibre is likely to accord with the currently recommended TLV and he is otherwise protected (*see* Preventive Measures). A young man with family commitments should not lightly be advised to change his job.

When the diagnosis is first made, reassurance which is realistic and seen by the patient to be founded on careful clinical and investigative examination should be given. Because both asbestosis and smoking may cause bronchial carcinoma he should be strongly advised to stop smoking permanently. Patients with troublesome paroxysmal cough require an appropriate antitussive drug, and if sputum is viscid and difficult to raise, the simple remedies of an expectorant and inhalation of steam in the mornings after rising (or whenever else necessary) give considerable relief.

Therapeutic measures for cor pulmonale, respiratory failure and bronchial carcinoma may ultimately be necessary.

MALIGNANT MESOTHELIOMA OF PLEURA AND PERITONEUM

This tumour arises from multi-potential coelomic mesothelial cells of the pleura or peritoneum and, until recently, was regarded as an excessively rare (Willis, 1967) but nevertheless authentic entity (Sano, Weiss and Gault, 1950). Wyers, in 1946, first noted the association of malignant 'endothelioma of the pleura' (that is, mesothelioma) and asbestosis, and in 1960 tumours of similar appearance were reported in individuals who had had industrial or residential contact with crocidolite asbestos more than twenty years earlier in the North-West Cape Province of South Africa (Wagner, Sleggs and Marchand, 1960). Since then the number of recorded cases of pleural and peritoneal tumours associated with past asbestos exposure has been steadily increasing in South Africa (Webster, 1970b), the United Kingdom (Enticknap and Smither, 1964; Wagner *et al.*, 1971), the United States of America (Lieben and Pistawka, 1967; Selikoff, Hammond and Churg, 1970), Germany (Anspach, Roitzch and Clausnitzer, 1965) and elsewhere. By 1970, in the United Kingdom alone, some 800 cases were on record. In Canada, by contrast, mesothelioma occurs rarely among workers in the chrysotile mines and mills (McDonald *et al.*, 1971). The diagnosis has been made either by biopsy or post-mortem examination, but chiefly the latter as diagnosis made by biopsy alone is not reliable (International Union against Cancer, 1965).

The tumour occurs in both sexes and the pleural site is more common than the peritoneal. On present evidence its occurrence appears to be related significantly to asbestos exposure—commonly crocidolite, but amosite (Selikoff, Hammond and Churg, 1972) and chrysotile (Wagner *et al.*, 1971) have also been implicated—in the distant past; that is, twenty or more years earlier and, in most cases, about forty years. In the United Kingdom, only 10 or 15 per cent of cases are said to be unrelated to asbestos exposure (Wagner *et al.*, 1971). In addition to a long latent period or development the 'attack rate' of the tumour in exposed populations seems to be very low

(Lieben and Pistawka, 1967) being, on present evidence, about 5 per cent (Wagner, 1973). The tumour sometimes occurs in brothers and sisters with

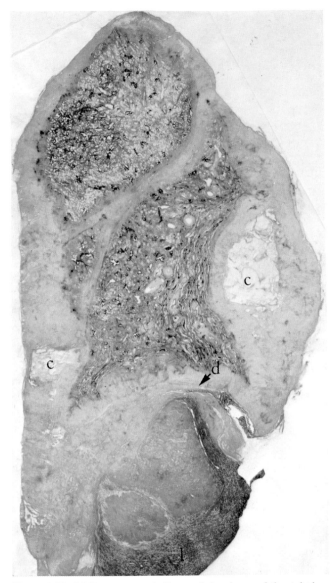

Figure 9.18. Malignant mesothelioma of the pleura of the right lung in a man exposed to an asbestos hazard for eighteen months twenty-five years before his death. Note the encasement and compression of the lung by the tumour, its extension into the fissures with necrotic cavitation (c) in the tumour mass. The tumour has spread through the diaphragm (d) into the liver (l)

past occupational exposure to asbestos but its site of origin and histological features are not necessarily similar.

Pathology

Macroscopic features

The tumour is ivory-white to grey-yellow in colour and varies in extent from a hard sheet about 0·5 to 1·0 cm thick covering a limited part of the surface of the lung and showing a tendency to spread along the interlobar fissures to a thick rubbery mass totally encasing one lung and invading it in lobulated fashion (*Figure 9.18*). All lobes of the lung are then much compressed and may be virtually obliterated. Both the pulmonary and the parietal pleura are involved and frequently there is massive continuous spread along interlobar and interlobular fissures, into and around the pericardium (when the tumour is on the left side), and sometimes into the liver and contralateral pleura. Plaques may be present in the parietal pleura on both sides.

The cut surface of the tumour may be glutinous (due to the production of hyaluronic acid); in places there may be necrotic cavities which contain either viscid and sometimes haemorrhagic fluid or a fibrinous material, and may be quite large.

This encasement of lung is most unusual in other types of growth although extension of an adenocarcinoma sometimes produces an identical appearance and a slimy surface.

In the peritoneum and mesentery the tumour has a similar appearance although symphysis of visceral and parietal peritoneum is unusual and a variable quantity of glutinous ascitic fluid is frequently present. Invasion of the gut wall beyond the muscularis propria is rare (Hourihane, 1964).

Metastasis to lymph nodes (hilar or abdominal) is not uncommon (Hourihane, 1964; Whitwell and Rawcliffe, 1971) but is unusual in other organs although, contrary to the opinion held until recently, it may occur, for example, in the contralateral lung, liver, suprarenals, thyroid, bone (Hourihane, 1964; Whitwell and Rawcliffe, 1971) and brain. Distant metastasis appears to follow disturbance of the growth during investigation or treatment. Spread of the pleural tumour to the chest wall may cause rib erosion, and invasion of aspiration needle tracks and thoracotomy incisions is common.

Microscopic features

There is much diversity of appearance not only from tumour to tumour, but also in the same tumour because both epithelial and connective tissue elements are present. Hence, there may be close similarity to either carcinoma or sarcoma. The histology of pleural and peritoneal tumours is essentially similar.

The tumour can be classified into four types (Whitwell and Rawcliffe, 1971): (1) tubulo-papillary; (2) sarcomatous; (3) undifferentiated polygonal; (4) mixed. However, it must be said that definitive segregation into one of these categories is often impossible.

Tubulo-papillary type (Figure 9.19).—The dominant pattern consists of glandular tubules (or acini), often of serpiginous form, lined by low columnar or cuboidal cells which are regularly ordered and, as a rule, contain few mitotic figures; in some places, however, the cells are flat, in others they may lie close in the lumen, and in yet others appear as branching papillary projections covering a fine reticulin core (Whitwell and Rawcliffe, 1971). In the lung or lymph nodes tumour cells occasionally contain dust particles; a feature rarely exhibited by carcinoma cells (Whitwell and Rawcliffe, 1971). There may be a variable amount of more or less acellular collagen.

In general, this is the commonest form of mesothelioma and, in many cases, is very difficult to distinguish from a secondary adenocarcinoma originating in lung, breast, stomach, prostate or ovary if the primary tumour is not identified; but the features just described are more likely to be associated

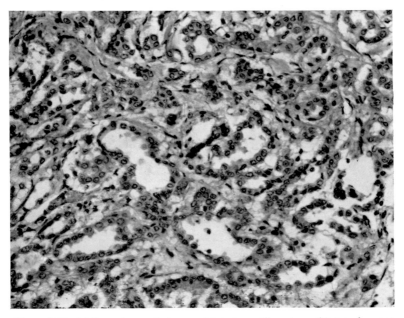

Figure 9.19. Malignant mesothelioma of tubulo-papillary type. (Original magnification, × 380, reproduced at × 960; H and E stain; by courtesy of Dr J. C. Wagner)

with mesothelioma than with carcinoma. A small proportion of these tumours exhibit a predominance of cystic spaces. Special staining techniques for hyaluronic acid may help in differentiation.

Sarcomatous type (Figure 9.20).—The pattern here varies from that of a very cellular fascicular fibrosarcoma to virtually acellular areas of collagen. But cell nuclei tend to be regular and mitotic figures are few. It can be seen that the acellular form may resemble a benign fibrous plaque very closely and an extensive search of the tumour may be required before the fibrosarcomatous character is identified.

Secondary fibrosarcoma must be excluded, and in general this is not difficult because the primary tumour, with the exception of uterine fibromyosarcoma, is usually clinically obvious.

Undifferentiated polygonal (epithelial) type.—The cells are polygonal (sometimes spheroidal) in shape, have a foamy cytoplasm and large nuclei in which mitosis is uncommon; they resemble the cells which line tubulopapillary structures (McCaughey, 1965). They occur in the other tumour

314

types but may constitute a pure, unmixed, epithelial tumour in which sheets of these cells are often supported by a more intricate framework of reticulin fibres (demonstrated by silver stains) than is usually to be found in similar areas of a carcinoma (McCaughey, 1965). They appear almost benign and this may be a source of misdiagnosis when examination of tissue is limited to small samples for biopsy.

Mixed type.—This consists of a mixture of the other three types although one is usually predominant. Thus, widespread examination of the tumour and metastatic deposits (for example, in lymph nodes) may be necessary before its mixed nature is evident. After the tubulo-papillary type it seems to be the

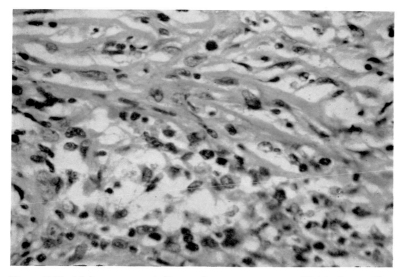

Figure 9.20. Malignant mesothelioma of sarcomatous type. (Original magnification × 380; reproduced at × 960; H and E stain; by courtesy of Dr K. F. W. Hinson)

most common of the mesotheliomas which is fortunate in that its pleomorphism makes it the easiest to diagnose.

Staining reactions

The mucopolysaccharide substance of mesotheliomas is hyaluronic acid which is usually extracellular and stains blue with alcian blue and Hale's colloidal iron (Pearce, 1968), but not with periodic acid Schiff (PAS) or mucicarmine. Adenocarcinomas occasionally give the alcian blue reaction but usually stain with PAS. In some cases the tumours can be differentiated by removing the hyaluronic acid from the mesothelial tissue with the enzyme hyaluronidase after which staining with alcian blue and colloidal iron becomes negative (Wagner, Munday and Harington, 1962). However, as this reaction is only produced consistently by the cystic type of tubulo-papillary mesothelioma which is comparatively rare in the United Kingdom accounting, possibly, for less than 15 per cent of all the malignant mesotheliomas seen (Wagner, 1972a), it is of limited value in the diagnosis of these tumours.

Asbestos bodies are found in the lungs of all cases in which there is

315

established past exposure to asbestos and in a proportion of those in which no known exposure can be traced. Asbestos bodies and fibres have been found in hilar and mediastinal lymph nodes, in the spleen, in the wall of the small bowel and in abdominal tumours; and asbestos bodies have also been recovered from abdominal lymph nodes and the peritoneum (Godwin and Jagatic, 1970).

Asbestosis accompanies malignant mesotheliomas (*Figure 9.21*) of the pleura in only very few cases, and then only to a minor degree, but is not uncommon with peritoneal tumours. This anomaly remains to be explained.

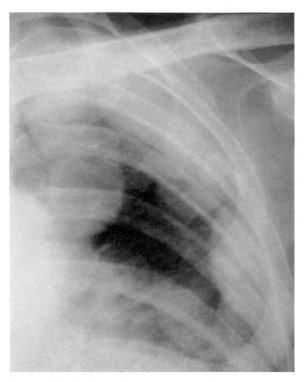

Figure 9.21. Radiographic appearances which may be presented by malignant mesothelioma. In some cases the appearances are those of pleural effusion

The authenticity of malignant mesotheliomas as a separate entity has been challenged over the years and recently by no less an authority than Willis (1967) who pointed, among other things, to the inadequacy of post-mortem examination in many cases of alleged 'mesotheliomas' so that primary tumours—especially 'small visceral carcinomas'—could have been overlooked. There is no doubt that this has been, and may still be, the case and that an unknown proportion of tumours has probably been wrongly classed under the diagnosis of mesothelioma. But apart from there being evidence for the pleural histogenesis of the tumour its macroscopic appearances are, if not pathognomonic, remarkably consistent although an adenocarcinoma may occasionally produce an identically gross appearance. In short, malignant mesothelioma is now accepted as a genuine entity. The diagnosis, however, must rest, not only upon evidence of past exposure to asbestos and careful histological study, but also upon stringent standards of post-mortem examination (*see* Diagnosis). Accordingly, epidemiological studies of the tumour, in order to be valid, must be based on these standards and not upon biopsy material.

Pathogenesis

Crocidolite has been most associated with the development of malignant mesothelioma (Wagner, Sleggs, and Marchand, 1960; Gilson, 1966) but the problem is far from straightforward, for not all crocidolite exposure is related to an unusually high incidence of these tumours. In two areas of South Africa, 400 miles apart, in which crocidolite is mined they have been fairly common in one (North-West Cape Province), but rare in the other (the Transvaal) where, however, asbestosis is common. In both cases the chemical composition is the same, but the average diameter of North-West Cape fibre is about three times less than in the Transvaal fibre so that its aerodynamic properties are thought to enable it to penetrate deeply to the periphery of the lung whereas Transvaal fibre is largely intercepted at bronchiolar level (Wagner *et al.*, 1971). This may explain the discrepancy. Against this, however, Webster (1973) has observed crocidolite fibres and bodies in the subpleural region in cases of asbestosis from the Transvaal mines. Curly shaped chrysotile fibres would also be expected to be intercepted at bronchiolar level and to reach the pleura in only minute quantities.

Mesotheliomas are most commonly related to brief and usually, but not necessarily, light asbestos exposure and an evident pattern of 'dose' response is lacking (Wagner, 1972b). Where exposure has been wholly or partly to chrysotile these tumours are in general very rare (Elwood and Cochrane, 1964; McDonald *et al.*, 1971), but a significant number have occurred in the United States of America in insulation workers who appear to have been exposed mainly to this type of fibre (Selikoff, Hammond and Churg, 1970), and a few have been observed in workers exposed only to amosite (Selikoff, Hammond and Churg, 1972). Webster (1973) has suggested that some other factor—possibly mineral—must be associated with asbestos before malignancy can occur.

Mesothelioma with similar histological patterns to human tumours have been induced in experimental animals by intrapleural inoculation of various samples of crocidolite, chrysotile, amosite and anthophyllite, but, by contrast, inhalation of dust clouds of the same samples resulted in very few of these tumours possibly because of failure of most of the inhaled fibres to reach the mesothelial surface (Wagner, 1972c). Crocidolite in tissue culture with human parietal pleura causes a pronounced proliferation of mesothelial cells and an increase of collagen in the underlying tissue (Rajan, Wagner and Evans, 1972). Under experimental conditions it appears that glass and aluminium oxide fibres may also induce mesotheliomatous changes (Maroudas, O'Neill and Stanton, 1973).

It has been suggested that polycyclic aromatic hydrocarbons which occur naturally in crocidolite in higher concentrations than in other forms of asbestos may be the cause of the tumours (Harington and Roe, 1965); however, Wagner and Berry (1969) found no difference in tumour-producing effect between natural and oil-extracted forms of crocidolite after intrapleural injection into rats. The chance of a tumour developing at a given age in animals appears to be proportional to the 'dose' of fibre received (Wagner, Berry and Timbrell, 1970).

Clearly, the pathogenesis of malignant mesothelioma in man is far from understood, but on present evidence crocidolite (or some factor associated with it) must be regarded as the fibre type most likely to give rise to both the pleural and peritoneal growths, although other types may be responsible for some cases. It appears likely that a longer period of exposure to amosite than to crocidolite is required before the tumour develops (Harington, Gilson and Wagner, 1971).

There is no evidence that mesotheliomas arise in pre-existing pleural plaques.

Clinical features

Symptoms

The pleural tumour.—There is a gradual and insidious onset of increasing breathlessness on effort which may or may not be associated with pain and, perhaps, tenderness or a heavy sensation on one side of the chest. If pain is present it is usually of 'nagging' type and not affected by respiration; later it becomes severe and persistent. Sometimes dyspnoea is of sudden onset due to the development of a large quantity of pleural fluid which, if removed, rapidly re-accumulates. In most cases weight loss and lassitude occur, but cough is not a constant feature. Some patients complain of frequent drenching and distressing night sweats.

The peritoneal tumour.—Once again, onset is insidious and symptoms vague and variable. There may be painless, diffuse swelling of the abdomen with early loss of weight. Increasing abdominal girth which is attributed to gaining weight may be the first symptom. In other cases, there may be symptoms indicative of upper and lower intestinal obstruction which may or may not be associated with pain, but acute obstruction is rare. Lethargy and loss of appetite are common.

Physical signs

The pleural tumour.—In the absence of coexistent asbestosis (which, as indicated earlier, is the rule) there is no finger clubbing. When the disease is advanced the patient is emaciated and ill, and dyspnoeic at rest.

On the affected side there are all the signs of pleural effusion in greater or lesser degree, and the chest wall may be painful or tender when palpated; in advanced disease the chest wall is flattened and almost immobile. Persistent basal crepitations indicative of asbestosis may be heard on the opposite side but are exceptional. For reasons which are not clear the tumour occasionally presents with ipsilateral spontaneous pneumothorax.

In some cases the liver, when invaded by tumour, may be palpable well below the costal margin, but is not often tender.

Evidence of local lymph node involvement is extremely uncommon.

The peritoneal tumour.—The patient is usually thin and ill. His abdomen is often distended and its girth may increase rapidly; the signs of ascites may then be elicited. In other cases distension may not be evident but indefinite, irregular, firm masses can be felt in the upper or lower abdomen; it is not possible to relate them to any abdominal organ. The signs of asbestosis may also be present.

Investigations

Radiographic appearances

The appearances of pleural mesotheliomas on the chest radiograph vary according to the stage at which the disease is first seen. The most important changes are as follows:

(1) Irregular, protuberant opacities on one chest wall extending into the lung field to a greater or lesser degree and surrounding much of it, but sometimes localized to one area only (*Figure 9.21*). At an early stage these opacities are indistinguishable from those of hyaline pleural plaques. Rarely, these appearances are bilateral.

(2) The appearances may be those of a unilateral pleural effusion, and extension of well-demarcated opacities along the sites of the greater or lesser fissures may suggest loculation but are often due to tumour mass alone. Tomography may help to decide this point by demonstrating uniform density of opacity at different levels. When pleural fluid is present and is aspirated irregular opacities of tumour masses on the chest wall are usually clearly visible on a subsequent radiograph.

(3) Erosion of ribs in the vicinity of the tumour may be observed at a late stage in some cases.

In the case of the peritoneal tumour radiographs of the abdomen give little help and show only generalized opacity of variable density. Signs of intestinal obstruction are rarely present.

Examination of pleural and peritoneal fluid

The fluid is clear, yellow, sometimes blood tinged, and sterile; it is frequently glutinous and to such a degree as to make aspiration difficult.

Aspiration of fluid may be necessary to relieve discomfort and dyspnoea but for diagnostic purposes it is usually more helpful in excluding other diseases than establishing the presence of mesothelioma, for it is often impossible to distinguish benign and 'atypical' mesothelial cells so that no clear dividing line between normal and malignant cells may be discernible and the one may be mistaken for the other (Klempman, 1962; Spriggs and Bonnington, 1968). The presumptive diagnosis of malignant mesothelioma on exfoliative cytology depends upon identifying malignant cells which still possess the characteristics of mesothelial cells (Klempman, 1962) and should be made only if cells of this type can be clearly recognized (Roberts and Campbell, 1972). Detection of hyaluronic acid in the fluid may provide corroborative evidence in favour of malignant mesothelioma (Harington, Wagner and

Smith, 1963) but it may also be found with other malignant tumours of the pleura.

Biopsy of tumour

Specimens of pleural tumour may be obtained by needle techniques or thoracotomy but examination of such limited material cannot establish the diagnosis with certainty; this can only be done after a searching post-mortem examination. Because of this and the propensity for mesothelial tumours to advance along needle and incision tracks and spread within the chest wall, these investigations should be avoided if possible. In some cases, however, a treatable disorder cannot confidently be excluded in any other way.

In the case of the peritoneal tumour laparotomy may be unavoidable but, like the pleural tumour, biopsy can only suggest the probability of mesothelioma.

Diagnosis

During life this can only be presumptive in most cases. The important features are:

(1) A history of past exposure to asbestos—especially to crocidolite.

(2) A latent period of twenty or more years between exposure and development of the tumour.

(3) Asbestos bodies in the sputum or lung tissue.

(4) The appearances of the chest radiograph in the case of pleural disease.

(5) The presence of hyaluronic acid in fluid and the microscopical appearances of the tumour.

But as already indicated it is often impossible to be certain that the tumour does not represent metastasis from an unidentified primary.

After death the diagnosis is made on the additional conditions that:

(1) The tumour exhibits a tendency to spread diffusely along serosal membranes. This may sometimes be established in life at thoracotomy or laparotomy.

(2) A searching necropsy fails to reveal a primary growth from which it could have originated.

(3) It possesses the histological features described.

Distant secondary deposits from malignant mesothelioma are exceptional, but if the other diagnostic criteria of the tumour are fulfilled their presence does not invalidate the diagnosis; however, multiple metastasis in various organs virtually excludes mesothelioma. The tumour which is most likely to be mistaken for mesothelioma is adenocarcinoma of pulmonary or abdominal origin.

Prognosis

The outlook is inevitably fatal, and the majority of patients with either pleural or peritoneal tumours die within twelve to eighteen months of the presumptive diagnosis being made. The time of survival from the onset of symptoms of the pleural tumour, however, may be as long as four to five years (Whitwell and Rawcliffe, 1971).

As the disease progresses there is increasing loss of weight and, in the case of pleural tumours, progressive dyspnoea and often severe, persistent chest pain. Death usually occurs from respiratory failure or bronchopneumonia but, occasionally, is due to extensive spread of tumour to the pericardium. In the case of peritoneal tumours there may be increasing ascites, and malnutrition and electrolyte imbalance resulting from anorexia and frequent vomiting. Intestinal obstruction is exceptional. Bronchopneumonia often ensues and causes death.

Treatment

There is no effective specific treatment. The tumour is resistant to radiotherapy and cytotoxic drugs.

Palliative treatment includes control of pain, and when night sweats are distressing in spite of light and absorptive personal and bed clothing, resort to the anhidrotic effect of belladonna may give relief. Periodic removal of pleural or ascitic fluid may be necessary to relieve dyspnoea or discomfort. The instillation of nitrogen mustard following aspiration may help to slow down re-accumulation of fluid and, after thoracotomy, may possibly reduce the likelihood of the tumour growing through the line of incision (Thompson, 1965).

PREVENTIVE MEASURES

In the first place, asbestos may be replaced by some other material. This has already been done by substituting glass wool and other harmless substances for use in some types of insulation and spraying work; and in the United Kingdom crocidolite has largely been replaced by amosite or chrysotile since 1970. Substitution is the only wholly satisfactory solution to the problem, but no substitute is available for some of the uses of asbestos—for example, the use of crocidolite as a reinforcing filler with high acid resistance and tensile strength in the pitch employed for moulded lead battery boxes.

But asbestos, being a uniquely valuable and in some respects life-saving mineral, will continue to have wide industrial applications. Hence, it is vital that safe conditions for its use and codes of practice are established. These can be briefly reviewed from three standpoints: conveyance and storage of asbestos fibre, factory conditions, and other occupational conditions. In the United Kingdom they are controlled by the Asbestos Regulations 1969 which came into force in May 1970 (Department of Employment and Productivity, 1970). Detailed code of practice instructions for different circumstances of asbestos exposure, including waste disposal, are provided in booklet form by the Environmental Control Committee of the British Asbestos Research Council.

(1) *Conveyance and storage of fibre.*—Fibre is now kept in sealed polythene or impermeable paper bags which prevent exposure to spillage previously experienced by dockers, truck loaders and factory workers.

(2) *Factory conditions.*—Where wet processes are used, as in the production of asbestos cement products, there is very little dust. But dusty dry processes (such as milling) can be effectively controlled by total or partial enclosure with effective exhaust ventilation and, where enclosure is not possible (as in

machining and sawing asbestos products), by hoods subjected to 'low-volume high velocity' exhaust ventilation.

Exhaust ventilation, both local and general, must carry the dust-laden air away and filter out the dust efficiently so that it does not return to the factory or escape to the outside air. Filtered dust is sealed in polythene bags.

Where a worker is likely to be exposed to an asbestos-dust risk, personal protective equipment must be worn. This consists of standard respirator masks, positive-pressure respirators powered by a portable mechanism, air-line breathing apparatus and also closely fitting overalls of synthetic fibre to which little dust adheres.

Dust on floors and other surfaces is regularly removed by specially designed cleaning plant.

The level of airborne dust must be monitored. This can be done in two ways: by the use of personal sampling instruments worn by the worker in his 'breathing zone', and by instruments designed to sample the general factory air. Sampling may be carried out for short specified periods or continuously over prolonged periods.

Recommendations for evaluating asbestos exposure in the working environment have recently been published in the United States of America (Recommendation Commission and International Association on Occupational Health, 1972). Under industrial conditions it is usual to determine the number of fibres per cubic centimetre but in urban surroundings a gravimetric method has been used with some success (Selikoff, Nicholson and Langer, 1972).

(3) *Other occupational conditions.*—Air-line respirators and impervious suits which are decontaminated in a shower before being removed are now used in British naval dockyards for work in the heavy dust concentrations encountered during removal of old lagging, acoustic board and sprayed asbestos in ships and submarines: for lower dust concentrations, nylon overalls and positive pressure power respirators are used. The area of operation is thoroughly vacuum cleaned after completion.

Where possible, old lagging should be soaked with water before it is removed to suppress liberation of dust and, when removed, put into polythene bags which are then sealed for disposal. Under conditions where the wet method is not practicable air-line breathing apparatus must be employed in addition to protective equipment. De-lagging should be done when other workers are not in the vicinity but, if this is impossible, they too should wear protective equipment. After completion of the operation, the area should be vacuum cleaned. Asbestos is now largely substituted by other insulating materials.

The dust produced by the spraying of asbestos for thermal and acoustic insulation and other purposes can be greatly reduced by wetting the fibre before it is fed into the spray-gun, and by confining the work area by plastic sheeting to prevent dissemination by wind and draughts. Approved respirators and protective clothing should be worn throughout the operation. Spraying of asbestos for fireproofing is now forbidden by law in New York City because of widespread neighbourhood contamination by asbestos containing materials during the treatment of sky-scraper buildings (New York City Department of Air Resources, 1971).

Drilling, sawing and shaping of asbestos cement sheeting should be segregated and the workers should wear protective equipment.

Threshold limits values

In the United Kingdom the average concentration of chrysotile, amosite and fibrous anthophyllite over a ten-minute period should not exceed 2 fibres per cm³ or 0·1 mg/m³ for fibres between 5 μm to 100 μm in length. If this value is exceeded, special sampling procedures are laid down; if fibre concentration is greater than 12 per cm³, protective clothing and approved respiratory protective equipment must be worn. In the case of crocidolite, breathing equipment must be worn if the dust concentration in the 'breathing zone' is in excess of 0·2 fibres/cm³ or 0·01 mg/m³ over a ten-minute period. (For details of these values and of sampling equipment and strategy, the reader is referred to Technical Data Note 13, Department of Employment and Productivity, 1970.) Standards for chrysotile were put forward by the British Occupational Hygiene Society in 1968.

In the United States of America the TLV for all types of asbestos is an 8-hour time-weighted average of 5 fibres/cm³ longer than 5 μm, and from July 1976 will be 2 fibres/cm³ (Utidjian, 1973).

Medical examination of workers

Medical examination of healthy asbestos workers should be done every one to two years and include a good quality, full-size chest radiograph and a record of VC, FVC and FEV_1. Ideally, details of current dust-count levels should be included in these records.

Employment of young persons

Special provisions applying to 'young persons' are laid down by the British Asbestos Regulations 1969.

'TALC' PNEUMOCONIOSIS

'Talc' pneumoconiosis was first described by Thorel (1896), since when it has not always been clear to what type of lung pathology this term has referred. It has sometimes been said that 'talc' does not cause pneumoconiosis although there is no doubt that pneumoconiosis may result from exposure to talc-associated minerals. Radiographic appearances may be either those of a nodular disease (such as silicosis, coal pneumoconiosis or sarcoidosis) or of diffuse interstitial fibrosis; both may be present in the one individual. The reason for much of this uncertainty is that in industry and commerce the term 'talc' often embraces a variety of minerals other than talc itself. The associated minerals differ according to the geological environment and the purity of the ore. Furthermore, the susceptibility of similarly exposed workers to develop pneumoconiosis appears to vary significantly.

'Talc' pneumoconiosis, in fact, appears to consist of three different basic lesions—irregular quasi-nodular fibrosis, diffuse interstitial fibrosis (fibrosing 'alveolitis') and foreign body granulomas—depending upon the dominant composition of dust inhaled. The often-used term 'talcosis' is, therefore, not appropriate.

323

Definition of talc

Talc is a hydrated magnesium silicate with the formula $Mg_3Si_4O_{10}(OH)_2$ although calcium, aluminium and iron are always present in variable amounts. Talc is usually formed in one of two ways: either by low-grade metamorphism of siliceous dolomites (*see* Chapter 2) or by hydrothermal alteration— frequently accompanied by dynamic metamorphism—of magnesium-rich ultrabasic rocks. In consequence, other minerals are almost invariably present in intimate association with talc, the most common being chlorite and magnesite, but serpentine minerals, tremolite, anthophyllite, dolomite, calcite and quartz may also be present. Tremolite and anthophyllite, of course, belong to the amphibole group of asbestos minerals—a fact which has an important bearing on the pathogenesis and pathology of some forms of 'talc' pneumoconiosis.

TABLE 9.3

VARIETIES OF COMMERCIAL 'TALCS' FROM NEW YORK STATE
(GOUVERNEUR DISTRICT)
By courtesy of Johns-Manville Research and Engineering Center, New Jersey

	1	2	3	4	5	6	7	8	9	10
Tremolite	68	98	17	–	78	38	29	15	88	46
Anthophyllite	–	–	20	–	–	–	45	78	4	39
Talc	–	1	63	–	4	–	–	7	1	5
Serpentine*	–	1	–	80	18	54	26	–	4	4
Quartz	31	–	–	–	–	–	–	–	2	4
Others	1	–	–	20	–	8	–	–	1	2

Figures indicate percentage composition.
Dashes indicate no determination made.
* Either massive or fibrous.

High-grade talcs from the Italian Alps, Pyrenees, China and India were formed from siliceous dolomite and dolomitic limestones and contain little or no quartz although this mineral may be encountered in trace amounts in the mining of Italian talc. Domestically-produced Norwegian talc is, however, of fairly low grade and usually contains chlorite, magnesite and, possibly, trace amounts of quartz. The 'talc' from the famous mines of St Lawrence County in New York State frequently contains as much as 50 per cent or more tremolite and less than 25 per cent talc—indeed, talc proper may be entirely absent from some grades; anthophyllite and significant amounts of quartz may also be present—an average content of 7·5 per cent of quartz having been observed in some mill samples (Weiss and Boettner, 1967). The variable composition of some New York State 'talc' samples is shown in Table 9.3. Californian 'talc' is also associated with tremolite, serpentine and calcite. Talc from the Vermont area, on the other hand, is associated with magnesite and dolomite, and quartz is either absent or of negligible amount. Canadian 'talc', which comes mainly from the Madoc district of Ontario, has a somewhat similar geological origin to that of St Lawrence County, and contains considerable quantities of tremolite and

324

dolomite, and some quartz which may remain in variable amount in the final product. In the United Kingdom only a very small quantity of talc is produced, mainly in the Shetlands; it is of low grade and the chief accessory mineral is magnesite.

It is evident, therefore, that significant amounts of quartz, tremolite and anthophyllite may be present in some lower grades of 'talcs'. Where talc is associated with substantial quantities of tremolite and anthophyllite it is

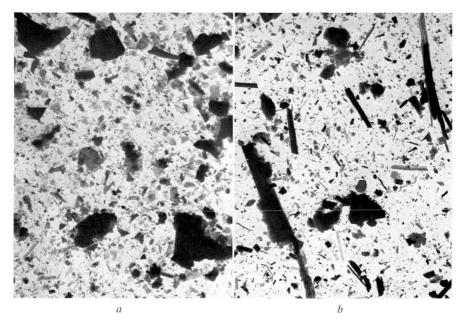

a   *b*

Figure 9.22. (a) Talc plates, good quality cosmetic talc. (b) Talc plates and tremolite, the acicular crystals and fibres of which are evident by their long axes. This is typical of industrial grade talc used in the United States of America. (Electron micrographs; original magnification × 5,000, reproduced at × 4,000; by courtesy of Johns-Manville Research and Engineering Center, New Jersey)

often known as *asbestine*. The presence of chrysotile is occasionally possible in some low-grade talcs.

Under the microscope, talc appears as flat polygonal plates (that is, platy, non-fibrous talc) whereas tremolite and anthophyllite consist both of prismatic, acicular crystalline and fibrous forms, and when either of these minerals predominate it is known as fibrous 'talc' (*Figure 9.22*). Talc and tremolite are strongly birefringent, but anthophyllite is only weakly so.

Steatite is the term used to describe the massive, fine-grained (cryptocrystalline) variety of talc; *soapstone* is a term loosely applied to impure talcose rocks containing variable amounts of talc and other minerals.

Pyrophyllite (*see* Chapter 2) is sometimes wrongly referred to as 'talc' in industry. It is an hydrated aluminosilicate with very similar properties to talc but, except in its purest form, contains quartz in abundance.

Most of the talc used for industrial purposes in the United Kingdom since (and before) World War II comes from Norway, France and Italy, and a substantial amount of Chinese and Indian talc is also imported. However, during the war all these sources of supply were cut off and were apparently replaced mainly by Canadian and, possibly, by some American 'talc'; This may well have an important bearing on the type of 'talc' pneumoconiosis which has been observed sporadically in some 'talc'-exposed workers in the United Kingdom following the war.

The qualities possessed by talc which are so useful in industry are extreme softness, whiteness (when in pure form), good hiding power, high surface area, lubricating (or high slip) property, good retention for filler purposes, chemical inertness, high oil absorption, high specific heat, low conductivity for heat and electricity, and high refractoriness.

Uses of talc

Because of the remarkably versatile properties of talc it has a vast array of uses and the grades employed are numerous. Only the most important uses are described.

Paints.—In the United Kingdom the greatest consumption of talc is in the paint industry as a filler and inert extender, for which high-grade talcs are valuable because of their whiteness and laminar form. But fibrous (asbestine) 'talc' is used as a suspending agent to reduce settling in ready-mixed paints.

Pharmaceutical and cosmetic industries.—High grade talcs are used in large quantities in pharmaceutical and cosmetic powders: for example, face powders, talcum powder, other cosmetic preparations and dermopaediatric powders. Particle size of good cosmetic talc is between 10 to 40 μm, which reduces the risk of penetration into the lungs to a minimum. Quartz must be absent and the only impurities should be calcium carbonate, magnesium carbonate and calcium sulphate. The best cosmetic talcs come from Italy and France.

Ceramics.—Both talc and steatite are employed in the ceramics industry for electronic equipment such as condenser end-plates, stand-off insulators, valve-holder bases, ignition insulators, rheostat blocks and the like. In combination with clay and alumina, talc is used to manufacture saggars for the pottery industry. In some countries—most notably the United States of America—talc is employed as a substitute for feldspar in the manufacture of earthenware bodies, especially wall tiles.

Roofing industry.—Here its lubricating and high-slip properties are used for dusting roofing felts to prevent the layers from sticking when rolled, and to increase resistance to fire and weather. Low-grade talcs have been, and are used for this purpose.

Rubber industry.—Again, the lubricant properties are made use of to prevent adhesion of the rubber in the moulds and to provide smooth extrusion. It is also used as a filler in hard-rubber goods such as accumulator cases and valves, and as an inert filler in some plastic compounds.

Refractory materials.—'Talc' finds a wide application as a refractory filler for mould and core castings in both ferrous and non-ferrous foundry castings. Steatite fired at about 900°C is used for refractory and electrical insulating materials.

Textile industry.—Finely ground french talc is used for loading and bleaching cotton sacks, cordage, string and rope.

Miscellaneous.—It is used as a dusting agent for glass moulds, and a polishing medium for chocolate, pea-nuts and chewing gum; as a filler and loading material for paper (for which fibrous American 'talc' has been favoured) and, until the beginning of the 1950s, was employed to dust moulds for the manufacture of lead accumulator plates before coating. It is used in large quantities annually as a carrier for pesticides and frequently appears to be associated with amphiboles in samples taken from the atmosphere and on land over a world-wide area (Speil and Leinewerber, 1969); it has also found a use in shoe manufacture to prevent the adherence of layers of leather.

Sources of exposure

Mining is carried out by both open-pit and underground methods. The milling operations involve jaw and roll crushers, screens and pebble mills. Cases of diffuse interstitial fibrosis have been recorded in miners and millers of New York State 'talc' (Siegel, Smith and Greenburg, 1943; Greenburg, 1947; Kleinfeld *et al.*, 1964a). Bagging of the milled material is also a potential risk.

A survey of the New York State mines and mills in 1954 revealed a much reduced concentration of airborne dust compared with 1940 due to dust suppression measures (Messite, Reddin and Kleinfeld, 1959).

Radiographic appearances consistent with silicosis have been reported in Italian talc-miners mainly in ILO category 'q' (Pettinati *et al.*, 1964), but the quartz content falls progressively during milling and preparation for factory use in which there appears to be no risk of silicosis (Dettori, Scansetti and Gribano, 1964). Some workers milling and bagging high-grade, apparently quartz-free, talc in the Hamata area of Egypt have been found to have either 'nodular' or conglomerate opacities (El-Ghawabi, El-Samra and Mehasseb, 1970).

Industrial applications.—Important sources of exposure have been in the roofing felt and shingle industry where talc is distributed liberally on the felt (often in an enclosed space) prior to rolling to prevent adhesion, and is sometimes used as a filler in the asphalt coating; in the rubber industry where the powder is blown on to the tacky rubber surface (for example, during extrusion of tubes and sheets) or dusted on to rubber goods prior to storage; in the moulding of accumulator plates; in leather finishing; and in preparing the mix for tiles, electrical porcelain and kiln saggar bodies. In all these processes only low-grade talc is required and, therefore, accessory minerals may be present.

Exposure to tremolite and quartz in industries normally using low-grade talc probably occurred to some extent in the United Kingdom during, and possibly for a time after, World War II (while stock piles lasted), due to substitution by Canadian and American 'talc' and pyrophyllite. The roofing felt industry has been further complicated by the fact that ground flint, quartzite sand and slate powder have been used as asphalt fillers or as surfacing materials; and that, to produce fire-resistant material, asbestos fibre has sometimes been employed as an asphalt filler and has caused significant dust exposure during addition to the mix.

327

Before and during the last war women worked in the rubber trade, especially at tyre extruding.

It is worth noting that, because talc is expensive, substitute minerals are often used for some processes. These include quartz, china clay and mica. Mica is a common substitute in the roofing felt industry because of its good weathering and slip qualities.

Talc heated above a temperature of 1,000°C (which is required in the manufacture of some ceramics) yields clinoenstatite and cristobalite, which is strongly fibrogenic (*see* Chapter 7).

Exposure to tremolite dust may occur in the manufacture of some types of paint.

As already noted, talc used for cosmetic preparations is of high grade and purity, and would not normally be expected to contain accessory minerals capable of causing lung fibrosis; certainly in the United Kingdom cosmetic and pharmaceutical talc does not contain asbestos minerals. Nevertheless, significant amounts of free silica and fibrous minerals (tremolite and anthophyllite) have been reported in occasional samples of talcum powder in the United States of America, the fibres being a possible source of 'ferruginous bodies' (Cralley *et al.*, 1968b). Dust-control measures have been employed in this industry at least since the 1950s, but men emptying bags of talc and pulverizing, weighing and mixing it have often been exposed to high concentrations of dust in the past. A probable case of pneumoconiosis with small discrete lesions from this source was recorded by Millman (1947).

It is evident, therefore, that 'talc workers' may be exposed to dusts of talc proper but also of tremolite, anthophyllite and quartz in various proportions.

Domestic.—It is unlikely that talcum and cosmetic powders offer any risk of pneumoconiosis even though innumerable people have been exposed to them from the cradle on for many years past, because the talc used is commonly of high grade and its particle size is large.

Epidemiology
There is little statistical information concerning 'talc' pneumoconiosis. Controlled studies of exposed populations have not been done. In cases where disease appears to have been due to past exposure to talc, details of the types of 'talc' and other minerals used are often lacking, and lung-dust analyses correlated with details of past occupations and histological features have rarely been carried out. However, radiological evidence of disease has been absent in some exposed workers (Scansetti, Gaido and Rasetti, 1963), and of widely varying prevalence and severity in others. Compositional differences in the 'talc' used may largely explain this.

In 1954 the prevalence of pneumoconiosis in mill men in New York State had not changed significantly from that of 1940 in spite of the introduction of dust-suppression measures but the severity and progression of disease was reduced; furthermore, severity of disease was appreciably less among men exposed mainly to non-fibrous 'talc' as opposed to fibrous 'talc' (Messite, Reddin and Kleinfeld, 1959).

Ten of 50 Egyptian talc workers had radiographic evidence of pneumoconiosis (El-Ghawabi, El-Samra and Mehasseb, 1970).

Mortality figures among talc-miners and millers in New York State who had more than 15 years' exposure revealed that the average age of death was 60·4 years (Kleinfeld *et al.*, 1967).

Pathology

Macroscopic appearances

Fibrous adhesions of the pleural surfaces are normally present, and in some of the tremolite- and anthophyllite-exposed cases in New York State, hyaline and calcified plaques have been observed in the diaphragmatic and costal parietal pleura. The cut surfaces of the lungs reveal areas of grey-white fibrosis which may be separated roughly into two types. In some cases it consists of small, ill-defined nodules, somewhat softer than silicotic nodules and lacking their compact concentric arrangement, scattered throughout the lungs but showing some partiality for their middle zones. Occasionally, coalescent fibrotic masses are large and may be the seat of ischaemic cavitation (Hunt, 1956) similar to that seen in the 'progressive massive fibrosis' of coal pneumoconiosis (*see* Chapter 8). In other cases it has the appearance of diffuse interstitial fibrosis (fibrosing 'alveolitis') which is dominant in the lower parts of the lungs. Both types of lesion may be present in the same lung. Silicotic nodules may sometimes be seen when there has also been exposure to significant amounts of quartz.

Microscopic appearances

The primary reaction to talc consists of an accumulation of macrophages and proliferation of fibrocytes around blood vessels in the vicinity of respiratory bronchioles forming a small stellate lesion which contains some reticulin fibres but negligible collagen (Schepers and Durkan, 1955a). Strongly birefringent acicular particles are often present in the lesion, both within and outside macrophages.

Three types of lesion are encountered:

(1) Ill-defined nodular lesions.
(2) Diffuse interstitial fibrosis.
(3) Foreign body granulomas.

The ill-defined nodular lesions consist of irregular acellular collagenous tissue (*Figure 9.23*) which sometimes shows incomplete whorling in places, resembling the arrangement of immature silicotic nodules. Numerous macrophages containing birefringent particles surround the lesions but fewer particles are present in the lesions themselves. Necrotic areas consist of amorphous, finely granular material which stains yellow with van Gieson's stain (Hunt, 1956).

The interstitial fibrosis, which originates around respiratory bronchioles, is similar in appearance to asbestosis and may obliterate alveolar spaces and lung architecture in many places (*Figure 9.24*). In some areas the alveolar walls are very cellular and birefringent particles are present in macrophages or are free in the interstitium; cells and particles are also common in the alveolar spaces. Other areas of fibrosis are acellular but usually contain some particles. Cystic spaces in areas of dense fibrosis consist of dilated bronchioles containing many desquamated cells and are lined by cuboidal cells (Kleinfeld *et al.*, 1963).

Endarteritis with intimal hyperplasia is common in the vicinity of both

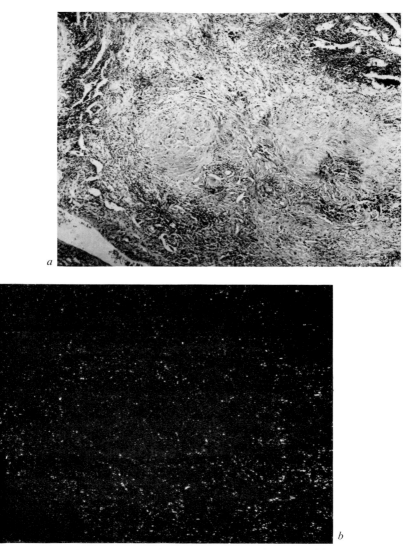

Figure 9.23. (a) Ill-defined nodular lesions in a rubber worker exposed for many years to 'talc' dust. The fibrosis is relatively acellular and shows only a suggestion of the concentric pattern of typical silicotic nodules. (Original magnifications × 55, reproduced at × 36; H and E stain.) (b) Right side of the field seen through crossed polarizers reveals the strong birefringence of numerous talc plates

types of fibrosis and 'talc bodies' are often found in close association with the diffuse interstitial fibrosis. These 'bodies' resemble asbestos bodies very closely under the optical microscope and, like them, give a positive Prussian blue reaction and are best demonstrated in 30 μm sections (*Figure 9.24*).

330

Foreign body granulomas accompany, and are often intimately associated with, the fibrotic lesions in some cases (Hunt, 1956; Kleinfeld *et al.*, 1963), and may also be present in the pulmonary pleura. Rarely they are the sole or dominant lesion (*Figure 9.25*). They consist of epithelioid cells and foreign body giant cells which sometimes contain asteroid inclusions (Kleinfeld *et al.*, 1963) and birefringent particles.

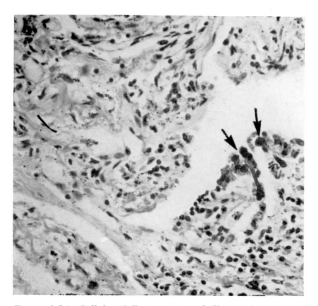

Figure 9.24. Cellular diffuse interstitial fibrosis from a man who worked with cosmetic talc. Numerous birefringent platy crystals were revealed by polarized light, but tremolite bodies (arrowed) are also present. Fibrosis, which contains small 'honeycomb' cysts, is widespread (see Figure 9.28). (Original magnification × 380, reproduced at × 285; H and E stain)

The birefringent, needle-shaped particles present in and around all these lesions can usually be identified as platy talc crystals or tremolite by electron microscopy. Many talc plates lie sideways on to the line of vision. Crystals visible by light microscopy vary from 0·5 to 5 μm in length, but many are less than 0·5 μm and thus, being optically invisible, are only identified by electron microscopy (Miller *et al.*, 1971). This is important in that light microscopy may fail to reveal the presence of talc crystals in the lesions of some cases.

Analysis of the lungs of talc-miners and millers in New York State showed that lungs with the quasi-nodular type of lesions contained significant quantities of talc but negligible amounts of quartz and little tremolite or anthophyllite; lungs with diffuse interstitial fibrosis and more extensive areas of fibrosis, however, contained appreciable quantities of tremolite and, occasionally, anthophyllite in addition to talc. Fairly large amounts of quartz present in some cases were attributed to other mining experience (Schepers and Durkan, 1955a).

331

In summary therefore, 'talc' pneumoconiosis consists of three different types of lesion which may occur alone or in various combinations in the lungs of one individual according to the composition of the dust to which he has been exposed. None of these lesions is pathognomonic.

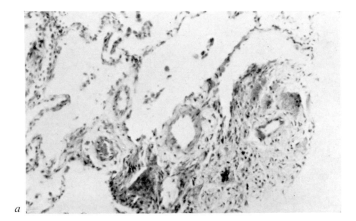

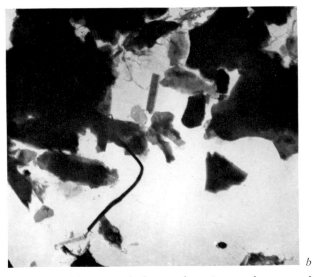

Figure 9.25. (a) Foreign body granuloma in a worker exposed to talc in the rubber industry. Biopsy specimen (original magnification ×50, reproduced at ×100; H and E stain, by courtesy of Drs A. Hanson and S. Steel). (b) Electron micrograph of this lesion reveals the presence of talc and mica-like plates. (Magnification ×3,000; by courtesy of Dr F. D. Pooley, Cardiff)

Pathogenesis

Because typical silicotic nodules are only rarely present in 'talc' pneumoconiosis even when men have been previously exposed to a free silica risk from other sources, it has been suggested that talc modifies the lung reaction to quartz (Schepers and Durkan, 1955a). This is supported by the observation in experimental animals that the fibrogenic effect of quartz when combined with talc appears to be reduced, although granulomatous lesions may result (Schepers and Durkan, 1955b). Quartz does not appear to enhance the pathogenicity of tremolite or anthophyllite.

Experimentally, talc alone produces no fibrosis or, at most, a very mild peribronchial fibrosis; this correlates with the apparent absence of collagenous lesions in the lungs of workers exposed to virtually pure talc (*see* last section). However, talc calcined at 1,200°C produces intense collagen fibrosis in rats, due to the cristobalite content (Lüchtrath and Schmidt, 1959), and talc with quartz also causes fibrosis (Schepers and Durkan, 1955b).

Tremolite particles 3 μm or less in size produce only small localized lesions of cellular perivascular infiltration, but fibres 20 to 50 μm in length produce a progressive, fibrocellular, diffuse interstitial fibrosis in experimental animals (Schepers and Durkan, 1955b). Anthophyllite also appears to cause cell proliferation and fibrogenesis in animals. Schepers and Durkan (1955b) showed that 20 to 50 μm tremolite fibres provoke the formation in animals of ferruginous bodies identical to those seen in 'talc' pneumoconiosis in man; hence, these are more appropriately referred to as 'tremolite bodies' than as 'talc bodies'.

Foreign body granulomas are probably caused by talc itself. Similar granulomas have been observed in the peritoneum, fallopian tubes and ovaries contaminated by talc in surgical glove dusting powder (German, 1943; Roberts, 1947). They may also occur in pulmonary arteries and arterioles due, not to inhalation, but to the intravenous introduction of talc from contaminated tablets (talc is employed for dusting tablet moulds in manufacture) and other materials used by drug addicts (Hopkins and Taylor, 1970); birefringent particles of talc crystals and cotton fibres may be seen in the lesions through crossed polarizers.

Calcified pleural plaques, which appear to occur mainly in workers exposed to tremolite-associated talc and asbestine, may be causally related to the anthophyllite content.

In short, although the pathogenesis of 'talc' pneumoconiosis is not completely understood, it appears certain that tremolite produces a diffuse interstitial fibrosis closely similar to asbestosis and probable, for similar reasons, that talc together with quartz gives rise to more localized fibrocellular lesions, and that talc alone may cause foreign body granuloma formation. The case of a man, seen by the author, who had spent all his working life with cosmetic grade talc is surprising in that there was extensive diffuse interstitial fibrosis which contained both talc plates and tremolite bodies (*see Figure 9.28*).

The variable incidence of pneumoconiosis in similarly exposed 'talc' workers suggests that individual susceptibility (possibly immunologically determined) may play a part in its development. But this aspect of pathogenesis does not appear to have been investigated.

Clinical features

Symptoms

There may be no symptoms for years but ultimately dyspnoea on effort, cough and sputum are complained of in most cases and are more commonly associated with the diffuse interstitial fibrosis type of disease than with the quasi-nodular form. In the latter type of disease these symptoms are usually associated with radiographic evidence of confluent massing. In general, symptoms develop gradually after about 15 to 20 years' exposure to 'talc' dust. Occasionally, when dust concentrations have been very high, severe dyspnoea and productive cough have developed within two years with rapidly progressive 'nodular' type disease (Alivisatos, Pontikakis and Terzis, 1955). In advanced disease, loss of weight has been reported.

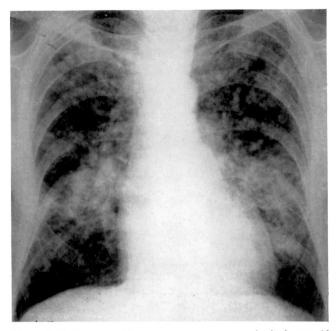

Figure 9.26. Radiographic appearances in a man who had spent 12 years in the roof felting industry exposed to 'talc' dust and smaller amounts of china-clay dust. The histology of the lesions was similar to that shown in Figure 9.23

Physical signs

There are no abnormal physical signs in the early stage nor in many cases of the later stages of predominantly 'nodular' disease. When large confluent masses are present, chest expansion may be impaired (being greater on the side of the major mass) and breath sounds reduced locally. Finger clubbing is not a feature of this type of talc pneumoconiosis.

When disease is of the diffuse fibrotic type the range of abnormal physical signs is the same as that observed in asbestosis. Finger clubbing is present in more than half of these cases.

Investigations

Lung function

The 'nodular' form of the disease (as in the case of silicosis) causes little if any abnormality in its early stages, but later a restrictive defect develops with decreased compliance, ventilation–perfusion imbalance, impaired gas transfer and hypoxia on effort with oxygen desaturation. In advanced cases oxygen desaturation may be present at rest (Alivisatos, Pontikakis and Terzis, 1955). In the diffuse interstitial fibrotic form the functional abnormalities are similar to those seen in asbestosis. In general, abnormal values are appreciably greater in persons with diffuse fibrosis who have been exposed to tremolite than in those with 'nodular' disease (Kleinfeld *et al.*, 1964a, b), although the correlation between functional abnormalities and the radiographic appearances is poor and impairment of the same parameters of lung function which mark the earliest stages of asbestosis may be observed before radiographic evidence of this type of 'talc' pneumoconiosis is apparent (Kleinfeld *et al.*, 1965).

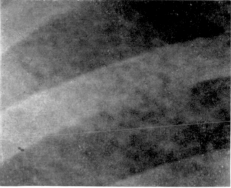

Figure 9.27. Miliary-type opacities in a rubber worker exposed to talc. Appearances due to foreign body granulomas. Biopsy findings in this case are shown in Figure 9.25. Investigations for tuberculosis and sarcoidosis were negative. (By courtesy of Drs. A. Hanson and S. Steel)

Radiographic appearance

As might be anticipated from the different types of lesion which occur, the appearances due to 'talc' pneumoconiosis are various:

(1) *Nodular*.—This consists either of discrete opacities some 3 to 5 mm diameter and resembling those of silicosis, or of appearances similar to 'mixed dust fibrosis' (*see* Chapter 7). They tend to favour the middle zones of the lung fields, but may be distributed throughout all zones (*Figure 9.26*). Rarely, opacities may be small and widely distributed, resembling 'idiopathic' sarcoidosis or miliary tuberculosis, and are due to multiple foreign-body granulomas (*Figure 9.27*). Occasionally there are massive opacities similar to those caused by confluent masses of coal pneumoconiosis with evidence of cavitation (Hunt, 1956; Kipling and Bech, 1960).

(2) *Diffuse interstitial fibrosis* (fibrosing 'alveolitis').—Here the picture is the same as that of asbestosis or any other type of diffuse interstitial fibrosis ('fibrosing alveolitis') in which the abnormal appearances predominate in the lower and mid-zones (*Figure 9.28*)—rarely in the upper and mid-zones (*Figure 9.4*).

(3) *Mixed*.—Both types of appearance occur in combination.

Evidence of pleural fibrosis—mainly in the lower halves of the lung fields and obliterating the costophrenic angles—may also be present, and it is important to note that calcified pleural and pericardial plaques of identical appearance and location to those associated with past exposure to asbestos may be seen in men who have worked mining and milling 'talc' (as in the New York State mines) and in some industrial processes (Smith, 1952) in all of which exposure to tremolite has undoubtedly occurred.

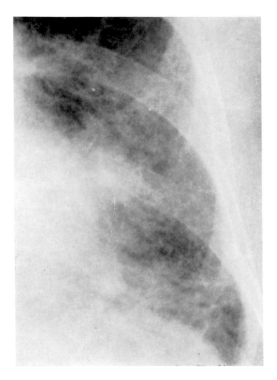

Figure 9.28. Appearance of severe diffuse interstitial fibrosis in a man whose occupational exposure had been to cosmetic talc and innocuous dusts for about 20 years. Histology seen in Figure 9.24; no rheumatoid arthritis; latex fixation test negative

Diagnosis

This rests upon the past occupational history and a known exposure to 'talc', and on the appearances of the chest radiograph. However, it is often impossible to obtain precise details of the type (or types) of 'talc' used in an industry twenty or more years ago, although this is sometimes available from the manufacturer's or supplier's records. It should be borne in mind that a worker may speak of having handled 'french chalk' (talc) when in fact the material may have been powdered slate or china clay, and that some industries which employed talc may also have used asbestos or quartz-containing minerals (as, for example, in roofing felt manufacture). It is also to be remembered that women have sometimes been exposed to talc in various industries (chiefly rubber) in the past.

The diagnosis can be made in the majority of cases without lung biopsy but, if this proves necessary, sufficient tissue should be taken (preferably by thoracotomy) to enable electron microscopy and x-ray diffraction to be done for positive identification of talc and tremolite. The differential diagnosis lies chiefly between quiescent tuberculosis, silicosis, asbestosis or some other type of diffuse interstitial fibrosis.

After death, the diagnosis is rendered virtually certain by the combination of an accurate history of industrial exposure, the presence of lung fibrosis and, sometimes, foreign-body granulomas, and the distribution of strongly birefringent particles of platy and acicular form. When tremolite bodies are present, diffuse interstitial fibrosis may be indistinguishable from asbestosis, but identification of numerous talc plates and of foreign body granulomas helps to resolve the problem.

Prognosis

As a rule, talc pneumoconiosis progresses very slowly and although a variable degree of respiratory disability may occur it appears that life expectancy is rarely significantly shortened. However, in those cases where there is massive confluent fibrosis or extensive diffuse interstitial fibrosis, pulmonary hypertension and subsequently cor pulmonale may develop and cause death in congestive heart failure. Among New York State miners and millers the time between first exposure to 'talc'-mine dust and death from the pneumoconiosis or its complications is, on average, about 26 years (Kleinfeld et al., 1967).

Occasionally, when a worker has been exposed to high concentrations of talc dust (possibly associated with significant amounts of quartz) progression to massive fibrosis with severe disability occurs within a very few years (Alivisatos, Pontikakis and Terzis, 1955).

Complications

There is no evidence that 'talc' pneumoconiosis predisposes to the development of tuberculosis.

Although Kleinfeld et al. (1967) found that the proportional mortality of New York State 'talc'-miners and millers from carcinoma of the lung and pleura was four times greater than that of a control population, Van Ordstrand (1970) appears unconvinced that there is an increased incidence of lung cancer. Further investigation of the problem is obviously necessary. An increased risk of malignant mesothelioma in talc workers does not appear to have been reported.

Treatment

In general, no treatment is effective apart from that required for concurrent lung disease or, in cases of advanced pneumoconiosis, for cor pulmonale. But when the pneumoconiosis consists predominantly of foreign-body granulomas, a substantial degree of regression appears to be possible with prednisone in large doses (30 to 40 mg daily) for two weeks (Moskowitz, 1970). Whether or not improvement of this sort is permanent remains to be determined. This observation may justify lung biopsy for diagnostic confirmation in those cases in which the chest radiograph suggests mainly granuloma formation.

Prevention

Dust suppression measures have been applied to the mining, crushing and milling of 'talc' for some years past. Finely milled 'talc' has a particle size which may range from 0·5 to 20 μm. Exhaust ventilation and enclosure of dusty processes have been introduced into most of the larger industries but some small factories still remain very dusty. Good housekeeping is essential to prevent dust accumulation, and monitoring of airborne dust in the worker's area is obviously desirable.

A record of the type and source of 'talc' and of relevant non-talc minerals used in an industrial process should be kept.

Threshold Limit Values recommended by the American Conference of Governmental Industrial Hygienists (1971) are as follows:

Talc
Soapstone $\Big\}$ 20 mppcf

Tremolite 5 fibres per cm³ greater than 5 μm in length (that is the TLV for asbestos).

For a mixture containing 80 per cent talc and 20 per cent quartz the TLV for 100 per cent of the mixture is given by:

$$\text{TLV} = \frac{1}{\dfrac{0·8}{20} + \dfrac{0·2}{2·5}} = 8·4 \text{ mppcf}$$

For a mixture of 25 per cent quartz, 25 per cent 'amorphous silica' and 50 per cent talc:

$$\text{TLV} = \frac{1}{\dfrac{0·25}{2·5} + \dfrac{0·25}{20} + \dfrac{0·5}{20}} = 7·3 \text{ mppcf}$$

Pneumoconiosis Associated with Other Silicates

KAOLIN (CHINA CLAY)

Description of disease
Mainly nodular or massive fibrosis of the lungs and occasionally mild diffuse interstitial fibrosis associated with past exposure to kaolin dust which is apparently free of accessory quartz or contains small amounts.

Nature and origin of kaolin
The kaolin, or china clay, group of clay minerals consists predominantly of *kaolinite* which is a hydrous aluminium silicate (approximate composition $2H_2O.Al_2O_3.2SiO_2$) with a platy pseudohexagonal morphology under the electron microscope.

Kaolinite is formed by the hydrothermal alteration of aluminosilicates such as feldspars in granites (as in Cornish china clay which may contain up to 3 per cent quartz), by residual weathering of granites and by erosion of kaolinized granite and its subsequent deposition (as in the large sedimentary kaolin deposits of South Carolina and Georgia which are virtually free of quartz).

Cornish kaolin is obtained by means of directing a high-pressure jet of water on to the walls of the open pit and subjecting it to differential sedimentation in water so that impurities such as grit, sand and mica are removed while the kaolin remains suspended. The water is largely removed either by the use of filter presses or by drawing it off, and the plastic residue transferred to drying kilns. The moisture content is thus reduced to about 10 per cent and the clay residue is either shovelled or conveyed on a moving belt to storage hoppers. Spray drying of high-grade clays is increasingly being used. It is then either bagged mechanically (but, until recent years, this was done by hand shovel) or bulk-loaded into trucks for transportation. Some quartz may remain in lower grade clays.

In North Carolina and Georgia, kaolin is obtained from the mines in moist lumps. Until the 1940s it was pulverized and then passed by a dry flotation process into classifying chambers. Subsequently, however, refining has been done by wet methods. The finished product is bagged or loaded into trucks. Other producing countries include Western Germany, India, France, China and Czechoslovakia.

Uses of kaolin

Kaolin is used as a filler to give body to paper pulp, for coating paper to produce a smooth surface, and in the manufacture of china (or whiteware) and stoneware. Residual kaolin is used for these purposes in the United Kingdom, and secondary kaolin of high purity in the United States. Kaolin also has important uses as a filler in rubber, paints, plastics and insecticides; in the manufacture of refractory bricks, crucibles, saggars and glass, and a refractory grog is produced by calcining it at high temperatures. It is employed as a mild abrasive in soaps and toothpaste and as a stiffener of textiles. Kaolin of high purity and small particle size is used for medicinal and cosmetic purposes.

Sources of exposure

Exposure has occurred mainly in the china-clay industry. After the clay left the driers all parts of the process were dusty; and, although ventilation and, in certain cases, enclosure methods now do much to reduce the dust, brushing the clay spilt from conveyors, cleaning the driers, bagging and bulk loading may still be very dusty (Sheers, 1964).

In the United States of America the flotation method of preparation used in the past was extremely dusty but, as noted, this was discontinued some thirty years ago; bagging and loading, however, remain a source of dust exposure.

Other sources of significant exposure have been, and may still be, found in the manufacture of paper, rubber and plastics. In the pottery and refractory industries exposure may also occur to dusts of other minerals—such as flint, feldspar, graphite and quartzite sand; in the rubber industry it is extensively employed.

Prevalence

In a radiographic survey of 553 Cornish kaolin-processing workers there was evidence of pneumoconiosis in 9 per cent (Sheers, 1964) and among 1,130 similar workers in Georgia, in 3·7 per cent (Edenfield, 1960). Of 914 processing workers in Ayyat, United Arab Republic, six had pneumoconiosis—two with confluent masses (Warraki and Herant, 1963).

Duration of exposure to the dust was found to be of significance in the Cornish workers in that 23 per cent of men exposed to high dust concentrations in milling, bagging and loading for more than 15 years had pneumoconiosis by contrast with 6 per cent of men similarly exposed for 5 to 15 years (Sheers, 1964). Among all these cases there were 12 with confluent masses and 30 with ILO Category 2 or 3 opacities.

Hence, only a small minority of similarly exposed workers have developed pneumoconiosis and then only after a prolonged period.

Pathology

Macroscopic appearances

The pulmonary pleura of lungs which contain massive lesions is usually thickened.

Lesions which simulate immature silicotic nodules have been found in some cases (Lynch and McIver, 1954; Hale *et al.*, 1956), but as a rule there are dust macules like those of coal pneumoconiosis although of a greyish hue.

Massive confluent lesions, which favour the upper parts of the lungs, are well circumscribed, grey to blue-grey in colour, and although firm to the touch, are not as hard as conglomerate silicotic masses.

Microscopic appearances

Numerous dust-laden macrophages and extracellular dust particles are present around bronchiolar arteries and fill adjacent alveolar spaces. Proliferation of reticulin fibres supports both cells and dust particles.

Nodules and massive confluent lesions consist of randomly distributed collagenous fibres, some of which are hyalinized, and large quantities of dust in similar fashion to the P.M.F. of coal and carbon pneumoconiosis; they are infiltrated and surrounded by innumerable dust-laden macrophages. Evidence of tuberculosis does not seem to have been found (Hale *et al.*, 1956; Edenfield, 1960), but obliterative endarteritis is prominent in the vicinity of the lesions and is responsible for the necrosis which is sometimes observed in them.

Lynch and McIver (1954) noted 'conspicuous fibrosis of alveolar walls' in one of their cases, and a photomicrograph they produced showed diffuse interstitial fibrosis. Diffuse interstitial fibrosis with much cellular infiltration (desquamative type of fibrosing 'alveolitis') including dust-containing macrophages has also been observed in a few cases of Cornish china-clay workers both in the presence and absence of nodular or massive fibrotic lesions, but it is of mild degree (Hinson, 1972; Wagner, 1972a)

(*Figure 9.29*). However, it remains to be proved that this is, in fact, caused by the kaolin dust.

Analysis of lung-dust in a Cornish case revealed a large amount of kaolin but only about 1 per cent of quartz; and in a case from Georgia with confluent masses the lungs contained some 98 per cent kaolin and no trace of quartz (Hale *et al.*, 1956). The size of kaolin particles in the Cornish case ranged from 1·0 to 2·0 μm and in the case from Georgia, from 0·5 to 1 μm.

Kaolinite is weakly birefringent.

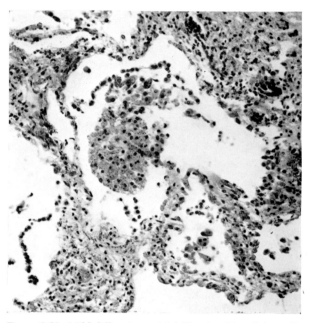

Figure 9.29. Mild diffuse interstitial fibrosis with cellular infiltration in a china-clay worker. Groups of dust containing macrophages are present in some alveolar spaces. (Original magnification, ×40, reproduced at ×20; H and E stain; by courtesy of Dr J. C. Wagner)

Pathogenesis

The problem is whether kaolin is wholly or partly responsible for these lesions or whether other causative factors are involved.

Although it has been claimed that some quartz always accompanies particles of kaolin (Policard and Collet, 1954) it is either absent from the lungs or present in small amount even, apparently, in those where the lesions simulate immature silicotic nodules, but there is a large quantity of kaolin dust. This is analogous to the situation in carbon and coal pneumoconiosis. The high concentrations of dust experienced by some workers and the predominantly small size and low density of kaolin particles favours the accumulation of dust in the lungs.

Tuberculous infection has been suggested as the factor which, in combination with kaolin dust, determines the development of these lesions (Edenfield,

1960). And, although no support for this has been found in human disease, extensive lesions have been produced in the lungs of experimental animals by a combination of kaolin and chromogenic opportunist mycobacteria (Byers and King, 1959) or *Mycobacterium tuberculosis* (Byers *et al.*, 1960).

Kaolin alone does not cause collagen fibrosis in the lungs of rats or guinea-pigs (Kettle, 1934; King, Harrison and Nagelschmidt, 1948; Attygalle *et al.*, 1954; Schmidt and Lüchtrath, 1958) but gives rise to a diffuse accumulation of cells—many of which are giant cells—in the alveolar walls and spaces; some coalescence of cells occurs with a mild proliferation of supporting reticulin fibres, but no nodulation; on the other hand, greater reticulin proliferation is produced by a mixture of kaolin and killed tubercle bacilli (King *et al.*, 1955) and pronounced collagen fibrosis by kaolin and quartz (Schmidt and Lüchtrath, 1958).

Kaolin particles actively adsorb antigens and are known to be a good adjuvant to immune reactions. Thus, it has been proposed that antigen attached to retained dust particles might localize an antigen-antibody reaction (Vigliani and Pernis, 1958). There is no evidence that this occurs in man, although analysis of the protein composition of the hyaline tissue of one of the cases reported by Hale *et al.* (1956) showed it to be rich in globulins (73 per cent) and relatively lacking in collagen (27 per cent) (Vigliani and Pernis, 1958).

Kaolin has the property of causing haemolysis of red cells *in vitro* which is increased by heating it to 200 or 350°C, lost at 500 to 650°C but re-established with much greater intensity at 900° to 950°C when some cristobalite is formed. The extent of haemolysis (which is an index of cell membrane damage and, therefore, probably of cytotoxicity) apparently depends upon changes in crystal structure and surface hydration (Mányai *et al.*, 1970). It would be interesting to determine if there is any difference in the ability (or inability) of kaolin to cause lung damage according to whether it is unheated, kiln dried or calcined at high temperature.

To summarize; the pathogenesis of kaolin pneumoconiosis is far from clear. It may be due—if kaolin alone is responsible—to the effect of a large dust load in the lungs as is believed to be the case in artificial graphite pneumoconiosis (Chapter 8), but it is likely that quartz or tuberculous infection are important (at least in some cases), and immunological factors may also play a part though this remains to be defined.

Clinical features

Symptoms
There are no symptoms associated with discrete lesions but breathlessness on effort, cough and sputum may be present when there are confluent masses, and in some of these cases disability is severe (Edenfield, 1960). There is no conclusive evidence that disability was caused by pneumoconiosis attributed to kaolin in the English cases reported by Sheers (1964).

Physical signs
The same conditions apply as in the case of coal and carbon pneumoconiosis (*see* Chapter 8).

Investigations

Lung function

No comprehensive studies of kaolin workers have been reported; but in the majority of cases without confluent massing, normal values are to be expected unless coincidental lung disease is present. In the case of confluent masses the situation is the same as that encountered with the similar lesions of coal pneumoconiosis.

Radiographic appearances

These are similar to the range of abnormal opacities seen in coal pneumo-coniosis. Some cases with confluent massing have signs of bullous emphysema (Hales *et al.*, 1956; *Figure 9.4*). Signs of diffuse interstitial fibrosis do not seem to have been recorded.

Prognosis

In the absence of masses, the prognosis for health and life span appears to be normal but, when these are present, slowly increasing respiratory disability occurs, and cor pulmonale may develop and ultimately cause death.

Treatment

No treatment, other than for concomitant lung disease, is effective.

Prevention

In the kaolin industry, wet methods, exhaust ventilation, enclosure of some sections, vacuum cleaning of the factory floor and other surfaces where dust accumulates have been introduced in the United Kingdom and similar measures have been applied in the United States of America. Control of dust in the bagging areas, however, is difficult.

Kaolin is classed among the 'Inert' or Nuisance Particulates by the ACGIH provided that the quartz content is less than 1 per cent. Otherwise a TLV of 50 mppcf or 15 mg/m³—whichever is smaller—is considered appropriate.

BALL CLAYS AND STONEWARE CLAYS

Ball clays consist essentially of kaolinite and, like china clay, they originated by natural decomposition of feldspathic rocks but were subsequently transported from their site of origin by rivers. During this journey the ratio of quartz to kaolin increased on account of loss of clay so that a larger quantity of quartz is present than in primary china clay.

These clays are mined by opencast and underground methods in Dorset and Devon in the United Kingdom, and in Tennessee and Kentucky in the United States of America. The 'free silica' content of Devon and Dorset ball clays has been reported to range from 5 to 29 per cent (Thomas, 1952). Their main use is for china or whiteware, sanitary pottery ware and electrical porcelain.

Pneumoconiosis has occurred among workers milling and preparing these clays (Thomas, 1952) and because of their fairly high quartz content it is of silicotic type although poorly formed immature silicotic nodules may be present. The radiographic appearances are similar to those of silicosis.

FULLER'S EARTH

Very few cases of pneumoconiosis supposedly caused by fuller's earth have been reported and most of those that have been were incompletely studied.

Fuller's earth is a very fine-grained adsorbent clay which consists mainly of the clay mineral calcium montmorillonite. Large deposits occur at Nutfield in Surrey and in Mississippi, Illinois, and Arkansas in the United States of America. In Georgia and Florida there are large deposits of fuller's earth which are extensively worked and consist essentially of attapulgite, a clay mineral with similar adsorptive properties to calcium montmorillonite. Fuller's earth is mined by opencast methods. After mining, lumps of clay are milled before being kiln dried and processed further. Until recent years the vicinity of the kilns, mills and bagging areas was very dusty.

The quartz content of Nutfield fuller's earth is extremely low, being about 0·8 per cent of the milled product with only a trace amount in elutriated fractions which have a particle size of less than 5 μm (Bramwell, Leech and Dunstall, 1940). By contrast, quartz is more abundant in the montmorillonite deposits in Illinois (Grim, 1933) and, although it may be present in mill dust, it is removed by subsequent air flotation purefying processes. Appreciable amounts of quartz—up to about 20 per cent—may, however, be found in some deposits.

The word 'fuller' derives from the verb 'to full' which means the cleaning and thickening of cloth or wool. The highly adsorbent property of fuller's earth enables it to remove grease and oily material with great efficiency. It has a wide variety of uses: to decolorize mineral, vegetable and animal oils; as an adsorbent of insecticides, alkaloids and vitamins; as a binder in foundry sands; as a filtering agent; as a stabilizing agent in emulsion paints; and as a filler in cosmetics, toilet and baby powders.

Only three post-mortem studies appear to have been recorded and these upon men who had been exposed to Nutfield fuller's earth. The fundamental lesions are round, firm—but not hard—black 'nodules' varying from 2 to 7·5 mm diameter and more in the upper than the lower parts of the lungs (Campbell and Gloyne, 1942; Tonning, 1949; Sakula, 1961); in one case they tended to run into small confluent masses in the upper lobes. Hilar lymph nodes are black.

The lesions are situated mainly around bronchiolovascular bundles and consist of aggregations of macrophages containing brownish particles some of which are extracellular; they are enmeshed by a network of reticulin fibres. Foreign body giant cells are absent. There is, therefore, a close resemblance to the lesions of kaolin pneumoconiosis and the non-collagen macules of coal pneumoconiosis. Mild collagenous fibrosis is present in the nodules and some extension into contiguous alveolar walls has been described (Tonning, 1949). Numerous birefringent particles may be seen in the nodules (Sakula, 1961) and are probably montmorillonite which is moderately birefringent. X-ray and electron diffraction studies in Sakula's (1961) case showed the patterns of montmorillonite but no evidence of quartz.

In a radiological survey of 49 fuller's earth workers in Illinois there were two (apparently occupied mainly in milling and bagging) whose films showed large confluent shadows indistinguishable from those which occur in coal-miners and some cases of silicosis. No post-mortem examinations were done (McNally and Trostler, 1941). Discrete opacities were observed in a small group of fuller's earth workers in Germany but various proportions of quartzose sand had been added to the clay in the past and there was also a significant content of naturally occurring quartz (Gattner, 1955).

It seems possible that montmorillonite may cause pneumoconiosis in some cases but quartz probably played an important part in the Illinois and German cases. Tuberculous infection has not been observed. The problem of pathogenicity remains unsolved as post-mortem studies have been so few, and recorded animal experiments inconclusive and not related to the lungs (McNally and Trostler, 1941; Campbell and Gloyne, 1942). If fuller's earth itself has a fibrogenic potential it appears to be of a low order.

In general, this pneumoconiosis occurs only after long exposure to high concentrations of fuller's earth dust; it is represented by small, discrete, low-density opacities (which occasionally show some tendency to confluence) mainly in the upper halves of the lungs; it runs a benign course, and does not shorten life expectancy. Respiratory disability without radiographic evidence of pneumoconiosis has been reported in some fuller's earth workers and was apparently due to non-specific chronic airways obstruction.

Exposure to fuller's earth in industrial processes and from cosmetic preparations is probably harmless.

BENTONITE

Bentonite consists of fine-grained clays containing not less than 85 per cent montmorillonite and the name originates from the occurrence of such clay at Fort Benton in Wyoming in the United States of America. There are two main forms, sodium and calcium montmorillonite (but, less commonly, beidelite), which have a greater capacity for water adsorption and base exchange than other plastic clays. Similar clays are found in Italy, Greece, Spain and elsewhere.

The bentonite clays were deposited as airborne volcanic ash and were later subjected to alteration by sea and ground water. The Wyoming clay is associated with sandstone and siliceous shale and is reported to have a 'free silica' content varying from less than 1 per cent to about 24 per cent (Phibbs, Sundin and Mitchell, 1971).

Mining is carried out by the opencast method, which is not a source of dust hazard, and the clay is then crushed and milled. Crushing and milling is done indoors and is a very dusty process. After crushing the clay is dried in oil-fired cylindrical driers. The 'free silica' in airborne and settled mill-dust has been found to consist of 'appreciable amounts of cristobalite' (Phibbs, Sundin and Mitchell, 1971) which is likely to have been formed by high-temperature conversion of quartz during the volcanic period rather than by the heat of the driers. Bentonite from Wyoming (which is the world's largest producer) is imported into the United Kingdom in the crude form and milled and processed here.

The chief uses of bentonite are in oil-well drilling muds and oil refining, as a bonding material for foundry sands, in various adsorbents, in insecticides and fungicides, in ceramics and as a fire retardant.

Bentonite by itself is not fibrogenic in the lungs of experimental animals but causes local accumulations of large cells with foamy cytoplasm which stains strongly positive with periodic acid Schiff, and a mild proliferation of reticulin (Timár, Kendrey and Juhasz, 1966). When mixed with quartz, however, collagen fibrosis occurs but is not as severe as that produced by quartz alone (Timár, Kendrey and Juhasz, 1966).

The pneumoconiosis of bentonite millers is undoubtedly due to quartz and cristobalite—the latter probably being responsible for the rapidity of development and severity of the disease in some cases. In short, it is silicosis.

THE MICA FAMILY

The nature of the mica family is referred to in Chapter 2. In addition to muscovite and biotite there is phlogopite which is a bronze-coloured magnesium mica.

Muscovite is widely used in the electrical industry, in the windows of furnaces and stoves. In crushed form it is put to the same use as talc to prevent adhesion in the roof felt and rubber industries, and is also employed in paints and other decoration materials. *Biotite* is used to a minor extent in the crushed state as a filler and coating in the rubber and roofing industries. *Phlogopite* is employed for electrical insulation at high temperatures.

It is very doubtful that a pneumoconiosis is caused by exposure to dust of the mica group of minerals alone. Certainly silicosis has occurred in Indian muscovite-miners owing to the high quartz content of associated pegmatite rocks (Government of India Ministry of Labour, 1953), and this remains a potential risk. When crude mica is crushed and milled, quartz is usually present in the dust and is not separated out until the later stages of refinement. However, remarkably little radiographic evidence of silicosis was found in one survey of muscovite- and pegmatite-miners in North Carolina (Dreesen et al., 1940), although in another survey of 79 men in the same region who were milling mica which was not thought to contain 'free silica', seven were reported to have definite pneumoconiosis (Vestal, Winstead and Joliot, 1943).

Only very few workers exposed to mica dusts have been reported to have radiographic appearances consistent with pneumoconiosis and of these the abnormalities have usually been of a minor order and alternative causes not excluded. Radiographic appearances similar to asbestosis were observed in one muscovite-grinder in North Carolina (Dreesen et al., 1940), and evidence of pleural calcification on chest films has been regarded in some cases as being due to mica (Smith, 1952; Kleinfeld, 1966), but in these the possibility of additional exposure to asbestos or tremolite was not adequately excluded.

Diffuse pigmented fibrosis was found at autopsy in the lungs of a man who had prolonged exposure to dusting powders in the rubber industry; the fibrotic areas contained numerous birefringent crystals (the mica minerals are all strongly birefringent) which on x-ray diffraction proved to be biotite, and 'free silica' was absent (Vorwald, 1960). But Vorwald concluded that there

346

was 'considerable uncertainty' that biotite was responsible and was unable to eliminate other possible causes.

In experimental animals, biotite, muscovite and sericite produce only local macrophage accumulation and mild proliferation of reticulin fibres (King, Gilchrist and Rae, 1947; Vorwald, 1960; Tripsa and Rotura, 1966; Goldstein and Rendall, 1970), and the changes are those of a foreign-body response to an inert dust which resolves in about twelve months (Vorwald, 1960). Hence, under these conditions these minerals are apparently innocuous.

The available evidence (which has rarely included satisfactory details of past occupational dust exposures), therefore, gives little support to the view that these mica minerals cause fibrotic pneumoconiosis, and the demonstration and doubtful significance of biotite in Vorwald's (1960) case can hardly be regarded as proof of a causal relationship

The ACGIH (1971) TLV for mica with 'less than 1 per cent crystalline silica' is 20 mppcf and other values are in operation in the Argentine, Finland, Poland, Romania and U.S.S.R. (ILO, 1970).

Vermiculite is the name given to a family of micaceous magnesium-aluminium silicates derived from hydrothermally altered biotite and is often classed with the clay minerals. It is of light weight and has the property of expanding—or 'exfoliating'—to some twelve times its original size when heated. It is obtained in various parts of the world by mining, after which the ore is crushed and shipped generally in the unheated—that is, unexpanded—form which is less bulky than the expanded form. When received by the expanding plant, prepared vermiculite is subjected to a furnace temperature of about 1,100°C, cooled, passed over separators to remove any impurities and packed in paper bags.

Expanded vermiculite is a good lightweight thermal insulator, is fireproof and resists decomposition, and has the properties of a mineral sponge. Its uses in industry include insulation granules for industrial and domestic buildings, as an aggregate for fireproof concrete, refractory bricks and pipe-lagging and, combined with gypsum, for fireproof building plasters; it is also used in soil conditioners, fertilizers and pesticides. Hence, for some purposes expanded vermiculite is a valuable substitute for the asbestos minerals.

It is important, therefore, that there appears to be no evidence of any harmful effect to the lungs resulting from mining and crushing vermiculite or from the preparation and use of expanded vermiculite. Furthermore, vermiculite does not cause fibrosis of the lungs (Goldstein and Rendall, 1970) nor, in particle size of less than 10 μm, mesothelioma of the pleura (Hunter and Thomson, 1973) in experimental animals.

THE SILLIMANITE GROUP OF MINERALS

These consist of andalusite, kyanite and sillimanite, all of which have the same aluminium silicate composition ($Al_2O_3.SiO_2$) but different crystal structures; they occur in such metamorphic rocks as gneisses and schists.

They are invaluable for the manufacture of high-grade refractories which are chemically inert under acid or basic conditions, and capable of withstanding higher temperatures than fireclay bodies. Hence, they are used in the manufacture of porcelains for laboratory ware, sparking plugs and

347

thermocouple tubing, and in special refractory bricks with high resistance to wear and temperature required, for example, in glass-making, non-ferrous metallurgy and forging furnaces.

Raw sillimanite minerals are calcined at 1,500°C for twenty-four hours, dry crushed and then milled with water in cylindrical mills. The resulting slip is mixed with varying amounts of clay for processing whatever type of ware is required. The calcination and crushing processes are potentially very dusty, and calcination converts these minerals into mullite ($3Al_2O_3 . 2SiO_2$), some cristobalite and glass.

No case of pneumoconiosis authentically demonstrated to be caused by these silicates appears to be on record. The abnormality of chest radiographs reported by Middleton (1936) in four sillimanite workers is of dubious significance. However, Gärtner (1947) believed that sillimanite can cause disease akin to silicosis, and described small irregular nodules in a portion of lung from a smelting-oven worker manufacturing corundum. X-ray analysis of lung ash revealed corundum, bauxite, 'amorphous silica' and mullite. It hardly seems justifiable to regard this case as being one of lung fibrosis due to sillimanite.

Animal experiments with uncalcined sillimanite have produced perivascular and peribronchiolar collections of macrophages, dust particles, fibroblasts, reticulin fibre proliferation and early collagen fibrosis; and also some diffuse interstitial fibrosis, but no evidence of nodules of silicotic type (Jötten and Eickhoff, 1944; Gärtner and von Marwyck, 1947).

It is difficult to know how to interpret the available evidence; sillimanite—or mullite, as suggested by Gärtner (1947)—may be capable of producing mild fibrosis, but the cristobalite which may be present in variable quantity in calcined sillimanite would seem to be more important. In practice, however, pneumoconiosis, even of the mildest order, does not appear to occur in workers exposed to either raw or calcined sillimanite dust alone; nevertheless, periodic medical surveillance of exposed workers is probably desirable.

REFERENCES

Alden, H. S. and Howell, W. M. (1944). 'The asbestos corn.' *Archs Derm. Syph.* **49**, 312–314

Alivisatos, G. P., Pontikakis, A. E. and Terzis, B. (1955). 'Talcosis of unusually rapid development.' *Br. J. ind. Med.* **12**, 43–49

Anjilvel, L. and Thurlbeck, W. M. (1966). 'The incidence of asbestos bodies in the lungs of random necropsies in Montreal.' *Canad. med. Ass. J.* **95**, 1179–1182

Anspach, M., Roitzsch, E. and Clausnitzer, W. (1965). 'Ein Beitrag zur Ätiologie des diffusion malignen Pleura-Mesothelioms.' *Arch. Gewerbepath. Gewerbehyg.* **21**, 392–407

Anton, H. C. (1968). 'Multiple pleural plaques.' Part 1. *Br. J. Radiol.* **41**, 341–348

Attygalle, D., Harrison, C. V., King, E. H. and Mohanty, G. P. (1954). 'Infective pneumoconiosis 1. The influence of dead tubercle bacilli (B.C.G.) on the dust lesions produced by anthracite, coal mine dust, and kaolin in the lungs of rats and guinea pigs.' *Br. J. ind. Med.* **11**, 245–259

Bader, M. E., Bader, R. A. and Selikoff, I. J. (1961). 'Pulmonary function in asbestosis of the lung; an alveolar-capillary block syndrome.' *Am. J. Med.* **30**, 235–242

— — Tierstein, A. S. and Selikoff, I. J. (1965). 'Pulmonary function in asbestosis: serial tests in a long term prospective study.' *Ann. N.Y. Acad. Sci.* **132**, 391–405

Bader, M. E., Bader, R. A., Tierstein, A. S., Miller, A. and Selikoff, I. J. (1970). 'Pulmonary function and radiographic changes in 598 workers with varying duration of exposure to asbestos.' *J. Mt Sinai Hosp.* **37**, 492–499

Bamber, H. A. and Butterworth, R. (1970). 'Asbestos hazard from protective clothing.' *Ann. occup. Hlth* **13**, 77–79

Beattie, J. and Knox, J. F. (1961). 'Studies in mineral content and particle size distribution in the lungs of asbestos textile workers.' In *Inhaled Particles and Vapours*, pp. 419–433. Ed. by C. N. Davies. Oxford and New York; Pergamon

Becklake, M. R., Fournier-Massey, G., McDonald, J. C., Siemiatycki, J. and Rossiter, C. E. (1970). 'Lung function in relation to chest radiographic changes in Quebec asbestos workers.' In *Pneumoconiosis. Proceedings of the International Conference, Johannesburg, 1969*, pp. 233–236. Ed. by H. A. Shapiro. Cape Town; Oxford University Press

— — Rossiter, C. E. and McDonald, J. C. (1972). 'Lung function in chrysotile asbestos mine and mill workers of Quebec.' *Archs Envir. Hlth* **24**, 401–409

Berry, G., Newhouse, M. L. and Turok, M. (1972). 'Combined effect of asbestos exposure and smoking on mortality from lung cancer in factory workers.' *Lancet* **2**, 476–479

Bramwell, A., Leech, J. G. C. and Dunstall, W. S. (1940). 'Montmorillonite in fuller's earth.' *Geol. Mag.* **77**, 102–112

British Occupational Hygiene Society Committee on Hygiene Standards (1968). 'Hygiene standards for chrysotile asbestos dust.' *Ann. Occup. Hyg.* **11**, 47–69

British Thoracic and Tuberculosis Association and the Medical Research Council Pneumoconiosis Unit (1972). 'A survey of pleural thickening: its relation to asbestos exposure and previous pleural disease.' *Envir. Res.* **5**, 142–151

Buchanan, W. D. (1965). 'Asbestosis and primary intrathoracic neoplasms.' *Ann. N.Y. Acad. Sci.* **132**, 507–518

Burilkov, T. and Michailova, L. (1970). 'Asbestos content of soil and endemic pleural asbestosis.' *Envir. Res.* **3**, 443–451

Byers, P. D. and King, E. J. (1959). 'Experimental and infective pneumoconiosis with coal, kaolin and mycobacteria.' *Lab. Invest.* **8**, 647-664

— — and Harrison, C. V. (1960). 'The effect of triton, a surface active polyoxethylene ether, on experimental infective pneumoconiosis.' *Br. J. exp. Path.* **41**, 472–477

Byrom, J. C., Hodgson, A. A. and Holmes, S. (1969). 'A dust survey carried out in buildings incorporating asbestos based materials in their construction.' *Ann. occup. Hyg.* **12**, 141–145

Campbell, A. H. and Gloyne, S. R. (1942). 'A case of pneumonokoniosis due to the inhalation of fuller's earth.' *J. Path. Bact.* **54**, 75–79

Cartier, P. (1965). 'Discussion on pleural plaques.' *Ann. N.Y. Acad. Sci.* **132**, 387–388

Cauna, D., Totten, R. S. and Gross, P. (1965). 'Asbestos bodies in human lungs at autopsy.' *J. Am. med. Ass.* **192**, 371–373

Cooke, W. E. (1924). 'Fibrosis of the lungs due to the inhalation of asbestos dust.' *Br. med. J.* **2**, 147

Cralley, L. J., Keenan, R. G. and Lynch, J. R. (1967). 'Exposure to metals in the manufacture of asbestos textile products.' *Am. ind. Hyg. Ass. J.* **28**, 452–461

— — — and Lainhart, W. S. (1968a). 'Source and identification of respirable fibres.' *Am. ind. Hyg. Ass. J.* **29**, 129–135

— Key, M. M., Groth, D. H., Lainhart, W. S. and Ligo, R. M. (1968b). 'Fibrous and mineral content of cosmetic talcum products.' *Am. ind. Hyg. Ass. J.* **29**, 350–354

Davis, J. M. G. (1965). 'Electron-microscope studies of asbestosis in man and animals.' *Ann. N.Y. Acad. Sci.* **132**, 98–111

— (1972). 'The effects of polyvinyl pyridine-N-oxide (P204) on the cytopathogenic action of chrysotile asbestos *in vivo* and *in vitro*.' *Br. J. exp. Path.* **53**, 652–658

— Gross, P. and de Treville, R. T. P. (1970). ' "Ferruginous bodies" in guinea pigs.' *Archs Path.* **89**, 364–373

Department of Employment and Productivity (1970). *Asbestos: Health Precautions in Industry*. Health and Safety at work, 44. London; H.M.S.O.

Dettori, G., Scansetti, G. and Gribando, C. (1964) 'Relievi sull' uiquinamento ambientale nell' industria del talco.' *Medna Lav.* **55**, 453–455

Doll, R. (1955). 'Mortality from lung cancer in asbestos workers.' *Br. J. ind. Med.* **12**, 81–86

— (1971). 'The age distribution of cancer. Implications for models of carcinogenesis.' *J. R. Statist. Soc.* **134**, 133–155.

Donna, A. and Cappa, A. P. M. (1967). 'Contributo sperimentale allo studio della pneumoconiosi da asbesto altivata pneumoconiotica dell'asbesto di chrisolito nel ratto.' *Medna Lav.* **58**, 1–12

Dressen, W. C., Dallavalle, J. M., Edwards, T. I. and Sayers, R. C. (1940). *Pneumoconiosis among Mica and Pegmatite Workers.* U.S. Pub. Hlth Serv. Publ. Hlth Bull. No. 250, Washington

Edenfield, R. W. (1960). 'A clinical and roentgenological study of kaolin workers.' *Archs Envir. Hlth* **1**, 392–406

Eisenstadt, H. B. (1964). 'Asbestos pleurisy.' *Dis. Chest* **46**, 78–81

— (1965). 'Benign asbestos pleurisy.' *J. Am. med. Ass.* **192**, 419–421

El-Ghawabi, S. H., El-Samra, G. H. and Mehasseb, H. (1970). 'Talc pneumoconiosis.' *J. Egypt. med. Ass.* **53**, 330–340

Elmes, P. C. (1966). 'The epidemiology and clinical features of asbestosis and related diseases.' *Postgrad. med. J.* **42**, 623–635

Elwood, P. C. and Cochrane, A. L. (1964). 'A follow-up study of workers from an asbestos factory.' *Br. J. ind. Med.* **21**, 304–307

Enterline, P. E. (1965). 'Mortality among asbestos products workers in the United States.' *Ann. N.Y. Acad. Sci.* **132**, 156–165

Enticknap, J. B. and Smither, W. J. (1964). 'Peritoneal tumours in asbestosis.' *Br. J. ind. Med.* **21**, 20–31

Fahr, T. and Feigel, F. (1914). 'Kristallbildung in der Lunge.' *Dt. med. Wschr.* **40**, 1548–1549

Fletcher, D. E. and Edge, J. R. (1970). 'The early radiological changes in pulmonary and pleural asbestosis.' *Clin. Radiol.* **21**, 355–365

Gaensler, E. A. and Kaplan, A. I. (1971). 'Asbestos pleural effusion.' *Ann. intern. Med.* **74**, 178–191

Gärtner, H. (1947). 'Über Lungenbefunde bei einem Korundschmelzer.' *Z. ges. Inn. Med.* **2**, 761–764

— (1955). 'Die Bleicherde-Lunge.' *Arch. Gewerbepath. Gewerbehyg.* **13**, 508–516

— and von Marwyck, C. (1947). 'Lugenfibrose durch Sillimanit.' *D. med. Wschr.* **72**, 708–710

Gerber, M. A. (1970). 'Asbestosis and neoplastic disorders of the hematopoietic system.' *Am. J. clin. Path.* **53**, 204–208

German, W. M. (1943). 'Dusting powder granulomas following surgery.' *Surgery Gynec. Obstet.* **76**, 501–507

Gilson, J. C. (1966). 'Health hazards of asbestos. Recent studies on its biological effects.' *Trans. Soc. occup. Med.* **16**, 62–74

Gloyne, S. R. (1931). 'Presence of asbestosis bodies in faeces in case of pulmonary asbestosis.' *Tubercle* **12**, 158–159

— (1932–33). 'The morbid anatomy and histology of asbestos.' *Tubercle (Edin.)* **14**, 445–451; 493–497; 550–558

Godwin, M. C. and Jagatic, J. (1970). 'Asbestos and mesotheliomas.' *Envir. Res.* **3**, 391–416

Gold, C. (1967). 'A simple method of detecting asbestos in tissues.' *J. Clin. Path.* **20**, 674

— and Cuthbert, J. (1966). 'Asbestos—a hazard to the community.' *Publ. Hlth, Lond.* **80**, 261–270

Goldstein, B. and Rendall, R. E. G. (1970). 'The relative toxicities of the main classes of minerals.' In *Pneumoconiosis. Proceedings of the International Conference, Johannesburg, 1969*, pp. 429–434. Ed. by H. A. Shapiro. Cape Town; Oxford University Press

Government of India Ministry of Labour (1953). *Silicosis in Mica Mining in Bihar.* Report No. 3. Office of the Chief Adviser Factories

Governa, M. and Rosanda, C. (1972). 'A histochemical study of the asbestos body coating.' *Br. J. ind. Med.* **29**, 154–159

Graham, J. and Graham, R. (1967). 'Ovarian cancer and asbestos.' *Envir. Res.* **1**, 115–128

Greenburg, L. (1947). 'The dust exposure in tremolite talc mining.' *Yale J. Biol. Med.* **19**, 481–501

Greenburg, M. (1970). 'Asbestos release from battery boxes.' *Ann. occup. Hlth* **13**, 79–80

Grim, R. E. (1933). 'Petrography of fuller's earth deposits, Olmstead, Illinois, with a brief study of some non-Illinois earths.' *Econ. Geol.* **28**, 344–363

Gross, P., Cralley, L. J. and de Treville, R. T. P. (1967). ' "Asbestos" bodies: their non-specificity.' *Am. ind. Hyg. Ass. J.* **28**, 541–542

— de Treville, R. T. P. and Haller, M. N. (1969). 'Pulmonary ferruginous bodies in city dwellers.' *Archs Envir. Hlth* **19**, 186–188

Hale, L. W., Gough, J., King, E. J. and Nagelschmidt, G. (1956). 'Pneumoconiosis of kaolin workers.' *Br. J. ind. Med.* **13**, 251–259

Harington, J. S. and Roe, F. T. C. (1965). 'Studies of carcinogenesis of asbestos fibres and their natural oils.' *Ann. N.Y. Acad. Sci.* **132**, 439–450

— Gilson, J. C. and Wagner, J. C. (1971). 'Asbestos and mesothelioma in man.' *Nature, Lond.* **232**, 54–55

— Wagner, J. C. and Smith, M. (1963). 'The detection of hyaluronic acid in pleural fluid of cases of diffuse pleural mesotheliomas.' *Br. J. exp. Path.* **44**, 81–83

Harries, P. G. (1971a). 'Asbestos dust concentrations in ship repairing: a practical approach to improving asbestos hygiene in naval dockyards.' *Ann. occup. Hyg.* **14**, 241–254

— (1971b). *The Effects and Control of Diseases Associated with Exposure to Asbestos in Devonport Dockyard.* Gosport; Institute of Naval Medicine

Heard, B. E. and Turner Warwick, M. (1973). Personal communication.

— and Williams, R. (1961). 'The pathology of asbestosis with reference to lung function.' *Thorax* **16**, 264–281

Hendry, N. W. (1965). 'The geology, occurrences and major uses of asbestos.' *Ann. N.Y. Acad. Sci.* **132**, 12–21

Hickish, D. E. and Knight, K. L. (1970). 'Exposure to asbestos during brake maintenance.' *Ann. occup. Hyg.* **13**, 17–21

Hill, I. D., Doll, R. and Knox, J. F. (1966). 'Mortality among asbestos workers.' *Proc. R. Soc. Med.* **59**, 59–60

Hinson, K. F. W. (1971). Personal communication

— (1972). Personal communication

— Otto, H., Webster, I. and Rossiter, C. E. (1972). *Working Group on the Biological Effects of Asbestos.* In the press

Hodgson, A. A. (1966). 'Fibrous Silicates.' Lecture Series, 1965, No. 4. London; The Royal Institute of Chemistry

Holt, P. F., Mills, J. and Young, D. K. (1966). 'Experimental asbestosis in the guinea pig.' *J. Path. Bact.* **92**, 185–195

Hopkins, G. B. and Taylor, D. G. (1970). 'Pulmonary talc granulomatosis.' *Am. Rev. resp. Dis.* **101**, 101–104

Hourihane, D. O'B. (1964). 'The pathology of mesotheliomata and an analysis of their association with asbestos exposure.' *Thorax* **19**, 268–278

— and McCaughey, W. T. E. (1966). 'Pathological aspects of asbestosis.' *Postgrad. Med. J.* **42**, 613–622

— Lessof, L. and Richardson, P. C. (1966). 'Hyaline and calcified pleural plaques as an index of exposure to asbestos. A study of radiological and pathological features of 100 cases with a consideration of epidemiology.' *Br. med. J.* **1**, 1069–1074

Hunt, A. C. (1956). 'Massive pulmonary fibrosis from inhalation of talc.' *Thorax* **11**, 287–294

Hunt, R. (1965). 'Routine lung function studies of 830 in an asbestos processing factory.' *Ann. N.Y. Acad. Sci.* **132**, 406–420

Hunter, B. and Thomson, C. (1973). 'Evaluation of the tumorigenic potential of vermiculite by intrapleural injection in rats.' *Br. J. ind. Med.* **30**, 167–173

International Labour Office (1970). *Permissible Levels of Toxic Substances in the Working Environment.* Occup. Safety and Hlth Series. No. 20. Geneva; I.L.O.

International Union Against Cancer (1965). 'Working group on asbestos and cancer.' *Archs Envir. Hlth* **11**, 221–229

Jacob, G. and Anspach, M. (1965). 'Pulmonary neoplasia among Dresden asbestos workers.' *Ann. N.Y. Acad. Sci.* **132**, 536–548

Jodoin, G., Gibbs, G. W., Macklem, P. T., McDonald, J. C. and Becklake, M. R. (1971). 'Early effects of asbestos exposure on lung function.' *Am. Rev. resp. Dis.* **104**, 525–535

Jones, B. M., Edwards, J. H. and Wagner, J. C. (1972). 'Absorption of serum proteins by inorganic dusts.' *Br. J. ind. Med.* **29**, 287–292

Jones Williams, W. (1958). 'The pathology of the lungs in five nickel workers.' *Br. J. ind. Med.* **15**, 235–242

Jötten, K. W. and Eickhoff, W. (1944). 'Lungenveränderungen durch Sillimanistaub.' *Arch. Gewerbepath. Gewerbehyg.* **12**, 223–232

Kazantzis, G. (1972). 'Chromium and nickel.' *Ann. occup. Hyg.* **15**, 25–29

Keal, E. E. (1960). 'Asbestosis and abdominal neoplasms.' *Lancet* **2**, 1211–1216

Kettle, E. H. (1934). 'Infective pneumoconiosis: infective silicatosis.' *J. Path. Bact.* **38**, 201–208

King, E. J., Gilchrist, M. and Rae, M. V. (1947). 'Tissue reaction to sericite and shale dusts treated with hydrochloric acid: an experimental investigation.' *J. Path. Bact.* **59**, 324–327

— Harrison, C. V. and Nagelschmidt, G. (1948). 'Effect of kaolin on the lungs of rats.' *J. Path. Bact.* **60**, 435–440

— — Mohanty, G. P. and Nagelschmidt, G. (1955). 'The effect of various forms of alumina on the lungs.' *J. Path. Bact.* **69**, 81–93

Kipling, M. D. and Bech, A. D. (1960). 'Talc pneumoconiosis.' *Trans. Ass. ind. med. Offrs* **10**, 85–93

Kiviluoto, R. (1960). 'Pleural calcification as a roentgenologic sign of non-occupational anthophyllite-asbestosis.' *Acta radiol.*, Suppl. 494

Kleinfeld, M. (1966). 'Pleural calcifications as a sign of silicatosis.' *Am. J. med. Sci.* **251**, 215–224

— Giel, C. P., Majeranowski, J. F. and Messite, J. (1963). 'Talc pneumoconiosis.' *Archs Envir. Hlth* **7**, 101–115

— Messite, J., Kooyman, O. and Sarfaty, J. (1966). 'Effect of asbestos dust inhalation on lung function.' *Archs Envir. Hlth* **12**, 741–746

— — — and Shapiro, J. (1964a). 'Pulmonary ventilatory function in talcosis of the lung.' *Dis. Chest* **46**, 592–598

— — — and Zaki, M. H. (1967). 'Mortality among talc miners and millers in New York State.' *Archs Envir. Hlth* **14**, 663–667

— — Shapiro, J. and Swencicki, R. (1965). Effect of talc dust inhalation on lung function. *Archs Envir. Hlth* **10**, 431–437

— — — Kooyman, O. and Swencicki, R. (1964b). 'Lung function in talc workers.' *Archs Envir. Hlth* **9**, 559–566

Klempman, S. (1962). 'The exfoliative cytology of diffuse pleural mesothelioma.' *Cancer (Philad.)* **15**, 691–704

Knox, J. F., Doll, R. S. and Hill, I. D. (1965). 'Cohort analysis of changes in incidence of bronchial carcinoma in a textile asbestos factory.' *Ann. N.Y. Acad. Sci.* **132**, 526–535

— Holmes, S., Doll, R. and Hill, I. D. (1968). 'Mortality from lung cancer and other causes among workers in an asbestos textile factory.' *Br. J. ind. Med.* **25**, 293–303

Langer, A. M., Rubin, I. and Selikoff, I. J. (1970). 'Electron microprobe analysis of asbestos bodies.' In *Pneumoconiosis. Proceedings of the International Conference, Johannesburg, 1969*, pp. 57–69. Ed. by H. A. Shapiro. Cape Town; Oxford University Press

— Baden, V., Hammond, E. C. and Selikoff, I. J. (1971). 'Inorganic fibres, including chrysotile in lungs at autopsy; preliminary report.' In *Inhaled Particles, 3*, pp. 683–692. Ed. by W. H. Walton. Woking; Unwin

Langlands, J. H. M., Wallace, W. F. M. and Simpson, M. J. C. (1971). 'Insulation workers in Belfast. 2. Morbidity in men still at work.' *Br. J. ind. Med.* **28**, 217–225

Leatheart, G. L. (1960). 'Clinical, bronchographic, radiological and physiological observations in ten cases of asbestosis.' *Br. J. ind. Med.* **17**, 213–225

— (1968). 'Pulmonary function tests in asbestos workers.' *Trans. Soc. occup. Med.* **18**, 49–55.

Leiben, J. (1966). 'Malignancies in asbestos workers.' *Archs Envir. Hlth* **13**, 619–621

— and Pistawka, H. (1967). 'Mesothelioma and asbestos exposure.' *Archs Envir. Hlth* **14**, 559–563

Lüchtrath, H. and Schmidt, K. G. (1959). 'Uber Talkum und Steatit, ihre Beziehungen zum Asbest sowie ihre Wirhung beim intrachealer Tierrersuch an Ratten.' *Beitr. Silikosforsch.* **61**, 1–60

Lumley, K. P. S. (1971). 'Asbestos dust levels inside firefighting helmets with chrysotile asbestos covers.' *Ann. occup. Hyg.* **14**, 285–286

— Harries, P. G. and O'Kelley, F. J. (1971). 'Buildings insulated with sprayed asbestos: a potential hazard.' *Ann. occup. Hyg.* **14**, 255–257

Lynch, K. M. and McIver, F. A. (1954). 'Pneumoconiosis from exposure to kaolin dust.' *Am. J. Path.* **30**, 1117–1127

— and Smith, W. A. (1935). 'Pulmonary asbestosis: carcinoma of the lung in asbesto-silicosis.' *Am. J. Cancer* **24**, 56–64

Mackenzie, F. A. F. and Harries, P. G. (1970). 'Changing attitudes to the diagnosis of asbestos disease.' *J. R. nav. med. Serv.* **56**, 116–123

McCaughey, W. T. E. (1965). 'Criteria for diagnosis of diffuse mesothelial tumours.' *Ann. N.Y. Acad. Sci.* **132**, 603–613

McDonald, J. C., McDonald, A. D., Gibbs, G. W., Siemiatyski, J. and Rossiter, C. E. (1971). 'Mortality in chrysotile asbestos mines and mills in Quebec.' *Archs Envir. Hlth* **22**, 677–686

McNally, W. D. and Trostler, I. S. (1941). 'Severe pneumoconiosis caused by inhalation of fuller's earth.' *J. ind. Hyg. Toxicol.* **23**, 118–126

McNulty, J. C. (1968). 'Asbestos mining Wittenoom, Western Australia.' In *First Australian Pneumoconiosis Conference, 1968*, pp. 447–474. Sydney; Joint Coal Board

Mancusa, T. F. (1965). Discussion. *Ann. N.Y. Acad. Sci.* **132**, 589–594

Mányai, S., Kabai, J., Kis, J., Süveges, E. and Timář, M. (1970). 'The effect of heat treatment on the structure of kaolin and its *in vitro* haemolytic activity.' *Envir. Res.* **3**, 187–198

Maroudas, N. G., O'Neill, C. H. and Stanton, M. F. (1973). 'Fibroblast anchorage in carcinogenesis by fibres.' *Lancet* **1**, 807–809

Mattson, S. B. (1971). 'Caplan's syndrome in association with asbestosis.' *Scand. J. resp. Dis.* **52**, 153–161

Merewether, E. R. A. (1949). *Annual Report Chief Inspector of Factories, 1947.* London; H.M.S.O.

— and Price, C. W. (1930). *Report on Effects of Asbestos on the Lungs and Dust Suppression in the Asbestos Industry.* London; H.M.S.O.

Messite, J. G., Reddin, G. and Kleinfeld, M. (1959). 'Pulmonary talcosis, a clinical and environmental study.' *Archs ind. Hlth* **20**, 408–413

Meurman, L. (1966). 'Asbestos bodies and pleural plaques in a Finnish series of autopsy cases.' *Acta path. microbiol. scand.* Suppl. 181

— Hormia, M., Isomäki, M. and Sutinen, S. (1970). 'Asbestos bodies in the lungs of a series of Finnish lung cancer patients.' In *Pneumoconiosis. Proceedings of the International Conference, Johannesburg, 1969*, pp. 404–407. Ed. by H. A. Shapiro. Cape Town; Oxford University Press

Middleton, E. L. (1936). 'Industrial pulmonary disease due to the inhalation of dust.' *Lancet* **2**, 59–64

Miller, A., Teirstein, A. S., Bader, M. E., Bader, R. A. and Selikoff, I. J. (1971). 'Talc pneumoconiosis. Significance of sublight microscopic mineral particles.' *Am. J. Med.* **50**, 395–402

Millman, N. (1947). 'Pneumoconiosis due to talc in the cosmetic industry.' *Occup. Med.* **4**, 391–394

Ministry of Labour (1967). *Problems Arising from the Use of Asbestos.* H.M. Factory Inspectorate. London; H.M.S.O.

Morgan, A. and Holmes, A. (1970). 'Neutron activation techniques in investigations of the composition and biological effects of asbestos.' In *Pneumoconiosis. Proceedings of the International Conference, Johannesburg, 1969*, pp. 52–56. Ed. by H. A. Shapiro. Cape Town; Oxford University Press

Morgan, W. K. C. (1964). 'Rheumatoid pneumoconiosis in association with asbestosis.' *Thorax* **19**, 433–435

Moskowitz, R. (1970). 'Talc pneumoconiosis: a treated case.' *Chest* **58**, 37–41

Muldoon, B. C. and Turner Warwick, M. W. (1972). 'Lung function studies in asbestos workers.' *Br. J. Dis. Chest* **66**, 121–132

Murphy, R. L., Levine, B. W., Faio, J. A. B., Lynch, J. and Burgess, W. A. (1971). 'Floor tile installation as a source of asbestos exposure.' *Am. Rev. resp. Dis.* **104**, 576–580

Murphy, R. L. H., Jr., Gaensler, E. A., Redding, R. A., Keelan, P. J., Smith, A. A., Goff, A. M. and Ferris, B. G. (1972). Low exposure to asbestos. Gas exchange in ship pipe coverers and controls.' *Archs envir. Hlth* **25**, 253–264

Murray, M. (1907). Report, Department, Commission on Compensation of Industrial Disease. Cd. 3496, pp. 127–128. London; H.M.S.O.

Nagelschmidt, G. (1965). 'Some observations of the dust content and composition in lungs with asbestosis, made during work on coal miner's pneumoconiosis.' *Ann. N. Y. Acad. Sci.* **132**, 64–76

Newhouse, M. L. (1969). 'A study of the mortality of workers in an asbestos factory.' *Br. J. ind. Med.* **26**, 294–301

— and Thompson, H. (1965). 'Mesothelioma of pleura and peritoneum following exposure to asbestos in the London area.' *Br. J. ind. Med.* **22**, 261–269

— Berry, G., Wagner, J. C. and Turok, M. E. (1972). 'A study of the mortality of female asbestos workers.' *Br. J. ind. Med.* **29**, 134–141

New York City Department of Air Resources (1971). 'Spraying of asbestos prohibited, local law 49.' In *Air Pollution Control Code of the City of New York*, sect. 1403, 2–9. 11(B)

Nice, C. M. and Ostrolenk, D. G. (1968). 'Asbestosis and nodular lesions of the lung.' *Dis. Chest* **54**, 226–229

Noro, L. (1968). 'Occupational and "non-occupational" asbestosis in Finland.' *Am. ind. Hyg. Ass. J.* **29**, 195–201

Pearce, A. G. E. (1968). *Histochemistry. Theoretical and Applied.* London; Churchill

Pernis, B., Vigliani, E. C. and Selikoff, I. J. (1965). 'Rheumatoid factor in serum of individuals exposed to asbestos.' *Ann. N. Y. Acad. Sci.* **132**, 112–120

Pettinati, L., Coscia, G. C., Francia, A. and Ghemi, F. (1964). 'Aspetti radiologie clinici della pneumoconiosi nell' industria estrattwa del talco.' *Medna Lav.* **55**, 58–63

Phibbs, B. P., Sundin, R. E. and Mitchell, R. S. (1971). 'Silicosis in Wyoming betonite workers.' *Am. Rev. resp. Dis.* **103**, 1–17

Policard, A. and Collet, A. (1954). 'Étude experimentale des effets pathologique du kaolin.' *Schweiz. Zr. allg. Path. Bakt.* **17**, 320–325

Pooley, F. D. (1972). 'Electron microscope characteristics of inhaled chrysotile asbestos fibre.' *Br. J. ind. Med.* **29**, 146–153

— Oldham, P. D., Chang-Hyun Um and Wagner, J. C. (1970). 'The detection of asbestos in tissues.' In *Pneumoconiosis. Proceedings of the International Conference, Johannesburg, 1969*, pp. 108–116. Ed. by H. A. Shapiro. Cape Town; Oxford University Press

Rajan, K. T., Wagner, J. C. and Evans, P. H. (1972). 'The response of human pleura in organ culture to asbestos.' *Nature, Lond.* **238**, 346-347

Recommendation of sub-Committee on Asbestosis of the Permanent Commission and International Association on Occupational Health (1972). 'Evaluation of asbestos exposure in the working Environment.' *J. occup. Med.* **14**, 560–562

Rickards, A. G. and Barrett, G. M. (1958). 'Rheumatoid lung changes associated with asbestosis.' *Thorax* **13**, 185–193

Rickards, A. L. and Badami, D. V. (1971). 'Chrysotile asbestos in urban air.' *Nature, Lond.* **234**, 93–94

Roberts, G. B. S. (1947). 'Granuloma of the fallopian tube due to surgical glove talc. Siliceous granuloma.' *Br. J. Surg.* **34**, 417–423

Roberts, G. H. (1971). 'The pathology of parietal pleural plaques.' *J. clin. Path.* **24**, 348–353

— and Campbell, G. M. (1972). 'Exfoliative cytology of diffuse mesothelioma.' *J. Clin. Path.* **25**, 577–582

Roe, F. J. C., Walters, M. A. and Harington, J. S. (1966). 'Tumour initiation by natural and contaminating asbestos oils.' *Int. J. Cancer.* **1**, 491–495

Ross, J. G. (1931). *'Chrysotile Asbestos in Canada*, pp. 128–130. Ottawa; Canada Dept of Mines

Rossiter, C. E. (1972). 'Evidence of dose-reponse relation in pneumoconiosis.' *Trans. Soc. occup. Med.* **22**, 83–87

— Bristol, L. J., Cartier, P. H., Gilson, J. C., Grainger, T. R., Sluis-Cremer, G. K. and McDonald, J. C. (1972). 'Radiographic changes in chrysotile asbestos mine and mill workers in Quebec.' *Archs envir. Hlth* **24**, 388–400

Rous, V. and Studený, J. (1970). 'Aetiology of pleural plaques.' *Thorax* **25**, 270–284

Sakula, A. (1961). 'Pneumoconiosis due to fuller's earth.' *Thorax* **16**, 176–179

Sano, M. E., Weiss, E. and Gault, E. S. (1950). 'Pleural mesothelioma.' *J. Thorac. Surg.* **19**, 783–788

Sayers, R. R. and Dreesen, W. C. (1939). 'Asbestosis.' *Am. J. Publ. Hlth* **29**, 205–214

Scansetti, G., Gaido, P. C. and Rasetti, L. (1963). 'Sulla pneumoconiosi del talcatori.' *Medna Lav.* **54**, 680–682

Schepers, G. W. H. and Durkan, T. H. (1955a). 'The effects of inhaled talc-mining dust on the human lung.' *Archs ind. Hlth* **12**, 182–197

— and Durkan, T. M. (1955b), 'An experimental study of the effects of talc dust on animal tissue.' *Archs ind. Hlth* **12**, 317–328

Schmidt, K. G. and Lüchtrath, H. (1958). 'Die Wirkung von frischen und gebranntem Kaolin auf die Lunge und das Bauchfell von Ratten.' *Beitr. Silikosforsch.* **58**, 1–37

Selikoff, I. J. (1965). 'The occurrence of pleural calcification among asbestos insulation workers.' *Ann. N.Y. Acad. Sci.* **132**, 351–367

— and Hammond, E. C. (1970). 'Asbestos bodies in the New York City population in two periods of time.' In *Pneumoconiosis. Proceedings of the International Conference, Johannesburg, 1969.* Ed. by H. A. Shapiro. Cape Town; Oxford University Press

— Churg, J. and Hammond, E. C. (1964). 'Asbestos exposure and neoplasia.' *J. Am. med. Ass.* **188**, 22–26

— Hammond, E. C. and Churg, J. (1968). 'Asbestos exposure, smoking and neoplasia.' *J. Am. med. Ass.* **204**, 106–112

— — — (1970). 'Mortality experiences of asbestos insulation workers.' In *Pneumoconiosis. Proceedings of the International Conference, Johannesburg, 1969*, pp. 180–186. Ed. by H. A. Shapiro. Cape Town; Oxford University Press

— — — (1972). 'Carcinogenicity of amosite asbestos.' *Archs envir. Hlth* **25**, 183–186

— Nicholson, W. J. and Langer, A. M. (1972). 'Asbestos air pollution.' *Archs envir. Hlth* **25**, 1–13

Sheers, G. (1964). 'Prevalence of pneumoconiosis in Cornish kaolin workers.' *Br. J. ind. Med.* **21**, 218–225

— and Templeton, A. R. (1968). 'Effects of asbestos in dockyard workers.' *Br. med. J.* **3**, 574–579

Siegal, W., Smith, R. A. and Greenburgh, L. (1943). 'The dust hazard in tremolite talc mining including roentgenological findings in talc workers.' *Am. J. Roentg.* **49**, 11–29

Simson, F. W. (1930). Annual Report, 1929, p. 64. Johannesburg; South African Institute for Medical Research

Skikne, M. I., Talbot, J. H. and Rendall, R. E. G. (1971). 'Electron diffraction patterns of U.I.C.C. asbestos samples.' *Envir. Res.* **4**, 141–145

Sluis-Cremer, G. K. (1970). 'Asbestosis in South African asbestos miners.' *Envir. Res.* **3**, 310–319

Smith, A. R. (1952). 'Pleural calcification resulting from exposure to certain dusts.' *Am. J. Roentg.* **67**, 375–382

355

Smither, W. J. (1965). 'Secular changes in asbestosis in an asbestos factory.' *Ann. N.Y. Acad. Sci.* **132**, 166–181

Solomon, A. (1969). 'The radiology of asbestosis.' *S. Afr. med. J.* **43**, 847–851

— (1970). 'Radiology of asbestosis.' In *Pneumoconiosis. Proceedings of the International Conference, Johannesburg, 1969*, pp. 243–247. Ed. by H. A. Shapiro. Cape Town; Oxford University Press

— Goldstein, B., Webster, I. and Sluis-Cremer, G. K. (1971). 'Massive fibrosis in asbestosis.' *Envir. Res.* **4**, 430–439

Speil, S. and Leineweber, J. P. (1969). 'Asbestos minerals in modern technology.' *Envir. Res.* **2**, 166–208

Spriggs, A. I. and Boddington, M. M. (1968). *The Cytology of Effusions*, 2nd Edn, pp. 23 and 31. London; Heinemann

Steel, S. J. and Winstanley, D. P. (1968). 'Trephine biopsy of the lung and pleura.' *Thorax* **24**, 576–584

Sundius, N. and Bygdén, A. (1938). 'Der Staubinhalt einer Asbestosis-lungen und die Beschaffenheit der sogennter Asbestosis-korperchen.' *Arch. Gewerbepath. Gewerbehyg.* **8**, 26–80

Suzuki, Y. and Chung, J. (1969). 'Formation of the asbestos body. A comparative study with three types of asbestos.' *Envir. Res.* **3**, 107–118

Technical Data Note 13 (1970). *Standards for Asbestos Dust Concentration for use with the Asbestos Regulations, 1969*. Department of Employment Productivity, H.M. Factory Inspectorate

Tellesson, W. G. (1961). 'Rheumatoid pneumoconiosis (Caplan's syndrome) in an asbestos worker.' *Thorax* **16**, 372–377

Thomas, R. W. (1952). 'Silicosis in the ball-clay and china-clay industries.' *Lancet* **1**, 133–135

Thompson, V. C. (1965). 'Clinical aspects of diffuse mesothelial tumours.' *Thorax* **20**, 248–251

Thomson, J. G. (1970). 'The pathogenesis of pleural plaques.' In *Pneumoconiosis. Proceedings of the International Conference, Johannesburg, 1969*, pp. 138–141. Ed. by H. A. Shapiro. Cape Town; Oxford University Press

— Kaschula, R. O. C. and MacDonald, R. R. (1963). 'Asbestos as a modern urban hazard.' *S. Afr. Med. J.* **37**, 77–82

Thomson, M. L., Pelzer, A. M. and Smither, W. J. (1965). 'The discriminant value of pulmonary function tests in asbestosis.' *Ann. N.Y. Acad. Sci.* **132**, 421–436

Thorel, C. (1896). 'Die Specksteinlunge.' *Beitr. path. Anat.* **20**, 85–101

Timár, M., Kendrey, G. and Juhasz, Z. (1966). 'Experimental observations concerning the effects of mineral dust on pulmonary tissue.' *Medna Lav.* **57**, 1–9

Timbrell, V. (1965). 'The inhalation of fibrous dusts.' *Ann. N.Y. Acad. Sci.* **132**, 255–273

— (1970). 'The inhalation of fibres.' In *Pneumoconiosis. Proceedings of the International Conference, Johannesburg, 1969*, pp. 3–9. Ed. by H. A. Shapiro. Cape Town; Oxford University Press

— Pooley, F. and Wagner, J. C. (1970). 'Characteristics of respirable asbestos fibres.' In *Pneumoconiosis. Proceedings of the International Conference, Johannesburg, 1969*, pp. 120–125. Ed. by H. A. Shapiro. Cape Town; Oxford University Press

Tobacco Research Council (1970). Personal communication

Tonning, H. O. (1949). 'Pneumoconiosis from fuller's earth.' *J. ind. Hyg. Toxicol.* **31**, 41–45

Tripsa, R. and Rotura, G. (1966). 'Recherches experimentales sur la pneumoconiose provoquée par la poussierre de mica.' *Medna Lav.* **57**, 493–500

Turner Warwick, M. and Haslam, P. (1971). 'Antibodies in some chronic fibrosing lung diseases 1. Non-organ-specific antibodies.' *Clin. Allergy* **1**, 83–95

— and Parkes, W. R. (1970). 'Circulating rheumatoid and anti-nuclear factors in asbestos workers.' *Br. med. J.* **3**, 492–495

Um, Chang-Hyun (1970). 'Study of the secular trend in asbestos bodies in lungs in London. 1936–1966.' *Br. med. J.* **2**, 248–251

Utidjian, H. M. D. (1973). 'Criteria documents.' *J. occup. Med.* **15**, 374–379

Utidjian, H. M. D., Gross, P. and de Treville, R. T. P. (1968). 'Ferruginous bodies in human lungs.' *Archs envir. Hlth* **17**, 327-333

Van Ordstrand, H. S. (1970). 'Talc Pneumoconiosis' (Editorial). *Chest* **58**, 2

Vestal, T. F., Winstead, J. A. and Joliot, P. V. (1943). 'Pneumoconiosis among mica and pegmatite workers.' *Ind. Med. Surg.* **12**, 11–14

Vigliani, E. C. and Pernis, B. (1958). 'Immunological factors in the pathogenesis of the hyaline tissue of silicosis.' *Br. J. ind. Med.* **15**, 8–14

Vorwald, A. J. (1960). 'Diffuse fibrogenic pneumoconiosis.' *Ind. Med. Surg.* **29**, 353–358

— Durkan, T. M. and Pratt, P. C. (1951). 'Experimental studies of asbestosis.' *Archs ind. Hyg. occup. Med.* **3**, 1–43

Wagner, J. C. (1963). 'Asbestosis in experimental animals.' *Br. J. ind. Med.* **20**, 1–12

— (1965). 'The sequelae of exposure to asbestos dust.' *Ann. N.Y. Acad. Sci.* **132**, 691–695

— (1971). 'Asbestos cancers.' *J. natn. Cancer Inst.* **46**, v–ix; 5

— (1972a). Personal communication

— (1972b). 'Current opinions on the asbestos cancer problem.' *Ann. occup. Hyg.* **15**, 61–64

— (1972c). 'The significance of asbestos in tissue.' In *Current Problems in the Epidemiology of Cancer and Lymphomas*, pp. 37–46. Ed. by E. Grundmann and H. Tulinius. London; Heinemann; Berlin, Heidelberg, New York; Springer

— (1973). Personal communication

— and Berry, G. (1969). 'Mesotheliomas in rats following inoculation with asbestos.' *Br. J. Cancer* **23**, 567–581

— Sleggs, C. A. and Marchand, P. (1960). 'Diffuse pleural mesothelioma.' *Br. J. ind. Med.* **17**, 260–271

— Munday, D. E. and Harington, J. S. (1962). 'Histochemical demonstration of hyaluronic acid in pleural mesotheliomas.' *J. Path. Bact.* **84**, 73–78

— Berry, G. and Timbrell, V. (1970). 'Mesothelioma in rats.' In *Pneumoconiosis. Proceedings of the International Conference, Johannesburg, 1969*, pp. 216–219. Ed. by H. A. Shapiro. Cape Town; Oxford University Press

— Gilson, J. C. Berry, G. and Timbrell, V. (1971). 'Epidemiology of asbestos cancers.' *Br. med. Bull.* **27**, 71–86

Walther, E. (1970). 'Dust problems in the use of asbestos products'. In *Pneumoconiosis. Proceedings of the International Conference, Johannesburg, 1969*, pp. 37–41. Ed. by H. A. Shapiro. Cape Town; Oxford University Press

Warraki, S. and Herant, Y. (1963). 'Pneumoconiosis in china clay workers.' *Br. J. ind. Med.* **20**, 226–230

Webster, I. (1970a). 'The pathogenesis of asbestosis.' In *Pneumoconiosis. Proceedings of the International Conference, Johannesburg, 1969*, pp. 117–119. Ed. by H. A. Shapiro. Cape Town; Oxford University Press

— (1970b). 'Asbestos exposure in South Africa.' In *Pneumoconiosis. Proceedings of the International Conference, Johannesburg, 1969*, pp. 209–212. Ed. by H. A. Shapiro. Cape Town; Oxford University Press

— (1972). 'The pathology of asbestosis.' In *Medicine in the Mining Industries*, pp. 39–55. Ed. by J. M. Rogan. London; Heinemann

— (1973). 'Asbestos and malignancy.' *S. Afr. med. J.* **47**, 165–171

Weiss, B. and Boettner, E. A. (1967). 'Commercial talc and talcosis.' *Archs envir. Hlth* **14**, 304–308

Whitwell, F. and Rawcliffe, R. M. (1971). 'Diffuse malignant pleural mesothelioma and asbestos exposure.' *Thorax* **26**, 6–22

Willis, R. A. (1967). *Pathology of Tumours*, pp. 181–183. London; Butterworths

Wood, W. B. and Gloyne, S. R. (1934). 'Pulmonary asbestosis.' *Lancet* **2**, 1383–1385

Wright, G. W. (1969). 'Asbestos and health.' *Am. Rev. resp. Dis.* **100**, 467–479

Wyers, H. (1946). Thesis presented to the University of Glasgow for the Degree of Doctor of Medicine

— (1949). 'Asbestosis.' *Postgrad. med. J.* **25**, 631–638

Zolov, C., Burilkov, T. and Babadjav, L. (1967). 'Pleural asbestosis in agricultural workers.' *Envir. Res.* **1**, 287–292

10—Beryllium Disease

Description of the Disease

This is a systemic disorder with predominantly pulmonary involvement occurring in a proportion of workers exposed to beryllium metal or its compounds, the development of which appears, in many cases, to be related to the total 'dose' of beryllium received. It has two forms: an *acute*, non-specific pneumonitis and a *chronic*, 'granulomatous pneumonitis' ending in fibrosis which may cause severe respiratory disability and, ultimately, death from respiratory failure and cor pulmonale. Rarely, death is due to renal failure.

Because it is a systemic disorder caused by beryllium fumes and mists as well as by dusts, and is sometimes confined to the skin alone, it cannot be classified solely as a pneumoconiosis. The term 'berylliosis' is undesirable because it has fostered the conception of a disease confined to the lungs. In view of the many similarities between the chronic form of the disease and 'idiopathic' sarcoidosis Scadding (1967) is content to call it 'beryllium sarcoidosis' and, while this is valid, 'beryllium disease' is an acceptable and more widely current term.

As a result of industrial hygiene measures since 1950 beryllium disease is now uncommon and should become rare. Nevertheless, the clinician must be well acquainted with its manifestations for these reasons: (1) the use of beryllium compounds has greatly increased since that date and will continue to increase; (2) accidental exposure to high concentrations of a compound is always possible; (3) the chronic form of the disease develops in many cases after a latent period of some years; (4) progression from acute to chronic disease may occur without further exposure to beryllium; (5) new cases are now likely to occur singly and their prompt treatment depends upon the disease being quickly recognized; and (6) the possibility that beryllium may be carcinogenic. Hence, it has an importance disproportionate to its rarity.

The acute form of the disease was originally described in Germany (Weber and Englehardt, 1933), Russia (Gelman, 1936) and the United States of America (Van Ordstrand, Hughes and Carmody, 1943) with the clinical features of dermatitis, conjunctivitis, rhinitis, bronchitis, bronchiolitis, pneumonitis and cyanosis. In the majority of cases it was believed to be

358

self-limiting after workers were removed from the source of exposure. But in 1946 Hardy and Tabershaw, in the United States of America, recognized both delayed onset and the chronic form of the disease in workers in the fluorescent lamp industry, and later Hardy (1948) recorded it in persons living adjacent to a factory manufacturing these lamps.

But there was scepticism at the time that beryllium compounds were responsible (Wright, 1948) and for a while the disease was incorrectly attributed to associated fluorides, beryllium being wholly exonerated (Hyslop et al., 1943; Shilen, Galloway and Mellor, 1944). The long time-lapse which frequently exists between exposure and development of disease added to the difficulty. However, beryllium metal or beryllium compounds are now established as the cause of the acute and chronic forms of this disease.

Acute disease is fairly rare today because, apart from accidental massive atmospheric contamination (as may occur in metallurgical processes), industrial hygiene control has greatly reduced the degree of exposure of workers to beryllium and its compounds. Only one such case has been recorded in the United Kingdom (Royston, 1949).

BERYLLIUM AND ITS COMPOUNDS

Metallic beryllium and its compounds are extracted from beryl ore—usually a granitic pegmatite, beryllium aluminium silicate ($3BeO.Al_2O_3.6SiO_2$). Beryl is mined in Brazil, Argentina, India, Rhodesia, South Africa and the United States of America, often as a by-product of mining mica and feldspar. Compounds used in industrial processes are the oxides, hydroxides, sulphates, fluorides, nitrates and synthetic silicates of beryllium.

There are other oxysalts and halides but these are seldom or never found under industrial conditions. All the compounds and the metal itself are potentially hazardous to health. Beryl ore, however, is not considered to be harmful, although prolonged exposure to its dust has apparently caused lesions consistent with beryllium disease in rats and monkeys (Stokinger, 1966).

Beryllium is extracted from the ore by the *sulphate or fluoride processes* in which ore is melted and treated either with concentrated sulphuric acid or with sodium silicofluoride. Both methods produce beryllium hydroxide from which the oxide can be derived by calcination. Chloride, fluoride and oxy-fluoride salts may be produced by electrolytic reduction. Beryllium extraction was not established in a large scale in Britain until the end of the 1950s, prior to which it was imported in the form of beryllium-copper master alloy.

Beryllium of metallurgical grade is vacuum cast and cut into small sections or milled to fine particle size.

Beryllium alloys

A 'master alloy' of beryllium and copper is produced by the reaction of beryllium oxide, carbon and copper in a carbon-arc furnace and usually contains 4 per cent beryllium. 'Industrial alloys' of copper and also steel, aluminium, manganese, nickel and zinc are prepared from the master alloy and contain 2 per cent or less beryllium.

Beryllium phosphors

A *phosphor* is a substance which phosphoresces when stimulated by external radiation. Until about 1950 in Britain (1949 in the United States of America)—when they were replaced by halophosphates—beryllium phosphors were used in fluorescent lighting tubes. Their preparation consisted of mixing oxides of beryllium, magnesium, manganese and zinc with silicic acid, milling the mixture and calcining it at a high temperature. The resulting zinc and manganese beryllium silicate contained a proportion of unreacted beryllium oxide and, apparently, small quantities of cristobalite.

Properties

Beryllium has the important properties of light weight (being the fourth lightest element) and low density yet with strength, hardness and high resistance to corrosion and heat. It is an efficient hardening agent of other metals to which it is added and heat treated; the commonest alloy, beryllium-copper, possesses non-magnetic and non-sparking qualities. Beryllium has a low neutron absorption and yields neutrons when bombarded by α particles; and its low atomic number, 4, renders it translucent to x-rays.

Beryllium oxide is most stable and is endowed with very high thermal conductivity (being superior to alumina in refractory properties especially at temperatures higher than 1,900°C), low thermal expansion, dielectric properties and low neutron absorption.

The vapour pressures of the halides are such that hazardous concentrations of all except the fluoride can be generated when they are subjected to temperatures as low as 158°C, and the volatilization of beryllium oxide is greatly increased in the presence of water vapour (Tepper, Hardy and Chamberlin, 1961). Vapour evolved condenses as fume.

Uses and sources of exposure

There are three situations in which exposure has occurred in the past and continue to be a potential risk today: occupational, para-occupational and neighbourhood. Beryllium or its compounds may become airborne in aerosol form as a dust, fume or mist according to the process involved.

Occupational exposure

Fume and dust are evolved during extraction of ore and the manufacture of master and industrial alloys; and one or other is produced by annealing furnaces, forging, casting, knocking-out and fettling castings; by hot-rolling industrial alloy in strip mills, and by heating, milling, and hot and cold pressing blocks of the metal. Any operation involving heat treatment of 2 per cent alloy is potentially dangerous, and chronic disease due to 1·8 per cent alloy has been recorded (Israel and Cooper, 1964).

Blocks of pure metal undergo corrosion in a humid atmosphere, which may be present under storage conditions, with the formation of a white powder containing beryllium oxide on their surfaces. The powder can be easily disturbed and become airborne.

Reclamation of non-ferrous scrap metals by melting down in a furnace can be particularly dangerous if an unsuspected beryllium alloy is included.

The most hazardous use of a beryllium until 1950 or thereabouts was in the fluorescent lamp industry, established commercially about 1940. It caused about half the cases of chronic beryllium disease up to 1966 (Hardy, Rabe and Lorch, 1967). All stages of manufacture were potentially dangerous from the preparation of the zinc and beryllium phosphor to coating the lamp tubes during which much phosphor dust contaminated with beryllium oxide was released, both naturally and accidentally, from spillage. Breakage of tubes by accident or during disposal also gave rise to dust. In Britain the manufacture, and certainly the disposal, of beryllium-containing fluorescent lamps continued for a few years after being stopped in the United States of America in 1949. But the use of phosphors in the manufacture of 'neon' sign tubes survived still longer. Many cases of disease from this source were not manifest until at least five to ten years after exposure ceased.

Beryllium silicate is used to coat high-energy cathode ray tubes for radar and similar installations, and may contain about 0·5 per cent beryllium oxide as an impurity.

Beryllium is employed in the manufacture of various non-ferrous alloys which have a wide application in modern technology: in electrical equipment (especially as beryllium-copper in integrated circuits), computers and other electronic devices; in aircraft and rocket parts including heat-shields used in the Apollo and other moon flights; in guidance systems, and in non-sparking tools, and the moving parts of engines. Beryllium metal and oxide are employed as reflectors to increase neutron flux in atomic reactors, and the metal was until recently an important constituent of encasement 'cans' in nuclear power systems, but is now replaced by stainless steel.

Machining and drilling operations of the metal and its alloys throw off metallic particles of mostly 'non-respirable' size, but a proportion may be less than 10 μm. When the amount of waste produced is substantial, dry machining is used to facilitate its recovery and much dust is then produced. Cutting oils are employed when the operation causes little waste and these capture most of the particles, but should the oils be re-used for other operations not involving beryllium they may present an unsuspected source of exposure. Wet grinding, honing and polishing, however, give rise to mists carrying beryllium particles. Deburring metallic components with high-speed burrs generates dust in close proximity to the operator's face (Benoit, 1967).

Welding of beryllium alloys produces beryllium oxide fume.

Beryllium metal finds other important uses in the windows of x-ray tubes, in optical systems employed by astronauts, and as a filler in moulded plastics. In the United States of America it has been employed—probably in powder form—in rocket fuels to increase their calorific value and, hence, increase the thrust of a given weight of fuel. This application appears to have been limited to the fourth stage of satellite launching vehicles in which there is about 140 lb of propellant containing approximately 12 per cent of beryllium. It has been used in a number of launchings since 1961. Static firing of rocket motors for experimental or ballistic assessment has also been carried out (Maxwell, 1971). Beryllium has not been used, however, for rocket propellants in Great Britain.

Analysis of rocket exhaust products indicates that about 50 per cent of the total beryllium is in the form of the oxide, 40 per cent the fluoride and the remainder mainly the chloride (Robinson and Schaffner, 1968).

Static firing of rocket motors would appear to present a significant risk, but as it is done in an enclosure which permits the exhaust to be scrubbed and filtered before discharge into the atmosphere, exposure should not occur. Firing has also been done in desert areas under favourable meteorological conditions with the operators sealed off from the atmosphere during firing and until the exhaust cloud has completely dispersed. The atmosphere and soil on the site and in the neighbourhood are monitored for beryllium, and the greatest care taken in handling and decontaminating the test stand and spent materials (Maxwell, 1971). Nonetheless, a potential risk of exposure would seem to exist.

Beryllium oxide is employed in technical ceramics (such as crucibles); in other refractories; in microwave windows and, combined with beryllium, in metal ceramics—or *cermets* (that is, materials consisting of a ceramic heat-bonded to a metal)—for rocket motor parts, nose cones, and in the manufacture of blading for jet engines. Technical ceramic shapes are slip-cast and pressed by cold and hot methods. These and other refractory shapes are fettled and finished by wet grinding. In the absence of good housekeeping and other hygienic measures it is evident that these processes could cause accumulation of dust on floors, benches and ledges.

Beryllium halides have some use as catalysts in certain organic chemical reactions.

The use of beryllium compounds by laboratory workers—chemists and physicists—has occasionally caused disease (Agate, 1948; McCallum, Rannie and Verity, 1961); cleaning exhaust ventilation ducts, dust collectors, cyclones and high-efficiency filters used for air-cleaning in dry beryllium processes, and the task of replacing filters may be a source of significant exposure.

Although many processes or operations are now totally enclosed or subjected to efficient exhaust ventilation, the possibility of hazardous airborne contamination exists wherever beryllium and its compounds are used. The importance of this is emphasized by the fact that, although there were in the United States of America at the end of the 1950s firms processing beryllium which were over-apprehensive of the hazard and applied excessive control measures, there were others which, while aware of the risk, used inadequate protection, and yet others which were wholly unaware of it (Cholak, 1961).

Accidental breakdown of dust and fume control systems or of storage containers may cause sudden high-level contamination of the atmosphere.

As a general principle it should be noted that because particles of beryllium metal or its compounds are so very light they readily become airborne.

Para-occupational

Men not involved in beryllium processes have sometimes been exposed to risk when working, for example, in the vicinity of furnaces melting non-ferrous metal scrap where factory arrangements have not been satisfactory. Spillage of powdered beryllium metal from container bags during transportation and subsequent brushing up are potential sources of concentrated exposure to dockers and other transport workers. Office staff and relatives visiting workers in beryllium factories have developed beryllium disease in the past (Sander, 1950).

Neighbourhood

Populations in the vicinity of a factory have been exposed indirectly to beryllium compounds in two ways; from the discharge of contaminated air from smoke stacks or from exhaust systems when not filtered or otherwise treated; and from workers' contaminated clothing taken home for cleaning or laundering. The latter was probably the more important of these two sources of exposure although cases have tended to occur in the direction of prevailing wind (Lieben and Metzner, 1959). Some neighbourhood cases with low exposure have suffered from more severe beryllium disease than beryllium workers themselves (Sterner and Eisenbud, 1951). This suggests the possibility of immunity being involved.

As the beryllium-containing fuel for satellite rockets already referred to operates at high altitudes it has been supposed that this does not offer any hazard to health, but the possibility that open-air experimental firings might do so cannot be excluded.

THE NATURAL HISTORY OF BERYLLIUM DISEASE

Beryllium metal and its compounds cause skin disease and conjunctivitis by direct contact, and respiratory and systemic disease by entry into, and absorption from, the upper respiratory tract and the lungs.

Acute disease has all the characteristics of a poisoning and is determined by the intensity of exposure. Contact dermatitis and conjunctivitis may result from the direct action of the soluble acid salts, and small ulcers of the skin, from the implantation of crystals of a soluble compound. Rhinitis, tracheitis, bronchitis and pneumonitis may be caused by inhalation of a mist of the soluble salts or of dust and fume of relatively insoluble compounds—chiefly the oxide—and pure beryllium metal (Aub and Grier, 1949). Skin disease may occur independently of respiratory disease but, after resolution, tends to recur earlier and more severely on second exposure when it may be associated with pneumonitis; this observation is consistent with acquired hypersensitivity playing a role in the causation of the disease.

As 'acute' disease (chemical 'pneumonitis') may sometimes be of insidious onset its definition is arbitrary and is taken to include manifestations of disease of *less than one year's duration* (Tepper, Hardy and Chamberlin, 1961). Acute disease has two forms: a fulminating illness occurring within about 72 hours of a brief, but massive, exposure and having a high mortality; and a more slowly developing disease following a longer period of exposure to lower concentrations of beryllium compounds. Illness similar to metal fume fever (*see* Chapter 12) was also described in Russia (Gelman, 1936) but has not been observed in the United States of America; it is likely that this was due to fumes other than those of beryllium compounds.

By contrast, *chronic disease* has none of the characteristics of an intoxication and has followed episodes of acute disease in about 6 per cent of cases after a variable length of time (Hardy, Rabe and Lorch, 1967). It exhibits some, but not all, of the characteristics of 'idiopathic' sarcoidosis and chiefly affects the lungs, although granulomas of skin may occur in the absence of disease of the lungs and other organs.

A record of all known cases of beryllium disease in the United States of America, established in 1952 and referred to as the United States Beryllium Case Registry (Tepper, Hardy and Chamberlin, 1961), has been, and is, an invaluable source of information. However, it and data from other countries are, in general, wanting in three important ways: the size of the populations which have been at risk are unknown; details of the degree of beryllium in the lungs and other organs of affected individuals are incomplete; and not all cases of the disease have been diagnosed or recorded. Hence, there is some uncertainty about the prevalence and behaviour of the disease.

Both sexes may be afflicted by either acute or chronic forms. In 'neighbourhood cases' chronic disease has been more common in women than in men,

TABLE 10.1

DELAY IN ONSET—CHRONIC DISEASE

Time	No. of cases
< 1 month	126
1 month–1 year	27
1–5 years	89
5–10 years	56
> 10 years	12
	Total 310

From Hardy *et al.*, 1967, by courtesy of Dr H. L. Hardy and the Editor of the *Journal of Occupational Medicine*

but it is not clear whether this has been due solely to the concentrations of the dust of beryllium compounds to which women were exposed when handling or cleaning contaminated clothing brought home from the factory or whether undue susceptibility played some part. The disease has also occurred in children (Hall *et al.*, 1959).

Data from the Beryllium Case Registry have shown that the early uncontrolled use of beryllium and its compounds produced a high incidence of disease but that, as the intensity of exposure has been reduced, the number of cases has fallen; and, at the same time, delay in onset of the disease has increased and its severity decreased (Hardy, 1965). Indeed, a continual decline in mortality has occurred over the years, confirming that the disease has become milder: for example, the fatality rate in Registry cases in 1943 was 8·5 per cent but in 1963 was 1·3 per cent (Hardy, 1965).

The latent period from last exposure or from an acute episode to the development of chronic disease may be more than fifteen years in some cases (Table 10.1), and the longer the period the milder it appears to be (Hardy, Rabe and Lorch, 1967). This, of course, means that persons with chronic disease are living longer than they did in the early 1950s.

This trend has been maintained since hygiene control measures were introduced in the 1950s and is strong evidence that, in most cases, the disease is dose related (Hardy, Rabe and Lorch, 1967). But individual susceptibility also appears to be an important determining factor in some cases for there is only a weak correlation between the attack rate of chronic disease and the duration of exposure, and it sometimes occurs after what has appeared to be trivial exposure to beryllium compounds, but this may be more apparent than real. Furthermore, lung analyses from routine autopsies of persons with no lung disease who lived near a beryllium plant have shown the presence of similar quantities of beryllium to those found in the lungs of patients with beryllium disease (Chamberlin, Jennings and Lieben, 1957). This aspect of the matter is discussed later in more detail.

Prevalence

By comparison with the United States of America few cases of beryllium disease have been recorded in Britain. There are probably a number of reasons for this. Beryllium compounds were introduced somewhat later into industry and ore extraction was not established until the 1950s when the health hazards were well recognized; beryllium phosphors were in use for only a brief period; some cases of acute and chronic disease probably escaped diagnosis especially in view of the delay in onset which may occur in both types of the disease—chronic in particular—after exposure, and also the failure of physicians to elicit the industrial history. There were 822 cases in the Beryllium Case Registry in the United States of America in 1972 (Hardy, 1972). In Britain at least 36 cases are known to have occurred since 1948, although it is certain that there have been others which remained unrecognized. The most recent cases of chronic disease were diagnosed in 1970.

Absorption and excretion of beryllium compounds

Information in man is incomplete but it appears that the soluble compounds are absorbed fairly readily from the lungs after inhalation although a variable quantity remains within them, whereas beryllium oxide is very slowly eliminated. Excretion occurs mainly via the kidneys and the amount excreted appears to depend upon the solubility of the compounds inhaled (Klemperer, Martin and Van Riper, 1951). A proportion which is not excreted, and is greater in acute than chronic disease, is stored in the skeleton, liver, spleen and lymph nodes (Tepper, Hardy and Chamberlin, 1961). There is no evident correlation between the presence or severity of disease and the quantity of beryllium excreted (Klemperer, Martin and Van Riper, 1951; Lieben, Dattoli and Vought, 1966).

Beryllium apparently crosses the placental barrier but no ascribable disease has been observed in infants (Tepper, Hardy and Chamberlin, 1961). Pregnancy, however, is apt to trigger off active disease, and women of childbearing age should not be subjected to the risk of beryllium exposure (Hardy, 1965).

Experimentally, beryllium salts are absorbed from the lungs at a rate which varies with the species of animal and are stored mainly in the skeleton (Stokinger, Steadman and Root, 1951; Van Cleave and Kaylor, 1955), but the relatively insoluble beryllium oxide is almost completely retained in the lungs (Stokinger, Steadman and Root, 1951). It has been suggested that this may be due to beryllium being complexed to lung tissue and only slowly released as the precipitates dissolve (Reeves, 1968).

Beryllium competes with magnesium and, experimentally, has been shown to inhibit the synthesis of desoxyribonucleic acid (Witschi, 1968), apparently by inhibiting the magnesium-dependent enzyme deoxythymidine kinase (Mainigi and Bresnick, 1969). But what significance this may have in human disease is not clear.

PATHOLOGY

As this book is concerned with lung disease the pathology and pathogenesis of beryllium disease of the skin and other organs will receive only incidental attention.

ACUTE DISEASE

Upper respiratory tract
The mucosa is oedematous and hyperaemic.

Lungs

Macroscopic appearances
In fatal cases, the lungs are heavy and have a firm, liver-like consistency. The pleura is not thickened although there may be some recent deposition of fibrin. Their cut surfaces have a pink to blue-grey colour, and a frothy, often bloodstained fluid can be expressed from them. The trachea, bronchi and bronchioles are oedematous and red, and hilar and bronchopulmonary lymph nodes are enlarged (Hazard, 1959).

Microscopic appearances
Alveolar spaces and walls are stuffed with fluid exudate which contains lymphocytes, large monocytes, plasma cells and cellular debris, but few neutrophil leucocytes (Vorwald, 1966); and foamy desquamated pneumocytes may be present in the spaces. A variable—often small—amount of protein-aceous material may also be seen adhering to alveolar walls. Organization of this exudate frequently occurs and is continuous with similar early organiza-tion within the walls.

Although occasional giant cells may be observed, granulomas (*see* next section) are uniformly absent (Freiman and Hardy, 1970).

The only abnormality to be found in the lungs of persons who have re-covered from the illness may be a very slight excess of connective tissue elements (Vorwald, 1966).

There is nothing characteristic in any of these appearances which are also seen in other chemical pneumonias.

Outside the lungs, centrilobular necrosis of the liver and coagulation necrosis of bone marrow have also been reported (Tepper, Hardy and Chamberlin, 1961).

CHRONIC DISEASE

Lungs

Macroscopic appearances
The visceral pleura is thickened and there may be extensive adhesion with the

parietal layer. In some cases there are thick-walled blebs on the lung surfaces similar to those seen in 'honeycomb' lungs. The lungs are heavy and their cut surfaces reveal grey-white interstitial fibrosis (*Figure 10.1*) and scattered nodules a few millimetres in diameter, and there may be thick-walled cysts— often quite large—associated with the fibrotic areas. No particular zones appear to be favoured by the lesions. Hilar lymph nodes are only slightly enlarged (Jones Williams, 1958).

None of these features is characteristic.

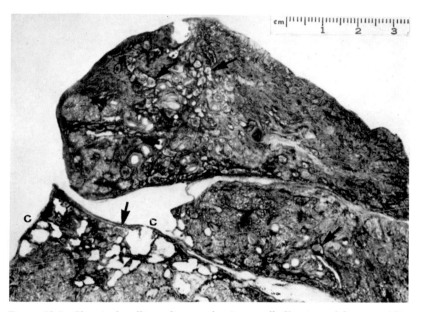

Figure 10.1. Chronic beryllium disease showing small fibrotic nodules resembling silicotic nodules (arrowed) and cystic areas ('c'). The upper and middle lobes are much contracted due to fibrosis and the pulmonary pleura is moderately thickened; this is particularly evident round the middle lobe and apex of lower lobe. (Paper-mounted lung section)

Microscopic appearances

In the majority of cases, the appearances are those of chronic interstitial pneumonitis with sarcoid-like granulomas, although these are not invariably present. The degree of cellular infiltration differs greatly in different cases; histiocytes predominate but there are also numerous lymphocytes and a variable number of plasma cells. The histiocytes tend to form into groups ranging from a few cells to large well-demarcated granulomas, but in some cases they are widely disseminated interstitially and are difficult to differentiate from lymphocytes.

The granulomas, which are also distributed in subpleural, peribronchial and perivascular sites, consist of epithelioid and Langhan's-type giant cells from which central necrosis is usually absent or only slight. There is often a surrounding infiltration of lymphocytes and plasma cells. Schaumann bodies (that is, conchoidal bodies and crystalline material) and asteroid bodies may

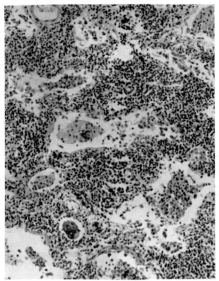

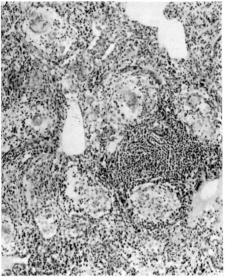

Figure 10.2. Chronic beryllium disease, Group IA. Extensive interstitial cellular infiltration without granuloma formation. (Magnification ×25)

Figure 10.3. Chronic beryllium disease, Group IB. Pronounced interstitial cellular infiltration and well-formed sarcoid-like granulomas with Langhan's giant cells. (Magnification ×25)

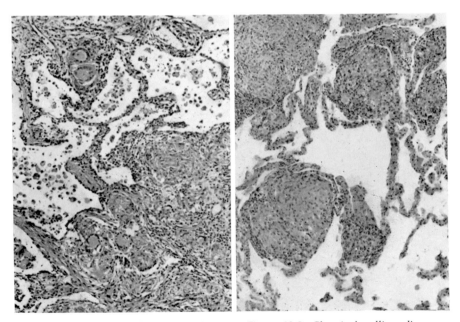

Figure 10.4. Chronic beryllium disease, Group II. Minimal interstitial cellular infiltration and well-formed sarcoid-like granulomas. (Magnification ×25)

Figure 10.5. Chronic beryllium disease, Group II. Appearances identical with idiopathic sarcoidosis. Prominent granuloma formation and negligible interstitial cellular infiltration (Magnification ×25)

Figures 10.2 to 10.5 inclusive are reproduced by courtesy of Drs Freiman and Hardy and the Editor of Human Pathology

be present in both epithelioid and giant cells in the same way as they are in 'idiopathic' sarcoid granulomas (Jones Williams, 1971). The birefringent, plate-like crystals in Schaumann bodies which consist of complex calcium mucoprotein and may precede their formation (Jones Williams, 1958) probably consist of calcite. Neither Schaumann nor chonchoidal bodies have diagnostic significance.

The evidence of light microscopy (Jones Williams, 1958), histochemistry (Jones Williams and Williams, 1967), the enzyme content (Williams, Jones Williams and Williams, 1969) and fine structure (Jones Williams, Fry and James, 1972) of beryllium granulomas indicates that their morphology is

TABLE 10.2

HISTOLOGICAL CLASSIFICATION OF CHRONIC BERYLLIUM DISEASE

Histological characteristics	Group I		Group II
	Sub-group IA	Sub-group IB	
Interstitial cellular infiltration	Moderate to marked		Slight or absent
Granuloma formation	Poorly formed or absent	Well formed	Numerous and well formed
Conchoidal bodies	Variable; frequently present and numerous		Few or absent

By courtesy of Freiman and Hardy, 1970, and the Editor of *Human Pathology*

identical to the granulomas of 'idiopathic' sarcoidosis, 'farmers' lung', Crohn's disease and non-caseating tuberculosis and can only be distinguished by chemical analysis of lung tissue (Jones Williams, 1971) (*see* Beryllium Content of the Lungs).

As a result of a study of the cases known to the United States Beryllium Case Registry, Freiman and Hardy (1970) have found that the histological features of chronic disease tend to fall naturally into one of three categories which they designate as Group I (which is subdivided into Sub-groups A and B) and Group II according to the relative degrees of interstitial cellular infiltration and granuloma formation and of the number of conchoidal and Schaumann bodies present. This classification is shown in Table 10.2 and the histological categories in *Figures 10.2 to 10.5*.

Cases which are difficult to classify usually fall into Sub-group IB.

Conchoidal bodies are found in about two-thirds of Group I cases but are relatively infrequent in Group II cases; and although they are not pathognomonic of chronic beryllium disease, they are not found with such frequency in any other disease (Freiman and Hardy, 1970)—apart from 'idiopathic' sarcoidosis (Jones Williams, 1967).

Granulomas are subsequently replaced by collagenous tissue and epithelioid cells are gradually obliterated by interlacing strands of hyaline material.

Well-demarcated fibrotic nodules which are partially or completely hyalinized are present in some 40 per cent of cases. These lesions vary from very few to large numbers, in which case they may be the predominant lesions (Freiman and Hardy, 1970). They are also found in hilar lymph nodes. The periphery of the nodules consists of a fairly narrow zone of fibrosis and the central hyalinized zone usually contains some black pigment and is sometimes necrotic; deposits of calcium are often present in the necrotic areas. The nodules may resemble silicotic nodules very closely although some exhibit peripheral granulomatous infiltration (*Figure 10.6*). The presence of these nodules in association with Group II lesions appears to be a valuable feature in distinguishing chronic beryllium disease from 'idiopathic' sarcoidosis (Freiman and Hardy, 1970). *Figure 10.1* shows an example of predominantly nodular lesions.

Diffuse interstitial fibrosis (chronic fibrosing 'alveolitis') of moderate to

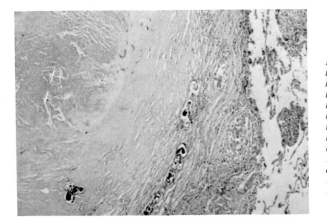

Figure 10.6. Chronic beryllium disease. Fibrotic nodular lesion with necrotic hyalinized central zone. Calcified inclusions (small densely black areas) are present in the fibrotic zone and granulomatous infiltration can be seen at the periphery. Magnification × 10; reproduced by courtesy of Drs Freiman and Hardy and the Editor of Human Pathology)

advanced degree is present in about half the cases. It is frequently found around granulomas some of which may also be partly or wholly fibrotic.

Endarteritis is sometimes found in the areas of fibrosis. Emphysema is not a characteristic feature of the disease although scar ('irregular') emphysema may occur in relation to fibrosis.

As the microscopical appearances are indistinguishable from those of 'idiopathic' sarcoidosis it is not possible to make an unequivocal diagnosis of chronic beryllium disease on these grounds alone (Jones Williams, 1967b).

Extrapulmonary
Granulomas may also be found in the skin, cervical, intrathoracic and abdominal lymph nodes, the kidneys, liver, spleen, bone marrow, skeletal muscle and myocardium. Skin granulomas may precede the lung disease (Jones Williams, 1971) but, unlike those of 'idiopathic' sarcoidosis, they may ulcerate (Jones Williams, 1967a). Although they contain particles of beryllium metal or phosphors when they are due to direct traumatic incursion of beryllium fragments, they may also occur in individuals who have been subjected only to respiratory exposure (Stoeckle, Hardy and Weber, 1969); in which case beryllium particles are not present.

BERYLLIUM CONTENT OF THE LUNGS

There have been many quantitative determinations of beryllium in lung tissue, but only a few of levels in other organs. The content of beryllium in the lungs bears no relationship to the type and severity of disease, nor, indeed, to its presence; and it varies greatly in different parts of the lungs without exhibiting any consistent pattern of distribution (Tepper, Hardy and Chamberlin, 1961). Levels in the hilar lymph nodes are generally higher than those in the lungs. Analyses of other organs—liver, kidney, spleen, bone—have revealed much smaller quantities of beryllium than the lungs but, once again, there was wide variation.

Beryllium disease is rarely seen without a measurable amount of beryllium in the lungs, the detection of which depends upon sensitive techniques and an adequate amount of tissue for analysis. In chronic disease the beryllium content of the lungs has been found to range from 0·3 to 28 μg per 100 g of tissue (Tepper, Hardy and Chamberlin, 1961) and as much as 1,842 μg per 100 g of lung tissue has been found in the lungs of beryllium-exposed workers in the absence of disease (Metzner and Leiben, 1961). With recently developed techniques it is possible to locate beryllium within lesions (*see* later under Diagnosis).

However, small quantities of beryllium may sometimes be found in the lungs of persons with no known industrial exposure to beryllium compounds and when conventional spectrographic methods of analysis are employed, the largest amount which has been detected is 1·98 μg per 100 g of tissue—the average value being 0·33 μg per 100 g of tissue (Cholak, 1959). Under these circumstances the presence of beryllium may have been due to contamination in some of the earlier estimations, but urban air may contain significant amounts of beryllium in the form of beryl in the ash of certain fossil fuels. Air samples from some thirty metropolitan areas in the United States of America have been found to contain from 0·0001 to 0·003 μg per m^3 (Chambers, Foster and Cholak, 1955). Spectrographic methods do not, of course, distinguish beryl from beryllium compounds.

Failure to detect beryllium in the lungs of exposed persons is due to faulty analytical technique.

At this point it is appropriate to summarize the relationship which beryllium in the tissues and urine may have to the presence of disease. (The means of determining of beryllium in the urine is mentioned under Other Investigations.)

(1) Beryllium may be present in the urine of ex-beryllium workers with no detectable disease years after exposure has ceased.

(2) The presence of beryllium in the lungs or urine implies only that there has been past exposure to beryllium; it is not proof of disease.

(3) There is no correlation between the quantity of beryllium in the lungs and urine and the severity of chronic disease.

(4) Beryllium may be absent from the urine in the presence of chronic disease.

(5) Beryllium may be absent from the lungs in some cases of chronic disease although present in significant amount in other tissues.

(6) The distribution of beryllium in the lungs with chronic disease is quite irregular and it may be absent from some areas.

371

BIOCHEMICAL ABNORMALITIES

There is often an increase in urinary calcium in patients with chronic beryllium disease, and, if renal function is impaired, hypercalcaemia occurs. The underlying reason for the high urinary calcium is obscure but as beryllium is known to be excreted by the tubules (Underwood, 1951) cellular intoxication at this level is a possible explanation; it is not attributed to immobilization of the patient or to prolonged treatment with steroids (Tepper, Hardy and Chamberlin, 1961). Renal failure is, however, rare unless nephrolithiasis occurs (*see* later—Complications). It is believed that increased urinary excretion of calcium may be related to activity of the disease (Stoeckle, Hardy and Weber, 1969). Steroid therapy results in return to normal of urinary calcium levels (Hardy, 1972).

Serum alkaline phosphatase has generally been reported as normal (Tepper, Hardy and Chamberlin, 1961). This does not appear to be consistent with an inhibiting effect of beryllium on this enzyme observed *in vitro* (Bamberger, Botbol and Cabrini, 1968). But extrapolation of *in vitro* to *in vivo* observations is not necessarily valid. In animals beryllium has been shown both to activate and to depress this enzyme (Aldridge, Barnes and Denz, 1950; Du Bois, 1950); or, again, to have no significant effect upon it (Vorwald, Reeves and Urban, 1966).

Hyperuricaemia, which is observed in 36 to 50 per cent of patients with 'idiopathic' sarcoidosis, is also found in 40 per cent who have chronic beryllium disease (Kelley, Goldfinger and Hardy, 1969). This appears to be due to reduced renal clearance rather than to an increased production of uric acid, but the cause of this is not understood. There is no correlation between hyperuricaemia and the type and duration of exposure to beryllium, severity of disease, or the presence of beryllium in the urine (Kelley, Goldfinger and Hardy, 1969).

CHANGES IN IMMUNOGLOBULINS

Increase in serum globulin levels is almost always present at one stage or another of symptomatic disease (Tepper, Hardy and Chamberlin, 1961). In the majority of patients with cutaneous or chronic lung disease this is due to an increased concentration of IgG, and not IgA or IgM. In some workers who have been in contact with the metal or its compounds for years, but who have shown no evidence of beryllium disease, IgG is also significantly raised (Resnick, Roche and Morgan, 1970). These observations are consistent with an allergic response and are, of course, in no way specific to chronic beryllium disease. Hypergammaglobulinaemia is also observed in 'idiopathic' sarcoidosis due mostly to IgG, although IgA is found in almost a third of cases and IgM occasionally (Sharma *et al.*, 1971).

The possibility of immune reactions occurring in the pathogenesis of beryllium disease is discussed in the next section.

PATHOGENESIS

The site and intensity of reaction to beryllium depends upon aerosol particle size, solubility of the salts and duration of exposure. The soluble salts are the chief cause of both upper and lower respiratory disease, but beryllium metal, oxides and phosphors are also an important cause of lung disease. Atmospheric concentrations of beryllium compounds which cause acute disease have been much greater than those which give rise to chronic disease.

Beryllium oxide and the soluble salts cause an acute pneumonitis in various species of experimental animals identical to that which occurs in man (Hall *et al.*, 1950; Stokinger *et al.*, 1950), and the fluoride is potentially more toxic than other beryllium compounds (Stokinger *et al.*, 1953). Chronic disease, with granulomas similar to human disease, has been produced in animals by beryllium oxide (Policard, 1950; Spencer *et al.*, 1968) and sulphate (Vorwald, Reeves and Urban, 1966). However, extrapolation of animal observations to human disease requires critical appraisal in relation to occupational features.

Although acute disease appears to be a direct result of intoxication, chronic disease has some features which are consistent with, but not conclusive evidence of, an immunological reaction:

(1) Only a small proportion of persons exposed to low concentrations of beryllium appear to develop disease, suggesting host susceptibility, although this may become less evident if detailed occupational and clinical information is available (Hardy, 1972).

(2) Recurrence of skin lesions following initial resolution sometimes in association with pneumonitis, after a second exposure to beryllium.

(3) A positive delayed-type skin response may follow the beryllium patch test (q.v.), and patients with beryllium disease have developed sarcoid-like granulomas at the site of a positive patch test after about three weeks (Norris and Peard, 1963).

(4) Lack of correlation between the amount of beryllium in the lungs and the severity of the disease. It appears that beryllium may move in and out of the lungs (Hardy, 1972).

(5) Elevation of serum IgG.

Furthermore, repeated intradermal injection of beryllium oxide into a human volunteer has resulted in epithelioid cell granulomas after as little as 1 μg of the oxide, and this is regarded as evidence of 'granulomatous hypersensitivity' by Epstein (1967).

Experimental work in animals indicates that beryllium can induce delayed hypersensitivity (Chiappino, Cirla and Vigliani, 1969). Beryllium has a high affinity for proteins and when in combination may form an antigenic stimulus at local sites in the lungs and elsewhere (Belman, 1969). Beryllium sulphate has been shown to be a potent adjuvent in increasing antibody response to antigen (*Maia squinado haemocyanin*) after its uptake by mouse macrophages, and this effect does not require antigen and beryllium to be present in the same macrophage (Unanue, Askonas and Allison, 1969).

Observations in guinea-pigs have also shown that passive transfer of lymphocytes, but not of serum, from beryllium-sensitized to normal guinea-pigs resulted in the transfer of skin sensitivity (Cirla, Barbiono di Belgiojoso and Chiappino, 1968); furthermore, the pulmonary response to beryllium (the severity of which depends upon the extent of exposure) can be alleviated by previous repeated intradermal injections of beryllium (Reeves *et al.*,

1972) a situation which appears to be analagous to the difference in severity of disease which may occur in human beings with 'neighbourhood' and occupational exposure to beryllium.

Perhaps the most significant support for an immunological hypothesis lies in the *in vitro* observation that macrophages from human subjects with apparent 'granulomatous hypersensitivity' to beryllium when exposed to beryllium oxide and then incubated with autologous sensitized lymphocytes, cause the lymphocytes to undergo rapid blastogenic transformation, whereas lymphocytes from unresponsive subjects remain unaffected (Hanifin, Epstein and Cline, 1970). By contrast with skin 'granulomas' caused by the injection of quartz (which form in all subjects tested irrespective of previous sensitization and consist of perivascular clusters of macrophages containing quartz particles), beryllium salts cause organized epithelioid cell granulomas in sensitized subjects only (Hanifin, Epstein and Cline, 1970). Blood lymphocytes from subjects with beryllium granulomas when cultured with beryllium oxide liberate a factor which inhibits macrophage migration, whereas those from normal persons do not. This may prove to be a valuable test in the diagnosis of beryllium disease (Henderson *et al.*, 1972). It is possible that a macrophage inhibitory factor may play a role in the formation of beryllium granulomas.

The experimental evidence, therefore, gives some support to the suggestion that delayed hypersensitivity is related to the pathogenesis of chronic beryllium disease in man, and that it may be a cell-mediated (Type IV) reaction.

Carcinoma of the lung has been caused in rats and monkeys following the inhalation or intratracheal injection of beryllium compounds (Vorwald, Reeves and Urban, 1966). Although there is some suggestion that exposure to beryllium may be associated with the development of bronchial carcinoma in man, this has not been established with any certainty (*see* section on Complications). Beryllium also causes rickets and osteosclerosis in experimental animals (Vorwald, Reeves and Urban, 1966), but these diseases have not been observed in man (Collins, 1966); and, although periosteal thickening has been noted, it is not believed to be of significance (Tepper, Hardy and Chamberlin, 1961).

CLINICAL FEATURES

Symptoms

The Beryllium Case Registry figures have shown that respiratory disease is the commonest mode of presentation (Hardy, Rabe and Lorch, 1967).

In *acute disease*, depending upon the magnitude of exposure, there is irritation of the nose and pharynx with copious mucoid nasal discharge and mild epistaxis; paroxysmal cough which raises bloodstained sputum when pneumonitis is present, but is non-productive in its absence; a burning, tight sensation in the centre of the chest, and moderate breathlessness on effort. These symptoms commence within about 72 hours of heavy exposure. In persons who have worked with soluble acid salts there may also be irritation of the eyes, and, in some cases, an itching, burning skin rash of exposed parts of the body, without respiratory symptoms. When the onset is slower, or subacute (usually within a few weeks of first exposure), there is cough of gradually increasing severity which is frequently paroxysmal and small quantities of sputum which may be bloodstained, progressively increasing breathlessness on exertion, and pronounced lassitude with anorexia and loss of weight. If these symptoms persist for more than twelve months the disease is said to be chronic.

In *chronic disease* symptoms develop insidiously, commonly within a month to some five years—rarely as much as twenty-four years (Freiman and Hardy, 1970)—after last exposure, but, as previously stated they may become established after the patient has partly recovered from acute disease. The most common is dyspnoea on exertion which is, in some cases, the only symptom. The next most common is an irritating, usually unproductive, cough which is worse in the mornings and after exertion and may be paroxysmal, ending in retching and vomiting; it is possible that this may be due to granulomas in bronchial walls (Tepper, Hardy and Chamberlin, 1961). Occasionally there is mucoid, or less often, purulent sputum, and, though haemoptysis has been recorded, it is rare. There is progressive, unremittent breathlessness on effort, and air hunger or orthopnoea develops in advanced disease in which anorexia, malaise, lassitude and severe loss of weight are usual. Sudden worsening of dyspnoea with chest pain may occur as a result of spontaneous pneumothorax (*see* section on Complications).

However, chronic disease may be symptomless or associated with only slight cough and mild breathlessness on effort, but sudden exacerbation may occur (possibly due to mobilization of tissue-stored beryllium) in relation to respiratory infection, surgery, pregnancy and re-exposure to beryllium compounds.

Physical signs

In *acute disease* there is low-grade fever, central cyanosis, rapid heart and respiratory rates, and widespread crepitations over the lungs. Contact dermatitis which may result from exposure to the acid salts is of papulovesicular type, sometimes weeping and oedematous, on the hands, arms, trunk, head and neck. Conjunctivitis is often associated with pronounced conjunctival oedema.

In cases of mild *chronic disease* there may be no abnormal signs but in more advanced disease, finger clubbing is present in about 20 per cent of cases (Stoeckle, Hardy and Weber, 1969), there may be central cyanosis, and pleural friction with crepitations (which predominate in the upper or lower parts of the lungs according to the distribution of the disease) are usual. In uncomplicated disease the liver is sometimes slightly enlarged, but not tender, (Hall *et al.*, 1959).

During exacerbation or rapid progression of chronic disease there may be fever up to about 38·9°C (102°F) with rigors, and in advanced disease there are signs of congestive heart failure. Pronounced cachexia was also a feature of the disease in the past but is now rarely seen.

Skin granulomas, indistinguishable from those of 'idiopathic' sarcoidosis, may develop at some stage of the illness but, unlike the persistent lesions caused by local traumatic implantation of particles of beryllium compounds,

375

resolve with steroid therapy or remission of disease. Lupus pernio and erythema nodosum do not occur.

INVESTIGATIONS

Lung function

The functional abnormalities of acute disease are those associated with pneumonia or pulmonary oedema and they consist of hypoxaemia and hyper-capnoea resulting from uneven distribution of ventilation and perfusion (*see* Chapter 1), and airways obstruction. The severity of these changes depends upon the extent of disease. Unless resolution is incomplete and the disease becomes chronic, function subsequently returns to normal.

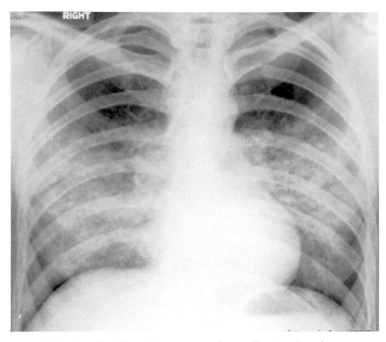

Figure 10.7. Acute beryllium disease in a male metallurgist. Complete recovery and clearing of the radiograph followed. (By courtesy of Dr Harriet Hardy)

The typical changes in chronic disease are those of diffuse interstitial fibrosis (chronic fibrosing 'alveolitis'): that is, the 'restrictive syndrome', hyperventilation and impairment of gas transfer. In the granulomatous stage of the disease, before fibrosis has occurred and when reduction in gas transfer is due mainly to impaired diffusion across the alveolar-capillary membrane, function may be improved towards normal by treatment with corticosteroids (*see* section on Treatment); but when fibrosis is established progressive impairment occurs. Gas transfer shows less deterioration than other functional parameters in patients tested serially over a period of five years (Andrews.

376

Kazuni and Hardy, 1969), although in one case followed for sixteen years the decline in gas transfer was virtually parallel with the fall in VC (Redding, Hardy and Gaensler, 1968).

The 'obstructive syndrome' (*see* Chapter 1) has not been regarded as a

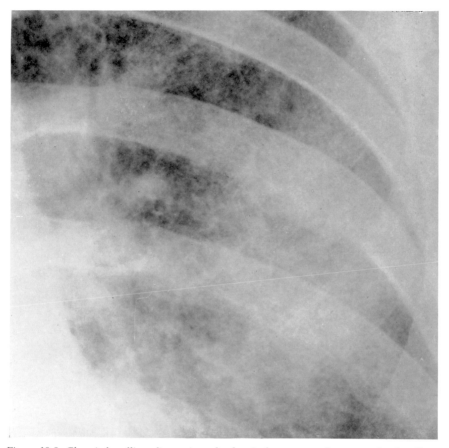

Figure 10.8. Chronic beryllium disease in male chemical process worker exposed to beryllium. For 3 years in the late 1940s in a laboratory manufacturing zinc aluminium silicate for fluorescent lamps and screens. Appearances of right lung field similar. Beryllium in the urine; loss of weight, moderate clubbing of the fingers and toes, central cyanosis and persistent crepitations in lower halves of the lungs; severe respiratory disability. Little response to corticosteroids. Died, aged 41 years, from cor pulmonale and respiratory failure 4 years after onset of the disease. Diagnosis histologically confirmed

feature of chronic disease but slight, though significant, airways obstruction with an accompanying increase of RV and RV/TLC was observed by Andrews, Kazuni and Hardy (1969) in about a third of 41 cases, and the majority of these had never smoked. They regard this as probably due to involvement of bronchioles and small bronchi by granulomas or fibrosis. The same investigation also showed that patients with obstructive and restrictive defects had the most severe hypoxaemia and were the most disabled, whereas those with a predominant gas transfer defect were the least disabled over a five-year period.

Radiographic appearances

Acute disease

Abnormality of the lung fields lags behind the symptoms and clinical signs by some one to three weeks. Serial films show the development first of a diffuse

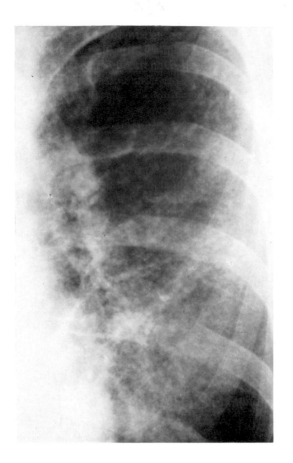

LUNG FUNCTION

	Observed	Predicted
	(litres)	(litres)
TLC	6·0	6·9
RV	2·8	2·1
FRC	4·1	4·3
VC	3·2	4·6
FEV₁	2·6	3·6
FEV₁/VC	81%	75%
T_L	16·2 ml/mmHg. per min	31·0 ml/mmHg. per min

Age 45 years: height 5 ft 10 in

Figure 10.9. Another appearance of chronic disease. Some of the lesions are apparently calcified. Exposure: machining and deburring non-ferrous metals containing beryllium for approximately 1 year in the mid 1950s. Disease diagnosed in 1966. Beryllium granulomas demonstrated on lung biopsy. Permanent corticosteroid treatment. Respiratory disability not severe. Working in a light job in 1971. Lung function tests same day as the film.

haziness and then large, irregular shadows which correlate with areas of consolidation. As the patient recovers the opacities clear and, in most cases, appearances return to normal in one to six months (*Figure 10.7*). In subacute disease very fine, discrete opacities appear throughout both fields but, with corticosteroid treatment, disappear within two to three weeks.

Chronic disease

There is a variety of abnormal appearances which occur within a few weeks of the onset of symptoms, but which are in no way pathognomonic. Abnormal opacities have been classified as 'granular' (discrete opacities up to 1 mm in diameter), 'nodular' (discrete opacities 1 to 5 mm in diameter) and 'linear' (Stoeckle, Hardy and Weber, 1969), and the following variations are seen (Weber, Stoeckle and Hardy, 1965):

(1) Fine, discrete ('granular'), widespread opacities which remain unchanged for years (*Figure 10.8*), and in some cases are unusually dense due to microscopic calcification in granulomatous lesions (*Figure 10.9*).

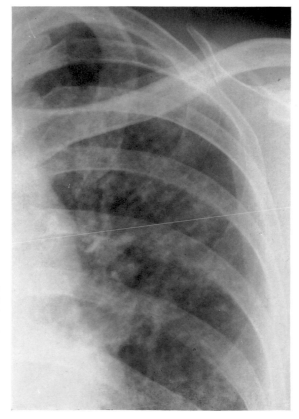

Figure 10.10. Chronic beryllium disease diagnosed in 1950 in a woman who worked in the fluorescent lamp industry. Severe respiratory disability by 1966 when this film was taken. Appearances similar on both sides. Receiving corticosteroids. (By courtesy of Dr Harriet Hardy)

(2) Similar type opacities confined mainly to the lower zones of the lung fields with subsequent development of condensed linear opacities in these zones and increased translucency in the upper zones. This evidence of lung contraction takes one to two years to appear.

(3) Small, discrete opacities in the upper and mid-zones which progress to linear shadows indicative of fibrosis with contraction of the upper zones and translucent areas of cyst formation (*Figure 10.10*).

(4) Widespread, discrete, larger ('nodular') shadows which increase progressively in size, and the subsequent development of numerous, translucent areas due to cysts and emphysematous bullae. Confluent opacities may appear later giving an appearance identical with nodular silicosis or coal

pneumoconiosis. In other cases, as the signs of fibrosis progress, 'nodular' opacities regress and disappear. Contraction and distortion of the upper halves of the lungs due to fibrosis may be severe and the trachea much displaced and deformed.

(5) 'Nodular' opacities with bilateral enlargement of hilar lymph node shadows. This enlargement is uncommon and very rarely more than moderate in degree and, unlike 'idiopathic' sarcoidosis, is not seen in the absence of abnormality in the lung fields. Occasionally the nodes become calcified (Stoeckle, Hardy and Weber, 1969).

(6) 'Nodular' opacities sometimes become strikingly dense and contrasted due to the presence of calcification. They are then similar to calcified silicotic lesions or the small, calcified lesions of the 'rheumatoid' variant of coal pneumoconiosis. These probably represent calcified hyaline nodules.

In some cases discrete opacities regress, decreasing both in number and density, but rarely disappear completely; in most, however, the abnormalities increase progressively, though often very slowly. A rapid deterioration in appearances is usually associated with exacerbation of disease. It is rare for no radiographic change to take place over a decade.

The commonest abnormal appearance consists of a mixture of 'granular', 'nodular' and 'linear' opacities, and the least common is that of 'granular' opacities alone (Stoeckle, Hardy and Weber, 1969).

Evidence of pleural thickening involving mainly the upper zones or of pneumothorax is seen in a small proportion of cases (*see* section on Complications).

The effect of corticosteroid treatment on radiographic appearances is referred to in the section on Treatment.

OTHER INVESTIGATIONS

The beryllium (Curtis) patch test

The observation that dermatitis developed in beryllium-exposed workers after a latent period of three to ten days and recurred more rapidly in some when they were re-exposed to beryllium suggested an allergic type reaction (De Nardi, Van Ordstrand and Carmody, 1949), and prompted the introduction of this test (Curtis, 1951).

A patch of gauze soaked with an unbuffered solution of 2 per cent beryllium sulphate or nitrate is applied to the skin of the forearm for 48 hours. A positive reaction consists of an acute inflammatory reaction which occurs within about 72 hours and persists for at least a week. An organized granuloma may appear at the site in about three weeks.

A positive reaction, however, only establishes a state of hypersensitivity to beryllium, and does not prove the existence of past or present disease.

The possibility that the test may provoke exacerbation of chronic disease is referred to by many writers and has resulted in the recommendation that it should be used with great caution or avoided altogether, although only one such case is on record (Sneddon, 1955). It is now rarely employed in the United States of America (Hardy, 1972). Certainly the test should not be used in the pre-employment examination of workers about to enter an industry in which beryllium may be encountered nor in the investigation of a previously exposed worker who may later return to the industry, as this may increase the likelihood of disease following exposure to low concentrations of beryllium.

In a minority of cases of chronic disease the test is negative (Stoeckle, Hardy and Weber, 1969).

Corticosteroids suppress a positive reaction in hypersensitive patients (Norris and Peard, 1963).

The Kveim test

This test has been found to be uniformly negative in chronic beryllium disease (Hardy, 1966) and is valuable, therefore, in distinguishing it from 'idiopathic' sarcoidosis (Stoeckle, Hardy and Weber, 1969).

Serology

Demonstration of hypergammaglobulinaemia and its Ig components may assist diagnosis when related to other criteria.

Urine

As has been pointed out already the presence of beryllium indicates only that at some time it has been assimilated into the body. A technique of analysis using gas chromatography which is sensitive, reliable, rapid and reproducible has recently been developed and can detect beryllium in a sample as small as 1 ml with a limit of detection as low as 1 ng per ml^{-1} (Foreman, Gough and Walker, 1970).

Measurement of excretion of urinary calcium may be of help in observing the course of chronic disease as transient hypercalcuria appears to be correlated with activity of the disease (Stoeckle, Hardy and Weber, 1969).

Lung biopsy and beryllium assay

In most cases it is unnecessary to remove lung tissue to establish the diagnosis, although biopsy is a helpful guide to prognosis. For biopsy an adequate amount of lung (10 g) should be obtained, preferably by thoracotomy; and for assay—which can been done on 1 g of tissue, but not less—it should be sent to the laboratory in a chemically clean borosilicate glass container.

Beryllium can be identified by conventional spectrography, and a technique employing both this and micro-emission spectrography has recently been described (Robinson et al., 1968). Another method which makes use of a laser microprobe and emission spectrography can identify beryllium in granulomas (Prine, Brokeshoulder and McVean, 1966). But the most reliable technique for general purposes is morin fluorimetric analysis of wet ashed tissue (Hardy, 1972)—see Tepper, Hardy and Chamberlin (1961). These techniques can also be applied to post-mortem material. There is a histochemical test which, although specific for beryllium (Deuz, 1949), detects only soluble compounds, and so has little practical value.

DIAGNOSIS

Acute disease

The diagnosis of acute nasopharyngitis, tracheobronchitis or pneumonitis depends mainly upon the recognition that a toxic beryllium compound has been inhaled—usually one to two days before the onset of symptoms. Other features supporting the diagnosis are low (not high) fever and rapid loss of weight. As described, the appearances of the chest radiograph are in no way characteristic, and laboratory tests cannot distinguish this disease from pneumonitis due to other causes except in the negative sense that evidence of bacterial or viral infection is lacking. Blood counts, E.S.R. serum protein levels and urinalysis do not help as they are near normal limits (Tepper, Hardy and Chamberlin, 1961).

Chronic disease

The criteria for diagnosis are:

(1) A history of significant past exposure to beryllium.

(2) Widespread opacities in the chest radiograph with or without respiratory symptoms, occasionally accompanied by granulomas of the skin.

(3) Reduction of gas transfer and hyperventilation initially only on exercise, and later, development of the 'restrictive syndrome'.

(4) A negative Kveim test.

(5) Demonstration in biopsy or post-mortem material of pulmonary lesions corresponding to one or other of the histological groups described earlier, often with diffuse interstitial fibrosis, and, occasionally, hyalinized nodules.

(6) The presence of beryllium in the lungs, other tissues or the urine.

The diagnosis can be made if at least the first four of these are fulfilled but the fifth is often required, and if past exposure to beryllium is uncertain the sixth is necessary. For reasons already stated the beryllium patch test is not a necessary criterion (Stoeckle, Hardy and Weber, 1969).

In taking the history the exact details of occupation and the nature of the materials and processes used, and the duration of exposure should be established, but when a patient is seen for the first time ten or more years after leaving the industry, this may be difficult or impossible. Should this be the case or if there is a possibility of exposure unsuspected by the patient (for example, reclamation of scrap alloys some of which may have contained beryllium) the employers should be asked for an analysis of the process and the conditions in which it was carried out. If there is no evidence of occupational exposure the possibility of para-occupational and neighbourhood exposure must be explored.

Other data which give support to the diagnosis are hyperglobulinaemia with a predominant increase in IgG. If these observations are added to the first four diagnostic criteria lung biopsy should not be necessary; but should these criteria be only partially fulfilled microscopical examination and beryllium assay are indicated. The presence of beryllium in lung tissue virtually excludes other causes of granulomatous lung disease and establishes the diagnosis beyond reasonable doubt.

Beryllium in the urine confirms past exposure and may, therefore, be of value in cases where a history of this cannot be established with any certainty; so that tissue assay may not be required. But as stated earlier the absence of beryllium does not exclude past exposure nor the existence of disease.

Hypercalcuria and hyperuricaemia are of no diagnostic assistance as they

382

occur in other diseases the most important of which in this context is 'idio-pathic' sarcoidosis.

'Idiopathic' sarcoidosis has invariably to be differentiated from chronic beryllium disease. The chief differences between the two—apart from the presence of beryllium in the tissues—are these. Uveitis, involvement of lachry-mal and salivary glands, cystic changes in the bones of the hands and feet, erythema nodosum and lupus pernio have not been observed in beryllium disease. Generalized peripheral lymphadenopathy is much rarer in beryllium disease than in 'idiopathic' sarcoidosis and radiographic enlargement of hilar lymph nodes without changes in the lung fields, or massive enlargement of these nodes with lung changes are not seen. But evidence of parenchymal calcification is more common than in 'idiopathic' sarcoidosis. The Kveim test is consistently negative in chronic beryllium disease but tuberculin reactivity is unaffected. And whereas circulating IgG is often increased in both diseases, IgA or IgM are prominent in a minority of cases of 'idiopathic' sarcoidosis but not in chronic beryllium disease (q.v.) The course of beryllium disease, unlike that of 'idiopathic' sarcoidosis, is usually slowly progressive although there may be long periods during which disability is unchanged.

Other diseases which may have to be excluded are:

(1) Tuberculosis of miliary, bronchopneumonic or fibrocavernous type.

(2) Histoplasmosis in endemic areas. This is excluded by the histoplasmin skin test, complement fixation test, cultures of *H. capsulatum* and biopsy of lung tissue.

(3) Pneumoconiosis. This includes siderosis, stannosis, silicosis and coal pneumoconiosis and, in most cases, the occupational history serves to make the distinction. Neither symptoms nor abnormality of lung function are associated with siderosis or stannosis.

(4) Chronic extrinsic allergic 'alveolitis' (farmers' lung and like disorders). Although this produces clinical, physiological, and radiographic features which are identical to chronic beryllium disease the occupational history and identification of beryllium in lung tissue make differentiation clear. Further-more, cellular, sarcoid-like granulomas, which are a feature of chronic beryllium disease are absent in chronic extrinsic allergic 'alveolitis' (*see* Chapter 11).

(5) Lymphangitis carcinomatosa. This may cause dyspnoea and radio-graphic changes similar to those of chronic beryllium disease but lack of exposure to beryllium and rapid deterioration in health should point to the diagnosis.

(6) Haemosiderosis. The youth of the patient, lack of occupational history, recurrent haemoptysis, iron deficiency anaemia, presence of sidero-phores in the sputum, and biopsy appearances make the diagnosis unequivocal.

PROGNOSIS

Acute disease

Recovery is the rule in the majority of cases within one to six months but fulminating disease (usually associated with accidental exposure) carries a risk of death in some 7 per cent of cases (Tepper, Hardy and Chamberlin.

1961). Episodes of pneumonitis may recur, however, following recovery if the subject is re-exposed to beryllium and, as has been described, a proportion of individuals may later develop chronic disease without further exposure to beryllium.

Occasionally, evidence of acute disease in the chest radiograph may persist for almost a year before finally disappearing.

Chronic disease

Prognosis in the individual cannot be predicted with certainty and different patterns of evolution of the disease occur, any one or all of which may be observed in the same patient.

The minority of individuals who experience no symptoms and in whom the only evidence of the disease, apart from beryllium assay and biopsy, is the chest radiograph may remain asymptomatic for a decade or more (Tepper, Hardy and Chamberlin, 1961), but at any time, symptoms and impairment of lung function may develop without evident change in the radiographic appearances.

The majority of persons have symptoms and the impaired pattern of lung function, described already, to the point of being slightly or moderately disabled though able to lead a fairly normal life for years. But should exacerbation of disease occur it is usually followed by increase of disability. When exacerbations are accompanied by fever and rigors the prognosis tends to be poor (Tepper, Hardy and Chamberlin, 1961). Severely disabling disease is of very variable duration—from about one to twenty years in corticosteroid-treated patients (Hardy, Rabe and Lorch, 1967). It may end in death from respiratory failure and cor pulmonale which, in some cases, may be precipitated by repeated episodes of spontaneous pneumothorax (*see* next section).

Although corticosteroids have a substantial ameliorating effect upon the course of chronic disease, complete resolution, either spontaneous or due to treatment, has not been reliably reported. But if it is not understood that long periods of remission occur in some cases these may be interpreted as a 'cure', and although susbtantial reduction of discrete radiographic opacities may occur during corticosteroid treatment they tend to reappear when it is stopped.

Freiman and Hardy (1970) have shown that the histological features (q.v.) afford a practical guide to clinical course and prognosis in that there is a distinct relationship between the histological features and the degree of morbidity and life expectancy. Prognosis is significantly worse in patients with Group I lesions than in those with Group II lesions.

COMPLICATIONS

Cor pulmonale

This is the commonest, but not necessarily inevitable, complication of chronic disease and is more often the cause of death than respiratory failure (Tepper, Hardy and Chamberlin, 1961).

Spontaneous pneumothorax

This is more an inherent part of chronic disease than a complication. It has

384

been observed in about 15 per cent of cases, may be recurrent and bilateral, and may be the immediate cause of death.

Carcinoma of the lung

It has already been noted that the carcinogenic effect of some beryllium compounds in experimental animals has not been detected with certainty in man and though there is some suggestion that there may be an excess of lung cancer among beryllium workers who have had pneumonitis in the past, the number of cases is small (Mancuso, 1970). Further epidemiological study of the problem is needed but, at present (1973), there is no satisfactory evidence that beryllium disease is associated with an increased risk of cancer of the lung.

Pulmonary tuberculosis

There is no increased tendency for persons with chronic disease to develop tuberculosis; on the contrary, it has been remarkably uncommon (Tepper, Hardy and Chamberlin, 1961).

Nephrolithiasis in chronic disease

In a small proportion of cases this leads to renal failure.

Gout

Gout has been recorded as a rare complication of the hyperuricaemia of chronic disease (Kelley, Goldfinger and Hardy, 1969).

Rheumatoid arthritis

An alleged association of rheumatoid arthritis with chronic disease is not supported by the available evidence (Tepper, Hardy and Chamberlin, 1961).

Effects of treatment

The complications of corticosteroid therapy have been recorded, but only in very few cases (Hardy, Rabe and Lorch, 1967).

TREATMENT

Administration of corticosteroids, which were first used to treat the disease between 1950 and 1952, is associated with a significant reduction in mortality and increased time of survival (Hardy, Rabe and Lorch, 1967), although it is difficult to be certain whether this is wholly due to their influence or partly to other causes (Freiman and Hardy, 1970).

Acute disease must be treated immediately with bed rest and prednisone 60 to 80 mg a day. If of fulminating type oxygen—preferably under positive pressure—will be necessary. Antibiotic agents are not indicated except in the event of secondary infection.

As soon as chronic disease is diagnosed on the basis of the foregoing criteria, prednisone should be commenced at an initial dose of 15 to 30 mg per day or 30 to 60 mg on alternate days (Stoeckle, Hardy and Weber, 1969) and later adjusted according to progress. This usually causes a reduction of symptoms and serum globulins, improvement in general health, gas transfer and, in some cases, radiographic appearances. Patients with Sub-group IA and Sub-group IB lesions respond equally well (Freiman and Hardy, 1970), but when fibrosis is established, no improvement can be expected. However, if corticosteroids are started early enough, fibrosis does not appear to progress, although deterioration in lung function may not be prevented.

When corticosteroids are discontinued there may, in some cases, be prolonged remission. In others, symptoms and abnormalities of lung function and chest radiographs quickly re-assert themselves; in which case life-long maintenance of these drugs may be necessary.

Chelating agents—such as aurintricarboxylic acid (ATA) and edathamil (EDTA)—are ineffective.

Supportive treatment of cor pulmonale, congestive heart failure and respiratory failure may ultimately be required.

When acute or chronic disease has been diagnosed the worker should never again return to any job which may incur the risk of exposure to beryllium in any form.

Skin ulcers must be curetted to remove the toxic particles, otherwise permanent healing will not occur; skin granulomas require early and wide excision.

PREVENTION

Preventive measures cannot be considered in any detail here—they are fully discussed by Breslin (1966)—but are summarized briefly.

Threshold limit value

The TLV for beryllium and its compounds recommended by the American Conference of Governmental Hygienists (1971) is 0·002 mg/m^3 of air as a time-weighted average over the period of an eight-hour day, and any isolated excursion above this level should not exceed a 'ceiling' of 25 μg/m^3. Rigorous control of the work environment and of methods of personal protection are required to achieve this.

Control of the work environment

The objective is to prevent contamination of the factory air and of the worker's skin and clothing. Routine beryllium processes should be segregated from the rest of the factory, preferably in a room subjected to a negative atmosphere.

Beryllium extraction, alloy production and reduction furnaces should be completely enclosed and ventilated, and beryllium liquids and slurries contained in closed vessels. Partial enclosure (for example, hoods) combined with low-volume high-velocity exhaust ventilation is required for grinding, deburring, drilling, machining and ceramic operations. General exhaust ventilation is applied to the factory or workroom atmosphere and the extracted air scrubbed and filtered by different methods according to whether the processes are dry or wet, so that no beryllium is discharged into the environmental air.

Rigid work practices are necessary to maintain a high standard of cleanliness and housekeeping. Any spillage must be dealt with promptly by wet mopping or a special vacuum cleaning system. Surfaces which are normally inaccessible (such as ventilation ducts, beams and lighting fixtures) should be cleaned at regular intervals. A specified code of practice is required for the maintenance of machinery (for example, lathes and grinders) and for entering enclosures.

Protection of personnel

All workers must be informed of the danger of beryllium, without causing apprehension. Special work clothes (overalls, caps, shorts, and underwear), must be worn and laundered on the factory site; they must never be taken home. An ideal arrangement consists of a locker room divided in the middle by showers or other washing facilities with the worker's work clothes housed on one side and his normal day clothes in the other. Special footwear should be provided and, for some processes (for example, handling soluble compounds and bulk materials or cleaning contaminated machines) gloves must also be worn.

Respirators of approved design must be used during the maintenance and cleaning of equipment and changing dust-collector bags. They may also be required in furnace operations, and should be easily accessible in areas where massive accidental contamination could occur.

An established emergency procedure must be in force for any process which carries a potential risk of massive contamination and should include a special alarm signal, prompt evacuation of the area and the donning of respirators by personnel who remain to deal with the emergency and by workers leaving the area if they have to walk any distance.

Air sampling

Both the general air and the worker's breathing zone should be sampled. To sample the general air a static sampling instrument is placed in a position which is representative of the conditions over the working area, usually at a height of four to six feet from the floor, and operates over a period of a day or more. And to sample the breathing zone the instrument may be placed in a fixed position near to the worker's nose or mouth, worn on his clothing or held in the zone by a technician for the required sampling time. Some four or five samples are collected and the results averaged.

Disposal of solid waste material

Any metal, wood, rags or paper which have been contaminated should be removed in sealed containers and buried in ground approved for the purpose.

Medical surveillance

(1) *Pre-employment examination.*—A careful clinical examination, with a good-quality full-sized chest film, must be done. Persons who already have respiratory tract disease should not be accepted for work in any process using beryllium for, although there is no evidence that they are more liable to develop beryllium disease than healthy persons, this would make later differential diagnosis extremely difficult. Hence, any chronic lung disease (including other occupational diseases), hay fever and asthma should

387

exclude the applicant, as should any evidence of past or present skin sensitization. And because of the effect which pregnancy is said to have, women of childbearing age should be excluded.

The beryllium patch test is contraindicated for any person likely to be accepted into the industry.

(2) *Routine examination of employees.*—Clinical examination, ventilatory function tests and a 17 × 14-inch postero-anterior chest radiograph should be carried out yearly in all workers. Workers in refinery, alloy or ceramic processes should be weighed and have their vital capacities measured monthly; an undue fall in either indicates the necessity for further investigation.

The skin should also be examined at regular intervals for evidence of contact dermatitis, granulomas and ulcers.

A detailed record of his work, the results of air sampling and medical examinations must be kept for each employee.

(3) *Medical examination after leaving employment.*—In between exposure and development of chronic disease, in many cases arrangements must be made for yearly medical supervision of ex-workers for at least 15 years after ceasing contact.

REFERENCES

Agate, J. N. (1948). 'Delayed pneumonitis in a beryllium worker.' *Lancet* 2, 530–533

Aldridge, W. N., Barnes, J. M. and Denz, F. A. (1950). 'Biochemical changes in acute beryllium poisoning.' *Br. J. exp. Path.* 31, 473–484

Andrews, J. L., Kazuni, H. and Hardy, H. L. (1969). 'Patterns of lung dysfunction in chronic beryllium disease.' *Am. Rev. resp. Dis.* 100, 791–800

Annotation (1951). 'The toxicity of beryllium.' *Lancet* 1, 1357–1358

Aub, J. C. and Grier, R. S. (1949). 'Acute pneumonitis in workers exposed to beryllium oxide and beryllium metal.' *J. ind. Hyg. Toxicol*, 31, 123–133

Bamberger, C., Botbol, J. and Cabrini, R. L. (1968). 'Inhibition of alkaline phosphatase by beryllium and aluminium.' *Archs Biochem. Biophys.* 123, 195–200

Belman, S. (1969). 'Beryllium binding of epidermal constituents.' *J. occup. Med.* 11, 175–183

Benoit, M. P. (1967). 'Open bench top deburring of metallic beryllium.' *J. occup. Med.* 9, 170–174

Breslin, A. J. (1966). *Occupational Health Aspects*, pp. 245–321. Ed. by H. E. Stokinger. New York and London; Academic Press

Chamberlin, G. W., Jennings, W. P. and Lieben, J. (1957). 'Chronic pulmonary disease associated with beryllium dust.' *Penn. med. J.* 60, 497–503

Chambers, L. A., Foster, M. S. and Cholak, J. (1955). 'A comparison of particulate loadings in the atmosphere of certain American cities.' In *Proceedings of 3rd National Air Pollution Symposium, Standard Research Institute, Pasadena, California*, p. 24

Chiappino, G., Cirla, A. and Vigliani, E. C. (1969). 'Delayed type hypersensitivity reactions to beryllium compounds.' *Archs Path.* 87, 131–140

Cholak, J. (1959). 'The analysis of traces of beryllium.' *Archs ind. Hlth* 19, 205–210

— (1961). 'The contamination of the atmosphere with beryllium operations concerned with handling and processing of the metal.' In *Workshop on Beryllium*, p. 39. Ohio; Kettering Laboratory, University of Cincinatti

Cirla, A. M., Barbiano di Belgiojoso, G. and Chiappino, G. (1968). 'La ipersensibilità ai composti di berillio; trasferimento passivo nella cavia mediante cellule linfoidi.' *Boll. Ist. sieroter. milan* 47, 663–668

Collins, D. H. (1966). *Pathology of Bone*, p. 96. London; Butterworths

Curtis, G. H. (1951). Cutaneous hysersensitivity due to beryllium. A study of 13 cases. *Archs Derm. Syph.* 64, 470–482

DeNardi, J., Van Ordstrand, H. S. and Carmody, M. G. (1949). 'Acute dermatitis and pneumonitis in beryllium workers. Review of 406 cases in an eight year period with follow-up on recoveries.' *Ohio St. med. J.* **45**, 567–575

Denz, F. A. (1949). 'The histochemical detection of beryllium.' *Q. Jl Microsc. Sci.* **90**, 317–321

Dubois, K. P. (1950). 'Studies on the biochemical effects of beryllium.' Massachusetts Institute of Technology Symposium

Epstein, W. L. (1967). 'Granulomatous hypersensitivity.' In *Progress in Allergy*, Vol. II, pp. 36–38. Ed. by P. Kallós and B. H. Waksman. Basel; Kayer

Foreman, J. K., Gough, T. A. and Walker, E. A. (1970). 'The determination of traces of beryllium in human and rat urine samples by gas chromatography.' *Analyst* **95**, 797–804

Freiman, D. G. and Hardy, H. L. (1970). 'Beryllium disease.' *Hum. Path.* **1**, 25–44

Gelman, I. (1936). 'Poisoning by vapours of beryllium oxyfluoride.' *J. ind. Hyg. Toxicol.* **18**, 371–379

Hall, R. H., Scott, J. K., Laskin, S., Stroud, C. A. and Stokinger, H. E. (1950). 'Acute toxicity of inhaled beryllium III. Observations correlating toxicity with physico-chemical properties of beryllium oxide dust.' *Archs ind. Hyg. occup. Med.* **2**, 25–48

Hall, T. C., Wood, C. H., Stoeckle, J. D. and Tepper, L. B. (1959). 'Case data from the Beryllium Register.' *Archs ind. Hlth* **19**, 100–103

Hanifin, J. M., Epstein, W. L. and Cline, M. J. (1970). '*In vitro* studies of granulomatous hypersensitivity to beryllium.' *J. Invest. Derm.* **55**, 284–288

Hardy, H. L. (1948). 'Delayed chemical pneumonitis in workers exposed to beryllium compounds.' *Am. Rev. Tuberc.* **57**, 547–555

— (1965). 'Beryllium poisoning—lessons in control of man-made disease.' *New Engl. J. Med.* **273**, 1188–1199

— (1966). Quoted by Jones Williams (1967). 'Skin granulomata due to beryllium oxide.' *Br. J. Surg.* **54**, 292–297

— (1972). Personal communication

— and Tabershaw, J. R. (1946). 'Delayed chemical pneumonitis occurring in workers exposed to beryllium compounds.' *J. ind. Hyg. Toxicol.* **28**, 197–211

— Rabe, E. W. and Lorch, S. (1967). United States Beryllium Case Registry (1952–1966). *J. occup. Med.* **9**, 271–276

Hazard, J. B. (1959). 'Pathologic changes of beryllium disease.' *Archs ind. Hlth* **19**, 179–183

Henderson, W. R., Fukuyama, K., Epstein, W. L. and Spitler, L. E. (1972). '*In vitro* demonstration of delayed hypersensitivity in patients with berylliosis.' *J. Invest. Derm.* **58**, 5–8

Hyslop, F., Palmes, E. D., Alford, W. C., Monaco, A. R. and Fairhall, L. T. (1943). *The Toxicity of Beryllium.* National Institute of Health Bulletin. No. 181. Washington, D.C.

Israel, H. L. and Cooper, D. A. (1964). 'Chronic beryllium disease due to low beryllium content alloys.' *Am. Rev. resp. Dis.* **89**, 100–102

Jones Williams, W. (1958). 'A histological study of lungs in 52 cases of chronic beryllium disease.' *Br. J. ind. Med.* **15**, 84–91

— (1967a). 'The pathology of sarcoidosis.' *Hosp. Med.* **2**, 21–27

— (1967b). 'The pathology of pulmonary sarcoidosis.' *Proc. R. Soc. Med.* **60**, 986–988

— (1971). 'The beryllium granuloma.' *Proc. R. Soc. Med.* **64**, 946–948

— and Williams, D. (1967). ' "Residual bodies" in sarcoid and sarcoid-like granulomas.' *J. clin. Path.* **20**, 574–577

— Fry, E. M. and James, E. M. V. (1972). 'The fine structure and nature of beryllium granulomas.' *Acta path. microbiol. scand.* **A80**, Suppl. 233, 195–202

Kelley, W. N., Goldfinger, S. E. and Hardy, H. L. (1969). 'Hyperuricaemia in chronic beryllium disease.' *Ann. intern. Med.* **70**, 977–983

Klemperer, F. W., Martin, A. P. and Van Riper, J. (1951). 'Beryllium excretion in humans.' *Archs ind. Hyg.* **4**, 251–256

Lieben, J. and Metzner, F. (1959). 'Epidemiological findings associated with beryllium excretion.' *Am. ind. Hyg. Ass. J.* **20**, 494–499

Lieben, J., Dattoli, J. A. and Vought, V. M. (1966). 'The significance of beryllium concentrations in urine.' *Archs envir. Med.* **12**, 331–334

McCallum, R. I., Rannie, I. and Verity, C. (1961). 'Chronic pulmonary berylliosis in a female chemist.' *Br. J. ind. Med.* **18**, 133–142

Mainigi, K. D. and Bresnick, E. (1969). 'Inhibition of deoxythymidine kinase by beryllium.' *Biochem. Pharmac* **18**, 2003–2007

Mancuso, T. F. (1970). 'Relation of duration of employment and prior respiratory illness to respiratory cancer among beryllium workers.' *Envir. Res.* **3**, 251–275

Maxwell, W. R. (1971). (Rocket Propulsion Establishment, Ministry of Defence.) Personal communication

Metzner, F. and Lieben, J. (1961). 'Respiratory disease associated with berylllium refining and alloy fabrication.' *J. occup. Med.* **3**, 341-345

Norris, G. F. and Peard, M. C. (1963). 'Berylliosis. Report of two cases with special reference to the patch test.' *Br. med. J.* **1**, 378–382

Policard, A. (1950). 'Histological studies of the effects of beryllium oxide (glucine) on animal tissues.' *Br. J. ind. Med.* **7**, 117–121

Prine, J. R., Brokeshoulder, S. F. and McVean, D. E. (1966). 'Demonstration of presence of beryllium in pulmonary granulomas.' *Am. J. clin. Path.* **45**, 448–454

Redding, R. A., Hardy, H. L. and Gaensler, E. A. (1968). 'Beryllium disease: a 16 year follow-up case study.' *Respiration* **25**, 263–278

Reeves, A. L. (1968). 'Über die Retention von eingeatmetein Beryllium sulfat— Aerosol in Rattenlungen.' *Arch. Gewerbepath. Gewerbehyg.* **24**, 226–237

— Krivanek, N. D., Busby, E. K. and Swanborg, R. H. (1972). 'Immunity to pulmonary berylliosis in guinea pigs.' *Int. Arch. Arbeitsmed.* **29**, 209–220

Resnick, H., Roche, M. and Morgan, W. K. C. (1970). 'Immunoglobulin concentration in berylliosis.' *Am. Rev. resp. Dis.* **101**, 504–510

Robinson, F. R., Brokeshoulder, S. F., Thomas, A. A. and Cholak, J. (1968). 'Microemission spectrochemical analysis of human lungs for beryllium.' *Am. J. clin. Path.* **49**, 821–825

Royston, G. R. (1949). 'Acute pneumonitis in a beryllium worker.' *Br. med. J.* **1**, 1030–1032

Sander, O. A. (1950). 'Clinical report of illness in the neon sign industry.' In *Symposium, Current Knowledge of Disease Encountered in the Handling of Beryllium and its Compounds: Clinical, Pathological and Engineering Data; USAEC. Report AECU—1921.* Massachusetts; Instit. Technol.

Scadding, J. G. (1967). *Sarcoidosis.* London; Eyre and Spottiswoode

Sharma, O. P., James, D. G., Bird, R. and White, E. W. (1971). 'Immunoglobulins in sarcoidosis.' *Fifth International Conference on Sarcoidosis, Prague, 1969,* pp. 171–173. Ed. by L. Levinský and F. Macholda. Praha; Universita Karlova

Shilen, J., Galloway, A. E. and Mellor, J. F. (1944). 'Beryllium oxide from beryl.' *Ind. Med.* **13**, 464–469

Sneddon, I. B. (1955). 'Berylliosis; a case report.' *Br. med. J.* **1**, 1448–1449

Spencer, H. C., Hook, R. H., Blumenshine, J. A., McCollister, S. N., Sadek, S. E. and Jones, J. C. (1968). *Toxicological Studies on Beryllium Oxides and Beryllium-containing Exhaust Products.* (AMRL-TR-68-148.) Ohio; Aerospace Medical Research Labs. Wright-Patterson Air Force Base

Sterner, J. H. and Eisenbud, M. (1951). 'Epidemiology of beryllium intoxication.' *Archs ind. Hyg.* **4**, 123–151

Stoeckle, J. D., Hardy, H. L. and Weber, A. L. (1969). 'Chronic beryllium disease.' *Am. J. Med.* **46**, 545–561

Stokinger, H. E. (1966). In *Beryllium. Its Industrial Hygiene Aspects,* p. 168. Ed. by H. E. Stokinger. New York and London; Academic Press

Stokinger, H. E., Spiegel, C. J., Root, R. E., Wall, R. H., Steadman, L. T., Smith, F. A. and Garder, D. F. (1953). 'Acute inhalation toxicity of beryllium IV, Beryllium fluids at exposure concentrations of one and ten milligrams per cubic metre.' *Archs ind. Hyg. occup. Med.* **8**, 493–506

Stokinger, H. E., Sprague, G. F., Hall, R. H., Ashenburg, N. J., Scott, J. K. and Steadman, L. T. (1950). Acute inhalation toxicity of beryllium, I. Four definitive studies of beryllium sulfate at exposure concentrations of 100, 50, 10 and 1 mg per cubic metre. *Archs ind. Hyg. occup. Med.* **1**, 379–397

Stokinger, H. E., Steadman, L. T. and Root, R. E. (1951). 'Retention of beryllium in animal tissues following inhalation of its salts.' *Archs ind. Hyg.* **3**, 422–423

Tepper, L. B., Hardy, H. L. and Chamberlin, R.'I. (1961). *The Toxicity of Beryllium Compounds.* Amsterdam; Elsevier

Unanue, E. R., Askonas, B. A. and Allison, A. C. (1969). 'A role of macrophages in the stimulation of airborne responses by adjuvants.' *J. Immun.* **103**, 71–78

Underwood, A. L. (1951). *Studies on the Renal Excretion of Beryllium.* (USAEC Report UR-171.) University of Rochester

Van Cleave, C. D. and Kayler, C. T. (1955). 'Distribution, retention, and elimination of ^{7}Be in the rat after intratracheal injection.' *Archs ind. Hlth* **11**, 375–392

Van Ordstrand, H. S., Hughes, R. and Carmody, M. G. (1943). 'Chemical pneumonia in workers extracting beryllium oxide.' *Cleveland Clin. Q.* **10**, 10–18

Vorwald, A. J. (1966). 'Medical aspects of beryllium disease.' In *Beryllium. Its Industrial Hygiene Aspects*, pp. 167–200. Ed. by H. E. Stokinger. New York and London; Academic Press

— Reeves, A. L. and Urban, E. C. J. (1966). 'Experimental beryllium toxicology.' In *Beryllium. Its Industrial Hygiene Aspects*, pp. 201–234. Ed. by H. E. Stokinger. New York and London; Academic Press

Weber, A. L., Stoeckle, J. D. and Hardy, H. L. (1965) 'Roentgenologic patterns in long-standing beryllium disease.' *Am. J. Roentg.* **93**, 879–890

Weber, H. H. and Engelhardt, W. E. (1933). Über eine Apparatur zur Erzeugung niedriger Staubkonzentrationen von grosser Konstanz und eine Methode zur mikrogravinctrischen Staubbestimmung. Anwendung bei der Untersuchang con Stauben aus der Beryllium gewinnung.' *Zentbl. GewHyg. Unfallerhüt.* **10**, 41–47

Williams, D., Jones Williams, W. and Williams, J. E. (1969). 'Enzyme histochemistry of epithelioid cells in sarcoidosis and sarcoid-like granulomas.' *J. Pathol.* **97**, 705–709

Witschi, H. P. (1968). 'Inhibition of DNA synthesis in regenerating rat liver.' *Lab. Invest.* **19**, 67–70

Wright, G. W. (1948). Discussion. *Am. Rev. Tuberc.* **57**, 555–556

391

11—Diseases due to Organic (Non-mineral) Dusts

Inhalation of organic dusts may cause 'asthma' or 'extrinsic allergic alveolitis'.

Asthma can be usefully defined 'in terms of a disorder of function as a disease characterized by variable dyspnoea due to widespread narrowing of peripheral airways in the lungs, varying in severity over short periods of time, either spontaneously or as a result of treatment' (Ciba Foundation Guest Symposium, 1959). This definition is widely used (Ciba Foundation Study Group, 1971) because it has practical advantages in the management of patients and conveys the concept, not of a 'disease', but of the response of a ' target organ' mediated by many different provoking factors via a variety of intermediate pathways.

As is well known, typical asthmatic reactions may be provoked either immediately or after an interval of some hours (so-called 'late' asthma) by a variety of inhaled materials including organic antigens. It has not been customary to regard *byssinosis* (that is, the syndrome of transient, ill-defined chest tightness and airways obstruction due to the organic dusts of cotton, flax, or soft hemp) as asthma but, if the definition is accepted, then it is logical to include byssinosis under the heading of non-reaginic mediated 'late' asthma.

Occupational asthma is discussed briefly in Chapter 12 because it is also caused by inorganic provoking agents, but byssinosis is described in greater detail in this chapter.

'*Extrinsic allergic alveolitis*' can be defined as a disorder related to the inhalation of organic material and characterized by the presence of specific precipitating antibodies (precipitins), and by lymphocytic infiltration and sarcoid-like granulomas in the walls of alveoli and small airways.

These histological features are characteristic of the acute stage of this disorder but a proportion of cases progress to irreversible (chronic) pulmonary fibrosis. The most common example of the extrinsic allergic alveolitis group of diseases is 'farmers' lung'.

Immediate (Type I) or late (Type III) allergic reactions (*see* Chapter 4) are the intermediate causes of allergic lung disease:

(1) An immediate, Type I, reaction mediated by reaginic, IgE non-precipitating, skin-sensitizing antibodies to a wide variety of inhaled antigens causes 'extrinsic' asthma in sensitive subjects and, in some, the development of hay fever or eczema. Persons in this group who are constitutionally predisposed to sensitization by ordinary every-day exposure to inhaled antigens have been referred to as 'atopic'. However, 'extrinsic', IgE mediated, asthma sometimes develops in non-atopic subjects (that is, those who do not readily become sensitized) if their exposure to allergens is unusually heavy or prolonged; and an Arthus (Type III) reaction involving IgG may also occur in such persons (Pepys, 1969).

(2) A late, Type III (Arthus) reaction mediated by precipitins in the walls of small bronchi, bronchioles and alveoli results in extrinsic allergic 'alveolitis'. Although this reaction is chiefly confined to non-atopic subjects it may occur in atopic subjects in addition to an immediate reaction.

The extrinsic allergic 'alveolitis' group of diseases will be discussed first.

TABLE 11.1

Spore type	Length (μm)	Width (μm)
Actinomycete	0·5–2·5	0·5–1·0
Aspergillus fumigatus	2·0–3·5	
A. clavatus	3·0–4·5	2·5–3·5
Cryptostroma corticale	4·0–6·5	3·5–4·0
Aureobasidium pullulans	4·0–14	2·0–7·0
Graphium	2·0–9·0	1·0–5·0
Cladosporium herbarum	4·5–15	4·0–7·0
Grass pollen	26–35	

EXTRINSIC ALLERGIC 'ALVEOLITIS'

Antigens of fungus and actinomycete spores are responsible for many of these diseases, but others may be caused by proteins from animal or insect sources. Since thermophilic actinomycetes were first recognized as the source of antigens in dust from mouldy hay causing farmers' lung disease (Pepys *et al.*, 1963) many more sources of organic antigens have been identified. The most important actinomycete was first thought to be *Thermopolyspora polyspora* (Corbaz, Gregory and Lacey, 1963), but was later identified as a new species, *Micropolyspora faeni* (Cross, Maciver and Lacey, 1968). It is likely that other sources of antigens remain to be discovered and that any organic dust may be a potential cause of a late, Type III reaction in the lungs (Pepys, 1969). Actinomycetes, incidentally, are now considered to be Gram-positive 'mycelial' bacteria rather than fungi.

The size of spores, and other particles, affects the site of their deposition in the lungs (*see* Chapter 3). Pollens and spores larger than 10 μm which are deposited mainly in the nose and bronchi, often cause immediate allergy, whereas smaller spores tend to cause a late, Type III reaction. Although alveolar deposition is maximal for particles smaller than 5 μm diameter (*see Figure 3.1*) and their removal from the alveoli is slow, Booker *et al.* (1967)

found that 5 μm particles were retained in decreasing number up to 300 days. Table 11.1 gives some examples of spore sizes.

Extrinsic allergic 'alveolitis' is most often associated with occupation, hobbies or therapeutic inhalations (for example, pituitary hormone snuff) rather than with casual exposure, because intensive or repeated exposure is required for sensitization of healthy, non-atopic subjects. The sources of antigens causing the chief forms of allergic 'alveolitis' are shown in Table 11.2. Other possible examples of extrinsic allergic 'alveolitis' which require authentication are listed later.

TABLE 11.2

TYPES OF EXTRINSIC ALLERGIC 'ALVEOLITIS'

	Origin of dust	Source of antigen
Farmers' lung	Mouldy hay	*Micropolyspora faeni* *Thermoactinomyces vulgaris*
Bagassosis	Mouldy sugar cane bagasse	*Thermoactinomyces sacchari*
Mushroom workers' lung	Mushroom compost	*M. faeni* and *T. vulgaris* (and possibly other components)
Malt workers' lung	Mouldy barley and malt	*Aspergillus clavatus* and *A. fumigatus*
Maple bark strippers' disease	Infected maple bark	*Cryptostroma corticale*
Suberosis	Mouldy oak bark in cork manufacture	*Penicillium frequentans*
Bird breeders' lung	Droppings of pigeons, budgerigars, parrots and hens	Serum proteins in droppings
Wheat weevil disease	Weevil infected wheat grain and flour	*Sitophilus granarius*
Pituitary-snuff takers' lung	Pituitary hormone snuff powder	Pig or ox pituitary extracts and serum proteins

Irrespective of the nature of the antigen causing extrinsic allergic 'alveolitis' the pathological, clinical, physiological and radiographical features are in general similar, but chronic disease is less prone to occur in some forms. Farmers' lung is the most extensively investigated form of the disease and is, therefore, described in some detail and the others more briefly.

FARMERS' LUNG

There is an old country tradition that mouldy hay has a harmful effect on the lungs. Over a hundred years ago Icelandic farmers already referred to it by name as Heymaedi ('hay-shortness-of-breath') (Björnsson, 1960). But it was not until 1932 that it was first recorded in the medical literature by Campbell at Carlisle in the United Kingdom. He accurately described the characteristic features of acute disease in a group of farm workers exposed to mouldy hay. Other descriptions then followed in England from Lancashire (Fawcitt, 1938), Yorkshire (Pickles, 1944), Devon (Fuller, 1953) and in Eire (Joyce and Kneafsey, 1955). Detailed study has also been done in the United States of America (for example, Dickie and Rankin, 1958; Emanuel *et al.*, 1964; Rankin *et al.*, 1967), Scandinavia (Törnell, 1946), Switzerland (Hoffman, 1946) and Australia (Cooper and Greenaway, 1961).

There is a tendency for the term 'farmers' lung' to be used in a general sense to embrace extrinsic allergic 'alveolitis' caused by other occupations than farming. This practice is confusing and ought to be avoided.

The disease takes two forms, acute and chronic. *Acute disease* follows in a few hours after exposure to mouldy hay or grain dust. It is potentially reversible with complete recovery. *Chronic disease* may occur after repeated episodes of acute disease which ultimately fail to resolve, or it may develop insidiously as a result of repeated exposure to small amounts of antigen over a long period; it is not reversible, and is usually progressive.

Epidemiology

Water is essential for the growth of fungi. Few can grow if the equilibrium relative humidity is less than 65 per cent (equivalent to 11 to 13 per cent water

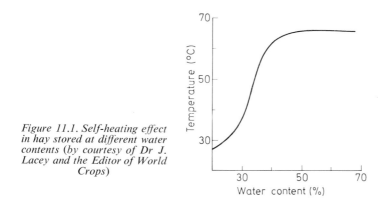

Figure 11.1. Self-heating effect in hay stored at different water contents (by courtesy of Dr J. Lacey and the Editor of World Crops)

content in hay) and many require more water. If hay, straw or cereal grains are stored damp because of poor harvesting conditions and insufficient drying, moulding will occur, often accompanied by heating. The initial heating of damp plant material may be caused by respiration of the plant cells, but subsequent respiration by micro-organisms plays an increasingly important part, until the plant cells are killed and heating is entirely microbial. The maximum temperature attained is related to water content, as shown for hay in *Figure 11.1*. Microbial heating is limited to a maximum of 65 to 70°C, but chemical processes may sometimes be initiated leading to further heating, and eventually to spontaneous ignition. Heating is ultimately limited by loss of water from the material, so that it cools to ambient temperature.

Successive stages in the heating process are caused by a sequence of different micro-organisms, of which fungi and actinomycetes are probably the most important. When water content is low, the *A. glaucus* group of fungi predominates and, due to respiration, increases the water content of the fodder. This permits other fungi to become established leading, in turn, to the proliferation of a succession of fungus and actinomycete species which favour increasing water content and temperature. Self-heating of fodder in this fashion encourages exuberant growth of such thermotolerant and thermophilic species as *T. vulgaris* and *M. faeni* (which are responsible for farmers' lung) and *A. fumigatus* when the water content exceeds 35 per cent and the temperature rises to 50°C or more (Festenstein *et al.*, 1965) (*Figure 11.2*). The characteristics of hay types is exemplified in Table 11.3.

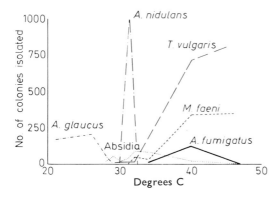

Figure 11.2. Growth of some fungi and actinomycetes in hay stored at different water contents (modified; by courtesy of Dr J. Lacey and the Editor of World Crops)

TABLE 11.3

CHARACTERISTICS OF DIFFERENT HAY TYPES

By courtesy of Dr J. Lacey and the Editor of World Crops

Hay type	Water content at baling (%)	Maximum temperature reached (°C)	Spore content (millions/g)	
			Fungi	Actinomycetes and bacteria
Very mouldy	35–50	50–65	10–100	350–1,200
Mouldy	20–30	35–45	2–60	3–250
Good	15–20	22–26	0·1–7	0·5–8

For storage with little or no moulding, the water content of hay must be less than 20 per cent, and of grain about 14 per cent. The spore content of good hay will usually be less than 5 million spores/g dry weight, compared with over 100 million spores/g in a mouldy hay, and sometimes in excess of 1,000 million spores/g in a farmers' lung type hay (Gregory, *et al.*, 1963).

When rainfall is high it is more difficult to make good hay without artificial drying, and the chances of moulding are therefore greater. This results in geographical and seasonal variations in the incidence of farmers' lung and other diseases related to hay moulding, e.g. mycotic abortion in cattle due to aspergillus or mucor infections (Hugh-Jones and Austwick, 1967).

The same principle relating water content and heating to fungal growth apply, in general, to bagasse and mushroom compost (*see* appropriate sections in this chapter).

Incidence and prevalence

In the British Isles, acute disease may occur sporadically throughout the year, but the incidence increases from September, reaching a peak from February to April, then declining rapidly. Sporadic cases may occur at any time. For obvious reasons more cases have been reported in men than in women, although as farmers' wives are recorded as farm workers in Britain their sex is not identified. Children have also acquired the disease (Staines and Forman, 1961; Barrowcliff and Arblaster, 1968). The highest 'attack rate' is between the ages of 41 and 60 years. Staines and Forman (1961) found that the regional incidence varied from 11·5 per 100,000 of the farming population

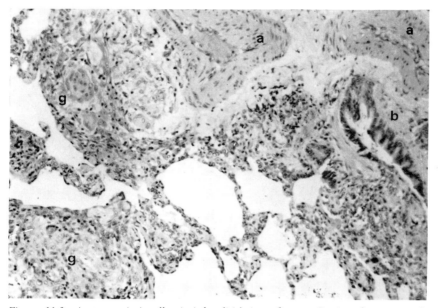

Figure 11.3. Acute extrinsic allergic 'alveolitis' in a farmer. Section shows sarcoid-like granulomas (g) and cellular infiltration of alveolar walls (by lymphocytes and plasma cells), arteritis (a) and involvement of the wall of a bronchiole (b) with narrowing of the lumen. (Original magnification × 150, reproduced at × 120, H and E stain. By courtesy of Dr R. M. E. Seal)

in East Anglia to 193·1 per 100,000 in Wales, and they computed that a conservative estimate of the annual incidence might be about 1,000. In Caithness (Scotland) the incidence of acute and chronic farmers' lung grouped together is 110 per 100,000 of the farming population (Boyd, 1971). In Orkney, Ayrshire and East Lothian the prevalence of precipitin-positive cases has been reported as 43, 36 and 0 per 1,000 respectively (Grant *et al.*, 1972).

Sources of exposure
Turning and stacking hay in the field and removing it to storage present little hazard. Exposure most often occurs when stored mouldy hay crops are handled during such operations as opening bales of hay and straw for animal feeding and bedding and poultry bedding, and when moving and threshing mouldy grain. Many of these activities may be carried out in poorly ventilated barns, sheds, shippens or partly open buildings so that the spore cloud— which may consist of up to 1,600 million spores, most of which are actino-

mycetes, per cubic metre of air (Lacey and Lacey, 1964)—is not diluted by clean air, and exposure is intense. The risk of exposure to mouldy material in these enclosed surroundings may occur at any time of the year. In addition to farm workers, stable hands, poultry workers and attendants of zoo and circus animals may also be at risk.

Pathology

Acute disease

Details of the pathology of acute disease have been obtained almost entirely from biopsy material taken at varying intervals after the onset of symptoms.

Microscopic appearances.—In the early stage there is oedema of the lungs with a predominantly lymphocytic infiltration and hence, thickening of alveolar walls; plasma cells are also—but not always—prominent. Within the first two weeks, non-caseating, epithelioid cell, sarcoid-like granulomas with Langhan's giant cells are usually present, but become less frequent as the time after exposure increases (*Figure 11.3*). These lesions have been called 'acute granulomatous interstitial pneumonitis' by Dickie and Rankin (1958).

The granulomas, which develop as oedema subsides, are very similar to those seen in 'idiopathic' sarcoidosis, Crohn's disease, chronic beryllium disease, tuberculosis without caseation, brucellosis and various fungal and protozoal infections (Jones Williams, 1967). They occur in alveolar walls and, to a significant extent, in the walls of terminal and respiratory bronchioles which they may almost obliterate (*Figures 11.3, 11.4*); changes tend to be greatest in the vicinity of respiratory bronchioles (Seal *et al.*, 1968). Brown, periodic acid Schiff-positive particles about 0·5 μm in diameter are often present in epithelioid cells, and are probably 'residual bodies'. Foreign body giant cells are also common, usually in alveolar spaces (Emanual and Wenzel, 1965), and often contain birefringent, ovoid-shaped foreign material of unknown significance. Small pulmonary artery branches are thickened due to swelling of their muscle fibres and proliferation of the intima (*Figure 11.3*) (Seal, Thomas and Griffiths, 1963).

Granulomas are not found in hilar lymph nodes.

In the case of disease of unusually acute onset numerous discrete, grey-coloured miliary nodules are seen throughout the lung on naked-eye examination. These consist of large numbers of lymphocytes, epithelial cells and early reticulin formation, but relatively few plasma cells and neutrophils, and no granulomas. In addition, there is acute vasculitis (Barrowcliff and Arblaster, 1968).

At a later stage of the disease, when the granulomas have resolved, substantial lymphocyte infiltration of alveolar walls with compact lymphoid follicles persists and, in addition, some collagen fibrosis may have occurred. The lesions closely resemble those of diffuse fibrosing 'alveolitis' of unknown cause or associated with collagen or other diseases; although healed granulomas may be found if carefully looked for.

No fungi can be identified by staining methods but thermophilic actinomycetes have been isolated from lung biopsy specimens (Wenzel and Emanuel, 1965).

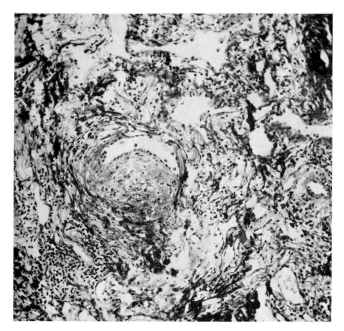

Figure 11.4. Chronic stage of extrinsic allergic 'alveolitis' in a worker exposed to avian antigens. A collagenized granuloma in the wall of a small bronchiole is partly obstructing its lumen. Severe interstitial fibrosis is also present. (Original magnification, × 160; reproduced at × 120; van Gieson stain. By courtesy of Dr K. F. W. Hinson and the Editor of Human Pathology)

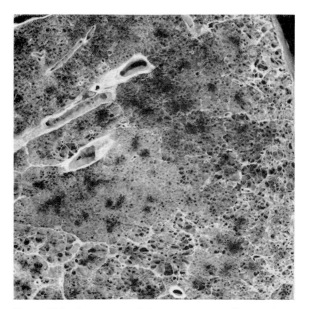

Figure 11.5. Appearance of chronic extrinsic allergic 'alveolitis' with honeycomb appearance. Natural size photograph from perfused lower lobe. (By courtesy of Dr R. M. E. Seal)

Chronic disease

Macroscopic appearances.—Thickening of the pleura is usual. The cut surface of the lungs reveal the appearances of diffuse interstitial fibrosis which, in places, may be confluent. The fibrosis contains smooth walled, 'honeycomb' cysts some of which may be as large as 2 to 3 cm in diameter (bronchiolectasis), and, characteristically, it involves the upper lobes more than the lower, although exceptions to this are seen. In some cases, the fibrosis is of fine type with very small cysts, and unless the lungs are prepared by formalin perfusion, it may not be identified (*Figure 11.5*).

Microscopic appearances.—There is diffuse collagenous fibrosis of alveolar walls and of peribronchiolar and perivascular areas. Foreign-body giant cells containing birefringent material are usually present. Active granulomas, however, are either absent, or very sparse, and are found only with difficulty—unless the interval since the acute attack is short. Healed granulomas are represented by small acellular nodules consisting of delicate (collagenous) fibrosis with groups of plasma cells—which identify the nature of the lesions—in close proximity. The presence of such lesions helps to establish that a diffuse interstitial fibrosis (fibrosing 'alveolitis') is of allergic rather than cryptogenic or other origin. Plasma cells are absent, or very occasionally found, in other parts of the lungs although, in some cases, substantial numbers are present in the medulla of the hilar lymph nodes (Seal *et al.*, 1968). In some fibrotic areas there is pronounced dilation of adjacent respiratory bronchioles characteristic of irregular (or 'scar') emphysema. The media of small pulmonary arteries may be thickened suggesting the presence of pulmonary hypertension (*See* Figure 11.4).

Pathogenesis and immunology

That farmers' lung is caused mainly by a late, Type III, Arthus reaction in the walls of non-respiratory and respiratory bronchioles and alveoli in response to particular antigens is supported by the following features which are broadly similar in other forms of extrinsic allergic 'alveolitis', but with different antigenic sources.

(1) There is a latent period of some few hours following exposure to mouldy hay dust before acute disease develops.

(2) Inhalation tests using aerosols of aqueous extracts of mouldy hay (or grain) provoke a reaction typical of acute disease (fever, malaise, basal crepitations and reduction of VC and gas transfer) a similar interval of a few hours in patients who have previously had acute disease, but not in control subjects (Williams, 1963) (*Figure 11.6*). Inhalation of extracts of *M. faeni* and, to a lesser extent, of *T. vulgaris* cause typical attacks of acute farmers' lung (Pepys and Jenkins, 1965) whereas extracts of *Aspergillus fumigatus* (and other aspergillus species), *Candida albicans*, Penicillium, Mucor, Alternaria, *Cladiosporium herbarum* and of good hay do not (Williams, 1963).

(3) Precipitating antibodies specific for the offending antigens are present in the patient's serum.

Precipitins arise as a result of previous exposure to antigen, and their capacity to mediate the reaction is closely related to the quantitative ratio of antigen to antibody. The most active complexes are formed when antigen is present in moderate excess (Ishazaka, 1963). However, a close correlation between the quantity of precipitins and their pathogenic effects does not necessarily exist and, when the amount of antigen is small, low precipitin levels may have greater pathogenic significance than high levels (Pepys, 1969). Precipitins may be present in the absence of detectable lung disease. These points are of significance when considering diagnosis. Spores of *M. faeni* are the most important source of farmers' lung antigens and the associated precipitins, but those of *T. vulgaris* may be of significance in a small

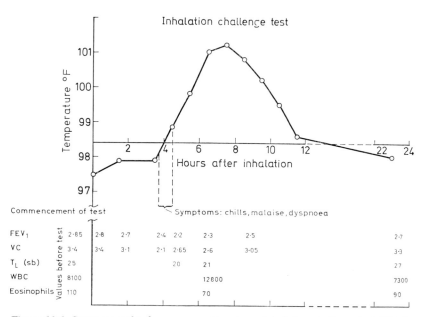

Figure 11.6. Systemic and pulmonary reactions to an inhalation challenge test. This is in fact a record of a challenge with avian antigen in a patient with bird-breeders' lung (q.v.), but the results with farmers' lung antigens are similar. (By courtesy of Professor J. Pepys)

number of cases. The antigens consist partly of glycopeptide and partly of polysaccharide (Pepys, 1969). Strains of *M. faeni* from four countries have been found to have little or no antigenic differences (Edwards, 1972a).

(4) *M. faeni* antigens have been demonstrated in bronchial walls and antibody-forming cells and vacuolated histiocytes which stain brilliantly for complement, found in the lesions in the lungs of patients with active farmers' lung (Wenzel, Emanuel and Gray, 1971).

(5) The pathological findings in hyper-acute disease (Barrowcliff and Arblaster, 1968), referred to already, are consistent with a late, Arthus type reaction.

(6) Pulmonary granulomas have been produced in both sensitized and unsensitized animals challenged with mouldy hay (Parish, 1961). Furthermore, typical lesions have been reported in a cow which became sick after being confined indoors and fed on poor quality hay during the winter months, and in which inhalation of an aerosol of *M. faeni* had caused a maximum

clinical respiratory response in eight hours (Pirie *et al.*, 1971). The term 'bovine farmers' lung' has been proposed to replace 'fog fever' in cattle (a disease with none of the features of extrinsic allergic 'alveolitis') but is, perhaps, capable of unhappy misinterpretation.

The presence of granulomas—an important feature of the pathology—has not been properly explained. It is not clear whether a cell-mediated, Type IV, reaction also participates. Experimental work in rabbits suggests that a cell-mediated reaction does take place (Jones, 1970), but there is no evidence of this in human disease.

When farmers' lung patients are skin tested with an appropriate antigen extract, oedema and erythema of the typical Arthus reaction may occur in four to six hours. However, skin tests have little practical value due to an irritant property of some antigens (notably *M. faeni*) and to false positive results.

Precipitins against *M. faeni* and *T. vulgaris* are demonstrated by standard double gel diffusion plate preparations; other fungi are also present but are probably only evidence of previous heavy exposure to those fungi and not of a pathogenic relationship as the lack of reaction to inhalation of their extracts confirms (Pepys, 1969). The antigens of *M. faeni* and *T. vulgaris* and mouldy hay extract are set up individually against the patient's serum.

Immuno-electrophoresis using Scheidegger's micro-method (1955) reveals a characteristic pattern of three arcs of constant position which have been termed A, B and C (*Figure 11.7*).These are derived mainly from the antigens of *M. faeni*: A and B are proteins and C is a glycopolypeptide. According to the intensity of the most consistent of these arcs the degree of reaction can be placed into three grades (Pepys, 1969). Altogether some 29 extracellular antigens of *M. faeni* have been identified (Fletcher, Rondle and Murray, 1970), but some of these are probably non-specific. Using special techniques Edwards (1972b) has shown that the major antigen in the C region—antigen 1 —is very heat stable whereas the major antigens in the A and B regions— antigens 2 and 3—are relatively thermolabile; other antigens are extremely thermolabile. Group I antigens, therefore, predominate in mouldy hay. Since antibodies to antigens which cannot be detected *in vitro* are present in some cases, it has been suggested that these antigens may be produced by a limited development of *M. faeni* spores within the lungs, and there is some circumstantial evidence to support this (Edwards, 1972b).

Precipitins against *M. faeni* are not present in the sera of populations which have not been exposed to mouldy hay or grain (or to mushroom compost—*see* mushroom workers' lung), but almost all persons with acute disease and about 18 per cent of apparently normal exposed workers give positive precipitin reactions (Pepys, 1969). In the case of 'normal' workers, however, probably all positive reactors should be regarded as potential candidates for farmers' lung disease. After exposure to antigen has ceased precipitin reactions gradually disappear so that a farmer with chronic disease is more likely to give a negative than a positive reaction. The higher the grade of the immuno-electrophoretic reaction the greater the number of attacks of acute disease which have occurred and the shorter, and more intense, the exposure that has been required to produce disease (Pepys, 1969).

Immunofluorescent studies of frozen sections of lung tissue of patients with

402

active farmers' lung suggest that *M. faeni* antigen can be found in the walls of small bronchi and that antibody-forming plasma cells and lymphocytes are present in the lesions. An important feature of all these cases was the presence of complement in large histocytes (Wenzel, Emanuel and Gray, 1971).

Circulating antinuclear factor (ANF) and rheumatoid factor (RF) are not a feature of *chronic* extrinsic allergic 'alveolitis' and their prevalence in this disease is no different from that in the general population (Turner-Warwick

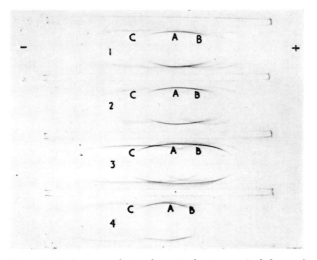

Figure 11.7. Immuno-electrophoresis showing typical farmers' lung hay reactions in the A, B and C regions given by farmers' lung serum. Test extracts (1) mouldy hay; (2) hay inoculated with a mixture of thermophilic actinomycetes; (3) hay inoculated with M. faeni; (4) culture filtrate extract of M. faeni. (By courtesy of Dr P. A. Jenkins)

and Haslam, 1971) (*see* Chapter 4). By contrast, rheumatoid factor may be present during acute disease and disappear when it has resolved (Banaszak, Thiede and Fink, 1970). The significance of this observation is not known, but might be related to the formation of intravascular immune complexes.

Clinical features

Acute disease

Symptoms.—Characteristically an acute attack occurs within four to twelve hours of exposure and often after the farm worker has retired to bed for the night. It consists of malaise, headache (frequently severe), rigors, sweating, fever, anorexia, nausea and vomiting. A cough which is either occasional or frequent and harassing is usual, but sputum is absent or of small volume, and mucoid in type. Haemoptysis may occur, but is rare. 'Tightness' of the chest is a common complaint and breathlessness on exertion is invariable and may be severe. Chest pain sometimes results from cough fracture of ribs but otherwise is absent. There is no rhinorrhoea or conjunctivitis.

The emphasis of symptoms, however, varies from patient to patient: in some the constitutional symptoms predominate, but in others, the respiratory; symptoms in general can vary from mild (of less dramatic onset) to very severe. In view of this and the similarity to the symptoms of various viral or bacterial diseases it is most important (as will be indicated in the section on Diagnosis) to obtain from the patient the appropriate history of exposure.

Acute symptoms usually subside in seven to ten days provided there has been no further exposure although some loss of weight often follows the attack and dyspnoea may persist for a few months in some cases. Many acute attacks may result from repeated exposures and, in a small proportion of patients, a point may be reached when a reaginic asthmatic response occurs immediately after exposure followed several hours later by typical symptoms of farmers' lung (Pepys and Jenkins, 1965).

Physical Signs.—Central cyanosis is sometimes present. There is tachycardia, fever which can be as high as 46°C (106°F) and dyspnoea at rest in patients whose symptoms are predominantly respiratory. Restlessness and apprehension may be prominent.

On auscultation there are heard fine crepitations towards the end of full inspiration distributed mainly in the lower halves of the lungs. Wheeze is not a feature of the disease but may be present in a small number of patients (Pepys, 1969). Rhonchi are absent and there are no signs of consolidation or pleural effusion.

Chronic disease

Symptoms.—After repeated acute attacks, cough and a variable amount of sputum and dyspnoea on effort become permanent, having increased progressively after each individual attack. In a few cases this occurs after a single episode of acute disease and in others, where there has been recurrent exposure to low concentrations of mould dust, symptoms develop insidiously without an antecedent acute episode. In most cases of chronic disease dyspnoea gradually worsens without further exposure to antigen. There are no constitutional symptoms but some patients complain of weakness in the legs on exertion.

Physical signs.—There are no characteristic physical signs. The patient is dyspnoeic on exertion, but not at rest until the disease has reached an advanced stage when central cyanosis may be observed. Finger clubbing is rarely seen. Signs of fibrosis of the lungs may be present: that is, deviation of the trachea, impairment of chest expansion on the more affected side, possibly with some flattening of the contour of the overlying chest wall. Crepitations in the lower halves of the lungs, so typical of acute disease, are not often heard and wheeze, in most cases, is conspicuous by its absence. The signs of cor pulmonale and congestive heart failure may be present in advanced disease.

Investigations

Acute disease

Lung function tests.—In the early stage some patients may be too ill to perform the tests.

Arterial oxygen desaturation and reduction in arterial carbon dioxide tension due to hyperventilation (caused, possibly, by the granulomatous lesions activating afferent nerve endings in the lungs) are the first changes to occur. These are soon followed by a fall in VC, TLC and compliance, and the decrease in gas transfer tends to be proportional to the reduction in VC. There is no evidence of airways obstruction. The degree of impairment of these functional parameters varies from mild to severe according to the severity of the disease.

These abnormalities resolve within six weeks in most patients treated with corticosteroids (Hapke *et al.*, 1968) and in twelve months in the majority not treated, but impairment of gas transfer and compliance can still be present after the chest radiograph has returned to normal (Williams, 1963). In a minority of patients VC and compliance do not return fully to expected normal values (*see* section on Prognosis). Lung function tests, therefore, are of help in assessing the response to treatment, but not in diagnosis.

Radiographic appearances.—In mild attacks there may be no abnormality. Otherwise abnormalities vary from barely detectable changes to widespread coarse opacities similar to the appearances of acute beryllium disease (*see Figure 10.5*).

The earliest changes consist of very fine, pin-point opacities in the central two-thirds or lower zones of the lung fields, and may be so slight as to be overlooked if the observer is not aware of the possibility of extrinsic allergic 'alveolitis'; even if he is, their presence may only be detected in retrospect by comparison with films taken after the patient has recovered. The use of an AP as well as a standard PA film viewed with a hand lens increases the accuracy of detection.

More definite abnormalities consist of discrete, well-defined opacities from pin-point to about 3 mm diameter in the middle and lower zones of the lung fields, but frequently sparing the costophrenic angles. In severe attacks larger, blotchy opacities are seen. The severity of symptoms, however, is poorly correlated with the degree of radiographic abnormality.

Larger opacities usually disappear within two or three weeks from the onset of disease, but the fine type may last up to six months before clearing. If fine opacities fail to disappear in six months to a year, they are unlikely to do so, and the appearances of chronic fibrotic disease may then develop (Hapke *et al.*, 1968).

Evidence of enlarged hilar lymph nodes is not seen.

Serology.—Serum should be examined for precipitins in all suspected cases of farmers' lung but it is important that antigens of acceptable standard are used.

Because of the lack of correlation between the quantity of precipitins and the presence or absence of lung disease it is not necessary, as a rule, to quantify precipitins by examining titres of serum (1:1 to 1:32), and they are simply recorded as being present or absent. But in the occasional patient who is strongly suspected of having acute farmers' lung although the standard test is negative, it may be reasonable to repeat the test with concentrated serum.

Precipitins against *M. faeni* or, less often, *T. vulgaris* are present in some 90 to 95 per cent of patients with acute disease but are not detectable in the remaining 5 to 10 per cent. Indeed, there are cases in which there is a typical history of exposure, but precipitins are persistently absent even on serum concentration, and it is probable that some other, unidentified, contaminating organic dust is responsible for the disease. Conversely, it must be emphasized that precipitins are evidence of exposure to antigens and not necessarily of lung disease. In general, it appears that failure to detect *M. faeni* antibodies in farmers' lung cases is due largely to lack of sensitivity in immuno-electrophoresis and, to a lesser extent, of immunodiffusion tests (Fletcher, Rondle and Murray, 1970).

Inhalation challenge tests.—Inhalation of the relevant antigens reproduces the features of the acute illness. However, in the majority of cases this challenge test is not necessary as the history, clinical signs and other investigations furnish the diagnosis; furthermore, it is not justifiable to risk increase of breathlessness in an already severely handicapped patient or the rare, but real, possibility of chronic disease which may follow the provocation of an acute attack. Nevertheless, the test may be of diagnostic value in patients in whom the history is equivocal or in whom no precipitins can be identified. If it is employed for this purpose it is most important that low dilutions must be used initially and subsequently increased in order to avoid undue reaction. It is absolutely contraindicated in patients with severe respiratory disability.

Challenge tests are helpful in other forms of extrinsic allergic 'alveolitis' for the identification of 'new'—that is, previously unsuspected—antigens, and for confirming the diagnosis of certain forms of the disease (for example, bagassosis, q.v.) in which the presence of precipitins may be erratic.

Lung biopsy.—This should only be necessary to verify the diagnosis in the uncommon cases which exhibit atypical features (*see* section on Diagnosis).

Skin tests.—These are not of practical value in diagnosis, because suitable extracts giving reliable results in patients and control subjects are not yet available.

Mycology.—Although culture of sputum for fungi in acute disease has yielded *M. faeni* (Lacey and Lacey, 1964), *Aspergillus* spp., *C. albicans* and *mucor* frequently grow, they are not of pathogenic or diagnostic significance being merely an indication of inhalation of the varied flora of mouldy hay.

Haematology.—There are no specific abnormalities. There may be a mild polymorphonuclear leucocytosis, but negligible eosinophilia.

Chronic disease

Lung function.—Patterns of impaired function are variable. In some patients there is reduction of gas transfer and compliance with or without decrease in lung volume, but no evidence of airways obstruction; in others—a minority—there is slight to moderate airways obstruction (reduced FEV_1/FVC per cent and increased RV) which is *not* reversed by inhalation of bronchodilator aerosols (Dickie and Rankin, 1958; Hapke *et al.*, 1968) and may be due to granulomatous or fibrotic involvement of terminal and respiratory bronchioles; and in yet others, there is a combination of both types of functional impairment (Hapke *et al.*, 1968). A small number of patients exhibit little or no abnormality. The airways obstruction found in some patients with extrinsic allergic 'alveolitis' can occur in non-smokers and is not reversed by bronchodilators.

A discrepancy sometimes exists between the symptoms complained of and the values of lung function tests at rest which may be near normal. This is analogous to the situation in early asbestosis and chronic beryllium disease.

Cardiac catheterization, incidentally, may reveal an increase in pulmonary artery pressure which is probably due to a permanent reduction in the vascular bed of the lungs (Bishop, Melnick and Raine, 1963).

Radiographic appearances.—Appearances vary according to the severity of the disease. They range from fine, linear or rounded, ill-defined opacities

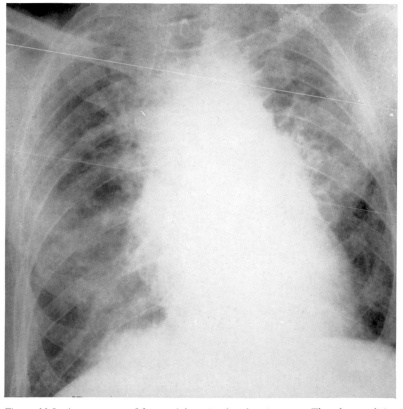

Figure 11.8. Appearances of farmers' lung in the chronic stage. The abnormalities predominate in the upper halves of the lung fields. Note the translucent cyst-like areas

to coarse linear opacities which tend to radiate from the hilar regions and, in advanced disease, are accompanied by tracheal deviation and distortion, lobar contraction, and by small translucent areas caused by cyst formation (*Figure 11.8*). By contrast with acute disease these appearances predominate in the upper and middle zones, and are often more pronounced on one side. They are indistinguishable from fibrosis and fibrocavernous tuberculosis. Undue translucency of the lower zones may be present. Occasionally fibrotic appearances are more evident in the lower than the upper halves of the lung fields.

Chronic disease may also be represented by small discrete opacities when these remain unchanged for about a year; they do not necessarily progress to the 'fibrotic' appearances just described. If serial chest films are not available these opacities could, in the presence of an acute respiratory illness, be interpreted as evidence of farmers' lung of acute type or of some unrelated disease.

Serology.—In the case of chronic disease the chance of demonstrating precipitins becomes less as the time since the last acute episode increases. Precipitins are still present in about 80 per cent of cases up to three years after an attack of acute disease, but in only about 20 per cent when the interval is longer than three years (Hapke *et al.*, 1968).

Lung biopsy.—In cases of diagnostic difficulty this can be of help, in association with other data, when healed granulomas are demonstrated.

Diagnosis

Farmers' lung has to be distinguished from many types of other respiratory diseases of fortuitous occurrence presenting with similar symptoms in farmers, such as influenza and lobar pneumonia. Chronic farmers' lung requires especially to be differentiated from other types of diffuse interstitial fibrosis (fibrosing 'alveolitis').

Acute disease

The most important diagnostic features consist of a detailed history of occupation and the mode of onset of disease, characteristic constitutional and respiratory symptoms and signs, the presence of precipitating antibodies and consistent radiographic appearances. Lung function tests are of no diagnostic help. It must be remembered that, in taking the history, the patient may not be aware, or may deny, that he has worked with mouldy hay or other material. In mild cases there are no dramatic symptoms.

The following diseases may need to be distinguished:

(1) *Influenza.*—Acute farmers' lung is most frequently confused with an influenzal illness, but the history of exposure and delayed onset of symptoms should lead to the correct diagnosis.

(2) *Acute bronchitis.*—Farmers' lung is distinguished by unproductive, or slightly productive cough; by rapidly developing breathlessness; by the presence of crepitations in the lower halves of the lung fields, and the absence of rhonchi; and by a lack of response to treatment with antibodies and bronchodilators.

(3) *Lobar pneumonia.*—The symptoms of two diseases are similar but the physical signs and radiographic signs of lobar consolidation are not present in farmers' lung.

(4) *Miliary tuberculosis.*—Differentiation here rests mainly upon the occupational and clinical history, and upon the presence of precipitins. Resolution of radiographic abnormalities after treatment with antituberculosis drugs is of no diagnostic assistance as in most cases acute farmers' lung recovers spontaneously.

(5) *Allergic bronchopulmonary aspergillosis.*—This occurs in atopic farm workers (who usually have a history of extrinsic asthma) after exposure to

mouldy hay with a high content of aspergillus spores. The features of this disease are entirely different from those of farmers' lung. They consist of a more rapid onset after exposure, an asthmatic attack with evident wheeze, expectoration of solid brown plugs of sputum which contain fungal mycelia, eosinophilia of sputum and blood, immediate (Type I) and late (Type III) skin responses to extracts of *A. fumigatus* which do not occur in farmers' lung, and radiographic evidence of lung consolidation or collapse.

(6) *'Idiopathic' sarcoidosis.*—In farmers' lung the work history, mode of onset of the illness, basal crepitations, absence of radiographic evidence of hilar lymphadenopathy and rapid recovery with resolution of radiographic changes all make confusion with sarcoidosis unlikely.

(7) *Cryptogenic diffuse interstitial fibrosis of rapid development (Hammon-Rich lung).*—The progressive nature of the disease, rapid deterioration of the patient's condition and absence of precipitins distinguish it from farmers' lung, but biopsy may be necessary to exclude precipitin-negative farmers' lung.

(8) *Silo-fillers' disease (see* Chapter 12).—Although the onset of symptoms may resemble that of farmers' lung it is usually more rapid, but in some cases it may be delayed for two to three weeks. In most cases the clinical and radiographical features are those of pulmonary oedema but, in some, the appearances of the chest film are identical with those of acute farmers' lung. However, the nature of the exposure should point to the diagnosis. But it is to be remembered that moulding of silo contents may ultimately occur and cause acute farmers' lung when they are disturbed after the silo is re-opened.

Chronic disease

If chronic disease does not follow single or repeated episodes of acute disease, or if these have passed unrecognized, diagnosis can be very difficult. The difficulty is emphasized by the fact that there are no characteristic physiological or radiographic features, and that farmers' lung precipitins are not only unlikely to be present more than three years after the last exposure, but may also be found in farmers who have remained in intermittent contact with mouldy hay and have lung fibrosis due to another cause.

Diagnosis depends upon a careful and detailed history of farm work and past respiratory illnesses and upon the exclusion of other causes of lung fibrosis. Biopsy may be necessary in disease of insidious onset but can be indecisive if epithelioid granulomas are not found, as is likely to be the case in disease that has been present for more than twelve months.

Differentiation may have to be made from the following diseases:

(1) *Fibro-cavernous tuberculosis.*—Past clinical, bacteriological and therapeutic history indicate the diagnosis in most cases, and in some *M. tuberculosis* can be cultured from the sputum.

(2) *'Idiopathic' sarcoidosis.*—Appearances of chest films in farmers' lung closely resemble these of sarcoidosis. The distinction rests upon the work history, absence of hilar lymphadenopathy and extra thoracic stigmata of sarcoidosis, a negative Kveim test and the presence of precipitins to *M. faeni* or *T. vulgaris*. It should be noted, however, that the reactivity of the tuberculin

test tends to be reduced in farmers' lung as it is in 'idiopathic' sarcoidosis (Scadding, 1967).

(3) *'Mixed dust fibrosis' (see* Chapter 7).—The different occupational history is decisive.

(4) *Chronic beryllium disease.*—The occupational history is usually sufficient to differentiate the two diseases. If this is not so, the identification of beryllium on biopsy of lung tissue will decide, but on histological grounds it is impossible to distinguish between the two.

(5) *Cryptogenic diffuse interstitial fibrosis (fibrosing 'alveolitis').*—In this disease the lack of a relevant occupational history and the fact that, in most cases, it favours the lower parts of the lungs distinguish it from chronic farmers' lung. The histological features of the two diseases are sufficiently similar in most cases to make differentiation on biopsy impossible.

(6) *Eosinophilic granuloma and Hand-Schüller-Christian disease.*—The systemic features and histological (biopsy) characteristics, which are most pronounced in the periphery of the lower lobes and do not resemble those of farmers' lung, are definitive; the comparative variety of these diseases make them unlikely contenders in differential diagnosis.

Prognosis and complications

Acute disease

After a single attack, complete recovery is the rule in from two to twelve weeks if the patient ceases to be exposed, but there are exceptions to this. After repeated attacks it is increasingly less likely, and the possibility of chronic disease greater. Corticosteroids hasten the rate of recovery.

Few follow-up statistics are available, but in one series of 44 patients who had acute disease, about 70 per cent were asymptomatic three or more years later and about 30 per cent were mildly or moderately dyspnoeic on effort (Barbee *et al.*, 1968).

Spontaneous pneumothorax is a rare complication.

Chronic disease

Dyspnoea on exertion steadily increases and, according to the severity of the disease, pulmonary hypertension may develop and eventually lead to fatal congestive heart failure. In the later stages emaciation may be a prominent feature.

There are as yet no epidemiological surveys of the natural history of chronic disease. It is probable that some cases of pulmonary fibrosis which may be encountered in farm workers (as well as mushroom and bagasse workers) represent the end-point of unrecognized episodes of extrinsic allergic 'alveolitis' in the past.

Treatment

Acute disease

As soon as the diagnosis is made, the patient must be removed from exposure, and this alone results in improvement. If the attack is severe he should be reassured and corticosteroids—the only treatment of any value—administered

in the form of prednisone in adequate dosage (about 40 mg/day) for two weeks followed by 20 mg daily until resolution of clinical and radiographic signs is complete.

Chronic disease

There is, of course, no treatment for fibrotic disease, but in some cases of moderately advanced disease acute lesions may also be present as a result of the most recent exposure to mouldy material and, in these, trial of corticosteroids is worth while.

Prevention

The chief aim is to dry hay or grain sufficiently by natural or artificial means (such as barn drying) and to prevent re-wetting during storage so that no moulding or heating can take place. Good ventilation of barns and storage buildings is required. Dust respirators of special design effectively prevent the inhalation of spores (Gourley and Braidwood, 1971), and should be worn by farm workers known to have had a previous attack of farmers' lung and are likely to be exposed to mouldy material.

One per cent of concentrated propionic acid, well mixed with grain before it is loaded into the silo for storage, prevents the growth of fungi and bacteria, and hence a rise in temperature favouring the growth of thermophilic organisms. A practical method of treating hay in this manner, however, has not yet (1973) been developed.

Substitution of silage for hay has been advocated as a preventive measure and is employed by some farmers.

Ideally, a farm worker who has had more than one acute attack should change his occupation, but usually he has no inclination or little aptitude for other work; and, if he is self-employed, change may be impossible.

BAGASSOSIS

Bagasse is the fibrous cellulose residue of sugar-cane stalk after it has been crushed and the juice extracted. It consists of tough 'true fibre' and soft 'pith' tissue from the inner stalk. Pith absorbs water readily and, if present in any quantity, hinders drying. It is fibrous, tough and has good insulating qualities for heat and sound.

Sugar-cane is grown in the West Indies, India, Pakistan, Brazil, Cuba, Argentina, the southern United States of America, South Africa, Australia and Mexico. After the extraction of sugar, bagasse may be baled for storage.

Baling is done in a press similar to a hay baler. The bales are bound by steel wire and stacked in the open in such fashion as to allow ventilation. Stacks may be protected against rain by a covering of asbestos or plastic sheeting. The bagasse is stored for about twelve months, when it may be transferred to another plant for compression into smaller compact bales for transportation. The baling plant only operates during the few months in the year when the crop is gathered.

An experimental batch of fresh bagasse, stored in bales, heated spontaneously to 54°C in five days and then cooled to 40°C before the temperature rose again to 49°C after thirty-three days. Bagasse with a 27 per cent water content heated to 49°C in three days (Lacey, 1969). Hence, the growth of many different species of fungi and thermophilic and mesophilic actinomycetes is favoured. Fermentation of the residual sugar by yeasts probably assisted the initial heating.

Since the late 1950s a system—the Ritter system—of bulk sorting unpithed or partly depithed bagasse has been used in some industrial plants. It consists of keeping piles of bagasse wet with a 'biological' liquor containing molasses and lactic acid-producing bacteria until required for use. An important advantage of this system is the elimination of dust from the bagasse (Paturau, 1969).

Mouldy bagasse contains enormous numbers of fungal spores—probably as many as 500,000,000 per g dry weight (Buechner, 1968)—and, although these were identified as *T. vulgaris* (Seabury *et al.*, 1968), it is now known that they consist in fact chiefly of a much more abundant, but closely related, species of thermoactinomyces named *T. sacchari* ('sacchari' = of sugar cane).

Bagassosis has the same acute and chronic forms as farmers' lung, but is more often found in the acute form. It follows exposure to the dust of dry, mouldy bagasse but not of fresh or autoclaved bagasse. It was described in New Orleans (Jamison and Hopkins, 1941) and, although most of the reported cases have occurred in the southern states of the United States of America (Sodeman and Pullen, 1944; Buechner *et al.*, 1958, 1964), there have been many others in Britain (Castleden and Hamilton Paterson, 1942; Hunter and Perry, 1946; Hargreave *et al.*, 1968), Italy (Caugini, 1951), India (Ganguly and Pal, 1955; Viswanathan *et al.*, 1963), the Philippines (Dizon, Almonte and Anselmo, 1962), Spain (González de Vega *et al.*, 1966) and the West Indies (Hearn, 1968). It is apt to occur in sporadic outbreaks when workers are exposed to mouldy material.

Uses of bagasse

Bagasse has many possible uses and these are summarized in Table 11.4. Bagasse in briquettes is employed as a fuel to generate electricity in cane-producing areas, although it is now being replaced by oil. Charcoal is produced by carbonization, and methane by anaerobic fermentation of the cellulose fraction. Manufacture of different types of paper and board has become increasingly important in recent years; particle board can be moulded to any shape for the furniture, container, motor car and shipbuilding industries. Furfural, which is also known as furfuraldehyde and is produced by acid hydrolysis of the xylan in bagasse, is employed in the refining of lubricating oils and the manufacture of resins. Bagasse is also used in the production of viscose rayon and as a filler and extender in reinforced thermosetting plastics. For details of the uses of bagasse *see* Paturau (1969).

Sources of exposure

A potential risk of bagassosis exists in the following processes if bagasse is dry and mouldy: removing bales from stacks to the compressing plant, the compressing operation, opening or shredding of bales in the factory, milling bagasse to desired particle size, during various manufacturing operations (including the grinding of hardboard), and the moving of bagasse for cattle and poultry bedding. In a British factory before World War II, bales were

412

opened using a wet process, but when, in the altered circumstances of the war, they were opened dry, cases of bagassosis occurred (Hunter and Perry, 1946).

The growth of bacteria and fungi in bagasse can now be prevented, however, by treating it when fresh with 1 per cent of propionic acid before or after milling. This has greatly increased the potential of bagasse in manufacture.

Pathology and immunology

The pathology of acute disease has the same features as acute farmers' lung, including granulomas (Sodeman and Pullen, 1943; Buechner, Bradford, Bealock and Wascom, 1961, 1962); but some cases are remarkable for the presence of large numbers of plasma cells both in the alveolar walls and

TABLE 11.4

USES OF BAGASSE

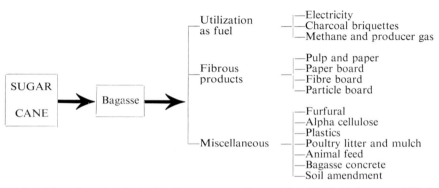

Adapted from *By-products in the Cane Sugar Industry* with permission of Dr J. M. Paturau and Elsevier Publishing Company.

spaces. Chronic disease consists of diffuse interstitial fibrosis with bronchiolectasis—mainly in the upper parts of the lungs—and pleural thickening (Buechner, 1962).

Precipitins are present in some two-thirds of patients during or shortly after an acute attack of bagassosis, but disappear within one to three years (Salvaggio *et al.*, 1969). *Thermoactinomyces vulgaris* was thought to be the chief, if not only, antigenic source (Seabury *et al.*, 1968), and inhalation of extract of *T. vulgaris*, but not of *M. faeni*, by men suffering from bagassosis appeared to reproduce the symptoms of the disease. However, Lacey (1971a) subsequently identified the organism as *T. sacchari*. This explains why precipitins to genuine *T. vulgaris* extracts have not been demonstrated (Hargreave, Pepys and Holford-Strevens, 1968; Hearn and Holford-Strevens, 1968). But when extracts of *T. sacchari* were tested by immuno-electrophoresis and agar-gel double diffusion against sera from patients with bagassosis in the United States of America and from exposed workers in Trinidad, characteristic precipitin reactions occurred (Lacey, 1971b). These reactions could not be altered by adsorption of the sera with *T. vulgaris* extracts (Holford-Strevens, 1971). However, one of the subjects who reacted to

413

extracts of *T. vulgaris* reacted similarly to extracts of *T. sacchari* (Lacey, 1971a) and immuno-electrophoresis suggests that the two species may contain some antigens in common.

Thermoactinomyces sacchari, therefore, appears to be the main cause of bagassosis and is the third actinomycete to be identified as responsible for extrinsic allergic 'alveolitis'. Inhalation tests with extracts of this organism and identification of precipitins against it should be helpful in the diagnosis of bagassosis.

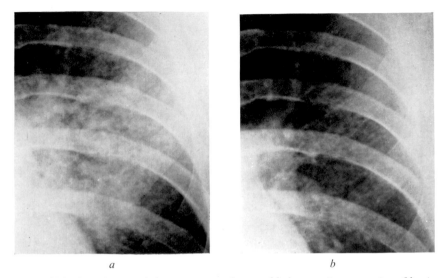

a   *b*

Figure 11.9. Acute bagassosis in a man exposed to mouldy bagasse in preparation of laminated boards. Initially, tuberculosis was suspected but was not substantiated and specific precipitins were demonstrated; (a) numerous small opacities in the mid-zone of the left lung seen after a few months' lassitude, breathlessness and loss of weight; (b) almost complete resolution six weeks later

Serum IgG and IgA, but not IgM, levels are raised in acute bagassosis (Salvaggio *et al.*, 1969).

Bagasse contains a small amount of quartz (about 0·1 to 0·2 per cent) derived from the soil and, because of this, some authorities believed bagassosis to be a form of silicosis. There is no foundation for this belief and it is evident that the pathogenesis and pathology of the disease do not resemble silicosis in any way.

Clinical features

The symptoms, physical signs and radiographic appearances of both acute and chronic disease are similar to those of farmers' lung (*Figure 11.9*), but in a number of acute cases there is no evident abnormality of the chest film.

Lung function tests during acute disease reveal some reduction of TLC, VC and gas transfer which subsequently return to normal in most cases (Weill *et al.*, 1966). Vital capacity in exposed workers without disease may be significantly lower than in unexposed workers, but the reason for this has not been ascertained (Hearn, 1968). However, a single episode of bagassosis can produce dyspnoea on effort, permanent reduction of lung volume and gas transfer, and hyperventilation on exercise (Miller, Hearn and Edwards, 1971).

Treatment

As in the case of farmers' lung, the majority of patients with acute disease recover spontaneously in four to twelve weeks after being removed from exposure. Corticosteroids in adequate dose may hasten clinical recovery, but do not appear to influence the rate at which lung function returns to normal (Pierce *et al.*, 1968).

Prevention

The application of 1 per cent of propionic acid to milled fresh bagasse before baling effectively prevents moulding even after bales are stored in the open for more than twelve months. If bagasse has not been treated in this way wet processes may be used for storage (Ritter process) or in the breaking open of bales. Exhaust ventilation and enclosure of machinery, when technically possible, are also employed. High-efficiency respirators may be worn, but are intolerable for work in hot and humid climates.

If more than one acute attack has occurred, the worker should be removed from further exposure to bagasse and should not transfer to agricultural work in which there could be contact with mouldy hay or fodder.

MUSHROOM WORKERS' LUNG

Mushroom workers' lung was first reported in the United States in 1959 (Bringhurst, Byrne and Gershon-Cohen, 1959) and is characterized by the same acute constitutional and respiratory symptoms and signs as farmers' lung, but only two cases of doubtful chronic disease appear to have been observed (Sakula, 1967; Jackson and Welch, 1970). It appears to be remarkably uncommon considering that mushroom cultivation is carried out on a large scale in Britain, the United States of America and European countries, but it is probable that the illness is more common than reports suggest and that it may often go unrecognized.

Intensive methods of cultivation have been used for some years. They involve the preparation of a compost consisting of wheat straw and fresh horse manure which is allowed to decompose in the open air for about three weeks, and is then subjected to a temperature of 55 to 60°C at 100 per cent humidity in boxes indoors, allowing exuberant growth of thermophilic and thermo-tolerant actinomycetes, including *M. faeni*, *T. vulgaris*, and various fungi (Fergus, 1964; Craveri, Guicciardi and Pacini, 1966). The compost is then tipped from the boxes, the spawn added and mixed mechanically, with the production of much dust which consists mainly of actinomycete spores. During growth of the mushrooms the temperature is kept at about 20°C and the humidity about 90 per cent. When the mushroom crop has been picked the growing sheds are heated to 60°C after which the compost is taken out and deposited on a dumping ground. The spawning operation and the removal of compost are, therefore, the chief sources of exposure to spores and of outbreaks of disease.

In six cases of typical acute extrinsic allergic 'alveolitis' in mushroom workers, precipitins against farmers' lung antigens were present in only two (Sakula, 1967; Jackson and Welch, 1970). With so rich a microflora as mushroom compost it is possible that organisms other than *M. faeni* and *T. vulgaris* may cause the disease. In Lacey's experience (1971b) thermomonospora-like actinomycetes are generally more abundant than *M. faeni* and *T. vulgaris*.

It has been suggested that nitrogen dioxide might be evolved by the compost (*see* silo-fillers' disease, Chapter 12) and cause the disease (Bringhurst, Byrne and Gershon-Cohen, 1959), but there is no evidence that significant concentrations of this gas occur and no reason to believe that it plays any part in the pathogenesis of mushroom workers' lung.

It is important to bear this form of extrinsic allergic 'alveolitis' in mind when a mushroom worker has an acute respiratory disease, especially as the illness is not necessarily severe. A worker who has more than one acute attack should be advised to leave the industry.

Preventive measures include efficient exhaust ventilation of the spawning houses and the use of dust respirators. Rapid cooling of compost after the initial heating has been recommended but is probably ineffective.

MALT WORKERS' LUNG

Although the feature of acute extrinsic allergic 'alveolitis' in malt workers were first recorded in 1928 (Vallery-Radot and Giroud) the significance of this observation has only recently been recognized (Riddel *et al.*, 1968; Channell *et al.*, 1969). The disease occurs in distillery maltsmen and brewery workers, but its prevalence is not known; a chronic form does not seem to have been recorded.

In the malting process barley from the farms is dried in hot-air kilns, stored in silos for at least eight weeks, and rehydrated in steeping tanks with hypochlorite used as a mild fungicide. It is then spread out on open floors and allowed to germinate. Traditionally the temperature of the grain is maintained at 18°C by turning and raking the grain periodically (which also releases carbon dioxide and water) or by varying the thickness of the layer. The heat is produced by the respiration of the barley during germination. When the process has reached the desired stage of germination, it is stopped by drying the malt at 82°C in a hot air kiln in which it is turned periodically to facilitate drying. It is then ready for the distillery.

The disease has been shown to be caused by *Aspergillus clavatus* (Riddle *et al.*, 1968; Channel *et al.*, 1969) and *A. fumigatus* (Vallery-Radot and Giroud, 1928). *A. clavatus* is a recognized contaminant of grain (Panasenko, 1967). Small amounts of inoculum may be present on grain in the field, but there are also many opportunities of infection in the malting process and the suitable conditions on the malt floor lead to rapid proliferation. The spores are present in husks and malt grist, suggesting that they can withstand the temperatures reached in the kilns (Channel *et al.*, 1969). Riddle *et al.* (1968) have suggested that the growth of fungi is encouraged by the presence of a large percentage of split corns, by maintenance of a higher floor temperature (24°C) assisted by spraying the grain with water to shorten the germination time, and that the hypochlorite treatment encourages the growth of *A. clavatus* by suppression of other organisms. Malt workers may be exposed to spore dust, therefore, when turning barley on the malt floor and malt in the malt kilns, and also when cleaning the kilns (Channell *et al.*, 1969).

A. clavatus is present in the sputum of all men exposed to the spores, and not only those who have disease (Channell *et al.*, 1969). Precipitins against *A. clavatus* are found in the serum of the sick men and in a proportion of healthy employees, but not in normal unexposed employees nor in patients with suspected farmers' lung (Channell *et al.*, 1969). Inhalation tests with *A. clavatus* spores have reproduced the disease in men who had previously suffered from it. In addition, some employees have precipitins against *Aspergillus fumigatus* and the rhizopus species which are also common contaminants of open malt floors, and might also be capable of inducing allergic pulmonary reactions (Channell *et al.*, 1969).

When contamination of a malting process with *A. clavatus* is discovered, clinical, radiographical and serological tests should be carried out on all exposed employees and the possibility of allergic 'alveolitis' considered in the event of acute respiratory disease.

The application of mechanical methods in some distilleries and breweries has greatly decreased the chance of workers inhaling spores, but their use is not yet general.

MAPLE BARK STRIPPERS' DISEASE

Acute respiratory disease in men who stripped the bark off maple trees was first reported by Towey, Sweany and Huron in 1932 since when a number of cases of allergic granulomatous 'alveolitis' have been reported (Emanuel, Lawton and Wenzel, 1962; Emanuel, Wenzel and Lawton, 1966; Wenzel and Emanuel, 1967). Although Towey, Sweany and Huron referred to the disorder as 'bronchial asthma' the clinical and radiographical features they described were typical of acute extrinsic allergic 'alveolitis'. The cause of the disease is inhalation of spores of *Cryptostroma* (*Coniosporum*) *corticale* which are ovoid and measure 4 to 5 μm in their greater axis. This fungus can produce disease under the bark of maples, hickories, bass woods and sycamores (Gregory and Waller, 1951). Wenzel and Emanuel (1967) found that *C. corticale* was not present in maples before they were felled but developed during prolonged storage afterwards. Exposure to the spores occurred mainly in paper mills during stripping of logs by hand or mechanical means, sawing, and shaking small long chippings through screens to remove bark fragments.

A chronic form of the disease does not seem to have been observed.

Precipitins specific for the spore extract are present in affected workers and also in exposed, but seemingly unaffected workers some of whom, however, have had subclinical disease (Emanuel *et al.*, 1966). Experimental work with *C. corticale* in rats supports the conclusion that delayed hypersensitivity plays an important role in maple bark disease (Tewksbury, Wenzel and Emanuel, 1968).

Biopsy of lung tissue during the illness reveals sarcoid-like granulomas and some degree of diffuse interstitial fibrosis, as in acute farmers' lung, and the presence of spores. The fungus can be grown from the tissue on Sabouraud's agar supplemented with an aqueous extract of maple wood (Emanuel, Wenzel and Lawton, 1966). The spores in the lungs closely resemble *Histoplasma capsulatum* but are distinguished by being stained black with Gomori's methenamine silver nitrate technique (Emanuel, Wenzel, and Lawton, 1966). Histoplasmin skin and complement fixation tests are negative.

Preventive measures consist of spraying logs during debarking with water containing detergent, remote control of some operations, the wearing of special respirators, monitoring of spore concentrations in the mill, and regular clinical, serological and x-ray examinations. The disease can be controlled by these means, but continual vigilance is necessary.

SUBEROSIS
(*suber, cork*)

Cork workers in Portugal—who number more than 20,000—are prone to lung disease which has been attributed to cork dust (Cancella, 1959). In atopic workers it has the features of bronchial asthma with transient opacities in the chest radiograph, but in non-atopic workers it is an extrinsic allergic 'alveolitis' with the same clinical, physiological and radiographic features as farmers' lung (Ávila and Villar, 1968; Pimentel and Ávila, 1973). Persons with acute or subacute 'alveolitis' appear to recover completely when removed from the working environment.

Cork bark (*Quercus suber* L.) may become mouldy after being boiled and stacked wet for straightening purposes in hot, damp warehouses. Dust which consists of cork and the spores of numerous different fungi, including *Penicillium frequentans* (Westling), is encountered in high concentrations during destacking and the preparatory manufacturing stages of discs and stoppers ('corks') (Lacey, 1973).

The pathology of acute disease consists of infiltration of alveolar walls with lymphocytes, histocytes and, later, fibroblasts, and by the appearance of sarcoid-like granulomas. In chronic disease there is dust pigmentation and nodular fibrosis with obliterative changes in small vessels (Ávila and Villar, 1968). The size of the spores of *P. frequentans* and some of the other airborne fungi will allow them to penetrate to alveolar level whereas cork particles tend to be larger (Lacey, 1973), although they are consistently present in lung lesions (Pimentel and Ávila, 1973).

Sera from cork workers with suberosis produce multiple precipitin arcs with extracts of mouldy—but not clean—cork dust (Ávila and Villar, 1968). And of the fungi isolated from the air of working areas *P. frequentans* appears to be the most important in this respect (Pimentel and Ávila, 1973); but whether sensitization is caused by the spores of this fungus or by cork dust particles contaminated by fungal metabolites and hyphae remains to be established (Lacey, 1973).

There is no evidence that the dust of clean, non-mouldy cork causes pulmonary disease.

BIRD BREEDERS' (FANCIERS') LUNG

This extrinsic allergic 'alveolitis', which is caused by avian protein antigens, is similar to farmers' lung in having acute and chronic forms with the same clinical, physiological, radiological and pathological features. It was first recorded in workers handling goose and duck feathers (Plessner, 1960) and in a budgerigar breeder (Pearsall *et al.*, 1960), and is now recognized to be related to exposure to the dust of the droppings of budgerigars (parakeets), pigeons, parrots and hens (Pepys, 1969). It has been reported in children as well as in adults (Stiehm *et al.*, 1967).

Exposure occurs during cleaning out pigeon lofts, bird cages and hen houses. People likely to be exposed, therefore, include those who breed budgerigars or pigeons professionally or as a hobby, pet shop workers, aviary attendants, and budgerigar fanciers who may only keep one bird. Among those looking after many birds who experience intermittent exposure to high concentrations of dust at one to two weekly intervals during cage cleaning, typical acute disease develops. Whereas those who keep a single pet bird at home are exposed more or less continuously to low concentrations of dropping dust, and in them the development of disease is gradual and insidious. These two modes of onset are, in fact, more clearly exemplified in this form of extrinsic allergic 'alveolitis' than in farmers' lung. However, typical acute disease appears to be rare among poultry farmers though it has been reported (Carreiro, Freitas e Costa and Teles de Araújo, 1969); tightness in the chest and cough are complained of by a minority after prolonged exposure (Elman *et al.*, 1968).

Many persons with bird breeders' lung give a history of repeated, acute, febrile respiratory illnesses from which they recover rapidly when they cease contact with the birds, but recur—sometimes after slight exposure—when they return to their bird houses. When all contact with the birds is stopped complete clinical recovery is the rule although in some patients—especially those who have had a number of previous acute atttacks—irreversible chronic disease may develop. When the onset is insidious and marked only by progressively increasing dyspnoea on effort, severe fibrosis of the lungs identical to that of chronic farmers' lung is likely to be established by the time the patient is first seen. But, as in the case in farmers' lung, not all persons exposed to avian antigens develop evidence of disease. The disease may occur in the children of pigeon and budgerigar enthusiasts and appears to be of more insidious onset than in adults (Chandra and Jones, 1972).

Lung biopsy in acute disease reveals infiltration of lymphocytes and plasma cells, reticulin proliferation and granuloma formation in alveolar walls; and in some cases the presence of foamy histocytes in alveolar walls and spaces (Nash, Vogelpoel and Becker, 1967; Hensley *et al.*, 1969). Mast cells have also been reported (Shannon *et al.*, 1969). In chronic disease, diffuse interstitial fibrosis, multinucleated giant cells, and sarcoid-like granulomas are seen, although foam cells are absent, and organizing bronchiolitis may be present (Fink *et al.*, 1968).

That avian antigens are causally responsible is demonstrated by the fact that acute respiratory and constitutional symptoms, basal crepitations and impaired gas transfer result about six hours after inhalation of a dilute aerosol of pigeon or budgerigar serum by patients who have previously had acute disease (Reed, Sosman and Barber, 1965; Hargreaves *et al.*, 1966). Precipitins and typical lesions of allergic 'alveolitis' with foam cells and

419

granuloma formation occur in rats after prolonged inhalation of pigeon dropping dust (Fink, Hensley and Barboriak, 1969). If inhalation tests are used in diagnosis (*see Figure 11.6*) the initial extracts must be weak in order to avoid prolonged respiratory symptoms which may require treatment with corticosteroids.

Precipitins against avian antigens are found in the serum of the majority of patients with acute pigeon breeders' disease and in some 16 per cent of pigeon fanciers with no evidence of disease (Barboriak, Sosman and Reed, 1965), but they are absent in unexposed persons. They are also present in a majority of unaffected poultry farmers (Elman *et al.*, 1968). In budgerigar fanciers the situation is remarkably different as precipitins are not found in exposed healthy subjects, although they are present in almost all those with allergic 'alveolitis' confirmed by inhalation tests (Faux *et al.*, 1971). These differences in clinical correlation may be due to differing potency of the various antigens, as well as to a variable intensity of individual exposures.

The precipitating antibodies in pigeon breeders' disease consist of pigeon serum albumin, β- and γ-globulins and an antigen (not present in the serum) which cross-reacts with pigeon γ-globulin. All are voided in the droppings but, due to subsequent enzyme activity, do not survive for more than a month (Edwards, Fink and Barboriak, 1969). All these antigens are apparently required to produce the disease and they exist together in the droppings, but not in the serum or feathers (Edwards, Barboriak and Fink, 1970).

Intradermal tests with avian serum or extracts of droppings usually cause an immediate, Type I, weal reaction followed later by an Arthus type reaction (Pepys, 1969). By contrast with farmers' lung the Arthus type skin reaction to avian antigens is closely associated with the presence of precipitins and may, therefore, be a useful pointer to diagnosis.

Lung function returns to normal in most patients when they cease contact with the birds, but may continue to deteriorate if they remain exposed. As in farmers' lung, irreversible airways obstruction is sometimes present but can later recover completely (Nash *et al.*, 1967; Dinda, Chatterjee and Riding, 1969). It is particularly important to identify the disorder in a child in whom permanent lung damage may develop unless he is removed from contact with the birds.

The diagnosis of acute disease is not likely to be confused with psittacosis for, although the symptoms may be somewhat similar, in psittacosis they develop after an incubation period of seven to fourteen—occasionally up to thirty days; lung consolidation may occur. Bedsoniae (which are sensitive to tetracycline) may be cultured from sputum or blood, and there is a rising titre in the complement fixation test.

The most important precept in the management of patients with acute (or subacute) disease is permanent avoidance of contact with the offending birds, but corticosteroids may be indicated to hasten resolution (*see* Treatment).

PITUITARY-SNUFF TAKERS' LUNG

Since the 1920s powdered extracts of pig and ox pituitary glands have been used as a snuff in the treatment of diabetes insipidus and, for short periods, in the treatment of enuresis in children. In atopic subjects this may cause rhinitis and extrinsic asthma (as has been long recognized) which is associated with the presence of reaginic IgE antibodies and an immediate skin reaction on intradermal injection of the offending material. But extrinsic allergic 'alveolitis' may also occur in both atopic and non-atopic subjects and can result in diffuse interstitial fibrosis (Mahon et al., 1967).

In contrast to the extrinsic allergic 'alveolitis' of farmers' lung, but like that of pigeon breeders' lung, a bronchial reaction—expressed by broncho-spasm and mild eosinophilia—tends to accompany the alveolar reaction. This is probably due to the range of particle size and the solubility of the antigens.

The pathological appearances of the lungs are similar to those of pigeon breeders' lung, and fibrosis may involve the walls of respiratory bronchioles as well as alveolar walls.

Precipitating antibodies against pig and ox serum proteins and pituitary antigens are present in patients with and without evidence of asthma, and intradermal tests with porcine and bovine sera provoke both Type I and Type III reactions (Pepys et al., 1966). Furthermore, due to cross reaction, such patients may develop auto-antibodies to antigens of human pituitary cells (Pepys et al., 1966).

Physiological and radiographic signs of 'alveolitis' usually resolve com-pletely after cessation of exposure (Harper et al., 1970), but evidence of irreversible fibrosis occurs in some cases (Mahon et al., 1967). It should be noted, however, that some patients with diabetes insipidus have pulmonary disease (Spillane, 1952) which is not associated with allergic 'alveolitis' and is usually present before pituitary snuff is used in treatment.

Acute 'alveolitis' should be treated with corticosteroids in view of the risk of lung fibrosis, and the pituitary snuff discontinued.

Synthetic lysine vasopressin administered by nasal spray is now available as a substitute for animal pituitary extracts, and should reduce the likelihood of allergic complications (Spiegelman, 1963), although rhinitis and asthma have been reported following its use (Mahon et al., 1967). If pituitary snuff is employed, preparations having a minimal particle size of 180 μm are recommended, but they are expensive. A 'control' chest radiograph should be taken before the treatment is started and repeated, together with tests for precipitins, at periodic intervals so long as it is continued.

RARE OR UNCERTAIN EXAMPLES OF EXTRINSIC ALLERGIC 'ALVEOLITIS'

(1) The features of acute and chronic extrinsic allergic 'alveolitis', including granulomas, have been observed in persons exposed to air from an air-conditioner contaminated with an organism closely resembling M. faeni with precipitins against it present in their serum (Banaszak, Thiede and Fink, 1970). Similarly authenticated disease of insidious onset which recurred during the central-heating season of the year has been shown to be caused by a M. faeni-like actinomycete growing in a forced air furnace (Fink et al., 1971). Aspergillus fumigatus deriving from an air-conditioning system has also caused an outbreak of lung disease (Wolf, 1969).

(2) Granulomatous 'alveolitis'—referred to as sequoiosis—has been

reported in a man exposed to mouldy sawdust of the giant redwood (*Sequoia sempervirens*) in whose serum precipitins against extracts of saw-mill dust were found (Cohen *et al.*, 1967). The responsible organisms have not been positively identified, but may be graphium or *Aureobasidium pullulans*.

(3) For many years it has been known that asthma may occur in sensitive granary or farm workers exposed to grain and flour dust (Frankland and Lunn, 1965; Lunn, 1966). This may be caused by a variety of mites and fungi, but the wheat weevil (*Sitophilus granarius*) can give rise, not only to a pronounced immediate (Type I) allergy, but also to precipitating antibodies (Jimenez-Diaz, Lahoz and Canto, 1947). Delayed (Type III) sensitivity with constitutional symptoms, basal crepitations and impairment of gas transfer have been produced in an atopic worker by an inhalation challenge test three hours after an immediate asthmatic reaction. Precipitins against weevil extract were found in his serum after concentration, and intradermal injection of weevil extract caused a delayed, Arthus-type reaction (Lunn and Hughes, 1967). The source of the antigen is weevil protein.

(4) Disease considered to be extrinsic allergic 'alveolitis' has been described after exposure to the following: fish meal used in the manufacture of animal foods (Ávila, 1971); animal hair in the course of work with furs—'*furriers' lung*' (Pimentel, 1970); and coffee bean dust (van Toorn, 1970). On present evidence, '*coffee workers' lung*' appears to be a doubtful entity and further investigation is required. Extracts of the coffee berry and the husk and its dust react specifically with the sera of coffee workers (Pepys, 1969), but the significance of this observation has not been elucidated.

(5) Lung disease having some of the features of acute extrinsic allergic 'alveolitis' with precipitins against *Penicillium casei* in their serum has been reported in Swiss cheese washers who clean the surface of mouldy, stored cheese blocks (DeWeck, Gutersohn and Butikofer, 1969). But there does not appear to be any strong correlation of intensity of symptoms with the presence of precipitins and although skin tests with *P. casei* extracts tend to give Type I reactions, Type III reactions are absent or inconclusive (Minnig and De Weck, 1972).

(6) Immediate allergy—asthma, hay fever, eczema—may occur in workers exposed to the dust of a proteolytic enzyme of *Bacillus subtilis* used in manufacturing 'biological' detergent laundering products. This, together with the nature of industrial exposure, is referred to in Chapter 12. However, although dyspnoea may not develop in many cases until some eight hours after exposure (Flindt, 1969) and precipitins against *B. subtilis* proteinase may be present (Pepys *et al.*, 1969), clear-cut examples of extrinsic allergic 'alveolitis' have not yet been identified; but there is suggestive evidence that it may occur (Flindt, 1969). Curiously, precipitins are more prevalent in healthy exposed workers than in those with allergy (Pepys *et al.*, 1969).

A potential health hazard to the housewife should also be considered (*see* Chapter 12).

OTHER TYPES OF LUNG DISEASE DUE TO FUNGI AND TO VIRUSES AND BACTERIA

It is appropriate to make brief mention of the most important of these specific infections and the occupational circumstances in which they may occur. Their pathology, clinical features and treatment can be found in textbooks of respiratory and mycotic diseases.

MYCOTIC DISEASES

Aspergillosis

The aspergillus species is ubiquitous in nature and is found in decaying vegetation, in grain, hay and straw and in farm buildings, and as it is a fairly common cause of disease in many species of birds, it may be present in their droppings. High levels of contamination by the spores may, therefore, be encountered by farm workers, threshers, millers, pigeon fanciers, poultry tenders, aviary workers and hair sorters. *A. fumigatus* is chiefly responsible but *A. niger*, *A. flavus*, *A. nidulans* and *A. clavatus* may also cause disease. Aspergillosis is the most common fungus disease of the lungs in Britain.

There are five varieties of aspergillosis, the first two of which occur in atopic subjects and the remainder in non-atopic subjects (Pepys, 1969).

(1) Asthma in which the fungus acts as an allergen in subjects with reaginic antibody.

(2) Asthma and pulmonary eosinophilia in patients with allergic bronchopulmonary aspergillosis who have both precipitating and reaginic antibodies.

(3) Saprophytic infection—aspergilloma—of lungs damaged by bronchiectasis, abscess, infarction, sarcoidosis, cystic fibrosis and various types of pneumoconiosis.

(4) Extrinsic allergic 'alveolitis'. This has already been referred to under the heading of 'malt workers' lung'.

(5) Disseminated aspergillosis which involves many organs in patients debilitated by neoplastic diseases and reticuloses, and those receiving corticosteroid or radiation treatment.

Histoplasmosis

The causal organism, *H. capsulatum*, is found in the soil and excreta of chickens, birds, bats and domestic and wild animals mainly in the east central area of the United States of America, in Canada, Central and South America and, to a minor degree, in Africa and Europe, but it is not indigenous to Britain. Inhalation of spores, which have a unique predilection for cells of the reticulo-endothelial system, may occur in farm workers, ditch diggers, construction workers, workers demolishing derelict buildings, and spelaeologists.

Both primary and progressive forms of the disease are seen. Calcified primary lesions have sometimes been mistaken for silicosis and may cause diagnostic difficulty in individuals of migrant habits.

Coccidioidomycosis (Friese, 1958)

Coccidioides immitis is an active saprophyte in the soil in the south-west of the United States of America, in Panama, Honduras and Cuba, and in South America. European countries, being an unsuitable climatic habitat, appear to be free of the organism. It is the arthrospores and chlamydospores of the fungus which when inhaled produce disease in man and animals, and

423

important factors in infection are long, dry summers, mild winters, a light soil productive of much dust and windy conditions to scatter the dust.

Persons at risk in endemic areas are agricultural workers (including tractor drivers), cotton pickers, cotton gin and compress operators, grape pickers, construction workers and, in particular, laboratory workers. However, it should be noted that transportation of contaminated materials and laboratory infection may cause isolated cases of the disease outside endemic areas. Negroes, Mexicans and Filipinos are especially susceptible to the disease.

North American blastomycosis

This is caused by *Blastomyces dermatitidis* which is endemic in the south-eastern United States of America and is probably due to inhalation of spores present in the soil and on vegetation. Rodents, dogs and horses may be infected and contaminate the soil with their faeces. Agricultural workers, nurserymen and construction workers are those mainly at risk (Veterans' Administration Cooperative Study on Blastomycosis, 1964).

The psittacosis-ornithosis group of viruses

These organisms, which cause pneumonia and pleural effusion, occur in pigeons, ducks, turkeys and other birds. Those potentially at risk are poultry, pet-shop and aviary workers, and pigeon fanciers.

Tuberculosis

Doctors, medical students, nurses, ward orderlies, physiotherapists, radiographers and laboratory workers comprise an occupational group particularly exposed to the possibility of tuberculous infection. B.C.G. inoculation is indicated in tuberculin-negative persons.

Anthrax

Spores of *B. anthracis* in wool and animal hides may cause pulmonary anthrax but nowadays it is virtually unknown in Britain owing to stringent hygiene controls. It occurs in butchers, veterinary surgeons, wool handlers, tanners and farmers.

BYSSINOSIS

The term 'byssinosis' ($\beta\acute{\upsilon}\sigma\sigma\sigma\varsigma$ = originally, flax and the linen made from it; later, Indian cotton), introduced by Proust in 1877, embraces a gradation of respiratory symptoms due to exposure to the dust of cotton, flax and soft hemp ranging from acute dyspnoea with cough and chest tightness (reversible by bronchodilators) on one or more days of a working week to chronic (that is, permanent) obstructive lung disease.

Although cotton and flax have been used in the manufacture of textiles since times of antiquity, byssinosis was first recognized by Ramazzini in the seventeenth century and seems to have affected cotton, flax and soft hemp workers in Europe during the eighteenth and nineteenth centuries (Patissier, 1822). It was described in Lancashire, where most of the British cotton industry is concentrated, in the first half of the nineteenth century (Kay, 1831) but was generally overlooked in Britain until surveys of the cotton industry were started about thirty years ago. The disorder was then thought to be mostly confined to Lancashire cotton workers (Schilling, 1956) and flax workers in Northern Ireland (Smiley, 1951) where it is commonly known as 'poucey chest' ('poucey' is a dialect word meaning dirty or nasty). But it is now known to occur in Scotland (Smith *et al.*, 1962), Holland, Germany, Sweden, the United States of America, Egypt, Greece, India and Taiwan (Bouhuys *et al.*, 1967a), Spain (Bouhuys *et al.*, 1967b), Belgium (Tuypens, 1961), Australia (Gandevia and Milne, 1965a) and Israel (Chwat and Mordish, 1963).

Sources of exposure

Cotton (Gossypium spp)
The chief sources of dust production occur in the ginnery where seeds are removed from the cotton after picking in a special machine, the 'gin'; in the 'mixing room' during opening of bales of cotton; in the 'blow room' where the cotton is beaten and blown to eliminate dust and short fibres; and in the 'cardroom' where carding engines comb the fibres and remove dirt and defective material. The fibres are then gathered and twisted into fine strands for spinning. Other dusty operations are 'stripping', which consists of removing dust and cotton fibre adherent to the wire teeth of the carding engine, and 'grinding' (sharpening) the teeth.

Airborne dust consists of broken cotton fibres, bracts (thin, brittle leaves surrounding the stem of the cotton boll which cannot be separated from the cotton), pericarps, bacteria, fungi and minerals. Particles vary from 3·8 cm ($1\frac{1}{2}$ inches) in length to less than 2 μm diameter. The larger airborne particles visible to the naked eye consist mainly of broken cotton fibres up to 2·5 cm in length—which are apparently innocuous—and fragments of plant debris too large to enter the lungs which are known as *fly*. 'Coarse' grade cotton produces more dust than the 'fine' grade when the fibres are long. Since the introduction of measures to suppress dust and of a TLV of 1 mg/m³ originally recommended by Roach and Schilling (1960), dust levels have been much reduced (*see* section on Prevention). And although, in general, there has been less dust in spinning rooms than in carding rooms there is a risk of increased concentrations in spinning rooms due to the introduction latterly of high-speed machinery.

Flax (Linum usitatissimum).
Although the industry is contracting owing to substitution of synthetic fibres, flax is still used (often with hemp, q.v.) to manufacture linen (an Old English word for flax) and yarn for rope, twine, thread, hosepipes, tarpaulins, fishing nets and clothing. In Britain this industry is confined to Northern Ireland and Scotland.

Bales of flax are first op ned and small bundles are separated out by hand, mixed, and then passed into a machine which combs out and straightens the fibres and eliminates dirt ('hackling'). Tow produced during 'hackling' or received in bales is passed through a carding machine to be opened and agitated. All these processes are dusty but carding is particularly so.

Fibres are next further straightened on 'drawing frames' and then formed into slivers of uniform thickness, twisted and wound on to bobbins. Much fine dust is produced. The yarn is then spun dry, half-dry or wet; only dry spinning gives off substantial amounts of dust. Winding, twisting and cabling of rope causes significantly smaller dust concentrations than opening, hackling, carding and spinning (Smith et al., 1969).

Hemp. (Soft hemp, *Cannabis sativa*; also known as English or Irish hemp. Hard hemp or Manilla hemp, *Musa textiles*; Mauritius hemp, *Furcraea gigantea*)

It appears that only soft hemp, which is a stem fibre unlike the others which are leaf fibres, is associated with the development of byssinosis. It is used in the manufacture of rope and yarn.

After the hemp plant is 'retted' (that is, subjected to a rotting process in water) it is dried, beaten (batted) to remove wood particles, 'hackled' (*see* previous section) and baled (Bouhuys et al., 1967b). Until recently this was a flourishing industry in Callosa de Segura in Spain, but is now in rapid decline due to the increased use of synthetic fibres.

Batting and hackling are very dusty activities, but dust concentrations during cabling, twisting and polishing rope are small (Smith et al., 1969).

Jute (Fibre from bark of *Corchorus capsularis* and *C. oliterius*)

This is grown mainly in India and Pakistan and is used in the manufacture of carpets, felt, wadding and, in combination with flax, in various types of cloth. Retted jute is received by the mill in bales, the opening of which is dusty; mixing grades of fibres, carding and drawing fibre are also dusty processes.

Sisal (Fibre from the leaves of *Agave sisalana*)

Sisal is employed chiefly in rope manufacture. The leaves are decorticated and brushed—a very dusty process—and the resulting fibre baled. Opening the bales and carding fibre also produce much dust.

Rayon (generic term for synthetic fibre produced from cellulose)

No untoward effects have been observed among workers in rayon spinning mills (Tiller and Schilling, 1958; Berry et al., 1972).

Natural history of byssinosis

As stated previously, byssinosis can be regarded as a form of asthma in that the lung airways are 'targets' of a bronchospasm-provoking factor initiated by the inhalation of cotton, flax or hemp dust which may result in chest tightness, breathlessness with objective evidence of airways obstruction over progressively longer periods during a working week, and which can usually be reversed by bronchodilator aerosols. The gradations of byssinosis are sufficiently well defined to allow of subdivision on clinical grounds.

Clinical grades

These, which were recommended by Schilling et al. (1963), may, for clarity, be prefixed by 'C' to distinguish them from the functional ('F') grades referred to in the next section.

Grade $C\frac{1}{2}$.   Occasional tightness of the chest on the first day of the working week.

Grade C1.   Tightness of the chest and/or difficulty in breathing on each first day only of the working week.

Grade C2.   Tightness of the chest and/or difficulty in breathing on the first and other days of the working week.

Grade C3.   Grade C2 symptoms accompanied by evidence of permanent respiratory disability from reduced ventilatory capacity.

Some workers do not develop symptoms for years after first exposure, others complain on first being exposed, and yet others never have respiratory symptoms.

Functional grades

Theoretically, the immediate, or acute, effect of exposure to dust can be determined by measuring FEV_1 before and at the end of a working shift on the first working day after a period (usually a weekend) away from work. The difference between these values—designated as Δ FEV_1—is the basis of the grading system suggested by Bouhuys, Gilson and Schilling (1970). An FEV_1 value below 80 per cent of predicted normal is taken as abnormal. When an abnormal value is recorded the test should be repeated after administration of a bronchodilator. It is, of course, necessary that the prediction data are valid for the populations examined. The grades are as follows.

Grade F0.   (F = Function.) No demonstrable acute effect of the dust on ventilatory capacity; no evidence of chronic ventilatory impairment.

Grade $F\frac{1}{2}$.   Slight acute effect of dust on ventilatory capacity; no evidence of chronic ventilatory impairment.

Grade F1.   Moderate acute reduction of ventilatory capacity; no evidence of chronic ventilatory impairment.

Grade F2.   Evidence of slight to moderate irreversible impairment of ventilatory capacity.

Grade F3.   Evidence of moderate to severe irreversible impairment of ventilatory capacity.

Data for each worker must also include his age, the nature and duration of his work, smoking habits and the presence of other respiratory disease.

It should be pointed out, however, that a grading system such as this has restricted practical value which is limited to specially controlled investigations. There are a number of reasons for this. For the purposes of routine medical examination in the clinic and factory, the error which may occur between repeated FEV_1 readings is likely to be significant and misleading; and it is impossible to estimate a residual acute effect due to exposure to cotton or similar dusts in the presence of chronic airways obstruction which is particularly likely to be present in smokers. Furthermore, it is not clear whether any difference is implied between 'chronic' and 'irreversible' ventilatory impairment in these grades.

A gradation of both symptoms and impairment of ventilatory capacity also occurs among flax workers and soft hemp workers (Mair *et al.*, 1960; Elwood *et al.*, 1965), but not in sisal workers in whom the effects are mild or absent (Velvart, 1971, 1972). Surveys of cotton, flax and jute workers have shown that tobacco smoking and atmospheric pollution increase the effects of inhaled dusts. This relationship is discussed in more detail in the section on Pathogenesis.

Prevalence

Cotton dust is the commonest cause of byssinosis. It has been said that jute does not give rise to the disease (Gilson *et al.*, 1962; Siddhu, Nath and Mehrotra, 1966) but mild functional changes have been found in workers milling the fibre (Gandevia and Milne, 1965b; Valic and Žuškin, 1971a);

TABLE 11.5

Average Dust Concentrations (mg/m^3)
in Five Cardroom Processes

Process	Mill	Respirable	Medium	Fly	Total
Cards	Medium	0·37	0·43	0·56	1·36
	Coarse	0·36	0·64	1·37	2·87
	Total	0·65	0·55	1·02	2·22
Drawframes	Medium	0·23	0·29	0·73	1·25
	Coarse	0·56	0·59	1·62	2·77
	Total	0·42	0·47	1·16	2·05
Speedframes	Medium	0·21	C·22	0·54	0·97
	Coarse	0·51	0·64	2·39	3·54
	Total	0·38	0·46	1·52	2·36
Combers	Medium	0·25	0·17	0·35	0·77
	Coarse	—	—	—	—
	Total	—	—-	—	—
Ring frames	Medium	—	—	—	—
	Coarse	0·42	0·49	1·83	2·74
	Total	—	—	—	—

(By courtesy of Drs M. K. B. Molyneux and J. B. L. Tombleson and the Editor of *Br. J. ind. Med.*)

sisal has been variously reported as having no effect (Gilson *et al.*, 1962) or only mild effects (Velvart, 1971).

Prevalence is often expressed as a percentage of the population exposed without distinction being made between different grades of byssinosis. It varies in different groups of workers in relation to the quality and quantity of cotton dust in their environment, and almost all workers exposed to large concentrations of coarse mill dust may be affected; these include, in particular, strippers, grinders, carders and undercarders. Table 11.5 shows the average dust concentrations recently observed in a group of Lancashire cotton mills, and Table 11.6, the prevalence of different clinical grades of byssinosis in operatives exposed to 'medium' and 'coarse' mill dust (Molyneux and Tombleson, 1970). In general, the prevalence of all grades of byssinosis is proportional to the total concentration of dust of medium and coarse cotton less the content of fly, and also to the duration of exposure (Žuškin and Valic, 1972). *Figure 11.10* shows the effect of exclusion of fly.

Prevalence among cotton ginnery workers in tropical countries has been reported as 20 per cent in the Sudan (Khogali, 1971) and 38 per cent in Egypt (El Batawi, 1962). In England, between 1963 and 1966 the total prevalence of byssinosis of grades $C\frac{1}{2}$ to C2 was 26·9 per cent, being higher in 'coarse' than 'medium' cotton-mills (Molyneux and Tombleson, 1970). Among cardroom workers in Holland the prevalence is 17 per cent (Lammers,

TABLE 11.6

BYSSINOSIS: PREVALENCE (%) IN 10 OCCUPATIONS IN MEDIUM AND COARSE MILLS

Occupation	Mill	Prevalence (%)				Total No.	Mean exposure (yr)
		Grade $\frac{1}{2}$	Grade 1	Grade 2	All grades		
Blowroom and cotton chamber (male)	Medium	6·0	12·0	6·0	24·0	50	9·7
	Coarse	6·4	4·3	3·2	13·8	94	11·8
Carder, undercarder (male)	Medium	5·3	23·7	7·9	36·8	38	19·1
	Coarse	14·5	14·5	10·9	40·0	55	19·2
Stripper and grinder (male)	Medium	9·2	22·4	17·1	48·7	76	18·5
	Coarse	9·9	34·1	14·3	58·2	91	17·0
Card tenter (female)	Medium	0·0	7·9	2·6	10·5	38	13·9
	Coarse	8·6	17·1	0·0	25·7	70	9·6
Drawframe tenter (female)	Medium	7·5	9·4	13·2	30·2	53	20·0
	Coarse	11·4	14·8	14·8	40·9	88	22·2
Speedframe tenter (female)	Medium	6·0	9·0	6·0	21·0	167	28·0
	Coarse	7·6	20·5	6·7	34·8	210	26·8
Comber tenter (female)	Medium	6·0	10·0	0·0	16·0	50	14·3
	Coarse	—	—	—	—	(0)	—
Ring spinner (female)	Medium	—	—	—	—	(0)	—
	Coarse	3·7	3·7	3·7	11·1	108	18·0
Labourer (male)	Medium	0·0	0·0	4·0	4·0	25	8·3
	Coarse	4·8	0·0	0·0	4·8	42	6·8
Wasteman (male)	Medium	—	—	—	—	(2)	—
	Coarse	15·4	0·0	7·7	23·1	13	14·5

(By courtesy of Drs M. K. B. Molyneux and J. B. L. Tombleson and the Editor of *Br. J. ind. Med.*)

Schilling and Walford, 1964) and in the United States of America, 25 per cent (Žuškin et al., 1969). By contrast, prevalence in spinners in England and Holland, is 1·5 per cent and 1·6 per cent respectively (Lammers, Schilling and Walford, 1964), and 12 per cent in the United States (Žuškin et al., 1969).

Although byssinosis in cotton workers is most prevalent in the blowing-room and cardroom, in flax workers it is equally prevalent in all parts of the mill (Mair et al., 1960). In Northern Ireland the lower grades of the disease are common in flax workers over 35 years of age (Carey et al., 1965).

Less is known about the frequency of byssinosis caused by dust from other

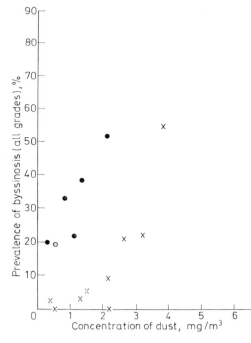

Figure 11.10. Prevalence of byssinosis (all grades); (●) plotted against total dust less fly, (×) plotted against total dust. (By courtesy of The British Occupational Hygiene Society)

TABLE 11.7

ANNUAL PRODUCTION OF COTTON YARN—PURE AND MIXED
(Thousand metric tons)

Selected countries		1953	1969
Argentine	(P)	76·2*	75·8
Australia	(P and M)	11·0	26·7
France	(P and M)	270·2	267·0
Germany (Fed. Repub.)	(P and M)	343·2	251·6
India	(P and M)	682·7	951·1
Italy	(P)	166·0	184·6
Mexico	(P)	—	145·4
Netherlands	(P)	64·5	54·7
Pakistan	(P)	53·7	303·3
Spain	(P)	—	104·4
U.A.R.	(P)	59·4	162·4
U.K.	(P)	359·2	166·2
U.S.A.	(P and M)	1,695·0	1,637·1
U.S.S.R.	(P and M)	898·7	1,437·7

(P, Pure; M, Mixed; * incomplete series)

ANNUAL WORLD PRODUCTION OF SYNTHETIC FIBRES
(Thousand metric tons)

	1953	1969
Rayon and acetate (continuous fibre)	935	1,420
Non-cellulosic (continuous fibre)	115	2,245

(Data from *United Nations Statistical Year Book*, 1970)

fibres, but substantially more chronic airways obstruction—known as *cannabosis*—has been found in Spanish hemp workers over 50 years of age (18·5 per cent of whom have severe respiratory disability) than in a control population none of whom has severe disability (Bouhuys *et al.*, 1969a). Chronic airways obstruction has also been reported in about 56 per cent of Czechoslovakian hemp workers (Velvart, 1971).

New cases diagnosed annually for compensation purposes in Britain are shown in Table 1.2, but these figures are a fairly crude index of prevalence.

Despite increased mechanization and dust control measures it is believed that, because of greater productivity, byssinosis in cotton mills may be increasing—at least, in the United States of America (Bouhuys *et al.*, 1967a). It must be remembered, however, that in mills with a low labour turnover workers will have had a longer exposure than those in mills with a high turnover.

Table 11.7 indicates the trends in production of cotton and synthetic fibres in certain countries of the world. Synthetic fibres which are produced chiefly by the major industrial countries (Europe and the United States of America), are used as a substitute for cotton but this is on too small a scale to reduce the general risk of byssinosis materially in the immediate future. Flax production is rapidly decreasing.

Pathology

No specific abnormalities have been identified. The lungs are often dust pigmented and, in individuals who have been diagnosed as having Grade C3 disease, there is some cellular infiltration of bronchial and bronchiolar walls, but no fibrosis. In cotton workers, cotton fibres, which are highly birefringent when viewed by polarized light, may occasionally be seen. Round or oval bodies up to 10 μm diameter which have a central black core surrounded by a yellowish coating and stain positively for iron may also be present, but they do not have any diagnostic significance.

Lesions characteristic of extrinsic allergic 'alveolitis' are not seen.

Pathogenesis

The byssinosis-producing potential of fibres varies from potent to negligible in this order: cotton, flax, soft hemp, jute and sisal.

Cotton and similar dust particles have been classified into size grades (Gilson *et al.*, 1962): 'coarse', greater than 2 mm; 'medium', 2 mm down to 7 μm; and 'respirable', less than 7 μm.

The ventilatory capacity of workers with symptoms of byssinosis falls when they are exposed to cotton dust during a working day, but it also falls— although to a lesser degree—under similar conditions in workers who do not have byssinosis (*Figure 11.11*) (Berry *et al.*, 1973). It was originally believed that byssinosis is closely related to overall dustiness (Roach and Schilling, 1960) but it has been shown more recently that the 'respirable' and 'medium' components of the total dust correlate most significantly with the prevalence of respiratory symptoms (Molyneux and Berry, 1971).

Because Bouhuys (1970) found that cotton and hemp workers who develop chest tightness and dyspnoea after exposure have reduced FEV_1, maximum expiratory flow rate and VC, but no significant fall of specific conductance

431

(the reciprocal of airways resistance per litre of thoracic gas volume), whereas men with no symptoms following exposure do not exhibit change in FEV_1, maximum expiratory flow rate and VC, but do have a significant reduction of specific conductance, it appears that the first type of response results from the action of the dust on smaller airways, and the second, from its action on larger airways.

An interesting feature of the production of the disorder is revealed by an observation in cotton cardroom workers. Those who have been away from dust exposure for longer than a weekend (that is, for two weeks) show a

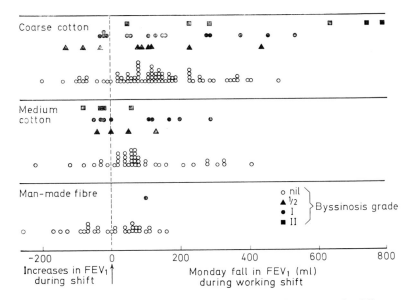

Figure 11.11. This shows the effect mill dust type has in determining the difference in Monday fall in FEV_1 among workers without byssinosis, the negligible mean fall in FEV_1 in man-made fibre mills and that the Monday fall of FEV_1, was related to symptoms of byssinosis only in the coarse-cotton mills. The relationship between Monday fall in FEV_1 and byssinosis is weak. (By courtesy of Berry et al., 1973, and the Editor of the British Journal of Industrial Medicine)

significantly higher first FEV reading and a significantly lower final FEV reading than is usual on the day of return to work; whereas, in workers without byssinosis, the first reading is little different from usual although the final reading is significantly lower (McKerrow and Molyneux, 1971) (*Figure 11.12*).

The mechanism by which cotton and the other vegetable fibre dusts cause narrowing of airways is not properly understood. There are three possibilities: (1) a local pharmacological effect; (2) an immunological reaction in the walls of the airways; (3) action of bacterial endotoxins.

Local pharmacological effect

Symptoms identical to the 'Monday feeling' may occur with similar changes in lung function when cotton dust is inhaled by healthy volunteers. These include decreased FEV_1 (sometimes lasting more than 24 hours) and VC, increased airways resistance, maximum expiratory flow/volume curves, RV, TLC and FRC, without any fall of gas transfer. Washed cotton dust, with similar physical properties, produces neither symptoms nor physiological changes on inhalation, suggesting that washing removes the causal agent (McDermott, Skidmore and Edwards, 1971). Bouhuys, Lindell and Lundin (1960) postulated that the agent might be a histamine-liberating substance in the cotton dust since histamine is a well-known powerful bronchoconstrictor.

However, there always appears to be no correlation between the response of individuals, or groups of individuals, and dust concentration when this exceeds about 1 mg/m^3. There are two possible explanations for this. First, low solubility of the bronchoconstrictive substance may allow it to be eliminated with the dust before it can be dissolved out; or second, the amount of the substance (histamine, for example) which can be released by the lungs may be limited in any one individual (McDermott *et al.*, 1971).

Aqueous extracts of cotton bracts inhaled by healthy volunteers cause

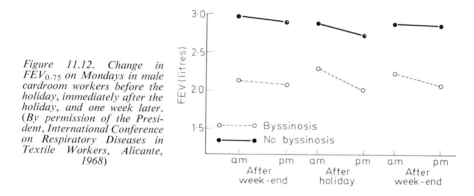

Figure 11.12. Change in $FEV_{0.75}$ on Mondays in male cardroom workers before the holiday, immediately after the holiday, and one week later. (By permission of the President, International Conference on Respiratory Diseases in Textile Workers, Alicante, 1968)

'Monday' symptoms, a reduction in the maximum expiratory flow rate and airways conductance; they also consistently release histamines from fresh slices of normal human lung (Douglas *et al.*, 1971). Flax and soft hemp also cause significant histamine-releasing activity in human lung (Nicholls, Nicholls and Bouhuys, 1966).

Just as the bronchoconstrictor effect of histamine aerosol inhaled by human volunteers is potentiated by the β-adrenergic receptor blocking agent, propranolol, and prevented by atropine, the effect of challenge inhalations of hemp dust is similarly potentiated and inhibited by these drugs (Bouhuys, 1971). Furthermore, estimation of twenty-four-hour excretion of the histamine metabolite 1-methyl-4-imidazole acetic acid in the urine is significantly increased in healthy volunteers following inhalation of cotton dust, but there is no increase after the inhalation of washed cotton dust (McDermott, Skidmore and Edwards, 1971).

These observations suggest that the acute changes of lung function provoked in normal persons might be due to histamine release from the lungs, and the unusually low final FEV values on the first day back at work after a holiday in workers without byssinosis are consistent with the possibility

2F   433

of an increase in histamine reserves during the holiday (McKerrow and Molyneux, 1971). But it is possible that the bronchoconstrictor effect is caused by a substance (or substances), the nature of which is not yet known, present in cotton bracts, flax and hemp. An unidentified contractor substance and 5-hydroxy-tryptamine have also been found in cotton dust (Davenport and Paton, 1962) although they appear to require too high a concentration to be the chief cause of airways narrowing *in vivo*. Evidently, further investigation of the problem is required. There is another possibility requiring investigation; that is, that a smooth muscle constrictor effect may also be exerted on the walls of small arteries.

Antigen-antibody reaction

Precipitating IgG antibody against an antigen in cotton is present in cotton workers and unexposed persons: its titre is highest in workers with byssinosis, lower in those without byssinosis and lowest in the unexposed subjects. It has been suggested that the symptoms of byssinosis are caused either directly by a late Arthus type reaction in the walls of airways or indirectly by the reaction liberating a pharmacologically active substance. The fact that symptoms of Grades C1 and C2 byssinosis disappear while the worker is still exposed to the dust was explained on the grounds that, as long as exposure continues, antibody is progressively removed from the circulation leaving insufficient to produce a reaction; whereas after a period away from the dust, during which antibody is not removed, its titre has increased by the time the worker is re-exposed (Massoud and Taylor, 1964). The presence of precipitins in control subjects may be due to antibodies to other antigens cross-reacting with cotton antigens.

Subsequently, Taylor, Massoud and Lucas (1971) demonstrated that the precipitin titre is greatest at the beginning of the working week than at the end, and is increased after returning from a week's holiday. Titration of precipitin before and after challenge inhalation of cotton antigen by byssinosis and non-byssinosis cardroom workers, revealed smaller titres six hours after inhalation than before. Although 'Monday' symptoms were reproduced by inhalation of antigen it is interesting that reduction in FEV_1 did not occur (Massoud, Taylor and Lucas, 1971).

Taylor, Massoud and Lucas (1971) claim to have identified the antigen as a polymer of leucocyanidin with smaller amounts of leucodelphinidin. Other observers (McDermott *et al.*, 1971), however, have been unable to confirm that cotton dust inhalation induces antibody production in normal subjects or that γ-globuin level increases ten days later (Popa *et al.*, 1969; Edwards *et al.*, 1970).

The fact that some workers similarly exposed to cotton or hemp dusts experience severe chest tightness with substantial reduction of FEV whereas others are in no way affected, appears to support the allergic hypothesis; but, on the other hand, the observations that raw cotton dust may produce an acute effect in a majority of healthy young persons (McKerrow and Molyneux, 1971) and that intradermal tests with cotton dust extracts are completely negative in some studies of workers with byssinosis (Voisin *et al.*, 1966) or have failed to establish a positive correlation with respiratory symptoms (Cayton, Furness and Maitland, 1952) would not suggest that byssinosis is simply an allergic phenomenon. However, a more recent investigation of cotton, flax, hemp and jute workers has shown that, although immediate skin reactions were seldom seen, delayed reactions were often present in those both with and without 'byssinotic' symptoms, but were generally absent in normal subjects in other industries (Popa *et al.*, 1969). The findings are summarized in Table 11.8.

Bacterial endotoxins
'Mill fever', which may occur in workers in cotton, flax and hemp mills and in granaries, consists of fever (37·8 to 39·4°C, 100 to 103°F), malaise, headache and dry cough (sometimes with vomiting) within twelve hours of first

TABLE 11.8

Points for and Against the Concept of Byssinosis as 'Late' Asthma Due to an Arthus Type Reaction

For	Against
Not all exposed persons have respiratory symptoms or fall in FEV	Recovery of symptoms and FEV on second or subsequent days while still exposed to dust
Symptoms and/or fall in FEV do not occur for some hours after exposure begins	Intradermal tests with cotton, flax and other extracts correlate poorly with symptoms
Precipitins present though of doubtful specificity	No specific precipitins

exposure, and is distinct from the 'Monday feeling' of byssinosis. It may recur on a few successive nights and then cease.

There is some evidence that the 'mill fever' group of diseases may be caused by the inhalation of endotoxins from bacteria which contaminate these materials (Pernis *et al.*, 1961) and, therefore, are not a form of extrinsic allergic 'alveolitis'. This has raised the question as to whether byssinosis might also be caused by endotoxins.

Cavagna, Foa and Vigliani (1969) found a better correlation between prevalence of byssinosis and concentration of airborne endotoxins than with the total amount of dust, and inhalation of an aerosol of purified endotoxin by healthy subjects and patients with chronic bronchitis caused a significant reduction of FEV_1 in a minority of both groups. Endotoxins are known to release histamine and serotonin (Hinshaw, Jordon and Vick, 1961; Davis, Bailey and Hanson, 1963). But if byssinosis is caused by endotoxins it is difficult to explain why two different syndromes—'mill fever' and byssinosis—should both be due to the same substance.

From this brief discussion it is clear that the pathogenesis of byssinosis is not properly understood but, on present evidence, the release of histamine caused by some unknown substance in cotton, flax, and soft hemp appears to be the most likely mechanism. By what means permanent airways obstruction is produced remains wholly unexplained.

Actinomycetes

Extrinsic allergic 'alveolitis' due to inhalation of spores of thermophilic actinomycetes in these materials does not seem to have been observed even though flax, hemp and jute fibres are wet when first removed from the retting process, and there appears to be no evidence as to whether microbial growth and, perhaps, heating occur if damp conditions persist.

Effect of smoking

Tobacco smoke potentiates the effect of cotton and the other fibre dusts in the production of byssinosis.

Byssinosis is more common and more severe among cotton operatives in Britain (Fox et al., 1973) and in the United States of America (Bouhuys et al., 1969b; Merchant et al., 1973) and among flax workers (Smith et al., 1962; Carey et al., 1965) who smoke than in their non-smoking fellow workers. Cotton and jute workers in Australia who smoke and have a productive cough show a greater and more consistent reduction of FEV_1 than similar workers who do not smoke (Gandevia and Milne, 1956a, b). Chronic respiratory symptoms are also more prevalent among smoking than non-smoking workers and ex-workers in the cotton industry.

However, in a Swedish survey 60 per cent of cotton cardroom workers who were non-smokers had respiratory symptoms (Belin et al., 1965). Spanish hemp workers aged 50 to 69 years who were moderate to heavy smokers have been found to have a significantly higher FEV_1 than their co-workers who were non-smokers or light smokers, although the values were lower than those of controls with similar smoking habits. The reason for this, it is suggested, is that men often affected by hemp dust (that is, those in whom the fall in FEV was most evident) stopped smoking, whereas those in whom the reduction in FEV was also less pronounced, did not; hence, the effect of lung dust in these men appeared to override that of smoking (Bouhuys, Schilling and van de Woestijne, 1969).

Effect of air pollution

Significantly more Lancashire cotton workers have been found to have respiratory symptoms than similar workers in Holland using the same grade of cotton; the smoking habits of the two groups did not appear to account for this, but the level of general air pollution which was substantially greater in Lancashire was thought to be the reason for the difference (Lammers, Schilling and Walford, 1964). However, the occurrence of byssinosis of all grades in countries with dry, hot climates and negligible atmospheric pollution makes it unlikely that pollution is an important contributing factor; indeed, in South Egypt where air pollution is less than in North Egypt byssinosis is more, and chronic bronchitis less, prevalent than in the North (El Batawi, 1962). A complicating factor, however, among Egyptian cotton workers which may influence such differences is their habit of smoking a highly irritating mixture of tobacco and a sugar-cane product.

Symptoms

The symptoms of byssinosis, which are distinct from those of 'mill fever', have already been summarized in Clinical Grades (q.v.). Acute symptoms resulting from exposure to cotton dust occur both in workers who have not been previously exposed as well as in those who have spent much of their working lives in dusty areas of the mills. Typically they consist of chest tightness and breathlessness (Grades $C\frac{1}{2}$ to C2) developing during the afternoon of work, although in severe cases they occur a few hours after starting work in the morning. Permanent breathlessness does not usually develop in cotton workers until they have had many years of exposure (ten or more) to the dust but may arise in a shorter period of time in flax workers (Carey *et al.*, 1965).

The 'Monday feeling' of Grade $C\frac{1}{2}$ consisting of chest tightness alone, occurs only on some Mondays (or first day back at work). Subsequently, breathlessness and fatigue, sometimes with cough, are complained of on every Monday in addition to chest tightness (Grade C1) but cease completely on the Tuesday. Grade C1 symptoms are best exemplified in the words of a cotton stripper and grinder who had been exposed to cotton dust for ten years (Schilling, 1950).

> Monday is a different day to me. Getting to 11 o'clock I feel tight in the chest and short of wind, but I have no cough. Towards 5.30 I feel done and struggle for breath and I can't walk at my ordinary speed. I am a dead horse on Mondays, but could fell a bull on Tuesdays.

In many workers there may be no further progression of symptoms during their work in the textile industry, and when they leave, symptoms cease completely leaving no residual disability.

Grade C2 is characterized by a gradual progression of symptoms. Chest tightness and breathlessness increase in severity and, although usually worse on Mondays, are present on other days of the week. There may be some cough. These symptoms, like Grade C1 symptoms, disappear when exposure to dust ceases. Once again, a cotton operative's own words are of interest (Schilling, 1950).

> I first noticed Monday feeling about 15 years ago, and at first I only got it on Mondays, but now I get it every day and I don't think there is much difference between my condition on Monday and other days of the week. Now I am always short of breath on exertion.

Some workers with Grade C2 symptoms gradually progress to Grade C3 in which chest tightness and breathlessness on effort are present every day and may be severe enough to prevent them continuing their work. Although some relief may be experienced when they leave the industry this is incomplete and respiratory disability is permanently established.

It is noteworthy that neither productive cough nor wheeze appear to be features of any grade of byssinosis. But chronic obstructive bronchitis may accompany byssinosis, and the problem of differentiation is discussed in the section on Diagnosis.

Physical signs
Apart from objective evidence of dyspnoea there are no abnormal signs in Grades C1 and C2 byssinosis, but breath sounds may be impaired in Grade C3. Curiously, wheeze does not seem to be reported.

Investigations

Lung function

There is a progressive reduction of ventilatory capacity (as indicated by FEV_1) and an increase of airways resistance throughout the working day in Grades C1 and C2 byssinosis, and also some unevenness of distribution of inspired gas (McKerrow *et al.*, 1958; Cotes, 1968). These changes are reversible on quitting exposure, but irreversible reduction in ventilatory capacity is present in some workers with Grade C2 (Grade F2) disease. Gas transfer remains within normal limits.

The changes which occur in maximum expiratory flow rate and specific conductance have been referred to already, but the FEV_1 remains the most informative and practical test for the assessment of exposed workers. After about six hours' exposure to cotton dust a significant fall in FEV_1 occurs in most individuals who have permanent (Grades F2 or F3), as well as those with transient (Grades $F\frac{1}{2}$ or F1), respiratory disability. The mean annual decline in FEV among cotton workers in one mill was 54 ml per year compared with 32 ml per year in workers in man-made fibre mills (Berry *et al.*, 1973).

Radiographic appearances

Byssinosis is not characterized by any abnormality of the chest radiograph, but the signs of emphysema may be evident in some cases of Grade 3 disease.

Intradermal tests

Intradermal prick tests are usually negative with the cotton extracts tried and are, therefore, of no help in identifying byssinosis in cotton workers.

Diagnosis

Ideally the diagnosis of Grades $C\frac{1}{2}$ to C2 rests on:

(1) A history of industrial exposure to cotton, flax or soft hemp dust
(2) A typical history of these clinical Grades
(3) Fall in FEV_1 during the working day or the working week.

In clinical practice the objective evidence of the FEV at the time of the symptoms is not always available and the diagnosis then depends entirely on the reliability of the patient's history. Hence, the technique of eliciting the history is all important. It is advisable, first, to allow him to relate his story without interruption and for the physician to ask leading questions only later in the examination; to start with leading questions ('Is your chest tight on Mondays?', for example) may result in false affirmative answers and wrong diagnosis. Every effort should be made to measure FEV_1 before, during and after a working shift.

Smokers may have chronic bronchitis distinguished as cough and sputum unrelated to periods of dust exposure for more than three months of the year (Smith *et al.*, 1962). In such patients byssinosis symptoms following exposure to dust may be differentiated, and an acute fall of the already impaired FEV_1 observed.

If chronic bronchitis can be excluded, the diagnosis of Grade C3 disease rests on the work history, a history of progressive development of the clinical grades of respiratory symptoms, and evidence of irreversible airways obstruction. But in patients with chronic obstructive bronchitis the diagnosis is impossible for, even if the patient's declared memory of having had Grade C1 and C2 symptoms is reliable, this cannot establish the co-existence of Grade C3 byssinosis. Although epidemiological evidence has shown that chronic respiratory disability is significantly more common among textile workers than among control subjects, this is of little practical help for diagnosis in individual patients. Grades $C\frac{1}{2}$ to C2 byssinosis cannot be confused with chronic bronchitis (MRC definition, 1965) although they may, of course, occur in chronic bronchitic subjects.

Prognosis

A recent survey has shown that cotton workers without byssinosis who have the greatest Monday fall in FEV are most likely to develop byssinosis subsequently (Berry *et al.*, 1972).

Complete symptomatic and functional recovery from Grade $C\frac{1}{2}$ and C1 disease occurs when the worker leaves the industry and, in general, this is often true of Grade C2 disease, although slight to moderate irreversible impairment of ventilatory capacity remains in some individuals (Grade F2). However, workers with Grade C1 disease appear to have an increased risk of developing chronic respiratory disability—compared with Grade 0 workers— if they remain exposed to dust.

Grade C3 (Grade F3) disease may ultimately end in pulmonary heart disease and congestive heart failure and detailed histology of the lungs is reported to be identical with the features of chronic bronchitis the presence of which may be fortuitous.

Prognosis of Grades C2 and C3 disease is worsened by cigarette smoking.

The incidence of chronic bronchitis is apparently increased in male and female workers with symptoms of byssinosis but is influenced by age and smoking (Molyneux and Tombleson, 1970). Chronic bronchitis also appears to be more common in non-smoking female hemp workers with byssinosis compared with those without byssinosis (Valic and Žuškin, 1971b).

Treatment

Workers with Grades C1 and C3 byssinosis should be moved away from areas of dust exposure.

The airways obstruction of Grades $C\frac{1}{2}$ to C2 can be reversed in most cases by inhalation of a bronchodilator aerosol (such as orciprenaline) and the Monday morning fall in FEV can be lessened by administration of antihistamines (Bouhuys, 1963). But such therapeutic measures are no substitute for prevention.

Prevention

Prevention depends upon the co-operation of engineering and medical disciplines, and involves:

(1) Dust control
(2) TLV and dust sampling
(3) Medical surveillance of workers.

439

Dust control

The most effective preventive measure is the replacement of natural by synthetic fibres. Although this has been achieved to some extent in Europe and the United States of America it is small by comparison with the world increase in cotton production; and, while the production of flax has declined that of hemp has not changed significantly.

Plant already in existence in established factories should be enclosed as far as is practicable and subjected to local exhaust ventilation; that is, cotton gins and opening and mixing and carding machines. But removal of dust is often inefficient due to unsatisfactory design, application and maintenance of equipment. The difficulty has been accentuated in recent years by rising production demands requiring a great increase in the speed of carding machines and, consequently, of the dust output. A proportionately greater demand, therefore, has been placed upon ventilation systems. In newly constructed mills it should be easier to achieve satisfactory results. Approved dust guards have been required fittings on carding engines in the United Kingdom since 1957 (Ministry of Labour, 1961).

General ventilation is also necessary and recirculated air must be efficiently filtered. It should keep concentrations of inhalable dust below the recommended TLV (*see* next section) in all processes which follow carding. Dust should be removed from machines, mill floors, ventilation equipment and other surfaces by vacuum cleaners.

Where sporadically large concentrations of dust occur (for example, stripping and grinding of carding machines) the operatives should wear efficient respirators.

TLV and dust sampling

Based upon the work of Roach and Schilling (1960) in Lancashire cotton mills the American Conference of Governmental Industrial Hygienists (1971) recommend a TLV of 1 mg/m³ of dust of all particle sizes. This, therefore, is a measurement of 'total' dust. But, as indicated earlier there is reason to believe that dust of 'medium' and 'respirable' size (that is, less than 7 μm) is more closely correlated with symptoms than the larger fractions. The Committee on Hygiene Standards of the British Occupational Hygiene Society (1972) has, therefore, recommended that the maximum average concentration should be 0·5 mg/m³, less fly. Nevertheless, it has been estimated that if the previous TLV for total dust were generally and consistently applied, the incidence of symptoms or of reduced FEV would probably be 5 per cent or less of all workers exposed.

Dust sampling should be systematic and carried out at regular intervals at relevant positions in the mill or factory, and, it is recommended, fly should be excluded from the total concentration of dust measured (British Occupational Hygiene Society, 1972). A permanent record of the results should be kept which will indicate the trends in dust levels over the years. Because cotton fibres are not the cause of byssinosis, sampling instruments of whatever type used, should be designed to exclude them.

Medical surveillance of workers

Pre-employment Examination.—It has been suggested (British Occupational

440

Hygiene Society, 1972) that all prospective employees in a textile industry using cotton (and flax or hemp) should answer a modification of the Medical Research Council's questionnaire on bronchitis adapted for byssinosis. This should assess chronic bronchitis, asthma, byssinosis, breathlessness, smoking history and occupational and past medical history. Details of the physical examination, FEV_1 and FVC are recorded, and PA and lateral chest radiographs taken.

This examination, of course, cannot prevent byssinosis but it should ensure that individuals with pre-existing lung disease are either excluded from working in the industry or are relegated to low- or no-risk areas, and it also provides the necessary basic information with which the results of later periodic medical examinations can be compared.

It is advisable that moderate to heavy cigarette smokers and persons with chronic or recurrent respiratory disease should be placed in low- or no-risk areas; but in practice, in the case of the smokers, there is probably little chance of achieving this. Individuals with a FEV_1 less than 60 per cent of the predicted normal value should not be exposed to dust.

There is no practical immunological method of detecting individual susceptibility.

Periodic medical examinations.—These serve two purposes: to identify workers who develop a pronounced reaction to the dust; and to provide a biological assessment of the efficiency of dust control and sampling in specific processes.

During the first month of his employment the worker's FEV_1 should be recorded before and after six hours of commencing his shift on the first day of a working week. If a significant decrease occurs he should be transferred to a less dusty area.

Systematic clinical examination and recording of FEV_1 and FVC should be done annually in all exposed workers. Those who are prone to develop substantial disability can be identified by comparing the annual fall of their FEV_1 with the predicted normal value after the effects of cigarette smoking are allowed for; they should be moved to a no-risk area as soon as this is recognized.

It must be emphasized that, although the pathogenesis of byssinosis is not fully understood, disability from the asthmatic phase can be prevented if it is recognized in its early stages.

REFERENCES

Ávila, R. (1971). 'Extrinsic allergic alveolitis in workers exposed to fish meal and poultry.' *Clin. Allergy* **1**, 343–346
— and Villar, T. G. (1968). 'Suberosis. Respiratory disease in cork workers.' *Lancet* **1**, 620–621
Banaszak, E. F., Thiede, W. H. and Fink, J. N. (1970). 'Hypersensitivity pneumonitis due to contamination of an air conditioner.' *New Engl. J. Med.* **283**, 271–276
Barbee, R. A., Callies, Q., Dickie, H. A. and Rankin, J. (1968). 'The long term prognosis in farmer's lung.' *Am. Rev. resp. Dis.* **97**, 223–231
Barboriak, J. J. Sosman, A. J. and Reed, C. E. (1965). 'Serological studies in pigeon breeder's disease.' *J. Lab. clin. Med.* **65**, 600–604

Barrowcliff, D. F. and Arblaster, P. G. (1968). 'Farmer's lung: a study of an early acute fatal case.' *Thorax* **23**, 490–500

Belin, L., Bouhuys, A., Hoekstra, W., Johansson, M.-B., Lindell, S.-E. and Pool, J. (1965). 'Byssinosis in card room workers in Swedish cotton mills.' *Br. J. ind. Med.* **22**, 101–108

Berry, G., McKerrow, C. B., Molyneux, M. K. B., Rossiter, C. E. and Tombleson, J. B. L. (1973). 'A study of the acute and chronic changes in ventilatory capacity of workers in Lancashire cotton mills.' *Br. J. ind. med.* **30**, 25–36

Bishop, J. M., Melnick, S. C. and Raine, J. (1963). 'Farmer's Lung: studies of pulmonary function and aetiology.' *Q. Jl Med.* **32**, 257–278

Björnsson, O. (1960). Quoted by Staines, F. H. and Forman, J. A. S. (1961). 'A survey of "farmer's lung".' *J. Coll. gen. Practnrs Res. Newsl.* **4**, 351–382

Booker, D. V., Chamberlin, A. C., Rundo, J., Muir, D. C. F. and Thomson, M. L. (1967). 'Elimination of 5 μ particles from the human lung.' *Nature, Lond.* **215**, 30–33

Bouhuys, A. (1963). 'Prevention of Monday dyspnoea in byssinosis: a controlled trial with an antihistamine drug.' *Clin. Pharmac. Ther.* **4**, 311–314

— (1970). Byssinosis in textile workers. In *Pneumoconiosis. Proceedings of the International Conference, Johannesburg, 1969*, pp. 412–416. Ed. by H. A. Shapiro. Cape Town; Oxford University Press

— (1971). 'Byssinosis.' *Archs envir. Hlth* **23**, 405–407

— Gilson, J. C. and Schilling, R. S. F. (1970). 'Byssinosis in the textile industry.' *Archs envir. Hlth* **21**, 475–478

— Lindell, S.-E. and Lundin, G. (1960). 'Experimental studies in byssinosis.' *Br. med. J.* **1**, 324–326

— Schilling, R. S. F. and van de Woestijne, K. P. (1969). 'Cigarette smoking, occupational dust exposure and ventilatory capacity.' *Archs envir. Hlth* **19**, 793–797

— Barbero, A., Schilling, R. S. F. and van de Woestijne, K. P. (1969a). 'Chronic respiratory disease in hemp workers.' *Am. J. Med.* **46**, 526–537

— Heaphy, L. J. Jr., Schilling, R. S. F. and Welborn, J. W. (1967a). 'Byssinosis in the United States.' *New Engl. J. Med.* **277**, 170–175

— Barbero, A., Lindell, S.-E., Roach, S. A. and Schilling, R. S. F. (1967b). 'Byssinosis in hemp workers.' *Archs envir. Hlth* **14**, 533–544

— Wolfson, R. L., Horner, D. W., Brain, J. D. and Žuškin, E. (1969b). 'Byssinosis in cotton textile workers: respiratory survey of a mill with rapid labor turnover.' *Ann. intern. Med.* **71**, 257–269

Boyd, D. H. A. (1971). 'The incidence of farmer's lung in Caithness.' *Scott. med. J.* **16**, 261–262

Bradford, J. K., Blalock, J. B. and Wascom, C. M. (1961). 'Bagasse disease of the lungs.' *Am. Rev. resp. Dis.* **84**, 582–585

Bringhurst, L. S., Byrne, R. N. and Gershon-Cohen, J. (1959). 'Respiratory disease of mushroom workers.' *J. Am. med. Ass.* **171**, 15–18

British Occupational Hygiene Society Committee on Hygienic Standards Sub-committee on Vegetable Textile Dusts (1972). 'Hygiene standards for cotton dust.' *Ann. occup. Hyg.* **15**, 165–192

Buechner, H. A. (1962). 'Bagassosis: a true pneumoconiosis.' *Ind. Med. Surg.* **31**, 311–314

— (1968). Quoted by Seabury *et al.* (1968), q.v.

— Aucoin, E., Vignes, A. J. and Weill, H. (1964). 'The resurgence of bagassosis in Louisiana.' *J. occup. Med.* **6**, 437–442

— Prevatt, A., Thompson, J. and Blitz, O. (1958). 'Bagassosis—a review, with further historical data, studies of pulmonary function and results of adrenal steroid therapy.' *Am. J. Med.* **25**, 234–247

Campbell, J. M. (1932), 'Acute symptoms following work with hay.' *Br. med. J.* **2**, 1143–1144

Cancella, de Carvalho (1959). 'Suberose. Alterações pulmonares relacionadas com a inalação de poeiras de cortiça.' Dissertação de Dontoramento, Lisboa

Cavagna, G., Foâ, V. and Vigliani, E. C. (1969). 'Effects in man and rabbits of inhalation of cotton dust or extracts and purified endotoxins.' *Br. J. ind. Med.* **26**, 314–321

Carey, G. C. R., Elwood, R. P., McAuley, I. R., Merrett, J. D. and Pemberton, J. (1965). 'Byssinosis in flax workers in Northern Ireland.' Government of Northern Ireland; H.M.S.O.

Carreiro, M. C., Freitas e Costa, M. and Teles de Araújo, A. (1969). 'Doença dos criadores de aves hum criador de galinhas.' *Rev. Post. Terap. Med.* **3**, 69–73

Castleden, L. I. M. and Hamilton-Paterson, J. L. (1942). 'Bagassosis. An industrial lung disease.' *Br. med. J.* **2**, 478–480

Caugini, G. (1951). 'Casi di bagassosi in Italia.' *Lotta c. tuberc.* **21**, 300

Cayton, H. R., Furness, G. and Maitland, H. B. (1952). 'Studies in cotton dust in relation to byssinosis. Part II. Skin tests for allergy with extracts of cotton dust.' *Br. J. ind. Med.* **9**, 186–196

Chandra, S. and Jones, H. E. (1972). 'Pigeon fanciers' lung in children.' *Archs Dis. Childh.* **47**, 716–718

Channel, S., Blyth, W., Lloyd, M., Weir, D. M., Amos, W. M. G., Littlewood, A. P., Riddle, H. F. V. and Grunt, I. W. B. (1969). 'Allergic alveolitis in maltworkers.' *Q. Jl Med.* **38**, 351–376

Chwat, M. and Mordish, R. (1963). 'Byssinosis investigations in two cotton plants in Israel.' *14th International Conference on Occupational Health, Madrid, 1963.* Int. Congr. Series, No. 62, pp. 572–573. Amsterdam; Excerpta Medica

Ciba Foundation Guest Symposium (1959). *Thorax* **14**, 286–289

— Study Group (1971). *Identification of Asthma.* Ed. by R. Porter and J. Birch. Ciba Foundation Study Group N. 38. Edinburgh and London; Churchill Livingstone

Cohen, H. I., Merigan, T. C., Kosek, J. C. and Eldridge, F. (1967). 'Sequoiosis.' *Am. J. Med.* **43**, 785–794

Cooper, I. A. and Greenaway, T. M. (1961). 'Farmer's lung: a case report.' *Med. J. Aust.* **2**, 980–981

Corbaz, R., Gregory, P. H. and Lacey, M. E. (1965). 'Thermophilic and mesophilic actinomycetes in mouldy hay.' *J. gen. Microbiol.* **32**, 449–455

Cotes, J. E. (1968). *Lung function. Assessment and Application in Medicine.* Oxford and Edinburgh; Blackwell

Craveri, R., Guicciardi, A. and Pacini, N. (1966). 'Distribution of thermophilic actinomycetes in compost for mushroom production.' *Ann. di Microbiol.* **16**, 111–113

Cross, T., Maciver, A. M. and Lacey, J. (1968). 'The thermophilic actinomyces in mouldy hay: *Micropolyspora faeni* sp. nov.' *J. gen. Microbiol.* **50**, 351–359

Davenport, A. and Paton, W. D. M. (1962). 'The pharmacological activity of extracts of cotton dust.' *Br. J. ind. Med.* **19**, 19–32

Davis, R. B., Bailey, W. L. and Hanson, N. P. (1963). 'Modification of histamine and serotin release after *E. coli* endotoxin administration.' *Am. J. Physiol.* **205**, 506–566

de Weck, A. L., Gutersohn, J. and Bütikofer, E. (1969). 'La maladie des laveurs de fromage ("Käsenwascherkrankheit"): une forme particulière du syndrome du poumon du fermier.' *Schweiz. med. Wschr.* **99**, 872–876

Dickie, H. A. and Rankin, J. (1958). 'Farmer's lung: an acute granulomatous interstitial pneumonitis occurring in agricultural workers.' *J. Am. med. Assoc.* **167**, 1069–1076

Dinda, P., Chatterjee, S. S. and Riding, W. D. (1969). 'Pulmonary function studies in bird breeder's lung.' *Thorax* **24**, 374–378

Dizon, G. D., Almonte, J. B. and Anselmo, J. E. (1962). 'Bagassosis and silicosis in the Philippines.' *J. Philipp. med. Ass.* **38**, 865–872

Douglas, J. S., Zuckerman, A., Ridgeway, P. and Bouhuys, A. (1971). 'Histamine release and bronchoconstriction due to textile dusts and their components.' In *International Conference on Respiratory Diseases in Textile Workers, Alicante, Spain, 1968*, pp. 148–155. Barcelona

443

Edwards, J. H. (1972a). 'The double dialysis method of producing farmer's lung antigens.' *J. Lab. clin. Med.* **79**, 683–688
— (1972b). 'The isolation of antigens associated with farmer's lung.' *Clin. exp. Immunol.* **11**, 341–355
— Barboriak, J. J. and Fink, J. N. (1970). 'Antigens in pigeon breeder's disease.' *Immunology* **19**, 729–734
— Fink, J. N. and Barboriak, J. J. (1969). 'Excretion of pigeon serum proteins in pigeon droppings.' *Proc. Soc. exp. Biol.* **132**, 907–911
— McCarthy, P., McDermott, M., Nicholls, P. J. and Skidmore, J. W. (1970). 'The acute physiological, pharmacological and immunological effects of inhaled cotton dust in normal subjects.' *J. Physiol.* **208**, 63–64P
El Batawi, M. A. (1962). 'Byssinosis in the cotton industry in Egypt.' *Br. J. ind. Med.* **19**, 126–130
Elman, A. J., Tebo, T., Fink, J. N. and Barboriak, J. J. (1968). 'Reactions of poultry farmers against chicken antigens.' *Archs envir. Hlth* **17**, 98–100
Elwood, P. C., Pemberton, J., Merrett, J. D., Carey, G. C. R. and McAuley, I. R. (1965). 'Byssinosis and other respiratory symptoms in flax workers in Northern Ireland.' *Br. J. ind. Med.* **22**, 27–37
Emanuel, D. A., and Wenzel, F. J. (1965). 'Clinical studies of farmer's lung.' *N. Y. St J. Med.* **65**, 3027–3032
— Lawton, B. R. and Wenzel, F. J. (1962). 'Maple bark disease. Pneumonitis due to *Coniosporium corticale*.' *New Engl. J. Med.* **266**, 333–337
— Wenzel, F. J. and Lawton, B. R. (1966). 'Pneumonitis due to *Cryptostroma corticale* (Maple bark disease).' *New Engl. J. Med.* **274**, 1413–1418
— — Bowerman, C. I. and Lawton, B. R. (1964). 'Farmer's lung. Clinical pathologic and immunologic study of twenty four patients.' *Am. J. Med.* **37**, 392–401
Faux, J. A., Wide, L., Hargreave, F. E., Longbottom, J. L. and Pepys, J. (1971). 'Immunological aspects of respiratory allergy in budgerigar (Melopsittacus undulatus) fanciers.' *Clin. Allergy* **1**, 149–158
Fawcitt, R. (1938). 'Occupational diseases of the lungs in agricultural workers.' *Br. J. Radiol.* **11**, 378–392
Fergus, C. L. (1964). 'Thermophilic and thermotolerant molds and actinomycetes of mushroom compost during peak heating.' *Mycologia* **56**, 267–284
Festenstein, G. N., Lacey, J., Skinner, F. A., Jenkins, P. A. and Pepys, J. (1965). 'Self heating hay and grain in Dewar flasks, and the development of farmer's lung antigens.' *J. gen. Microbiol.* **41**, 389–407
Fink, J. N., Hensley, G. T. and Barboriak, J. J. (1969). 'An animal model of a hypersensitivity pneumonitis.' *J. Allergy* **46**, 156–161
— Banaszak, E. A., Thiede, W. H. and Barboriak, J. J. (1971). 'Interstitial pneumonitis due to hypersensitivity to an organism contaminating a heating system.' *Ann. intern. Med.* **74**, 80–83
— Sosman, A. J., Barboriak, J. J., Schlueter, D. P. and Holmes, R. A. (1968). Pigeon breeder's disease. A clinical study of hypersensitivity pneumonitis.' *Ann. intern. Med.* **68**, 1205–1219
Fletcher, S. M., Rondle, C. J. M. and Murray, I. G. (1970). 'The extracellular antigens of *Micropolyspora faeni*: their significance in farmer's lung disease.' *J. Hyg., Camb.* **68**, 401–409
Flindt, M. L. H. (1969). 'Pulmonary disease due to inhalation of derivatives of *Bacillus subtilus* containing proteolytic enzyme.' *Lancet* **1**, 1177–1181
Fox, A. J., Tombleson, J. B. L., Watt, A. and Wilkie, A. G. (1973). 'A survey of respiratory disease in cotton operatives. Part II. Symptoms, dust estimations, and the effect of smoking habit.' *Br. J. ind. Med.* **30**, 48–53
Frankland, A. W. and Lunn, J. A. (1965). 'Asthma caused by the grain weevil.' *Br. J. ind. Med.* **22**, 157–159
Friese, M. J. (1958). *Coccidioidomycosis*. Springfield; Thomas
Fuller, C. J. (1953). 'Farmer's lung: a review of present knowledge.' *Thorax* **8**, 59–64
Gandevia, B. and Milne, J. (1965a). 'Ventilatory capacity changes on exposure to cotton dust and their relevance to byssinosis in Australia.' *Br. J. ind. Med.* **22**, 295–304

Gandevia, B. and Milne, J. (1965b). 'Ventilatory capacity on exposure to jute, dust, and the relevance of productive cough and smoking to the response.' *Br. J. ind. Med.* **22**, 187–195

Ganguly, S. K. and Pal, S. C. (1955). 'Early bagassosis.' *J. Indian med. Ass.* **34**, 253–254

Gilson, J. C., Stott, H., Hopwood, B. E. C., Roach, S. A., McKerrow, C. B. and Schilling, R. S. F. (1962). 'Byssinosis: the acute effect on ventilatory capacity of dusts in cotton ginneries, cotton, sisal and jute mills.' *Br. J. ind. Med.* **19**, 9–18

González de Vega, N., Zamora, A., Cano, M. and Fernández Castany, A. (1966), 'Nuestra experiencia personal sobre la bagazosis en España Enferm.' *Tórax* **15**, 215–237

Gourley, C. A. and Braidwood, G. D. (1971). 'The use of dust respirators in the prevention of recurrence of farmer's lung.' *Trans. Soc. occup. Med.* **21**, 93–95

Grant, I. W. B., Blyth, W., Wardrop, V. E., Gordon, R. M., Pearson, J. C. G. and Mair, A. (1972). 'Prevalence of farmer's lung in Scotland. A pilot survey.' *Br. med. J.* **1**, 530–534

Gregory, P. H. and Waller, S. (1951). *Cryptostroma corticale* and sooty bark disease of sycamore. (Acerpseudoplantanus.) *Trans. Br. mycol. Soc.* **34**, 579-597

— Lacey, J., Festenstein, G. N. and Skinner, F. A. (1963). 'Microbial and biochemical changes during moulding of hay.' *J. gen. Microbiol.* **33**, 147–174

Hapke, E. J., Seal, R. M. E., Thomas, G. D., Hayes, M. and Meek, J. C. (1968). 'Farmer's lung.' *Thorax* **23**, 451–468

Hargreave, F. E., Pepys, J. and Holford-Strevens, V. (1968). 'Bagassosis.' *Lancet* **1**, 619–620

— Pepys, J., Longbottom, J. L. and Wraith, D. G. (1966). 'Bird breeder's (fancier's) lung.' *Lancet* **1**, 445–449

Harper, L. O., Burrell, R. G., Lapp, N. L. and Morgan, W. K. C. (1970). 'Allergic alveolitis due to pituitary snuff.' *Ann. intern. Med.* **73**, 581–584

Hearn, C. E. D. (1968). 'Bagassosis: An epidemiological, environmental and clinical survey.' *Br. J. ind. Med.* **25**, 267–282

— and Holford-Strevens, V. (1968). 'Immunological aspects of bagassosis.' *Br. J. ind. Med.* **25**, 283-292

Hensley, G. T., Garancis, J. C., Cherayil, G. D. and Fink, J. N. (1969). 'Lung biopsies in pigeon breeder's disease.' *Archs Path.* **87**, 572–579

Hinshaw, L. B., Jordon, M. M. and Vick, J. A. (1961). 'Mechanism of histamine release in endotoxin shock.' *Am. J. Physiol.* **200**, 987-989

Hoffman, W. (1946). 'Die Dreschkranheit.' *Schweiz. med. Wschr.* **76**, 988–990

Holford-Strevens, V. (1971). Quoted by J. Lacey (1971), q.v.

Hugh-Jones, M. E. and Austwick, P. K. C. (1967). 'Epidemiological studies of bovine mycotic abortion.' *Vet. Rec.* **81**, 273–276

Hunter, D. and Perry, K. M. A. (1946). 'Bronchiolitis resulting from the handling of bagasse.' *Br. J. ind. Med.* **3**, 64–74

Ishizaka, K. (1963). 'Gamma globulin and molecular mechanisms in hypersensitivity reactions.' *Prog. Allergy* **7**, 32–106

Jackson, E. and Welch, K. M. A. (1970). 'Mushroom worker's lung.' *Thorax* **25**, 25–30

Jamison, C. S. and Hopkins, J. (1941). 'Bagassosis—A fungus disease of the lung.' *New Orl. med. surg. J.* **93**, 580–582

Jimenez-Diaz, C., Lahoz, C. and Canto, G. (1947). 'The allergens of mill dust. Asthma in millers, farmers and others.' *Ann. Allergy* **5**, 519–525

Jones, B. (1970). 'Experimental pathology relating to "farmer's lung".' *Tubercle, Lond.* **51**, 217–218

Jones Williams, W. (1967). 'The pathology of sarcoidosis.' *Hosp. Med.* **2**, 21–27

Joyce, J. C. and Kneafsey, D. (1955). 'Farmer's lung.' *J. Irish med. Assoc.* **37**, 313–315

Kay, J. P. (1831). 'Observations and experiments concerning molecular irritation of the lungs as one source of tubercular consumption; and on spinner's Phthisis.' *N. Engl. med. surg. J.* **1**, 348–363

Khogali, M. (1971). 'A population study in cotton ginnery workers in the Sudan.'

In *International Conference on Respiratory Diseases in Textile Workers, Alicante, Spain, 1968*, p. 79. Barcelona

Lacey, J. (1969). 'Bagassosis.' In *Rothamsted Experimental Station Report for 1968*. Part 1, p. 133

— (1971a). 'Thermoactinomyces sacchari sp. nov., a thermophilic actinomycete causing bagassosis.' *J. gen. Microbiol.* **66**, 327–338

— (1971b). Personal communication

— (1973). 'The air spora of a Portuguese cork factory.' (To be published.)

— and Lacey, M. E. (1964). 'Spore concentrations in the air of farm buildings.' *Trans. Br. mycol. Soc.* **47**, 547–552

Lammers, B., Schilling, R. S. F. and Walford, J. (1964). 'A study of byssinosis, chronic respiratory symptoms, and ventilatory capacity in English and Dutch cotton workers, with special reference to atmospheric pollution.' *Br. J. ind. Med.* **21**, 124–134

Lunn, J. A. (1966). 'Millworker's asthma. Allergic responses to the grain weevil (Sitophiles granaries).' *Br. J. ind. Med.* **23**, 149–152

— and Hughes, D. T. D. (1967). 'Pulmonary hypersensitivity to the grain weevil.' *Br. J. ind. Med.* **24**, 158–161

McDermott, M., Skidmore, J. W. and Edwards, J. (1971). 'The acute physiological, immunological and pharmacological effects of inhaled cotton dust in normal subjects.' In *International Conference on Respiratory Diseases of Textile Workers, Alicante, Spain, 1968*, pp. 133–136. Barcelona

McKerrow, C. B. and Molyneux, M. K. B. (1971). The influence of previous dust exposure on the acute respiratory effects of cotton dust inhalation. In *International Conference on Respiratory Diseases in Textile Workers, Alicante, Spain, 1968*, pp. 95–101. Barcelona

Mahon, W. E., Scott, D. J., Ansell, G., Manson, G. L. and Fraser, R. (1967). 'Hypersensitivity to pituitary snuff with miliary shadowing in the lungs.' *Thorax* **22**, 13–20

Mair, A., Smith, D. H., Wilson, W. A. and Lockhart, W. (1960). 'Dust disease in Dundee textile workers. An investigation into chronic respiratory disease in jute and flax industries.' *Br. J. ind. Med.* **17**, 272–278

Massoud, A. and Taylor, G. (1964). 'Byssinosis: antibody to cotton antigens in normal subjects and in cotton card-room workers.' *Lancet* **2**, 607–610

— and Lucas, F. (1971). 'Bronchial challenge with cotton plant antigen in byssinotics.' In *International Conference on Respiratory Diseases in Textile Workers, Alicante, Spain, 1968*, pp. 124–132. Barcelona

Merchant, J. A., Lumsden, J. C., Kilburn, K. H., O'Fallon, W. M., Ujda, J. R., Germino, V. H. and Hamilton, J. D. (1973). 'An industrial study of the biological effects of cotton dust and cigarette smoke exposure.' *J. occup. Med.* **15**, 212–221

Miller, G. J., Hearn, C. E. D. and Edwards, R. H. T. (1971). 'Pulmonary function at rest and during exercise following bagassosis.' *Br. J. ind. Med.* **28**, 152–158

Ministry of Labour (1961). *Dust in Card Rooms*. Report on Int. Advis. Comm. of the Cotton Ind. London; H.M.S.O.

Minnig, H. and De Weck, A. L. (1972). 'Die "Käsewascherkrankeit". Immunologische und epidemiologische Studien.' *Schweiz. med. Wschr.* **102**, 1205–1212; 1251–1257

Molyneux, M. K. B. and Berry, G. (1971). 'The correlation of cotton dust exposure with prevalence of respiratory symptoms.' In *Proceedings 2nd International Conference on Respiratory Diseases in Textile Workers (Byssinosis), Alicante, Spain*, pp. 177–183

— and Tombleson, J. B. L. (1970). 'An epidemiological study of respiratory symptoms in Lancashire mills, 1963–66.' *Br. J. ind. Med.* **27**, 225–234

Nash, E. S., Vogelpoel, L. and Becker, W. B. (1967). 'Pigeon breeder's lung—a case report.' *S. Afr. med. J.* **41**, 191–193

Nicholls, P. J., Nicholls, G. R. and Bouhuys, A. (1966). 'Histamine release by Compound 48/80 and textile dusts from lung tissue dusts from lung tissue *in vitro*.' In *Inhaled Particles and Vapours, II*, pp. 69–74. Oxford and New York; Pergamon

Panasenko, V. T. (1967). 'Ecology of microfungi.' *Bot. Rev.* **33**, 189–215

Parish, W. E. (1961). 'The response of normal and experimental animals to products of mouldy hay.' *Acta allerg.* **16**, 78–79

Patissier, P. (1822). *Traité des Maladies des Artisans.* Paris

Paturau, J. M. (1969). *By-products of the Cane Sugar Industry.* Amsterdam; Elsevier

Pearsall, H. R., Morgan, E. H., Tesluk, H. and Beggs, D. (1960). 'Parakeet dander pneumonitis. Acute psittaco-kerato-pneumoconiosis.' *Bull. Mason Clin.* **14**, 127–137

Pepys, J. (1969). *Hypersensitivity Diseases of the Lungs due to Fungi and Organic Dusts.* Basel; Karger

— and Jenkins, P. A. (1965). 'Precipitin (F.L.H.) test in farmer's lung.' *Thorax* **20**, 21–35

— — Lachman, P. J. and Mahon, W. E. (1966). 'An iatrogenic autoantibody: immunological response to "pituitary snuff" in patients with diabetes insipidus.' *Clin. exp. Immunol.* **1**, 377–389

— Longbottom, J. L., Hargreave, F. E. and Faux, J. (1969). 'Allergic reactions of the lungs to enzymes of *Bacillus subtilis.*' *Lancet* **1**, 1181–1184

— Turner Warwick, M., Dawson, P. L. and Hinson, K. F. W. (1968). *Proc. 6th Int. Congr. Allergy, Montreal.* Excerpt on Med. Int. Congr. Sc. 162, 221

— Jenkins, P. A., Festenstein, G. N., Gregory, P. H., Lacey, P. H. and Skinner, F. A. (1963). 'Farmer's lung: thermophilic actinomycetes as a source of "farmer's lung hay" antigen.' *Lancet* **2**, 607–611

Pernis, B., Vigliani, E. C., Cavagna, G. and Finulli, M. (1961). 'The role of bacterial endotoxins in occupational diseases caused by inhaling vegetable dusts.' *Br. J. ind. Med.* **18**, 120–129

Pickles, W. N. (1944). 'The country doctor and public health.' *Publ. Hlth* **58**, 2–5

Pierce, A. K., Nicholson, D. P., Miller, J. M. and Johnson, R. L. (1968). 'Pulmonary function in bagasse worker's lung disease.' *Am. Rev. Dis.* **97**, 561–570

Pimentel, J. C. (1970). 'Furrier's lung.' *Thorax* **25**, 387–398

— and Ávila, R. (1973). 'Respiratory disease in cork workers ("suberosis").' *Thorax* **28**, 409–423

Pirie, H. M., Dawson, C. O., Breeze, R. G., Wiseman, A. and Hamilton, J. (1971). 'A bovine disease similar to farmer's lung: extrinsic allergic alveolitis.' *Vet. Rec.* **88**, 346–350

Plessner, M. M. (1960). 'Une maladie des trieurs de plumes: la fièvre de canard.' *Archs Mal. prof. Méd. trav.* **21**, 67–69

Popa, V., Gavrilescu, N., Preda, N., Teculescu, D., Plecias, M. and Cîrstea, M. (1969). 'An investigation of allergy in byssinosis: sensitisation to cotton, hemp, flax and jute antigens.' *Br. J. ind. Med.* **26**, 101–108

Proust, A. (1877). *Traité d'Hygiène Publique et privée*, pp. 171–174. Paris; Masson

Rankin, J., Kobayashi, M., Barbee, R. A. and Dickie, H. A. (1967). 'Pulmonary granulomatoses due to inhaled organic antigens.' *Med. Clins N. Am.* **51**, 459–482

Reed, C. E., Sosman, A. and Barbee, R. A. (1965). 'Pigeon breeder's lung.' *J. Am. med. Ass.* **193**, 261–266

Riddle, H. F. V., Channell, S., Blyth, W., Weir, D. M., Lloyd, M., Amos, W. M. G. and Grant, I. W. B. (1968). 'Allergic alveolitis in a maltworker.' *Thorax* **23**, 271–280

Roach, S. A. and Schilling, R. S. F. (1960). 'A clinical and environmental study of byssinosis in the Lancashire cotton industry.' *Br. J. ind. Med.* **17**, 1–9

Sakula, A. (1967). 'Mushroom worker's lung.' *Br. med. J.* **3**, 708–710

Salvaggio, J., Arquembourg, P., Seabury, J. and Buechner, H. (1969). 'Bagassosis IV. Precipitins against extracts of thermophilic actinomycetes in patients with bagassosis.' *Am. J. Med.* **46**, 538–544

Scadding, J. G. (1967). *Sarcoidosis*, p. 160. London; Eyre and Spottiswoode

Scheidegger, J. J. (1955). 'Une microméthode de l'immuno-électrophorèse.' *Int. Archs Allergy appl. Immun.* **7**, 103–110

Schilling, R. S. F. (1950). 'Byssinosis.' *Br. med. Bull.* **7**, 52–56

Schilling, R. S. F. (1956). 'Byssinosis in cotton and other textile workers.' *Lancet* **2**, 261–265; 319–324

— (1964). 'Epidemiological studies of chronic respiratory disease among cotton operatives.' *Yale J. Biol. Med.* **37**, 55–74

— Vigliani, E. C., Lammers, B., Valic, F. and Gilson, J. C. (1963). *A Report on a Conference on Byssinosis.* (14th International Conference on Occupational Health, Madrid, 1963), pp. 137–144. Int. Congr. Series. No. 62. Amsterdam; Excerpta Medica

Seabury, J., Salvaggio, J., Buechner, H. and Kunder, V. G. (1968). 'Bagassosis III. Isolation of thermophilic and mesophilic actinomycetes and fungi from mouldy bagasse.' *Proc. Soc. exp. Biol. Med.* **129**, 351–360

Seal, R. M. E., Thomas, G. O and Griffiths, J. J. (1963). 'Farmer's lung.' *Proc. R. Soc. Med.* **56**, 271–273

— Hapke, E. J., Thomas, G. O., Meek, J. C. and Hayes, M. (1968). 'The pathology of the acute and chronic stages of farmer's lung.' *Thorax* **23**, 469–489

Shannon, D. C., Andrews, J. L., Recavarren, S. and Kazeini, H. (1969). 'Pigeon breeder's lung disease and interstitial pulmonary fibrosis.' *Am. J. Dis. Child.* **117**, 504–510

Siddhu, C. M. S., Nath, K. and Mehrotra, R. K. (1966). 'Byssinosis among cotton and jute workers in Kaupur.' *Ind. J. Med. Res.* **54**, 980–994

Smiley, J. A. (1951). 'The hazards of rope making.' *Br. J. ind. Med.* **8**, 265–270

Smith, D. H., Lockhart, W., Mair A. and Wilson, W. A. (1962). ' "Flax workers" byssinosis in East Scotland.' *Scot. med. J.* **7**, 201–211

Smith, G. F., Coles, G. V., Schilling, R. S. F. and Walford, J. (1969). 'A study of rope workers exposed to hemp and flax.' *Br. J. ind. Med.* **26**, 109–114

Sodeman, W. A. and Pullem, R. L. (1964). 'Bagasse disease of the lungs.' *Archs intern. Med.* **73**, 365–374

Spiegelman, A. R. (1963). 'Treatment of diabetes insipidus with synthetic vasopressin.' *J. Am. med. Ass.* **184**, 657–658

Spillane, J. D. (1952). 'Four cases of diabetes insipidus and pulmonary disease.' *Thorax* **7**, 134–147

Staines, F. H. and Forman, J. A. S. (1961). 'A survey of "farmer's lung".' *J. Coll. gen. Practnrs Newsl.* **4**, 351–382

Stiehm, E. R., Reed, C. E. and Tooley, W. H. (1967). 'Pigeon breeder's lung in children.' *Pediatrics* **39**, 904–915

Taylor, G., Massoud, A. A. E. and Lucas, F. (1971). 'Studies in the aetiology of byssinosis.' *Br. J. ind. Med.* **28**, 145–151

Tewksbury, D. A., Wenzel, F. J. and Emanuel, D. A. (1968). 'An immunologic study of maple bark disease.' *Clin. exp. Immunol.* **3**, 857–863

Tiller, J. R. and Schilling, R. S. F. (1958). 'Respiratory function during the day in rayon workers.' *Trans. Ass. ind. med. Offrs* **7**, 161–162

Törnell, E. (1946). 'Thresher's lung.' *Acta med. scand.* **125**, 191–219

Towey, J. W., Sweany, H. C. and Huron, W. H. (1932). 'Severe bronchial asthma apparently due to fungus spores found in maple bark.' *J. Am. med. Ass.* **99**, 453–459

Turner-Warwick, M. and Haslam, P. (1971). 'Antibodies in some chronic fibrosing lung diseases 1. Non-organ-specific auto-antibodies.' *Clin. Allergy* **1**, 83–95

Tuypens, E. (1961). 'Byssinosis among cotton workers in Belgium.' *Br. J. ind. Med.* **18**, 117–119

Valic, F. and Žuškin, E. (1971). 'A comparative study of respiratory function in female non-smoking cotton and jute workers.' *Br. J. ind. Med.* **28**, 364–368

— — (1971). 'Effects of hemp dust exposure on non-smoking female textile workers.' *Archs envir. Hlth* **23**, 359–364

Vallery-Radot, P. and Giroud, P. (1928). 'Sporomycose des pelleteurs de grains.' *Bull. Soc. méd. Hôp. Paris* **52**, 1632–1645

van Toorn, D. W. (1970). 'Coffee workers' lung.' *Thorax* **25**, 399–405

Velvart, J. (1971). 'Respiratory symptoms and changes in lung function in workers handling hemp, flax and sisal in Czechoslovakia.' In *Proceedings of the International Conference on Respiratory Diseases in Textile Workers (Byssinosis), Alicante, Spain, 1968*, pp. 55–58

Velvart, J. (1972). 'Schädigung der Atemwege durch Staubeinwirkung von Sisal.' *Int. Arch. Arbeitsmed.* **30**, 213–222

Veterans Administration Cooperative Study (1964). 'Blastomycosis. A review of 198 collected cases in Veterans Administration Hospitals.' *Am. Rev. resp. Dis.* **89**, 659–672

Viswanathan, R., de Monte, A. J. H., Shivpuri, D. N., Venkitasubramanian, T. A., Tandon, H. D., Chandrusekhars, S., Jain, S. K., Gupta, I. M., Singh, P., Gambhie, K. K., Randhawa, H. S. and Singh, V. N. (1963). 'Bagassosis.' *Indian J. med. Res.* **51**, 563–633

Voisin, C., Jacob, M., Furon, D. and Lefebre, J. (1966). 'Aspects cliniques et allergologiques des manifestations asthmatiques observées chez 114 ouvriers de filatures de coton.' *Poumon Cœur* **22**, 529–538

Weill, H., Buechner, H. A., Gonzales, E., Herbert, S. J., Aucoin, E. and Ziskind, M. M. (1966). 'Bagassosis: As study of pulmonary function in 20 cases.' *Ann. intern. Med.* **64**, 737–747

Wenzel, F. J. and Emanuel, D. A. (1965). 'Experimental studies of farmer's lung.' *N.Y. St J. Med.* **65**, 3032–3037

— and Emanuel, D. A. (1967). 'The epidemiology of maple bark disease.' *Archs envir. Hlth* **14**, 385–389

— — and Gray, R. L. (1971). 'Immunofluorescent studies of the lung in patients with farmer's lung.' *J. Allergy* **47**, 102–103

Williams, J. V. (1963). 'Inhalation and skin tests with extracts of hay and fungi in patients with farmer's lung.' *Thorax* **18**, 182–196

Wolf, F. T. (1969). 'Observations on an outbreak of pulmonary aspergillosis.' *Mycopath. Mycol. appl.* **38**, 359–361

Žuškin, E. and Valic, F. (1972). 'Respiratory symptoms and ventilatory function changes in relation to length of exposure to cotton dust. *Thorax* **27**, 454–458

— Wolfson, R. L., Harpel, G., Welborn, J. W. and Bouhuys, A. (1969). 'Byssinosis in carding and spinning workers.' *Archs envir. Hlth* **19**, 666–673

12—Miscellaneous Disorders

This chapter is concerned with some of the transient or permanent pulmonary disorders which may be caused by inhalation of a variety of dusts, fumes or gases. The number of these which cause or, rightly or wrongly, are thought to cause lung damage, is very large and an exhaustive discussion is not possible. Only those disorders which are likely to be of practical importance are described. In spite of their diversity the diagnosis of almost all rests primarily upon a careful and informed occupational history.

OCCUPATIONAL ASTHMA

A definition of asthma which has wide acceptance is given in Chapter 11 and the meaning of the term 'atopic' explained.

Asthmatic reactions may be of immediate or 'late' onset ('late' means some six hours following exposure), and may occur in non-atopic as well as atopic subjects. Reversible airways obstruction can be induced by a wide variety of inhaled agents—dusts, fumes and vapours—which on some occasions act as an irritant to the bronchial tree and, on others, as an antigen mediating an allergic response; hence, they may be antigenic or non-antigenic, and the underlying mechanisms respectively immunological or non-immunological.

Extrinsic allergens—usually in dust form—cause immediate, Type I, reaginic-mediated asthmatic reactions in atopic subjects. Precipitins are absent in the former but present in the latter. In some cases both types of allergic reaction occur so that immediate asthma is followed by 'late' asthma —the so-called dual reaction.

Specific dusts, fumes and vapours may cause a direct action on the smooth muscle of airways, local liberation of histamine or other effects not yet fully understood which may involve the release of some humoral substance. Here again asthma may be immediate or 'late'.

In some cases, a third asthmatic episode may occur some hours after a late reaction, and often during the night (Gandevia, 1970).

Occupational asthma falls into two broad groups: common and uncommon. The first group is common because it consists mainly of atopic subjects who may be readily sensitized to multifarious antigens; and the second is

450

uncommon because it consists of non-atopic subjects in whom asthma results after intensive exposure to antigens encountered in special circumstances. Byssinosis is discussed separately in Chapter 11.

Table 12.1 shows examples of some of the causes and types of occupational asthma.

TABLE 12.1

OCCUPATIONAL ASTHMA

Provoking agent	Examples	Type of asthma	Precipitin*
Organic dusts	Feathers, wool, furs, wheat grain	Immediate (Type I)	None
	Spores of: M. faeni S. granarius A. clavatus	†'Late' Type III	Specific
	Avian proteins		Specific
	A. fumigatus	Immediate and 'late'	†Specific
	B. subtilis enzymes	Immediate and 'late'	†Non-specific
	Cotton	†'Late' (direct histamine release?)	†Non-specific
	Gum acacia and karaya gum	†'Late'	None
	Red cedar wood (Thuja plicata)	†'Late'	None
	Piperazine	†'Late'	None
Fumes and vapours	Toluene diisocyanate	Immediate and †'late'	†Non-specific
	Complex platinum salts	Immediate and †'late'	None
	Alluminium soldering flux	Immediate and †'late'	None

* This table presents in an abbreviated form the main published immunological data at present available (1972), but much research is in progress and more complex precipitin patterns will undoubtedly be identified.
† 'Late' asthma is asthma whose onset is delayed about 4 to 6 hours after exposure to the provoking agent.

COMMON GROUP

Immediate Type I asthma may occur in atopic subjects whose work involves handling wool, feathers, furs and wheat or other grain. If the concentration of dust from such sources is high and exposure prolonged, non-atopic subjects may also develop immediate asthma. Asthma due to wheat, grain, or flour dusts—often called 'millworkers' asthma'—has more than one cause.

Millworkers' Asthma

Allergens in the wheat grain itself (Duke, 1935; Wolfromm, Gervais and Herman, 1966) or grain smuts, rust or mites (Wittich, 1940) may be responsible. But contamination by the wheat weevil (Sitophilus granarius) is also common (Frankland and Lunn, 1966; Lunn, 1966). However, although many mill workers may have positive skin reactions to mixed flour or weevil extracts, only a minority complain of asthma and few react to inhalation with weevil extract (Lunn, 1966).

Outbreaks of asthma have occurred among people exposed to a prevailing wind carrying grain dust from neighbouring mills (Cowan et al., 1963).

451

UNCOMMON GROUP

'Late' asthma may result from the inhalation of the spores of *Micro-polyspora faeni* in mouldy fodder or of *Aspergillus clavatus* in contaminated maltings and from the dust of avian proteins (budgerigars and pigeons in particular). Extrinsic allergic 'alveolitis' is usually, but not always, present in these cases. Specific precipitins are usually to be found.

The isocyanates

The production of polyurethanes for the manufacture of fibres, plastics, elastomers, adhesives, surface coatings and flexible and rigid foams involves isocyanates which react with a variety of compounds containing active hydrogen atoms. The isocyanates are made by the reaction of amines with phosgene, and the four most important are toluene diisocyanate (TDI), and diphenylmethane diisocyanate (MDI), naphthalene diisocyanate (NDI) and hexamethylene diisocyanate (HDI) (Buist and Lowe, 1965). Of these TDI is by far the most significant commercially and toxicologically, its major use being the manufacture of the foams. However, although the others have a more limited use, they have all been reported as occasionally causing respiratory symptoms (Report of the Isocyanate Sub-Committee, 1971).

TDI and HDI are highly volatile and vaporize readily, but the volatility of MDI used for urethane surface coatings is much lower. TDI in the undistilled form employed for polyurethane manufacture is a dark brown liquid.

Exposure to TDI vapour may occur in the following occupational situations: during its production; in the vicinity of foam-producing machines; during spraying and moulding operations; accidental leakage or spillage of liquid TDI during bulk or drum handling or drum emptying; leakage from pumps; during disposal of TDI waste and welding polyurethane-covered wires (Pepys *et al.*, 1972). It is encountered with increasing frequency in non-occupational circumstances: for example, when polyurethane products are burned or during the use of polyurethane varnish with a TDI activator (Pepys *et al.*, 1972).

High concentrations of vapour (as may occur in major accidental spillage) cause rhinitis, pharyngitis, breathlessness, chest tightness, cough, wheezing and crepitations (Hama, 1957) and in severe cases there may be pulmonary oedema or bronchopneumonia. More commonly, low concentrations are encountered. In the first few months of exposure many workers complain of upper respiratory tract irritation which is usually transient although some complain of cough and wheezing towards the end of the day and at night. As the cough may predominate and there is a small amount of sputum, 'bronchitis' is often diagnosed rather than asthma. Recovery usually occurs after about a week away from work and no further symptoms may occur on returning (Gandevia, 1970). However, a smaller, but important, number of workers develop 'late' asthma—often from very low concentrations of TDI—which seems to have little relation to their atopic status. The asthmatic episode, even when not unduly severe, may take some weeks to subside. Individual susceptibility varies greatly, but once sensitization has occurred, exposure even to minimal concentrations may provoke severe asthmatic reactions. Hence, TDI may cause the clinical features of primary irritation of mucous membranes or of sensitization which often follows several episodes of severe irritation (Bruckner *et al.*, 1968).

The underlying mechanism of the asthma is not yet clear but eosinophilia may occur (Avery *et al.*, 1969) and the presence of reaginic antibodies to TDI (Taylor, 1970) and the production of lymphoid cell transformation by TDI (Bruckner *et al.*, 1968) suggest that many immunological processes are involved. Heavy exposure of the respiratory tract of experimental animals to TDI increases its sensitivity to contact with TDI but this may not involve an allergic process (Stevens and Palmer, 1970).

Significant reduction of FEV_1 without asthmatic symptoms may occur in the afternoon of the first day following a break from work in workers exposed to very low concentrations of vapour, and this may persist to the following morning, or may continue through the working week (Peters, Murphy and Ferris, 1969). Smoking does not appear to contribute to this effect (Peters, 1970) nor to an apparently high rate of chronic bronchitis (M.R.C. definition) among workers exposed briefly to high concentrations of TDI (McKerrow, Davies and Jones, 1970). Acute changes in ventilatory capacity may occur in some workers exposed to TDI levels below the present (1971) recommended TLV (Peters, 1970).

There is no conclusive evidence that chronic effects occur as a result of long-term, low-dosage exposure, but prospective study is required to clarify this.

There are no related radiographic abnormalities in the asthmatic subjects.

Other reported effects of TDI exposure are dermatitis, euphoria and ataxia (McKerrow, Davies and Jones, 1970); thrombocytopenic purpura has occurred (Jennings and Gower, 1963) but is of doubtful significance.

Special preventive measures are required and, briefly, these include the following. Exhaust ventilation hoods of varying design according to the processes involved and the wearing of full-face respirators during bulk or drum handling and the disposal of waste when exhaust ventilation systems are not provided. The environmental atmosphere should be constantly monitored, not only at fixed points in the factory but also in the vicinity of workers open to potential exposure, and instruments are available for continuous automatic monitoring which sound an alarm when the TLV is exceeded (Parkes, 1970). All exposed personnel must receive detailed instructions about the source of potential risks and the routine for decontamination after accidents. Pre-employment and periodic medical examinations with assessment of ventilatory function are most important. A detailed code of practice is given in the Report of the Isocyanate Sub-committee (1971).

Threshold Limit Value   0·02 ppm or 0·14 mg/m³   (This is Ceiling Value.)

Proteolytic enzymes

The most important of these as a health hazard are enzymes derived from *Bacillus subtilis* (Alcalase and Maxatase) and used with the usual detergent ingredients in 'biological' washing powders. These powders were introduced to Britain and the United States of America in 1967.

Occupational exposure may occur among workers handling drums or paper sacks of the enzymes and during preparation and packing of the powders (Flindt, 1969; Pepys *et al.*, 1969; Greenburg, Milne and Watt, 1970), and the risk of sensitization may also be present during their industrial and (rarely) domestic use (Belin *et al.*, 1970). These enzymes are also used for certain processes in the baking, brewing, fish, silk and leather industries.

In some cases, asthma is of immediate type occurring within half an hour of exposure, but often is of 'late' type which can be severe and can sometimes last, with diminishing severity, for a few days (Mitchell and Gandevia, 1971). Skin rashes may occur but are normally of minor importance.

Using standardized prick-test antigens, How and Cambridge (1971) demonstrated that reagin-mediated, Type I, allergy was present in exposed factory workers but not in control subjects, and immediate prick-test reactions have been found to be approximately twice as common among 'atopic' workers (that is, those who react to common allergens) as the non-atopic (Greenburg, Milne and Watt, 1970; Newhouse *et al.*, 1970). But 'late' skin reactions following prick-tests do not seem to have been reported (How and Cambridge, 1971). However, Mitchell and Gandevia (1971) observed no significant correlation between immediate (prick) and five-hour (intradermal) skin reactions to the enzymes and immediate and 'late' asthma. Both immediate and 'late' asthma may be provoked by inhalation challenge tests with the enzymes (Pepys *et al.*, 1969). Non-specific precipitins may be present in both symptomatic and non-symptomatic exposed workers (How and Cambridge, 1971) but they correlate poorly with the asthma and have been found more often in asthmatic and healthy subjects who had not worked with the enzymes (Pepys *et al.*, 1969). It has been suggested, therefore, that some other unidentified factors in addition to allergy are involved in the causation of this form of occupational asthma but cigarette smoking does not appear to be one of them.

No evidence of permanent lung damage, as revealed by lung function tests, has been detected in exposed workers whether sensitized or not (Mitchell and Gandevia, 1971), but some reduction of gas transfer and increase in the alveolar-arterial oxygen tension, supposedly due to small airway obstruction, has been described in a small group of workers (Shore, Greene and Kazemi, 1971).

Chest radiographs show no relevant abnormality.

Asymptomatic workers should have regular medical surveillance including spirometry and skin-prick tests to common allergens, and atopic subjects should be excluded from exposure at pre-employment examination. Symptomatic workers should be removed from exposure. Exhaust ventilation of relevant processes and strict personal hygiene is required.

No TLVs are given; but in Great Britain, the Soap and Detergent Industry Association (1971) has recommended procedures for handling enzyme materials.

Gum and wood dusts
'Late' asthma has occurred due to the inhalation of gum acacia (gum arabic), (*Acacia senegal* Willd.) and karaya gum (Indian tragacanth) (*Sterculia ureus* Roxb.) (Bohner, Sheldon and Tronis, 1941; Fowler, 1952) which have a variety of uses in industry, in particular in colour printing (printers' asthma). It develops more readily in atopic subjects with multiple skin sensitivities

to common allergens than in non-atopic subjects (Turiaf, Marland and Tabart, 1966) and can be prevented by substitution of the gums by an inert material. No precipitins are found.

The dust of Canadian or Western red cedar wood (*Thuja plicata*) which is widely employed for window frames, panelling and garden sheds and furniture may cause asthma in carpenters and men working with them. This is usually of 'late' type, but occasionally there is a dual reaction (Gandevia, 1970). There are no precipitins and immediate and delayed skin reactions are either negative or only weakly positive (Gandevia, 1970). Iroko wood and 'Cedar of Lebanon' dusts have also been found to cause 'late' asthma especially in atopic subjects (Greenburg, 1972; Pickering, Batten and Pepys, 1972).

Complex salts of platinum

Exposure to various chloroplatinates may occur in platinum-refining workshops during the manufacture of chloroplatinic acid, and in laboratory workers (Parrot *et al.*, 1969). The effects, which occur after some period of exposure and are often referred to as *platinosis* (Roberts, 1951), consist of rhinopharyngitis, conjunctivitis, itching of the skin, dermatitis and asthma.

The asthmatic reaction may be of immediate, 'late' or dual type and can be reproduced by inhalation challenge tests; skin-prick tests with low concentrations of chloroplatinates give immediate positive reactions. No precipitins have yet been found. The asthmatic reactions are inhibited by inhalation of disodium chromoglycate (Pepys, Pickering and Hughes, 1972).

In animals the salts cause an immediate histamine release (Parrot *et al.*, 1969).

Piperazine

Exposure to piperazine dichloride and hexahydrate during the production of piperazine materials in the factory (as in the manufacture of sheep drench) or laboratory may cause 'late-type' asthma with productive cough, lachrymation, rhinorrhoea and, in some cases, cutaneous sensitization (McCullagh, 1968; Pepys, Pickering and Loudon, 1972); and the risk of sensitization is present in those who use these materials.

Delayed skin-prick tests are negative but asthmatic reactions can be provoked by inhalation challenge tests in sensitized subjects after three to four hours and may not resolve completely for thirty hours. Isoprenaline reverses the attack and disodium chromoglycate completely prevents its development (Pepys, Pickering and Loudon, 1972).

No antibodies have so far been demonstrated.

Aluminium soldering flux

A soldering flux containing aminoethyl ethanolamine for jointing aluminium has been introduced in recent years, particularly in cable jointing where aluminium has largely replaced copper. Fume containing ammonia and the amine vapour is evolved when solder at 320°C is poured over the flux (McCann, 1964).

Asthma may develop following exposure which often occurs in confined spaces. It is usually of 'late' type with wheeze, productive cough and dyspnoea on effort, and the symptoms may persist in milder form for two or three weeks; some degree of breathlessness may be present for months.

Inhalation challenge tests with aminoethyl ethanolamine vapour induce typical 'late' asthmatic reactions which are not prevented by disodium chromoglycate but are reversed by isoprenaline. In some subjects a 'dual' reaction may occur (Sterling, 1962; Pepys and Pickering, 1972). The tests must be done with great caution in view of the possible severity of the asthma.

The underlying mechanism of the asthma is not understood.

DIAGNOSIS

The diagnosis of asthma of occupational origin depends chiefly on a detailed clinical and work history and awareness of the possibility by the physician.

There may be difficulty in diagnosing 'late' occupational asthma because the time lag between its development and exposure to the provoking agent may obscure the relationship and lead to a diagnosis of 'intrinsic' asthma or 'bronchitis'. It must be established whether the subject is atopic or not, and, if immunological mechanisms are involved, it is necessary to distinguish clearly between demonstrable sensitization as revealed by skin tests or the presence of precipitins and specifically induced clinical symptoms (Turner Warwick, 1971).

In cases of doubt, inhalation challenge tests with carefully controlled aerosol concentrations of the suspected agent will establish the diagnosis. They should be done only under hospital conditions when the patient is symptom free, and most careful control of dosage is necessary if dangerous bronchial reactions are to be avoided.

TREATMENT AND PROGNOSIS

The most important step in treatment is to remove the patient from exposure to the reponsible process. In the majority of cases this is curative although occasionally it is not.

Symptomatic treatment with bronchodilator drugs is helpful during the attack but is only partially effective in 'late' type asthma. Corticosteroids may reverse the symptoms but must not be used for prolonged periods. The effectiveness or otherwise of disodium chromoglycate (Intal) in these cases is not yet known. Desensitization may sometimes work in cases of immediate-type asthma in atopic individuals with positive skin tests to common allergens and bronchial reactions to specific challenge.

GENERAL PREVENTIVE PRINCIPLES

(1) Pre-employment medical examination should include a record of FVC and FEV_1. Atopic subjects should not be allowed to come into contact with the hazardous dust, fume or vapour.

Periodic medical examination should be done annually.

(2) Substitution of the harmful material by a harmless one is usually and theoretically the ideal but may be impracticable and, in view of the fact that asthma can be provoked by a wide variety of irritant aerosols, ineffective.

(3) Efficient enclosure, exhaust ventilation and, under some conditions, close-fitting respirators of approved design.

(4) Environmental control by regular monitoring of the toxic agent. In the case of particulate aerosols all those which are capable of reaching the tracheobronchial region—that is, less than 10 μm—and not just those which penetrate to the alveoli, should be monitored. The results should be carefully recorded. But it should be noted that, in contrast to lung disease caused by fibrogenic dust, asthma may continue to occur in the presence of very minute quantities of an offending agent.

CADMIUM INHALATION POISONING

Cadmium metal or its compounds may either be inhaled or ingested, but only the results of inhalation which occur in industry are relevant here.

Freshly generated cadmium fumes are so toxic that at one time they were considered as a possible weapon of chemical warfare. Cadmium oxide fumes produced when the metal burns in air are orange-brown in colour and they tend to settle as a fine dust on cold surfaces. The metal melts at 321°C (610°F) and boils at 767°C (1800°F).

Uses and sources of exposure

Cadmium is highly resistant to corrosion and is used in antifriction metal alloys for engine bearings, for electroplating iron and steel, in the plates of nickel–cadmium storage batteries, in brazing and soldering alloys, wires and rods; in copper alloys for cables and trolley wires, in electrical capacitors, as cadmium sulphide and sulphoselenide in the preparation of pigments for paints, ceramics, glass, plastics and leather; in pesticides and veterinary medicines and as a neutron absorber in atomic reactors. It is worth noting that both cadmium and beryllium—the two most toxic metals to the lungs— are used in the manufacture of non-sparking tools.

Any of these processes is a potential source of exposure to dust or fume. Exposure to fume may also occur during the smelting and refining of zinc, lead and copper ores in which cadmium is present; during the recovery of scrap metal containing cadmium, and occasionally outside industry as in the use of cadmium alloys by sculptors in metal and by enthusiasts in metallist hobbies.

Oxyacetylene burning and welding of cadmium-plated metal and silver brazing have proved to be especially hazardous (Beton *et al.*, 1966; Blejer and Caplan, 1971) because they are often carried out in enclosed or ill-ventilated places, the fume is freshly generated and the risk is frequently unsuspected. Silver brazing is a form of high temperature welding in which metal is joined by the application of heat from 98 to 165°C (1800 to 3000°F) with a silver alloy filler (commonly containing cadmium) which melts at about 428°C (800°F). Cadmium-plated metals may resemble galvanized (zinc-plated) metals and be mistaken for them. A simple test for the detection of cadmium is to heat gently a *small* spot of the metal with the welding rod when the film formed in the presence of cadmium is golden-yellow but is smoky-grey if zinc is present (Blejer and Caplan, 1971).

The danger is heightened by the fact that concentrations of cadmium fume or dust sufficient to cause severe illness or death do not give rise to any early warning symptoms. Therefore, any process which may evolve cadmium fume or dust in the vicinity of a worker's 'breathing zone' must be regarded as potentially dangerous; that is, any form of heating, brazing, welding, soldering or grinding of cadmium-containing metals (Blejer and Caplan, 1971).

Smokers are exposed to low concentrations of cadmium because some 70 per cent of the cadmium content of tobacco passes into the smoke (Nandi et al., 1969) and, although many foods contain measurable amounts of cadmium which is poorly absorbed from the gastro-intestinal tract, tobacco smoke is probably the chief non-industrial source of cadmium accumulation in the body—chiefly in the liver and kidneys—especially in heavy smokers (Lewis et al., 1972).

Cadmium-induced disease is uncommon but, because it occurs unexpectedly and is potentially lethal, is important.

Absorption

Cadmium fume is readily soluble in slightly acid media and so is rapidly absorbed into the blood following inhalation. The dust tends to be of larger particle size, to be less soluble and to follow the routes of dust elimination from the lungs (see Chapter 3), although some solution evidently occurs. In the alkaline-battery industry only 20 per cent of particles were found to be of 'respirable' size (Adams, Harrison and Scott, 1969). These differences are reflected in the Threshold Limit Values (q.v.). The total amount of cadmium in the lungs, therefore, correlates poorly with its toxic effects but large quantities are found in the liver, kidneys, pancreas and thyroid of exposed persons (Lane and Campbell, 1954; Friberg, 1957).

PATHOLOGY

Acute poisoning

Acute poisoning is due chiefly to freshly generated fume.

Petechiae may be present in the pulmonary pleura. The lungs are voluminous and massively oedematous with blood-tinged fluid which is also found in the airways. Oedema is less pronounced if the patient has survived a week or more.

Microscopically, the alveoli and terminal airways are filled with protein-aceous fluid, and large areas of intra-alveolar haemorrhage may be seen. There may be partial hyaline membrane formation (Blejer and Caplan, 1971). The alveolar walls are thickened by oedema and may contain many lymphocytes and neutrophils and a number of fibroblasts. There are hyperplasia and metaplasia of alveolar epithelial cells with much desquamation, but in some cases many alveolar spaces are completely filled by masses of cuboidal cells (Patterson, 1947; Christensen and Olsen, 1957; Beton et al., 1966). The type of appearance varies according to the time the patient survives. If he recovers, these lesions probably resolve completely.

Acute cortical necrosis of the kidneys may occur in fatal cases (Beton et al., 1966).

Experimentally, cadmium has a similar effect to ozone (q.v.) in that desquamated Type I pneumocytes are replaced by a large number of Type II pneumocytes (Carrington and Green, 1970) and that it causes a striking increase in vascular permeability (Steele and Wilhelm, 1967).

Chronic poisoning

Chronic poisoning may result from repeated short exposures to moderate or low concentrations of cadmium oxide fumes, cadmium oxide, sulphide and stearate dusts over a prolonged period of time (Smith, Smith and McCall, 1960; Bonnel, 1965; Friberg, 1971).

Effect on the lungs

Emphysema, supposedly from this cause, has been described and in one group of cases appeared, in whole lung sections, to be of severe panlobular type (Smith, Smith and McCall, 1960) and, in another case, with repeated short exposures, to consist of severe centrilobular type (Lane and Campbell, 1954). A case reported by Baader (1952) also appears to be of panlobular type. However, Gough (1960, 1968) considers that 'cadmium emphysema' is a severe centrilobular emphysema. Mild peribronchiolar fibrosis has also been described (Baader, 1952).

Very few post-mortem studies of the lungs of men with long exposures to cadmium appear to have been reported.

Effects on the kidneys

Proteinuria which resembles that found in disorders characterized by renal tubular malabsorption occurs in workers who have been exposed to cadmium for about a decade or longer (Kazantzis *et al.*, 1963) and, initially, is insignificant. Its incidence correlates with the concentrations of cadmium in the air to which the men have been exposed (Adams, Harrison and Scott, 1969). The proteinuria persists when exposure ceases, and consists of low molecular weight proteins (10,000 to 30,000) with a small albumin fraction. Some thirty proteins appear to be present in the urinary colloids but there is none specific for cadmium poisoning (Piscator, 1966). Ultimately the complete Fanconi syndrome may develop. Cadmium is usually present in the urine and may be excreted for as long as ten years after last exposure (Blejer and Caplan, 1971). Its concentration is significantly higher in men with proteinuria than in those without, and is low among retired men with proteinuria (Adams, Harrison and Scott, 1969).

Diffuse interstitial fibrosis of the kidneys with atrophy of tubules and ischaemic atrophy of glomeruli has been described (Bonnell, 1955; Adams, Harrison and Scott, 1969).

Other effects

Mild hypochromic anaemia (Cotter and Cotter, 1951), osteoporosis with pseudofracture appearances on bone radiographs (Nicaud, Lafitte and Gros, 1942) and renal calculi (Ahlmark *et al.*, 1960) may occur. The anaemia is believed to be due to iron deficiency and increased red cell destruction (Friberg, 1957), and the osteoporosis and calculi to hypercalcuria and secondary hyperparathyroidism.

The underlying reason for the toxicity of cadmium is considered to be due to inhibition of enzyme systems (in the kidney those which regulate tubular reabsorption) dependent upon the presence of copper, cobalt and zinc ions (Kendrey and Roe, 1969; Mustafa *et al.*, 1971).

In spite of the concentration of cadmium in the liver, cirrhosis or other severe chronic effects do not seem to have been reported (Friberg, 1971).

The problem of 'cadmium emphysema'

Emphysema of panlobular or centrilobular type is common in the population at large. Hence, proof of a cause-and-effect relationship between cadmium exposure and emphysema requires particularly strict criteria which, unfortunately, have not always been applied. Most of the available information is based on clinical, physiological and radiological studies during life which, for the most part, have lacked epidemiological control, details of smoking habits and strict radiographic criteria. Although some observers have found evidence of emphysema in cadmium workers during life (Holden, 1965; Bonnell, Kazantzis and King, 1959) others have not (Potts, 1965; Townshend, 1968) and a more recent comprehensive study revealed none of the signs of emphysema, though proteinuria was present in some of the subjects (Teculescu and Stănescu, 1970). An unreported survey of some sixty cadmium workers did not reveal an unexpected excess of emphysema on radiographic criteria (Simon, 1972). Respiratory disease was not found to be an important cause of ill-health in workers in an alkaline accumulator factory after twelve years of exposure (Adams, Harrison and Scott, 1969).

On the other hand, as cadmium appears to inhibit the activity of some enzymes it is possible that it may exert this effect on α_1 antitrypsin which is known to be associated with some cases of panlobular emphysema (*see* Chapter 1). Indeed, the cadmium content of the liver has been found to be significantly higher in smokers with a diagnosis of bronchitis and emphysema than those without (Lewis, Lyle and Miller, 1969), but whether these are related to cadmium rather than to some other constituent of tobacco smoke has not been determined. Repeated injections of cadmium chloride into the lungs of guinea-pigs results in condensation of the parenchyma and 'generalized hyperinflation of remaining lung spaces' (Thurlbeck and Foley, 1963).

In short, more evidence than is at present available is needed before a cause-and-effect relationship between cadmium inhalation and emphysema can be regarded as proved.

CLINICAL FEATURES

Acute poisoning

There are no symptoms during exposure. They are delayed for several hours, commonly starting when the man has returned home and retired to bed, and are identical to those of 'metal fume fever' (q.v.) with the addition, in some cases, of abdominal cramps and diarrhoea. He may feel well enough to return to work the following day. But some twelve to thirty-six hours later there is dyspnoea, severe chest pain with a sense of precordial constriction (which may be mistaken for myocardial infarction), persistent cough with frothy sputum which may be bloodstained, wheeze, weakness and malaise (Beton *et al.*, 1966).

On examination of severely ill patients there is fever, central cyanosis,

460

restlessness and the signs of pneumonia or pulmonary oedema. There may be mild proteinuria and toxic liver damage may be suggested by increased serum glutamic oxylactic transaminase (SGOT) and bilirubin levels (Blejer and Caplan, 1971). Pronounced loss of weight occurs in patients who survive some days.

The chest radiograph reveals the appearances of pulmonary oedema which usually resolve in a week or two but may not disappear completely for two or three months (Townshend, 1968).

Complete recovery is usually rapid with appropriate treatment, although a mortality rate of 15 to 20 per cent due to respiratory failure has been reported (Bonnell, 1965). Following recovery, later deterioration of ventilatory function and diffusing capacity does not appear to occur (Townshend, 1968).

Chronic poisoning

Symptoms of chronic poisoning develop insidiously over a number of years.

There is tiredness and loss of weight sometimes with anaemic pallor. The typical presenting symptom is said to be breathlessness due to emphysema thought to be caused by cadmium, but with little cough or sputum (Bonnell, 1965). Later, bone pains and symptoms of nephrolithiasis, and ultimately of chronic renal failure, occasionally develop after prolonged exposure. Anosmia, sometimes with watery nasal discharge, may be complained of (Adams and Crabtree, 1961).

Lung function tests and the chest radiograph may or may not indicate the presence of emphysema.

Proteinuria which can be detected with a 3 per cent solution of sulpho-salicylic acid or 25 per cent trichloroacetic acid, but not by boiling, is usually present. There may be evidence of a multiple tubular reabsorptive defect which, as a rule, is slight and not associated with any disability, but in some cases there is significant renal glycosuria, abnormal aminoaciduria, hyper-calcuria, hyperchloraemic acidosis and impaired concentration of urine. Rarely, the clinical and radiographic signs of osteomalacia with multiple spontaneous fractures are seen.

The cause of death in some patients has been cor pulmonale and respiratory failure due to emphysema, which has been attributed to cadmium. Death due to renal failure appears to be very uncommon.

DIAGNOSIS

Acute poisoning

The two most important requirements are a detailed occupational history from the patient or a workmate, and an awareness by the physician of the existence of this disorder and the conditions which may give rise to it.

It is imperative that the diagnosis is made promptly and that the illness is not mistaken for harmless 'metal fume fever'. If symptoms persist—especially fever and severe chest pain—after twenty-four hours (when those of 'metal fume fever' have ceased) in a man with an appropriate or suspicious work history, acute poisoning must be suspected. A worker who has previously experienced 'metal fume fever' and is unaware of recent exposure to cadmium fume may wrongly attribute his symptoms to 'metal fume fever' and not seek medical advice until the delayed effects of cadmium are established. It should be noted that the other most commonly mistaken diagnoses are broncho-pneumonia, virus pneumonia, influenza and, possibly, myocardial infarction.

There are no specific diagnostic tests. With sensitive techniques cadmium can usually—though not always—be detected in the blood and urine; normally it is not present in either. But this merely confirms exposure to cadmium and is not proof of poisoning. Concentrations which indicate that a harmful level of exposure has occurred are given as follows (Blejer and Caplan, 1971):

$$\text{Blood} \quad 0.05 \ \mu g/g$$
$$\text{Urine} \quad 0.1 \ \ \mu g/ml$$

Chronic poisoning

Given, in a worker with long exposure to cadmium, that other cases of general ill-health, anaemia, weight loss and renal malabsorption with 'tubular' proteinuria are excluded, chronic poisoning can be diagnosed. Occasionally, the symptoms of renal calculi may draw attention to this. It is open to doubt that the presence of emphysema supports the diagnosis whether or not it is associated with renal damage or other abnormalities. Absent or little cough and sputum with emphysema are sometimes quoted as a feature of 'cadmium emphysema' but this is also true of primary or 'pure' emphysema.

Cadmium may be present in the blood and urine and, in reported cases, has been found in the following ranges (Blejer and Caplan, 1971):

$$\text{Blood} \quad 1.2 \text{ to } 3.8 \ \mu g/g$$
$$\text{Urine} \quad 0.1 \text{ to } 0.36 \ \mu g/ml$$

TREATMENT

Acute poisoning

First aid

    (1) Warmth, rest and reassurance;

    (2) Administration of oxygen;

    (3) The patient must be warned against the slightest exertion.

In hospital

    (1) Warmth and rest must be continued for several days over the period when delayed-onset pulmonary oedema may occur.

    (2) Oxygen administered by intermittent positive pressure ventilation in a concentration no greater than 70 per cent. In the event of respiratory failure mechanical assistance of respiration will be necessary.

    (3) Removal of bronchial exudates by suction tube. In many cases elective tracheostomy with a large cuff endobronchial tube is indicated.

    (4) Corticosteroids. Early administration greatly improves the prognosis. In severely ill patients they should be given intravenously for a few days and thereafter in the form of prednisone by mouth until recovery is established.

    (5) Chelating agents. Calcium ethylenediamine tetracetic acid (EDTA) by the intravenous route has been recommended by some authorities but is regarded by Friberg (1971) as undesirable. If it is used the dose must be

strictly controlled and renal function frequently checked. The reason for this is that it is nephrotoxic in combination with cadmium. The maximal recommended dose is 2·5 g per 4·5 kg bodyweight, and for each 4·5 kg is 170 mg per hour, 330 mg per day or 1,670 mg per week. No more than two such courses with a one-week interval should be given (Blejer and Caplan, 1971). Dimercaprol (BAL) is contraindicated.

(6) Analgesics may be required for chest pain but morphine or other respiratory depressants should be avoided or given only in small doses.

(7) A bronchodilator drug may give additional relief if wheezing is pronounced.

(8) A broad spectrum prophylactic antibiotic is probably desirable.

(9) Digitalis-type drugs and diuretics are contraindicated. The pulmonary oedema is not due to left ventricular failure.

(10) Therapeutic measures for toxic hepatitis may be required.

Chronic poisoning
The patient should be removed from exposure to cadmium and may require treatment for anaemia and renal malabsorption. The use of EDTA should be avoided as it may worsen the renal damage.

Prevention
(1) The potential hazard of cadmium exposure and the processes and materials which can cause it should be made clear to all likely to be concerned. A warning label should be firmly attached to all cadmium-containing materials and, whenever possible, cadmium-free silver-alloy fillers should be available for silver brazing.

(2) Efficient exhaust ventilation must be applied to alloying and refining furnaces, to all dusty operations and, whenever practicable, to welding and similar processes involving cadmium alloys. During oxyacetylene burning, welding or brazing in confined spaces where exhaust ventilation is impossible or when carried on outdoors (where dangerous concentrations of fume may still occur in workers' breathing zones) appropriate respirators must be worn. Men working in the vicinity of fume-producing processes should also have respirator protection.

(3) The concentration of cadmium dust or fume in environmental and 'breathing zone', air should be monitored periodically and the results recorded.

(4) Workers should not be allowed to eat, drink or smoke in workplaces where cadmium fume or dust may be present, and they should not take working clothes home.

(5) Men who are likely to be exposed routinely to cadmium should have a pre-employment medical examination which should include tests for proteinuria, anaemia and ventilatory function and a chest radiograph. Those who have evidence of anaemia or renal or cardio-respiratory disease should not be accepted.

Exposed workers should be similarly examined annually.

Threshold limit values

Cadmium oxide fume   0·1 mg/m^3 (Ceiling Value.)

This value which is a 'maximum allowable concentration' should not be exceeded and all fluctuations should occur below this level.

Cadmium (metal dust and soluble salts) 0·2 mg/m³

NOXIOUS GASES

I. OXIDES OF NITROGEN

The oxides of nitrogen include nitrous oxide (N_2O), nitric oxide (NO), nitrogen dioxide (NO_2), nitrogen trioxide (N_2O_3) and nitrogen tetroxide (N_2O_4). Nitrous oxide, of course, is a harmless anaesthetic gas. The other oxides which may be encountered in industry originate as NO. Nitric oxide is fairly stable having a half-life of about 10 parts per million per hour and, therefore, converts slowly to NO_2 (the situation in the case of explosions may be different) (Commins, 1972). Nitrogen dioxide may polymerize to N_2O_4 which is so unstable that it promptly dissociates to NO_2. These gases are often popularly, but incorrectly, referred to as 'nitrous fumes'. Nitrogen dioxide is a reddish-brown gas which is heavier than air and it is the oxide of medical importance.

Nitrogen dioxide may be encountered in a wide variety of industrial situations: during the manufacture and use of nitric acid, and the manufacture of explosives; during welding, electro-plating and engraving; in the exhaust from metal cleaning processes; in forage tower silos; during shot-firing in mines and other blasting operations; from slow burning of gun-cotton and cordite and from the exhaust of diesel engines. Nitrogen dioxide has been used as a constituent of jet engine fuel and has occurred as an accidental contaminant of nitrous oxide for anaesthesia (Clutton-Brock, 1967).

Metal welding and cutting
Nitrogen dioxide may be produced in significant concentrations by oxy-acetylene and electric arc welding and by oxygas cutting (Roe, 1959) due to the combination of oxygen and nitrogen caused by the high temperatures (3,000°C in an electric arc) and ultraviolet radiation. It is only harmful, however, when welding is done in enclosed and poorly ventilated spaces (Norwood *et al.*, 1966; Steel, 1968). The larger the current used in arc welding the more nitrogen dioxide is likely to be evolved, and electrodes with a high cellulose coating give rise to above average amounts of the gas. In general, there is little likelihood of hazardous concentrations of gas occurring when these processes are carried out in 'open shop' conditions. Gas-shielded welding, in which the electrode and molten weld are protected from the air by a stream of inert gas (such as argon, helium or carbon dioxide) from an orifice around the electrode, produces insignificant quantities of nitrogen dioxide (Roe, 1959; Morley and Silk, 1970).

In passing, it should be noted that the high welding temperatures also vaporize the electrode core and coating, the base and weld metal, and any paint, paint primer (Steel, 1964) or plastic with which the metal is covered. Therefore, the effects of welding, apart from those of nitrogen dioxide, depend upon the nature of the metal, the temperature and duration of the process and the ventilation and size of the welding area. Welding and flame

cutting of ferrous metals produce iron oxide fumes which may be of high concentration when iron powder is injected into the flame to facilitate cutting of heat-resistant steels (Roe, 1959) (*see* Siderosis, Chapter 6). Zinc or copper fumes are sometimes produced in sufficient quantity in enclosed spaces to cause 'metal fume fever' (q.v.). The asbestos or quartz contained in some electrode coatings are not a source of risk as they are decomposed by the high temperature of the arc (about 4,000°C). Welding of beryllium alloys is referred to in Chapter 10, and cadmium alloys in this chapter.

The term 'welders' lung' is often used without reference to specific pathology and should be avoided.

Forage tower silos

The need for a reliable supply of bulk fodder for cattle in winter months led to the adoption of ensilage of grass or other green crops. This began on

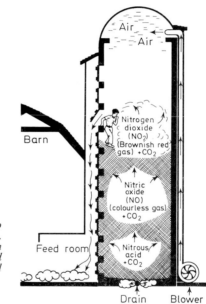

Figure 12.1. Diagram (not to scale) of a forage tower silo. (Adapted, with permission, from Ramirez and Dowell (1971) and the Editor of Annals of Internal Medicine)

the European continent in the mid-nineteenth century and spread to Britain (Jenkins, 1884). At first, lined pits or adopted barns were used but the method was a failure owing to lack of understanding of the biological processes involved. The tower silo was introduced to the eastern counties of England from the United States of America at the beginning of this century (Hall, 1923). However, it was not generally adopted because of the expense involved, and above-ground clamps, later with devices for self-feeding of cattle, were in common use until the 1950s (Turner, 1953). Then, a new type of American tower silo with mechanical loading and distributing equipment came to Britain in the late 1950s and has been installed increasingly since, its stark outline in the countryside being a mark of agricultural change (*Figure 12.1*).

Concentrations of nitrogen dioxide produced during the preparation of silage may be sufficiently high to cause death to a worker entering a silo (Grayson, 1956; Lowry and Schuman, 1956; Delaney, Schmidt and Stroebel, 1956; Desbaumes, 1968; *Farmer and Stockbreeder*, 1970).

Evolution of carbon dioxide—which is detected first (Commins, Raveney and Jesson, 1971)—and NO_2 begins a few hours after silo-filling commences, is maximal in one to two days and continues at a decreasing rate for a week or ten days (Lowry and Schuman, 1956). At the same time, the concentration of oxygen falls. The processes which underlie the production of these gases is not wholly understood but appears broadly to be as follows.

Carbohydrates in the crops yield acetic and lactic acids and CO_2 due to degradation by bacteria. The nitrate content of plants is derived chiefly from inorganic nitrates which are converted into nitrites by enzymatic action; it is increased by soils highly nitrated by fertilizers, by drought and by immaturity of the plants. The potential concentration of NO_2 is said to be roughly proportional to the amount of nitrate in the silage crop by some authors (Lowry and Schuman, 1956) but not by others (Commins, Raveney and Jesson, 1971). The nitrites react with the acids to form nitrous acid (HNO_2) which decomposes to water, NO and NO_2 as the temperature of the silage rises due to fermentation (Grayson, 1956). Temperatures $3\frac{1}{2}$ feet (105 cm) below the silage surface may range from 40·6°C to 57°C (Delaney, Schmidt and Stroebel, 1956). Initially the concentration of NO is higher than that of NO_2 but later this situation is reversed and the ratio NO_2/NO rises (Commins, Raveney and Jesson, 1971). Some N_2O_4 is also evolved but breaks down rapidly to NO_2. According to the type of crop, its pH and moisture content, bacterial activity may, in addition, give rise to free ammonia, butyric acid and free amines.

The presence and concentrations of the gases varies widely in different towers but there is no evidence that those made of concrete are less likely to develop potentially dangerous concentrations, due to their porosity, than steel towers (Jesson, 1972).

Both CO_2 and NO_2, being about one and a half times heavier than air, are concentrated at or near the silage surface and in depressions. Dangerous amounts of gas may be present, not only for a few days after filling, but some months later if the silo has remained unopened. The silage surface and silo wall may be stained yellow-red and a similar coloured vapour may be seen above the surface. An open door in the discharge (or feed) chute permits the gases to flow down into an attached barn (*Figure 12.1*). A man entering the silo does so normally through a chute door above the silage surface. He climbs the vertical chute ladder, opens one of the chute doorways at the appropriate height, climbs through the narrow opening and jumps on to the surface which may be a few feet below. If he becomes unwell due to the effects of accumulated gases he may be physically incapable of the effort necessary to retrace his path through the door and down the ladder. When the surface is convex he is more likely to encounter higher gas concentrations immediately on entry than when it is concave, but a concavity may also contain high concentrations (*Figure 12.2*). Levelling the silage surface, therefore, may be a dangerous procedure if the difference between its highest and lowest levels exceeds the height of a man (Jesson, 1972). When the surface is concave the peripheral concentration of gas may be too low at breathing level to be detected by smell and so cause a false sense of security on entry; while the higher concentrations at the surface and in depressions may make descent into a depression and its disturbance during levelling, or an accidental

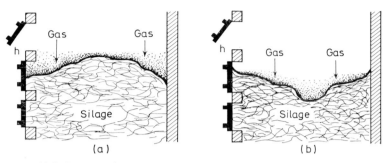

Figure 12.2. Diagram showing two different contours of the silage surface. Gas is likely to be encountered by the farm worker as he climbs on to a convex surface (a) from the hatch (h) or descends into a central concavity (b) disturbing pockets of NO_2 gas

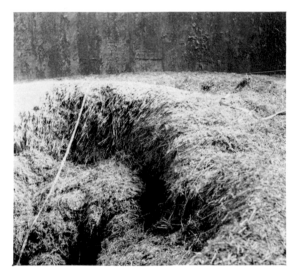

Figure 12.3. Photograph showing a concavity in the silage some five or six feet deep in the silage surface. The potential danger of the situation is evident. (By courtesy of Mr M. W. Jesson and the National Institute of Agricultural Engineering, Silsoe, Bedfordshire)

fall, especially hazardous (*Figure 12.3*). Furthermore, the movement of men in a tower disturbs the gases and may release gas trapped in the silage.

The presence of high CO_2 and low oxygen concentrations are important as they cause deep breathing which facilitates penetration of nitrogen dioxide to alveolar level and so enhances its effect (Commins, Raveney and Jesson, 1971). High concentrations of gas render a man helpless in two or three minutes (*Farmer and Stockbreeder*, 1970).

Respiratory illness due to nitrogen dioxide in silos is known as *silo fillers'*
disease. Although it does not yet appear to have been an important problem
in Britain its potential seriousness and the increasingly widespread use of
tower silos indicate the necessity for a general awareness of the risks involved.

Mining

Nitrogen dioxide is produced in varying degree by the firing of nitro-
explosive charges in mines and from the exhaust of diesel haulage locomotives.

The regular use of 'exhaust gas conditioners' on diesel engines in British
coal-mines greatly reduces the output of NO_2, and concentrations of the gas
in the vicinity of these engines and in the driver's cab are usually well below
the recommended TLV (q.v.). The average concentration of nitrogen
dioxide appears to be about 10 per cent of the nitrogen oxides in undiluted
exhaust gases (Godbert and Leach, 1970).

Concentrations of gas from shot-firing only reach dangerous levels under
conditions of imperfect detonation of charges or poor ventilation which
may exist, for example, in tunnelling operations. Ventilation in most areas
of coal-mines is good and serious pulmonary disease does not, therefore,
occur. However, as there is some speculation that shot-firing in coal-mines
might constitute a hazard to underground workers the matter must be discussed in a little more detail. If an effect were produced it would be most
likely to occur in men ('deputies' and shot-firers) working on headings and
in tunnels, although in British coal-mines it is the practice that they do not
return to the working place for at least ten minutes after firing more than
six charges, or at least five minutes after firing six or less.

Both NO and NO_2 are produced by the explosion, the former being present
in larger quantity, and the production of these gases varies little with the
different explosives used but those with a negative or near-negative oxygen
balance give rise to smaller quantities of gas. The gases are evolved in the
form of a bolus and the rate at which this travels away from the explosion
and is dispersed is determined by the velocity of the ventilating air. As the
bolus passes a given point the concentration of the gases rises rapidly and
then gradually falls, and the further it travels from source the more the gases
are diluted. Hence, peak concentrations are very brief and the men are not
likely to be exposed to them because they are outside the area. There is,
moreover, no evidence that such transient peak concentrations have any
medical significance.

Coal-miners, therefore, run no risk of developing acute lung disease—
unless, of course, they disregard shot-firing regulations (Kronenberger, 1959).

A variety of conditions influence the amount of oxides produced. They
include the nature and quantity of explosive, the method of stemming and
detonation, the area of the working place and the air volume. Therefore,
although the concentrations vary from place to place those to which miners
are subjected are uniformly low (Graham and Runnicles, 1943; Powell,
1961; Godbert and Leach, 1970). The average concentrations of mixed
oxides for a whole working shift at the return end of the coal-face has been
found to be 4 ppm (Graham and Runnicles, 1943), but may now be lower
since the introduction of power loading in the 1960s. There is no satisfactory
evidence to suggest that such concentrations are injurious to health, but

the problem is at present (1972) under investigation by the National Coal Board.

Mode of action of nitrogen dioxide and pathology

Experimental.—The severity of the effect of NO_2 depends mainly on its concentration and the duration of exposure to it, and is similar whatever its mode of origin. Unlike most water-soluble gases it is only feebly irritant to the upper respiratory tract. The reason for this is believed to be that, owing to its relatively low solubility, its conversion to HNO_2 and HNO_3—which are the cause of its harmful effects in the lungs—occurs slowly in water or humid air and is not maximal, therefore, until it reaches the peripheral airways and alveoli (Pattey, 1963). Nitric acid apparently dissociates in the lungs into nitrates and nitrites resulting in local tissue damage and the formation of methaemoglobulin (Clutton-Brock, 1967), and methaemoglobulinaemia is known to follow exposure to high concentrations of NO_2.

Short-term exposure of experimental animals to 7 to 16 parts per million (ppm) of NO_2 causes endothelial damage with transudation of fluid into alveolar and air spaces, impairment of surfactant activity and airway closure (Dowell, Kilburn and Pratt, 1971). Oedema, haemorrhage, hyperinflation, desquamation of the respiratory epithelium and bronchopneumonia are produced by the inhalation of the higher oxides of nitrogen (Shiel, 1967). Long-term exposure of animals to 12 to 26 ppm of NO_2 has been reported to cause bronchiolar hyperplasia and mild centrilobular dilatation of alveoli (Freeman and Haydon, 1964); and some partial closure of terminal bronchioles by fibrosis and occasional attenuation and fracture of alveolar walls has been described many weeks after prolonged exposure to an average of 15 ppm of NO_2 had ceased (Freeman, Crane and Furiosi, 1969). There is, however, no evidence that these and similar observations are applicable to human beings. Low-dose exposure to NO_2 results in increased susceptibility to bacterial and viral infections (Ehrlich and Henry, 1968; Valand, Acton and Myrvik, 1970) due to impairment of the activity of alveolar cells (Acton, Myrvick and Salem, 1972).

Human disease.—The gross appearances of the lungs in rapidly fatal cases following exposure to large concentrations of NO_2 are those of haemorrhagic oedema with watery blood-tinged fluid in the airways and patches of pneumonia; in patients who survive for a few weeks before finally succumbing there are small palpable nodules and haemorrhagic areas.

Microscopy of rapidly fatal cases shows, in addition to oedema, extensive damage of the respiratory epithelium which may be completely shed in the small bronchi and bronchioles (Spencer, 1968); and in the later cases, generalized infiltration of alveolar walls with lymphocytes, numerous macrophages in alveolar spaces and bronchiolitis obliterans in various stages of organization which is responsible for the palpable nodules (McAdams, 1955; Darke and Warrack, 1958; Moskowitz, Lyons and Cottle, 1964). If the patient recovers, these lesions usually resolve completely, especially if he has been treated with corticosteroids (Moskowitz, Lyons and Cottle, 1964).

Clinical features

The absence of immediate and pronounced irritation of the upper respiratory tract allows the worker to inhale gas for some time without distress. Irritation of the throat does not apparently occur until concentration of the oxides of nitrogen reaches 60 ppm, and cough, not until it is 100 ppm (Pieters and Creyghton, 1951). Severe headache and dizziness which have sometimes been complained of by magazine attendants, 'deputies' and shot-firers in coal-mines have been caused more by absorption of the nitroglycerin of explosives cartridges through the skin or by ingestion, or to the inhalation of carbon monoxide from an exploded charge than by nitrogen dioxide (Powell and Lomax, 1960). But dizziness may occur early in some cases of NO_2 exposure due to the production of systemic hypotension.

The onset of respiratory symptoms is delayed for 3 to 30 hours after exposure (although some transient choking and tightness in the chest, and sometimes central chest pain with profuse sweating may occur during exposure) so that, in some cases, a man may return to work before becoming ill. However, in the mixed gas conditions which may be encountered in a tower silo a man may rapidly be rendered senseless.

The patient becomes acutely ill with paroxysmal cough, wheeze, frothy bloodstained sputum, nausea, vomiting, increasing dyspnoea, restlessness and anxiety. He is feverish (38·3°C to 38·9°C) and centrally cyanosed and there are widespread crepitations and polymorpholeucocytosis. There may be systemic hypotension and evidence of haemoconcentration due to intrapulmonary fluid loss; and the chest radiograph reveals the ill-defined, wooly opacities characteristic of pulmonary oedema. Death from respiratory failure may occur at this stage.

Patients who recover may then pass into a latent period lasting two to six weeks during which they continue to improve and then suddenly relapse with a *second acute episode* of similar symptoms and physical signs and unremitting dyspnoea without having been re-exposed to gas. However, this does not occur in every case. Small opacities which have been mistaken for miliary tuberculosis (Becklake et al., 1957) or confluent shadows may be seen (*Figure 12.4*). This stage, the cause of which is not understood and during which the patient may die, is believed to correspond to the development of bronchiolitis obliterans. But with prompt corticosteroid treatment this is reversible and recovery is usual (Moskowitz, Lyons and Cottle, 1964; Milne, 1969), but irreversible bronchiolar fibrosis seems to have occurred in some untreated cases.

Hence, there are three distinct clinical stages:

(1) Acute oedema.
(2) A period of apparent recovery.
(3) Relapse in a second acute illness. This stage may develop even though the Stage 1 illness may have been mild.

Lung function during stages 1 and 3 shows variable abnormal patterns but vital capacity is much reduced, airways resistance increased, gas distribution uneven and gas transfer impaired. Although airways obstruction and reduction of gas transfer may be present for weeks or months after the chest radiograph has cleared it is rare to find any permanent abnormality of function (Becklake et al., 1957; Ramirez-R. and Dowell, 1971), although mild hyperinflation (Moskowitz, Lyons and Cottle, 1964) or airways obstruction

—possibly due to residual narrowing of small airways (Becklake *et al.*, 1957) —may persist in a few cases.

The chest radiograph clears quickly with treatment without evidence of residual lung damage.

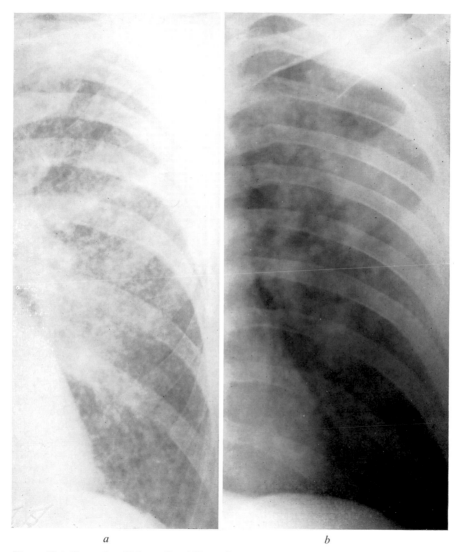

a   *b*

Figure 12.4. Examples of (a) small and (b) confluent opacities which developed in two men some three to four weeks after exposure to high concentrations of nitrogen dioxide in tower silos. Complete resolution subsequently occurred in both cases. (By courtesy of Dr R. H. Greenspan, Connecticut)

Possible long-term effects of frequent exposure to low concentrations of nitrogen dioxide
It is sometimes suggested that exposure of this sort may cause chronic obstructive bronchitis and emphysema and Kennedy (1972) has offered

471

evidence to support this contention in a group of coal-miners exposed inter-mittently to shot-firing gases underground. However, the following points concerning this study should be noted: the men do not appear to have been randomly selected and no control subjects are included, the effects of cigarette smoking are not analysed, and NO and NO_2 were not monitored separately. Although it appears that emphysema—which in most experiments has been of non-destructive type and possibly related to bronchiolitis and consequent air-trapping—can be produced in experimental animals by low doses of NO_2 over prolonged periods due, it is postulated, to induction of abnormalities in enzyme systems or the structural proteins of the lung (Hueter and Fritzhand, 1971), there is at present no satisfactory evidence that long-term intermittent exposure to low concentrations of NO_2 gives rise either to emphysema or to chronic obstructive bronchitis in man. It may be, of course, that there is a synergistic effect between cigarette smoke and NO_2 in low concentration, but this has not been demonstrated with any certainty in human beings. Evidently the results of comprehensive controlled studies in man must be awaited.

Diagnosis

Awareness of the pattern of illness caused by NO_2 and a detailed occupational and medical history will usually point to the diagnosis but it may be necessary to exclude myocardial infarction. It is important that diagnosis is made without delay and that a second acute episode is not mistaken for pneumonia because failure to use appropriate corticosteroid treatment at this stage may be fatal.

The place, nature and timing of exposure will usually differentiate silo fillers' disease from acute farmers' lung, though occasionally the latter may occur in a silo worker who has disturbed mouldy forage from the previous year's harvest. If there is difficulty in making the distinction during a severe initial illness the identification of methaemoglobulinaemia will help to resolve it.

Treatment

The principles are the same as those for the treatment of the respiratory effects of acute cadmium poisoning excepting EDTA. But the following additional measures may be required:

1. Reconversion of methaemoglobulin by an initial dose of methylene blue 2 mg/kg intravenously and subsequent doses titrated against the methaemoglobin concentration in the blood (Prys-Roberts, 1967).

2. Correction of haemoconcentration in some cases. Venesection is often recommended.

3. The use of a vasopressor drug if there is severe systemic hypotension.

Prevention

Good ventilation is the most important measure in any potential nitrogen dioxide hazard. Some welding processes can be subjected to exhaust ventila-tion techniques. Respirators used in enclosed spaces must be of approved type as some models are ineffective against NO_2.

Special measures apply to forage tower silos. These include:

1. Thorough ventilation of the tower by use of the blower (*Figure 12.1*) for at least half an hour before entry (Jesson, 1972).

2. A safety harness which can take a rope should be worn and two work-mates should be in attendance outside the tower.

3. If it is necessary to enter a silo during filling (for example, to level the silage by hand), this should be done immediately after the last load and not left until the following day when gas may already have been evolved.

It has also been recommended that, after opening a chute door, the worker should immediately climb above it in order to be higher than any remaining gas which might escape. However, Jesson (1972) has shown that this man-oeuvre cannot be relied upon and may be hazardous as the direction of air-flow after a chute door is opened varies with wind direction.

Threshold limit values

Nitrogen dioxide 5 ppm or 9 mg/m^3 (Ceiling Value.)
Nitric oxide 25 ppm or 30 mg/m^3

II. OZONE

Ozone is a highly toxic gas which is normally present in the atmosphere in minute quantities without any harmful effect, but it occurs in significant concentrations at high altitudes (Young, Shaw and Bates, 1962). It is produced in lightning and high-tension, non-sparking, electrical discharges in air or oxygen. It is used in industry for sterilizing water, bleaching paper, flour and oils and deodorizing organic factory effluents by masking, but not destroying, the odour (Pattey, 1963).

Ozone may be evolved in dangerous quantities from atmospheric oxygen due to ultraviolet radiation produced during inert gas-shielded welding with consumable or non-consumable electrodes and arc-air gouging (Sanderson, 1968). It is formed up to a distance of one metre from the source of radiation of 1800 Å in gas-shielded welding (Frant, 1963). However, insignificant amounts appear to be produced by manual arc-welding (Doig and Challen, 1964).

In experimental animals, ozone causes necrosis and sloughing of Type I pneumocytes which is followed by a remarkable increase in Type II cells (Carrington and Green, 1970); it lowers resistance to bacterial infection, impairs activity of alveolar macrophages (Huber *et al.*, 1971), attacks capillary endothelial cells and causes pronounced mural thickening of pulmonary arteries (P'an, Beland and Jegier, 1972), alters cell wall permeability leading to pulmonary oedema and reacts with proteins to produce a heterogeneous antigen which stimulates an antibody response in rabbits (Scheel *et al.*, 1959). The gas also appears to have a similar effect on animal cells to that exerted by ionizing radiation (Brinkman, Lamberts and Veninga, 1964) but the significance of this in man is still to be determined.

Clinical features
Ozone is 10 to 15 times more toxic than NO_2 (Stokinger, 1965).

473

Acute illness following exposure is either rapid in onset consisting of severe headache, substernal oppression and dyspnoea (suggesting myocardial infarction) or develops more slowly and consists of irritation of the nose and eyes which may last for a day or so, with severe cough, bloodstained sputum, dyspnoea and fever. Symptoms, physical signs and radiographic appearances are those of pulmonary oedema (Kleinfeld, Giel and Tabershaw, 1957), and, like the effects of nitrogen dioxide, may be delayed. Exposures of from 5 to 20 ppm from one hour or more are likely to be fatal (Stokinger, 1965).

Exposure to low concentrations of ozone (0·6 to 0·8 ppm) for two-hour periods causes a significant impairment in gas transfer and a less pronounced reduction of vital capacity and forced vital capacity which may be due to thickening of alveolar walls by oedema (Young, Shaw and Bates, 1964). These abnormalities disappear after a short time. Workers exposed to concentrations of about 1 ppm or less complain of upper respiratory tract irritation, headache and tightness in the chest and wheezing (Challen, Hickish and Bedford, 1958).

Treatment

In cases of acute illness this is similar to that required for the effects of nitrogen dioxide, but methaemoglobulinaemia does not occur.

Prevention

Local exhaust ventilation is necessary but is unlikely to be adequate unless measures to screen off the ozone-producing radiation are taken (Frant, 1963).

Threshold limit value

$$0·1 \text{ ppm or } 0·2 \text{ mg/m}^3$$

III. CHLORINE

Chlorine is a greenish-yellow gas, two and a half times heavier than air, the toxic qualities of which were exploited in World War I. It is used in the manufacture of innumerable chemicals varying from pharmaceuticals to plastics, and for disinfecting water. It is usually transported commercially by road, sea or rail as a liquid under pressure. Exposure can, therefore, occur at the place of manufacture (Jones, 1952); it may in the course of transport affect many people (Chasis *et al.*, 1957; Kowitz *et al.*, 1967; Weill *et al.*, 1969).

The injurious effects of the gas are thought to be due to its potent oxidative properties which liberate nascent oxygen—a protoplasmic poison—from water and to the fact that hydrochloric acid is formed (Kramer, 1967). The changes in the lungs may be those of oedema with some fibrin and the formation of hyaline membrane in alveoli (Spencer, 1968), and early bronchiolar damage and obstruction of small blood vessels by thrombi. Brief concentrations of 3 to 5 ppm of the gas appear to be tolerated without injury, but exposure to 5 to 8 ppm for a significantly long period may cause mild acute illness. Levels of 14 to 21 ppm are dangerous. The effects of exposure, however, depend on a number of factors: for example, the concentration of gas and duration of exposure; persons with pre-existing lung disease, the very young and the aged suffer more severely than healthy adults (Kramer, 1967).

Clinical features

Exposure to the gas concentrations which may be encountered in industry causes smarting of the eyes, lachrymation, rhinorrhoea, severe persistent cough, dyspnoea, retrosternal chest pain and a sense of constriction. Nausea, epigastric pain and vomiting may also occur. In spite of the severity of the symptoms the patient usually recovers quickly when removed from the area of contamination. But with higher concentrations of gas there is pink, frothy sputum, and restlessness, severe respiratory distress, central cyanosis, widespread coarse crepitations—often with wheezing—and low-grade fever (Beach, Sherwood Jones and Scarrow, 1969). The patient is critically ill for some 48 hours and, even with appropriate treatment it may be some weeks before dyspnoea on exertion finally ceases.

The chest radiograph of severely ill patients shortly after exposure shows the presence of pulmonary oedema which may be occasionally followed in a few days by bronchopneumonic consolidation (Beach, Sherwood Jones and Scarrow, 1969). However, although both oedema and secondary infection are uncommon complications (Flake, 1964), death may sometimes occur (Beach, Sherwood Jones and Scarrow, 1969).

After clinical recovery there are no residual respiratory symptoms and lung function returns to normal (Weill *et al.*, 1969).

The delayed-type illness characteristic of exposure to nitrogen dioxides is not seen.

Long-term exposure of chlorine gas workers to concentrations of less than 1 ppm is not associated with significant impairment of ventilatory function, but those who smoke have a lower maximum mid-expiratory flow rate than non-smokers (Chester, Gillespie and Krause, 1969).

Treatment

This is similar to that required for nitrogen dioxide poisoning with the exception of correction of methaemoglobulinaemia. A bronchodilator in nebulizer form is often recommended but may be unnecessary if corticosteroids are used. In healthy adults with mild poisoning, simple symptomatic treatment and oxygen at atmospheric pressure may be all that is needed. The case of intense exposure from which the individual could not immediately escape is a medical emergency which demands prompt treatment of shock, coma and respiratory arrest.

Pre-employment medical examination should be done on workers who may be exposed to a potential chlorine hazard to exclude those with respiratory or cardiovascular disease.

Threshold limit value

$$1 \text{ ppm or } 3 \text{ mg/m}^3$$

IV. OTHER GASES

Phosgene (carbonyl chloride)

This highly toxic gas may be encountered in the chemical industry and during gas-shielded welding processes if the components welded have been incompletely dried following degreasing with carbon tetrachloride or trichloroethylene which are decomposed and phosgene liberated by the heat, ultraviolet radiation and, possibly, ozone generated (Doig and Challen, 1964).

The effects of the gas develops some hours after exposure as there is little irritation of the upper respiratory tract. Low concentrations cause respiratory distress with cough, breathlessness and tightness in the chest; high concentrations result in a similar pattern of illness and changes in the lungs to those provoked by high concentrations of chlorine (Spencer, 1968).

Threshold limit value

$$0·1 \text{ ppm or } 0·4 \text{ mg/m}^3$$

Ammonia

Exposure may occur in the chemical and fertilizer industries and from accidental leakage from cylinders or tanks during transport, or from refrigeration plants.

In contrast to phosgene, the gas has an immediate irritant effect on the eyes, mouth, throat and upper respiratory tract which usually prompt the individual to escape from exposure. But if concentrations are sufficiently high, pulmonary oedema develops within a few hours and may be followed in two or three days by bronchopneumonia (Caplin, 1941).

Treatment

Treatment of respiratory illness due to either of these gases is similar to that for chlorine poisoning.

Threshold limit value

25 ppm or 18 mg/m³   (At present under review by the ACGIH.)

METAL FUME FEVER

This is a fairly common non-specific, benign, self-limiting acute illness which resembles an attack of malaria. In the past it has been variously known as *brass founders' ague, welders' ague, copper fever, Monday fever* and *the smothers*. It is caused chiefly by the fumes of zinc, copper or magnesium when heated above their melting points.

Examples of responsible sources—especially in enclosed or poorly ventilated conditions—are zinc smelting, galvanizing, and the welding or oxyacetylene cutting of galvanized iron; zinc fume from molten brass in brass founding, and copper fume from molten or red-hot copper and from the arc-air gouging process (Sanderson, 1968). Copper dust from the polishing of copper plates (Gleason, 1968) and from other sources may produce identical symptoms; hence, the term 'metal fume fever' is not wholly accurate.

The illness commences a few hours after exposure and consists of thirst, dry cough, dry throat, nausea, headache, shivering, profuse sweating, fatigue, aching in the chest and pains in the limbs. Temperature rises to 38·9°C (102°F) or higher, and there is polymorphonuclear leucocytosis.

Recovery is usually complete in 24 hours and the man is able to return to work.

A curious feature of this syndrome, which may have an immunological explanation, is that men who are continuously exposed acquire a tolerance which, however, is lost after a short period away from work—such as a week-end (Monday fever).

With a proper occupational history, the diagnosis should be evident, but the symptoms of acute cadmium inhalation poisoning are initially identical. As the prognoisis of the two disorders is quite different it is most important that cadmium poisoning should be suspected in welders in whom the symptoms persist with fever and severe chest pain after 24 hours (*see* Cadmium Inhalation Poisoning). Influenza may be wrongly diagnosed.

Treatment is symptomatic.

POLYMER FUME FEVER

The features of this syndrome are identical to those of 'metal fume fever' although of different origin. They are caused by fumes from thermal decomposition of polytetrafluoroethylene products (Teflon, Haflan, Fluon) when heated to temperatures above 300°C but are also associated with exposure to dust from machining these products when cold (Challen, Sherwood and Bedford, 1955; Sherwood, 1955). The simultaneous smoking of cigarettes appears to be a decisive determining factor of symptoms due to inhalation of the dust (Challen, Sherwood and Bedford, 1955; Harris, 1959), for the average temperature of the burning end of a cigarette is approximately 884°C (Touey and Mumpower, 1957)—more than sufficient to effect decomposition of the most stable polytetrafluoroethylene. The identity of the pyrolytic product responsible for the symptoms is not known. Epidemic episodes ascribed to smoking dust-contaminated cigarettes have occurred (Lewis and Kerby, 1965).

Polytetrafluoroethylene is one of the fluorine-containing polymers used extensively in the manufacture of thermoplastics and resins.

Tolerance of exposure, as observed in 'metal fume fever' (q.v.), does not occur (Malton and Zielhuis, 1964).

In general, there appear to be no lasting effects although radiographic appearances similar to those of pneumonic consolidation followed by impairment of ventilatory function and diffusing capacity after six months have been reported (Capodaglio, Monarca and de Vito, 1961).

Preventive measures
These include prohibition of smoking in factory areas where fluorine-containing polymers are produced; special local ventilation measures if the temperatures of processes exceeds 200°C to 250°C, instruction of workers regarding the necessary hygiene measures and the burning of all refuse in special furnaces.

Threshold limit values
None is recommended at present (1971) but air concentrations should be minimal.

HARD-METAL DISEASE

Cemented tungsten carbide, or *hard-metal*, is extensively used because of its extreme hardness, strength, rigidity and resistance to very high temperatures in drills for metal and rock cutting, other tools, dies, bearings and as an alloy in the aircraft and motor car industries. It was introduced in Germany in the 1920s and to England and the United States of America in the 1930s, and the possibility that respiratory disease might be related to this industry has been suggested in several countries since Jobs and Ballhausen described abnormal radiographic appearances in a small number of tungsten carbide workers in Germany in 1940.

Tungsten carbide is produced by blending and heating tungsten (wolfram) and carbon in an electric furnace. It is then mixed in a ball-mill with cobalt in quantities varying from 3 to 25 per cent in order to form a matrix for the tungsten carbide crystals, and other metals—such as chromium, nickel, titanium and tantalum—may be added according to the properties required in the final product. All these constituents are in a finely divided state having a mean diameter of about 1·5 μm (Coates and Watson, 1971). The powdered metal is next pressed into ingots or particular shapes. After pressing, it is fused (or sintered) in an electric furnace. All these processes and dry grinding, drilling and finishing of hard-metal products, and cleaning equipment are dusty if exhaust ventilation is inadequate.

It is computed that some 15,000 to 20,000 persons are potentially exposed to dust in the hard-metal industry throughout the world and this number is certain to increase. However, it is noteworthy that only a small proportion of exposed persons appears to develop evidence of respiratory disease—for example, in one industry in the United States of America, 9 out of 1,500 workers (Coates and Watson, 1971).

Both acute and chronic forms of illness seem to occur.

Acute disease

After a variable period of time in the industry, a small number of exposed workers may develop asthma with productive cough and chest tightness towards the end of the day's work or in the evening (Tolot *et al.*, 1970; Coates and Watson, 1971). This ceases during week-ends and holidays but recurs usually in the first day back at work; it is relieved by bronchodilators and cured by removal from exposure (Bruckner, 1967). The chest radiograph shows no abnormality and, as far as is known, no permanent bronchopulmonary damage occurs.

The mechanism responsible for the asthma, which has been reported in both non-atopic and atopic subjects has not been elucidated.

Another type of acute reaction may also occur. This consists of rapid onset of cough, sputum, dyspnoea on exertion, crepitations in the lung bases and linear or ill-defined rounded opacities with prominent hilar regions on the chest radiograph after one or two years in the industry; in some cases there is complete resolution and in others the process is arrested on removing the worker from exposure (Miller *et al.*, 1953; Lundgren and Öhman, 1954; Scherer *et al.*, 1970). The underlying lesion appears to be a desquamative type of fibrosing 'alveolitis' (Scherer *et al.*, 1970).

478

Chronic disease

Sporadic cases of progressive diffuse interstitial fibrosis (fibrosing 'alveolitis') have occurred in susceptible workers after some years in the industry; the period varies from 2 to 25 years but is usually in excess of 10 years. They have been reported in Britain (Bech, Kipling and Heather, 1962), Europe (Jobs and Ballhausen, 1940; Reber and Burckhardt, 1970; Sherer *et al.*, 1970), Sweden (Lundgren and Öhman, 1954; Ahlmark, Bruce and Nyström, 1960), Czechoslovakia and Russia (Bech, Kipling and Heather, 1962), Australia (Joseph, 1968) and the United States of America (Miller *et al.*, 1953; Coates and Watson, 1971).

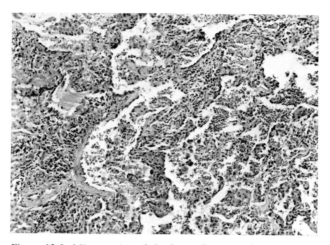

Figure 12.5. Microsection of the lung of a man who worked for two years in the final grinding process of tungsten carbide. There is pronounced interstitial cellular infiltration, fibrosis of alveolar walls and some metaplasia of alveolar lining cells. Large cells, many of which are multinucleated, lie free in the alveolar spaces. (Original magnification × 175, reproduced at × 87·5; H and E stain; courtesy of Dr E. Osborne Coates, Detroit, and the Editor of Annals of Internal Medicine)

The histological features range from mainly cellular to chiefly collagenous changes in the alveolar walls—the 'mural' type of fibrosing 'alveolitis' (*see* Chapter 4). In the one there is intense cellular infiltration of the walls with some collagen formation, cuboidal metaplasia and desquamation of alveolar cells; in the other, the amount of mural collagen is much greater and a moderate number of mononuclear cells—apparently Type II pneumocytes—and a number of multinucleated cells of histiocytic appearance may be present in the alveolar spaces (Coates and Watson, 1971) (*Figure 12.5*). Sarcoid-type or foreign body granulomas are not found. Electron microscopy reveals that Type I pneumocytes assume a cuboidal or columnar appearance with numerous microvilli and that normal appearing cells are absent. Hard crystals suggestive of tungsten carbide are present in alveolar septa and in macrophages and their lysosomes (Coates and Watson, 1971). The presence of tungsten, with or without cobalt, has been demonstrated on post-mortem analysis of the lungs in a few cases.

479

Pathogenesis

Cobalt is generally incriminated as the causal agent chiefly on the grounds that particulate cobalt metal is strikingly toxic to the lungs of experimental animals when inhaled or injected by the intratracheal route. It results in haemorrhagic oedema, obliterative bronchiolitis and proliferation and desquamation of alveolar cells (Harding, 1950; Schepers, 1955a), whereas particulate tungsten metal, tantulum and titanium alone are relatively innocuous (Schepers, 1955b, c; Kaplun and Mezencewa, 1960). Dust mixtures containing tungsten, titanium and cobalt cause a more pronounced effect than cobalt alone (Kaplun and Mezencewa, 1960). Finely divided cobalt, but not tungsten carbide, is toxic to normal human leucocytes *in vivo*, particularly in patients with fibrosing 'alveolitis' (Coates and Watson, 1971).

However, there is no correlation between the quantity of cobalt in human lungs and the severity of fibrosis (Coates and Watson, 1971) although tungsten and titanium are usually present (Bech, Kipling and Heather, 1962). But there is a similar lack of correlation in beryllium disease (Chapter 10) and Harding (1950) has suggested that the high solubility of cobalt in proteinaceous fluids allows it to escape rapidly from the lungs. If cobalt is responsible for the disease in man the reason for its effect is not known.

It is of interest that allergic dermatitis may be caused by metallic cobalt and that skin patch tests with the powdered metal are positive in affected persons (Schwarz *et al.*, 1945) but no evidence of an underlying immunological mechanism in the lung disease appears to have been described.

Although a causal relationship between exposure to dust in the hard-metal industry and fibrosing 'alveolitis' cannot be regarded as definitely established on all the available evidence, especially as the prevalence of cryptogenic fibrosing 'alveolitis' in the general population is not known, it seems likely on these grounds:

(1) Almost all the metallic particles are less than 10 μm in size and the average range is of the order of 1·2 to 1·9 μm (McDermott, 1971), hence a large proportion are capable of reaching the alveoli (*see Figure 3.1*). And tungsten and the associated metals may be found in affected lungs.

(2) Despite the fact that the number of cases recorded is very small relative to the numbers of workers exposed, the clinical features and pathology are similar in all.

(3) In the majority of cases the disorder develops in middle life after some years of exposure (Coates and Watson, 1971).

Evidently, careful, prospective epidemiological study of the hard-metal industry is necessary to clarify the matter.

Clinical features

The clinical, physiological and radiographic features are similar to those of diffuse interstitial fibrosis from other causes which is predominant in the lower halves of the lungs (*Figure 12.6*). In a few cases the disease has been fatal due to cardio-respiratory failure. As the atomic number of tungsten is 74 it might be expected that small dense radiographic opacities would be seen if sufficient dust is stored in the lungs but this does not seem to have been described. No investigations of circulating antibodies appear to have been reported but hyperglobulinaemia is recorded (Miller *et al.*, 1953).

Treatment

The early stage of the disorder—that of desquamative fibrosing 'alveolitis'—
responds to treatment with corticosteroids. Prompt diagnosis is therefore
paramount. On recovery, the worker should not return to exposure. The
later stage is not amenable to treatment.

Prevention

Dust from the various processes in the preparation of hard-metal and the
finishing of products should be reduced to a minimum by efficient exhaust

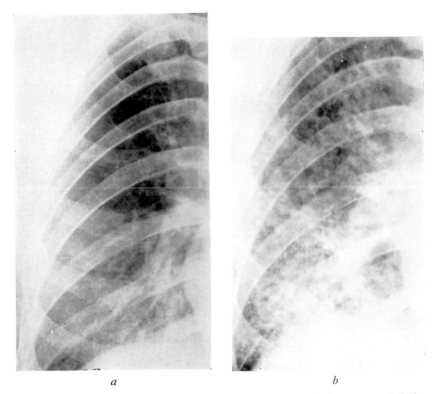

a	*b*

*Figure 12.6. Radiographs of a man who worked with soft and hard tungsten carbide for
four years. Fine linear opacities (ILO Category 's') are present in the lower half of the
lung field in (a). Film (b), taken 10 years later, shows coarse linear and round opacities
with some suggestion of 'honeycombing'. (By courtesy of Dr E. Osbourne Coates and
the Editor of Annals of Internal Medicine)*

ventilation of the high-velocity, low-volume type locally applied as in the
machining of beryllium alloys (Chapter 10) (McDermott, 1971). And
the environmental air, both breathing-zone and general, should be
monitored.

Periodic medical examination including chest radiographs and tests of
ventilatory function should be done yearly, and atopic subjects are probably
best excluded from work involving potential exposure to dust.

Threshold limit values

None is recommended at present (ACGIH, 1971) for hard-metal dust but air concentrations should be minimal.

The value for cobalt as fume or dust is 0·1 mg/m³ and that for insoluble tungsten compounds, 5 mg/m³ (both are time-weighted averages). Titanium dioxide is classed as an 'Inert' or Nuisance Particulate (ACGIH, 1971).

'ALUMINIUM LUNG'

This term refers to lung fibrosis attributed to two different inhalable materials: on the one hand, fumes from the smelting of *bauxite* (Al_2O_3), on the other, metallic aluminium dust. Unfortunately this and another commonly used term—'aluminosis'—beg the question of pathogenesis which has not been satisfactorily answered. Fibrosis related to bauxite fume is often known as *Shaver's disease*, after Shaver who jointly described the association in 1947.

Bauxite is the ore from which aluminium is smelted or extracted by electrolysis when *alumina* (aluminium oxide, Al_2O_3) is dissolved in molten *cryolite* (sodium aluminium fluoride, Na_3AlF_3). Quartz, clay minerals and iron oxide are present as impurities. *Corundum*, being a naturally crystallized oxide of aluminium, is not usually classed with bauxite. Artificial corundum —or synthetic emery—is manufactured from bauxite.

Aluminium is used not only in metal alloys (such as Duralumin), in wrapping foils and refractory materials, but in finely divided form for explosives and fireworks (when it is known as 'pyro'), and, in a coarser form, for paints and ink.

Sources of exposure

Artificial corundum production

Ground, calcined bauxite is the chief raw material. It is mixed with coke (to reduce some of the oxides) and iron and fused in an electric furnace with movable carbon electrodes at a temperature of about 2,000°C, although the temperature in the neighbourhood of the electrodes is nearer 4,000°C (Finlay, 1950). White fume which consists of alumina, non-crystalline (amorphous) silica—the crystalline and cryptocrystalline forms of silicon dioxide are decomposed below these temperatures (*see* Chapter 2)—and alumina-silica glass is evolved and is particularly dense when new raw material is added to the furnaces. The particle size of the fume is less than 1 μm and generally ranges from 0·5 μm to 0·02 μm (Hatch, 1950). Men who developed lung disease operated the furnaces or worked above them on overhead storage bins and cranes (Shaver and Riddell, 1947; Hagen, 1950).

During the electrolytic extraction of aluminium, incidentally, particulate and gaseous fluorides are evolved as well as other fumes and gases (Kaltreider *et al.*, 1972).

Preparation and use of aluminium powders

There are two sorts of powder: a flake type, the particle size of which may be as small as 0·6 μm, prepared in a stamp or ball-mill from the cold metal or foil, and a granular type made from molten metal. Stearin (a mixture of fatty acids prepared by hydrolysis of fats) or paraffin is usually added to the flake variety as a lubricant to permit separation of the particles.

Flake powder of small particle size ('pyro') is employed in the manufacture of explosives, incendiary devices and fireworks, and in Germany during and for some time after World War II stearin was not used owing to short supply. Many of the early cases of fibrosis attributed to aluminium exposure were reported from that country during this period (Goralewski, 1940; Goralewski and Jaeger, 1941; Barth, Frik and Scheidemandel, 1956). There have also been similar reports among workers in stamping-mills in the United Kingdom and Sweden where, for a period, stearin was either reduced in quantity or replaced by mineral oil (Ahlmark, Bruce and Nyström, 1960; Mitchell *et al.*, 1961; McLaughlin *et al.*, 1962). In the preparation of powder for paint manufacture fairly large quantities of stearin are added.

Pathology and pathogenesis

The pathology appears to be similar in workers who have been exposed to bauxite fume or aluminium dust.

The lungs are indurated and grey-black, and the pulmonary pleura is thickened, often with numerous underlying air blebs. Emphysematous bullae are common. When the lungs are cut, radiating bands or dense areas of grey-black fibrous tissue are seen predominantly in the upper and middle zones. Silicotic nodules are absent. In some cases scar emphysema may be severe.

Microscopically, there is cellular infiltration with thickening of alveolar walls, macrophages in the air spaces and interstitial alveolar wall fibrosis in which particles of dust may be evident. Giant cells with clefts, possibly occupied by cholesterol crystals, are fairly numerous. In places, the histological features are those of the 'mural' type of fibrosing 'alveolitis' (Wyatt and Riddell, 1949; Mitchell *et al.*, 1961). Obliteration of alveolar spaces by fibrosis may be widespread but the elastic framework of the walls can be recognized. Bronchioles and alveoli which survive in fibrotic areas are lined by epithelial cells and may be much dilated giving a 'honeycomb' appearance. Obliterative endarteritis and perivascular fibrosis may be present in or near the fibrosis (Wyatt and Riddell, 1949). No evidence of silicotic nodules, granulomas of foreign body or sarcoid type, or lipoid pneumonia has been found in recorded cases.

Ash of the lungs from some workers exposed to bauxite fume contains a high percentage of alumina and 'silica' of particle size as low as 0.02 μm and in proportions similar to those present in furnace fumes (Jephcott, 1950). Chemical analysis of the lungs of workers exposed to aluminium powders has confirmed the presence of aluminium, and specific staining for aluminium with auramine may identify particles of the metal (Mitchell *et al.*, 1961).

Turning now to pathogenesis, two questions arise. Does aluminium really cause fibrosis or is some other agent responsible? Is Shaver's disease due to amorphous 'silica'?

To take the dust first, there is, in general, a notable lack of lung fibrosis among exposed workers. No evidence of disease has been found in men in aluminium reduction plants (Medical Research Council, 1936; Kaltreider *et al.*, 1972), in potteries where alumina has replaced flint for biscuit placing (Posner and Kennedy, 1967), and in stamp-mills producing aluminium powders for paint and ink manufacture (Crombie, Blaisdell and McPherson, 1944), although in this case the authors did not state whether stearin was added or not. A survey of men polishing Duralumin aeroplane propellers discovered no evidence of fibrosis (Hunter *et al.*, 1944), but the dust they inhaled was chiefly that of the aluminium oxide abrasive employed and not metallic aluminium. The dust involved in these studies, therefore, was alumina. Granular metallic powder usually has a covering of aluminium oxide.

Where fibrosis has been ascribed to the dust this has, in most cases, been flake aluminium in which stearin has been wholly or partly replaced by mineral oil or wax (Goralewski, 1947; Ahlmark, Bruce and Nyström, 1960; Mitchell *et al.*, 1961), although an exception to this is to be found in the case described by McLaughlin *et al.* (1962). There is no evidence that the lubricants are fibrogenic.

It has frequently been suggested that an aluminium oxide covering of granular powder particles and a stearin covering of flake particles prevents metallic aluminium from exerting a fibrogenic effect. But when separate samples of stamped aluminium powder, one of which contained stearin, another mineral oil and a third which was defatted were administered by intratracheal injection to rats, all three caused pronounced fibrosis of equal severity, whereas granular aluminium powder had a negligible effect (Corrin, 1963). These findings appear to contradict the foregoing hypothesis and are at odds with the industrial experience. However, the large dose of dust administered may have allowed a sufficient concentration of aluminium to escape from the stearin and oil coatings to cause fibrosis (Corrin, 1963). It is noteworthy that there is a significant species difference in the fibrogenic action of metallic aluminium and hydrated alumina dust which is pronounced in rats but insignificant in rabbits, mice and guinea-pigs (Engelbracht *et al.*, 1959).

The suggestion has also been made that amorphous silica particles may be responsible (Hatch, 1950) but this seems unlikely as the quartz originally present would be converted to glass at the operating temperatures of the furnaces, and survival of tridymite or cristobalite in the fume does not seem to have been reported; furthermore, amorphous silicon dioxide smoke from a ferrosilicon smelting furnace was found to cause in the rat lung only minor fibrotic changes which are not progressive, and fine glass particles are non-fibrogenic in the lungs of rats and guinea-pigs (Gross, Westrick and McNerney, 1960). On the other hand, metallic aluminium burnt in air evolves γ Al_2O_3 (Finlay, 1950) which causes fibrosis in the rat lung, whereas α Al_2O_3 does not (Stacy *et al.*, 1959).

It may be that sensitization plays a part in human disease. Aluminium metal reacts with sodium chloride producing sodium aluminate and aluminium chloride which hydrolyse to aluminium hydroxide. Aluminium hydroxide, like silicic acid, is capable of polymerizing into giant molecules which can react with proteins (Holt, 1957). But no evidence of immunological reactions in aluminium workers with lung fibrosis appears to have been described.

So, to summarize, what part, if any, aluminium dust or fume plays in causing lung fibrosis appears uncertain and the variability of the results of animal experiments makes the validity of their application to human disease doubtful. On the one hand, innumerable workers have been exposed to both dust and fume but few have developed disease; on the other, in industries where disease has occurred it is notable that there have often been a number of cases having similar features (*see* next section) which have not been easily accounted for in other ways. It can be assumed, therefore, that aluminium may sometimes be responsible, and one possible—but speculative—causal explanation is immunological reactivity.

Clinical features

In most cases, fibrosis develops gradually over a period of years and respiratory symptoms are usually absent until it is well established, when breathlessness on effort and cough—often without sputum—are complained of. In advanced cases, dyspnoea is severe and chest pain, associated with spontaneous pneumothorax and loss of weight, may occur. In some instances, however, symptoms develop and disease advances with remarkable rapidity after only one or two years' exposure (Mitchell *et al.*, 1961), especially in workers exposed to fume among whom spontaneous pneumothorax, which may be bilateral and recurrent, is a common complication (Riddell, 1950).

The abnormal physical signs of established disease are those of fibrosis of the upper parts of the lungs, often with deviation and distortion of the trachea, and, possibly, pneumothorax.

Lung function tests reveal a restrictive pattern without significant fall in gas transfer (Mitchell *et al.*, 1961).

Radiographic abnormality precedes the onset of symptoms in most cases by some years. The earliest change appears to be widening of the mediastinal shadows at hilar level, although the reason for this is not clear. Fine linear and discrete opacities appear later in the upper zones and then throughout the lung fields. There may be evidence of spontaneous pneumothorax (Shaver, 1948; Riddell, 1950). In other cases, evidence of fibrosis commences in the apical regions and progresses to large irregular opacities with adjacent distortion of the trachea and, occasionally, the oesophagus when delineated by barium swallow (Goralewski, 1950; Mitchell *et al.*, 1961). These appearances are obviously indistinguishable from those of fibrocaseous tuberculosis. Signs of basal tractional emphysema with distortion of the diaphragm may be present.

It is worth noting that men who were exposed to fluoride dust or fume from the electrolytic production process during the 1940s may show the radiographic signs of fluorosis (that is, osteosclerotic density of ribs, spine and pelvis, and calcification of ligaments) which is symptomless. Under modern plant conditions this is no longer seen even after years of exposure (Kaltreider *et al.*, 1972).

There is apparently no increased liability to tuberculosis.

Treatment

If the chest radiograph reveals evidence suggestive of disease the worker should be removed from exposure. If this is done progressive fibrosis may not occur.

Prevention

Exhaust ventilation to remove fume and, in the case of dust, enclosure of machinery or if this is not practicable, personal protection of the worker in enclosed suits supplied with compressed air are required.

Threshold limit value

No value has been recommended by the ACGIH but aluminium oxide as the abrasive alundum is classed as an 'Inert or Nuisance Particulate'.

MANGANESE PNEUMONIA

Exposure to pyrolusite (MnO_2) dust or the dust and fumes of manganese which has many uses in metal alloys, bleaching of glass, printing, preserving wood and the manufacture of dry-battery boxes may be associated with an unduly high incidence of pneumonia (Lloyd-Davies and Harding, 1949; Morichau-Beauchant, 1964).

HAIR LACQUER SPRAYS

There are three basic types of hair lacquer:

(1) *Polyvinyl-pyrollidone (PVP) type.* PVP is combined with trichloro-fluoromethane and dichlorofluoromethane as aerosol propellants in metal dispensers.

(2) *Shellac type.* Dewaxed shellac mixed with castor oil and the same aerosol propellants.

(3) *Mixed type.* A mixture of the other two.

Lubricants such as castor oil, lanolin and wool wax may be added in various quantities to all of these.

The possibility that inhalation of such sprays may be responsible for lung disease was pointed out by Bergmann, Flance and Blumenthal in 1958 and the term '*thesaurosis*' ($\theta\eta\sigma\alpha\upsilon\rho\sigma\varsigma$ = treasure), in general currency to refer to storage of unusual quantities of normal or foreign substances in the body, used to describe it. But the existence of a cause-and-effect relationship has been disputed on the grounds that other causes of disease have not been excluded with certainty in individual cases and that surveys of exposed populations and animal studies have failed to confirm it.

Hairdressers, both male and female, are occupationally exposed but, in the home, women may frequently use, and children play with, hair sprays. Hence exposure is very widespread. The size of the majority of particles produced by hand nebulizers and pressurized containers is under 1 μm (McLaughlin, Bidstrup and Konstam, 1963).

Disease attributed to hair sprays has been variously described as diffuse interstitial fibrosis with hilar lymphadenopathy (Bergmann, Flance and Blumenthal, 1958; Bergmann *et al.*, 1962; McLaughlin, Bidstrup and Konstam, 1963), sarcoid-type granulomas (Bergmann *et al.*, 1962) and foreign body granulomas (Gowdy and Wagstaff, 1972). Intracytoplasmic, PAS-positive granules observed in macrophages in lung tissue and in lymph nodes have been thought to represent plastic particles (Bergmann *et al.*, 1962) but similar staining granules may be seen in sarcoid and other granulomas, and chemical analysis has failed to demonstrate PVP which is readily soluble in water and chemically inert. Brunner *et al.* (1963) discounted PVP as a cause of lung disease, but the possibility that lubricants in PVP and mixed sprays might give rise to granulomatous lesions or fibrosis does not appear to have been excluded. The patient described by McLaughlin, Bidstrup and Konstam (1963), in whom idiopathic sarcoidosis was apparently excluded, was exposed to shellac-based sprays. Inhalation of shellac is a known cause of fibrosing lung disease presumed to be due to its high fatty acid content (Hirsch and Russell, 1945). Shellac is obtained from the secretion on plants of an insect of the coccidae family, *Laccifer lacca*, and has a complex composition which may include insect proteins and, conceivably, therefore, could provoke extrinsic allergic 'alveolitis'. In all, only 29 cases have been described to date (1972) and the extrapulmonary stigmata of sarcoidosis have been absent in all (Gowdy and Wagstaff, 1972).

Radiographic surveys of a large number of hairdressers in the United Kingdom and Germany have shown no evidence of pulmonary disease which could be ascribed to sprays (John, 1963; McLaughlin, Bidstrup and Konstam, 1963; Haug, 1964) although a similar survey of 227 in the United States of America revealed an unexplained excess of increased 'bronchovascular markings' in comparison with the general population which did not correlate with respiratory symptoms (Gowdy and Wagstaff, 1972).

Rats, guinea-pigs and dogs exposed to PVP aerosols have not developed lung disease (Gowdy and Wagstaff, 1972), but granuloma formation has been reported in mice after prolonged exposure to four different types of commercial hair spray (Vivoli, 1966).

The average period of exposure before lung disease was diagnosed in human cases has been 2·9 years, ranging from six months to eight years, the youngest patient being eight years old; but the appearances of pulmonary infiltration have often occurred after starting, or increasing, the use of hair sprays (Gowdy and Wagstaff, 1972).

Affected individuals may complain of cough and breathlessness, sometimes with mild pyrexia, but others are symptomless. The chest radiograph may show patchy or fine linear opacities with occasional evidence of hilar node enlargement, or the appearance of lobar consolidation—the least frequently seen abnormality. After the use of sprays has ceased, radiographic appearances have returned to normal within six months in most cases (which suggests that the sprays may have been the cause) but, in a few it has taken about two years (Gowdy and Wagstaff, 1972).

It cannot be concluded, therefore, that hair lacquer sprays are an established cause of lung disease, although in some cases the evidence is suggestive and it is possible that this is another example of individual susceptibility. Hence, if known forms of pulmonary disease can be excluded in a patient who habitually employs hair sprays, a causal relationship should be suspected and their use discontinued.

FIBROUS GLASS PARTICLES

Brief reference must be made to glass fibre materials because they have been manufactured in increasing quantities since the 1930s and are now extensively used as a substitute for asbestos in thermal, electrical and acoustical insulation, and, therefore, it may be asked if they have a deleterious effect on the lungs.

Glass fibres are manufactured by subjecting thin streams of molten glass to a jet of steam or by spinning them off a centrifuge. A phenolformaldehyde resin may then be added as a binder in glass-wool insulation and filtration materials. In the manufacture of glass-fibre reinforced plastics for boats, car bodies, building panels, electrical components and the like a variety of thermosetting polyester resins is employed.

The production of glass wool may give rise to fibrous glass particles of inhalable size during the process, but they appear to form a small proportion of the total number of fibres. Their diameter ranges from 5 μm to 14 μm and the minimal lengths from 8 μm to 90 μm but only 6 per cent of all airborne fibres are less than 20 μm in length and only 40 per cent, less than 100 μm (Keane and Zavon, 1966). In the production of fibre glass reinforced plastics vapour from resin curing is evolved in addition to glass fibres, and finishing of moulded products releases both fibres and resin dust (Lim *et al.*, 1970).

Men working in the manufacture of fibre glass and in the production, packing and shipping of the finished products, and particularly insulation workers using glass wool which readily breaks down with handling and with impact may be exposed to fibres small enough to remain airborne for appreciable periods of time.

Irritation of the conjunctivae and nose and throat with sneezing may occur, but the most tiresome complaint is itching of the skin of the hands, wrists, neck, waist and ankles with punctate erythema. Skin sensitization is not induced. These symptoms usually cease promptly on leaving exposure, but in some cases not for one or two days (Keane and Zavon, 1966). Surveys of large numbers of workers exposed to fibre glass for many years have not revealed the presence of any form of disease of the lower respiratory tract, either clinically or radiographically, which can be attributed to inhalation of the fibres (Keane and Zavon, 1966; Wright, 1968; Hill *et al.*, 1973) nor has a post-mortem study of the lungs of workers with long exposures shown any specific disease or tissue alteration which could be related to their inhalation (Gross, Tuma and de Treville, 1971).

Similarly, glass flakes produced by the handling of foam glass—also an insulating material—are without harmful effect (Keane and Zavon, 1966).

Plastic dust and vapour present a complex problem and have not been completely exonerated as a possible cause of lung disease, although some samples of fibre glass reinforced plastics have not provoked fibrosis in experimental animals (Schepers, 1961).

In short, there is no evidence that exposure to glass fibres or flakes is associated with any acute or permanent lung damage, but in view of their irritating properties their concentration in the working environment should be reduced to a minimum.

Threshold limit value
The value is that of 'Inert or Nuisance Particulates', that is: 10 mg/m³ or 30 mppcf of total dust during a working day (ACGIH).

IONIZING RADIATION

RADIOACTIVE AEROSOLS IN MINING

This is a large and complex subject but a short and simplified discussion of its implications is relevant.

Prolonged inhalation of radioactive aerosols may result in the development of carcinoma of the lungs, and possibly other changes. Radioactivity may be encountered in certain types of mining, in tunnels and in thorium refining and metal production.

Uranium is widely distributed in the earth's crust but is concentrated in various areas. It gives rise to decay chain products of which uranium-238 is the first member through a series of solid elements to radium-226 which decays to the gas radon-222 which, in turn, when in air rapidly gives rise to other isotopes—radon 'daughters'. The important members of the series in the present context are those which emit α-particles: namely, radon-222 (half-life 3·8 days) and the three radon daughters, polonium-218 (half-life 3·05 minutes), polonium-214 (half-life 26·8 minutes) and polonium-210 (half-life 19·4 years). Radon-222 leaks from rocks, fallen ore and soil and escapes into the air although concentrations at ground level are very low (Morgan, 1970). But in enclosed areas, such as mines, concentrations may be high because the gas has less chance to diffuse away, it may be carried into the workings by mine-waters from which it escapes, and ventilation is limited.

Thorium, also fairly abundant in the earth's crust, is usually found in association with uranium. It decays into thoron gas and α-emitting isotopes thorium A, thorium B and thorium C, but most of the dose to the lungs is due to thorium B and thorium C (Albert, 1966).

When first formed, the decay products are single ionized atoms but they readily attach themselves to molecules of water vapour or to dust particles as 'cluster ions' (Chamberlain and Dyson, 1956). It has been calculated that their mean radioactivity diameter is about 0·25 μm in non-operational mines and about 0·4 μm diameter in operational mines (Davies, 1967). In this aerosol state, therefore, they can, on inhalation, penetrate to the trachea, bronchi and beyond, and be retained in the lungs.

Alpha-particles are positively charged helium nuclei with two protons and neutrons which have a greater mass than other radiation particles and great kinetic energy but, owing to their large mass and positive charge, have only feeble penetrating power. They cause dense ionization along the path of their traverse which is maximal when their energy is nearly spent; that is, when they have passed through the bronchial mucosa and reached the basal cells. Their average penetrability is about 50 μm (Lea, 1955). Beta particles, being electrons, have greater penetrating capacity but less ionizing power. It is believed that this ionizing process causes malignant change in living cells.

It is for this reason that inhaled α-particles are more important than β-particles—although high doses of the latter may induce lung tumours in experimental animals—and there is strong evidence that exposure of man to radon-222 and α-emitting radon daughters is responsible for a significantly increased risk of developing carcinoma of the lung. The radiation dose to the lungs of radon and thoron appears to be approximately similar (Albert, 1966).

Gamma rays are also emitted by some of the isotopes of the uranium decay series but their intensity in uranium mines is extremely low (Federal Radiation Council, 1967).

Uranium mining

This is carried on in Canada (Saskatchewan), Australia (Queensland, Northern Territory and South Australia), the United States of America (Colorado, Arizona, New Mexico and Utah), South Africa (Witwatersrand), Czechoslovakia (Joachimstal) and the U.S.S.R. and, like any other hard rock mining, the ore is extracted by either deep mining, or open pit methods. Dust production is sporadic but emanation of α-particles is continuous.

Airborne radon was suggested as the cause of an excess of carcinoma of the lung in Schneeberg metal miners and Joachimstal uranium miners (Ludewig and Lorensen, 1924; Šikl, 1930), and an increased frequency of undifferentiated bronchial carcinomas (Saccomanno et al., 1964) and mortality due to lung cancer in American uranium miners has been correlated with radiation exposure and was found to be greater as the level of exposure increased (Archer and Lundin, 1967; Donaldson, 1969; Lundin et al., 1969) above 120 Working Level Months (q.v.) (Archer, Wagoner and Lundin, 1973).

To control radiation levels in mines the United States Public Health Service introduced the *Working Level* (WL) unit which is defined as any combination of radon daughters in one litre of air that will result in the ultimate emission of 1.3×10^5 MeV of potential alpha energy (MeV = million electron volts. One electron volt is the energy acquired by an electron when accelerated through a potential difference of one volt); and a measure of total exposure of miners is expressed as a *Working Level Month* (WLM) which results from inhalation for one working month (170 hours) of air containing a radon daughter concentration of 1 WL, or from two months exposure to a concentration of 0.5 WL—and so on.

Saccomanno et al. (1971) have confirmed an increased incidence of undifferentiated lung carcinomas with increasing radiation exposure compared with a control population matched for age and smoking habits. Where radiation exposure was high (that is, more than 1,500 cumulative WLM) small cell undifferentiated tumours (WHO Classification 2B) accounted for more than half the total number. An average of 15.9 years elapsed from the commencement of mining to the development of cancer. The effect of radiation is to increase the small cell undifferentiated tumours in all age and cigarette smoking groups, but to decrease the squamous cell tumours which are related mainly to age. An excess of small cell tumours has also been observed in South African (Webster, 1970) and Joachimstal uranium miners (Horáček, 1969).

A striking synergistic, or co-carcinogenic, effect of cigarette smoke with radiation has been established, the lung cancer rate being ten times greater among smoking uranium miners than among non-smoking miners (Lundin et al., 1969). Doll (1972) considers that the data of this study are more consistent with a multiplicative causal hypothesis than that the two agents act independently.

Control of the radiation hazard

This rests essentially upon the amount of radon-222 and α-emitting radon daughters in air being kept at or below maximum permissible concentrations, but the level of these concentrations has not yet been generally agreed upon. There is no 'safe' level of exposure. At present the WL unit is accepted by most authorities although a 0·3 WL was suggested in 1959 (International Commission on Radiological Protection). In 1968 the United States Department of Labor issued regulations which require that no worker shall receive an exposure of more than 2 WLM in any consecutive three-month period and no more than 4 WLM in any consecutive twelve-month period which is equivalent to an average concentration of radon daughters of 0·3 WL over the working year (Duggan et al., 1970).

Periodic determination of the concentration of radon and the short-lived radon daughters in mine air is required and the frequency of sampling will depend upon the geological characteristics of the region. This involves special equipment and techniques. A personal film badge akin to the type worn by x-ray workers would express individual miners' exposure more accurately and is in process of development (Rock, Lovell and Nelson, 1969). Accurate records of radiation levels must be kept.

Efficient ventilation of the mine is imperative and is applied to working areas by portable air ducts or fans. Radon-bearing water must be prevented from flowing through mine workings.

Regular medical examination is necessary, including a full-size chest radiograph, yearly for the first few years of exposure and, possibly, more frequently in later years, but six-monthly sputum cytology in the hands of an experienced cytologist is more likely to detect pre-cancerous metaplasia. Class II, Stage III metaplasia (WHO classification) is said to be the last stage before malignancy supervenes (Saccomanno et al., 1965). If this change is observed, the worker must be removed from further exposure and should be advised to stop smoking. Miners, however, should be encouraged to give up smoking when they enter employment.

The methods of protection against radiation are described in booklets issued by the Department of Employment (1971) and the International Labour Office (1968); international arrangements for radiation protection have been summarized by the World Health Organization (1972).

Before leaving the topic of uranium mining it must be remembered that the quartz content of many uranium-bearing rocks is high, so that miners are also exposed to a risk of silicosis. Some uranium miners exhibit a pattern of impaired lung function compatible with fibrotic changes and it has been suggested that α-particles may increase the fibrogenic effect of quartz (Trapp et al., 1970); but this remains to be proved. Lung fibrosis has been induced in dogs by inhalation of an α-emitter (Sanders and Park, 1971).

Milling uranium ore

The crushing of the ore and the weighing and packing into drums of the extracted product carries a similar risk of airborne radioactivity and quartz-containing dust as mining the ore.

Preventive measures include enclosure of mills and weighing and packing machines, protective clothing, efficient exhaust ventilation, good 'housekeeping' and monitoring of the air. The ACGIH threshold limit value for uranium in the form of soluble or insoluble compounds is 0·2 mg/m³. As soluble compounds are absorbed into the blood, deposited in bone and excreted via the kidney the uranium level in the urine should be determined regularly as part of periodic medical examination.

The burden of natural uranium in the lungs of exposed workers may be high or low according to the physical and chemical properties of the uranium aerosol and, possibly, physiological idiosyncrasy (Donaghue et al., 1972). The methods for analysing uranium in the urine have been described in one of the Hygienic Guide Series (1969).

Other types of mining

It is now recognized that potential radioactivity may be present in any type of mining and periodic monitoring for radon-222 and its daughters is desirable.

Thorium mining

Thorium is largely obtained by surface digging of monazite sands and under these conditions radiation levels are low, but in underground workings (for example, in granite) fairly high concentrations of thoron daughters have been observed (Albert, 1966).

Fluorspar (fluorite) mining

Newfoundland fluorspar (CaF₂) miners, who have probably been exposed to radon and radon daughter levels of between 2·5 and 10 WL, have a lung cancer rate about 29 times greater than expected. But no radioactive ore bodies have been detected and it is probable that the radon is carried into the mine by water (de Villiers and Windish, 1964).

Metal mining

A threefold increased incidence of lung cancer attributed to radon daughters has been observed in a group of underground metal miners in the United States of America (Wagoner et al., 1963).

Hematite mining

Mortality from lung cancer among iron ore miners in West Cumberland hematite mines in which radon daughter levels have been found to be greater than 0·3 WL (Duggan et al., 1970) is apparently about 70 per cent higher than expected (Boyd et al., 1970). It has often been speculated that iron oxide dust may be the carcinogen but it is at least as likely that α-particles in the mine air are responsible (*see* Chapter 7). As in the case of Newfoundland fluorspar mines it appears that the source of radon-222 may be mine water as no unusual radioactivity has been detected in representative samples of exposed rock (Boyd et al., 1970).

Coal-mining

By contrast, the median concentration of radon in twelve coal-mines in England and Scotland is very low and the values recorded in Pennsylvania coal-mines are of similar order (Duggan, Howell and Soilleux, 1968). There is no evidence that the concentrations of radon of the magnitude found in British coal-mines is associated with an increased incidence of lung cancer; indeed, as pointed out in Chapter 8, the incidence of lung cancer in British coal-mines is appreciably below the national average (Doll, 1958; Goldman, 1965).

Some Other Sources of Exposure to Ionizing Radiation

Excessive levels of radon-222 may be present in the air of tunnels and underground chambers in some rock formations and necessitate an efficient ventilatory system, possibly steel plate or concrete barriers, and regular monitoring of radioactivity (Lloyd, Pendleton and Downard, 1968).

Alpha emitters may be present in thorium plants (where a risk of silicosis may also exist as the quartz content of monazite sands is high) and thorium refining, but little appears to be known of the concentrations occurring under various conditions. One survey of a thorium refinery did not reveal any evidence of radiation injury in a small number of long-term workers (Albert, 1966).

Potential exposure exists in the atomic energy industry, but elaborate precautions are taken to prevent this.

OTHER INDUSTRIES ASSOCIATED WITH BRONCHIAL CARCINOMA

An excess rate of bronchial carcinoma in iron oxide miners and in individuals with asbestosis has been referred to (*see* respectively Chapter 6 and Chapter 9). An estimated mortality rate from this tumour five times that of the general population has also been reported in workers refining nickel by the nickel carbonyl process (Doll, 1958); and an increased incidence— about three and a half times that expected—has occurred in workers in the chromate and chrome pigment-producing industries (Jafafer, 1953; Bidstrup and Case, 1956). The responsible carcinogens in these industries remain unidentified.

REFERENCES

Acton, J. D., Myrvik, Q. N. and Salem, W. (1972). 'Nitrogen dioxide effects on alveolar macrophages.' *Archs envir. Hlth* **24**, 48–52
Adams, R. G. and Crabtree, N. (1961). 'Anosmia in alkaline battery workers.' *Br. J. ind. Med.* **18**, 216–221
— Harrison, J. F. and Scott, P. (1969). 'The development of cadmium-induced proteinuria, impaired renal function and osteomalacia in alkaline battery workers.' *Q. Jl Med.* **38**, 425–443
Ahlmark, A., Bruce, T. and Nyström, A. (1960). *Silicosis and Other Pneumoconioses in Sweden*, pp. 361–365; 371–373. London; Heinemann
— Axelsson, B., Friberg, L. and Piscator, M. (1960). 'Further investigations into kidney function and proteinuria in chronic cadmium poisoning.' *Proc. 13th Internat. Congr. Occup. Hlth New York*, pp. 201–203
Albert, R. E. 1966). *Thorium. Its Industrial Hygiene Aspects.* New York and London; Academic Press
Archer, V. E. and Lundin, F. E., Jr. (1967). 'Radiogenic lung cancer in man: exposure-effect relationship.' *Envir. Res.* **1**, 370–383
— Wagoner, J. K. and Lundin, E. E. (1973). 'Lung cancer among uranium miners in the United States.' *Hlth Phys.* **25**, 351–371

Avery, S. B., Stetson, D. M., Pan, P. M. and Mathews, K. T. (1969). 'Immuno-logical investigation of individuals with toluene di-isocyanate asthma.' *Clin. Exp. Immunol.* **4**, 585–596

Baader, E. W. (1952). 'Chronic cadmium poisoning.' *Ind. Med. Surg.* **21**, 427–430

Barth, G., Frik, W. and Scheidemandel, H. (1956). 'Die Aluminiumlunge. Ver-laufsbeobachtungen und Neuerkrankungen in der Nachkreigszeit.' *Dt. med. Wschr.* **81**, 1115–1119

Beach, F. X. M., Sherwood Jones, E. and Scarrow, G. D. (1969). 'Respiratory effects of chlorine gas.' *Br. J. Ind. Med.* **26**, 231–236

Bech, A. O., Kipling, M. D. and Heather, J. C. (1962), 'Hard metal disease.' *Br. J. ind. Med.* **19**, 239–252

Becklake, M. R., Goldman, H. I., Boxman, A. R. and Freed, C. C. (1957). 'The long-term effects of exposure to nitrous fumes.' *Am. Rev. Tuberc.* **76**, 398–409

Belin, L., Hobarn, J., Falsen, E. and André, J. (1970). 'Enzyme sensitisation in consumers in enzyme-containing washing powder.' *Lancet* **2**, 1153–1157

Bergmann, M., Flance, I. J. and Blumenthal, H. T. (1958). 'Thesaurosis following inhalation of hair spray: A clinical and experimental study.' *New Engl. J. Med.* **258**, 471–476

— Flance, I. J., Cruz, P. T., Klam, N., Aronson, P. R., Joshi, R. A. and Blumenthal, H. T. (1962). 'Thesaurosis due to inhalation of hair spray. Report of 12 new cases including 3 autopsies.' *New Engl. J. Med.* **266**, 750–755

Beton, D. C., Andrews, G. S., Davies, H. J., Howells, L. and Smith, G. F. (1966). 'Acute cadmium fume poisoning.' *Br. J. ind. Med.* **23**, 292–301

Bidstrup, P. L. and Case, R. A. M. (1956). 'Carcinoma of the lung in workmen in the bichromates-producing industry in Great Britain.' *Br. J. ind. Med.* **13**, 260–264

Blejer, H. P. and Caplan, P. E. (1971). *Occupational Health Aspects of Cadmium Fume Poisoning.* 2nd Ed. California; Bureau Occup. Hlth and Environ. Epidemiol.

Bohner, C. B., Sheldon, J. M. and Trenis, J. W. (1941). 'Sensitivity to gum acacia with report of 10 cases of asthma in printers.' *J. Allergy* **12**, 290–293

Bonnell, J. A. (1955). 'Emphysema and proteinuria in men casting copper-cadmium alloys.' *Br. J. ind. Med.* **12**, 181–195

— (1965). 'Cadmium poisoning.' *Ann. occup. Hyg.* **8**, 45–50

— Kazantzis, G. and King, R. (1959). 'A follow-up study of men exposed to cadmium oxide fume.' *Br. J. ind. Med.* **16**, 135–147

Boyd, J. T., Doll, R., Faulds, J. S. and Leiper, J. (1970). 'Cancer of the lung in iron ore (haematite) miners.' *Br. J. ind. Med.* **27**, 97–105

Brinkman, R., Lamberts, H. B. and Veninga, T. S. (1964). 'Radiomimetic toxicity of ozonised air.' *Lancet* **1**, 133–136

Bruckner, H. C. (1967). 'Extrinsic asthma in a tungsten carbide worker.' *J. occup. Med.* **9**, 518–519

— Avery, S. B., Stetson, D. M., Dodson, V. N. and Ronayne, J. J. (1968). 'Clinical and immunological appraisal of workers exposed to di-isocyanates.' *Archs envir. Hlth* **16**, 619–625

Brunner, M. J., Giovacchini, R. P., Wyatt, J. P., Dunlap, F. E. and Calandra, J. C. (1963). 'Pulmonary disease and hair spray polymers; a disputed relationship.' *J. Am. med. Ass.* **184**, 851–857

Buist, J. M. and Lowe, A. (1965). 'The chemistry of polyurethanes and their applications.' *Ann. occup. Hyg.* **8**, 143–162

Caplin, M. (1941). 'Ammonia-gas poisoning.' *Lancet* **2**, 95–96

Capodaglio, E., Monarca, G. and de Vito, G. (1961). 'Sindrome respiratoria da inalazione di composti fuorati alifatici nella preparazione del politetra-fluoroetilene.' *Rass. Med. Ind.* **30**, 124–139

Carrington, C. B. and Green, T. J. (1970). 'Granular pneumocytes in early repair of diffuse alveolar injury.' *Archs intern. Med.* **126**, 464–465

Challen, P. J. R. (Ed.) (1965). *Health and Safety in Welding and Allied Processes* (Institute of Welding). 2nd edition. London and Woking: Unwin

— Sherwood, R. J. and Bedford, J. (1955). ' "Fluon" (polytetrafluoroethylene):

a preliminary note on some clinical and environmental observations.' *Br. J. ind. Med.* **12**, 177–178

Challen, P. J. R., Hickish, D. E. and Bedford, J. (1958). 'An investigation of some health hazards in an inert-gas tungsten-arc welding shop.' *Br. J. ind. Med.* **15**, 276–282

Chamberlain, A. C. and Dyson, E. D. (1956). 'The dose to the trachea and bronchi from the decay products of radon and thoron.' *Br. J. Radiol.* **29**, 317–325

Chasis, H., Zapp, J. A., Bannon, J. H., Whittenberger, J. L., Helm, J., Doheny, J. L. and MacLeod, C. D. (1947). 'Chlorine accident in Brooklyn.' *Occup. Med.* **4**, 152–176

Chester, E. H., Gillespie, D. G. and Krause, F. D. (1969). 'The prevalence of chronic obstructive pulmonary disease in chlorine gas workers.' *Am. Rev. resp. Dis.* **99**, 365–373

Christensen, F. C. and Olsen, E. C. (1957). 'Cadmium poisoning.' *Archs ind. Hlth* **16**, 8–13

Clutton-Brock, J. (1967). 'Two cases of poisoning by contamination of nitrous oxide with higher oxides of nitrogen during anaesthesia.' *Br. J. Anaesth.* **39**, 388–392

Coates, E. O. and Watson, J. H. L. (1971). 'Diffuse interstitial lung disease in tungsten carbide workers.' *Ann. intern. Med.* **75**, 709–716

Commins, B. T. (1972). Personal communication

— Raveney, F. J. and Jesson, M. W. (1971). 'Toxic gases in tower silos.' *Ann. occup. Hyg.* **14**, 275–283

Corrin, B. (1963). 'Aluminium pneumoconiosis II. Effect on the rat lung of intra-tracheal injections of stamped aluminium powders containing different lubricating agents and of a granular aluminium powder.' *Br. J. ind. Med.* **20**, 268–276

Cotter, L. H. and Cotter, B. H. (1951). 'Cadmium poisoning.' *Archs ind. Hyg.* **3**, 495–504

Cowan, D. W., Thompson, H. J., Paulus, H. J. and Mielke, P. W. (1963). 'Bronchial asthma associated with air pollutants from the grain industry.' *J. Air. Pollut. Control Ass.* **13**, 546–552

Crombie, D. W., Blaisdell, J. L. and MacPherson, G. (1944). 'Treatment of silicosis with aluminium powder.' *Can. med. Ass. J.* **50**, 318–328

Darke, C. S. and Warrack, A. J. N. (1958). 'Bronchiolitis from nitrous fumes.' *Thorax* **13**, 327–333

Davies, C. N. (1967). In *Assessment of Airborne Radioactivity*, pp. 3–20. Vienna; Internat. Atomic Energy Agency

Delaney, L. T., Schmidt, H. W. and Stroebel, C. F. (1956). 'Silofillers' disease.' *Proc. Staff Meet. Mayo Clin.* **31**, 189–198

Department of Employment (1971). *Code of Practice for the Protection of Persons Exposed to Ionising Radiations in Research and Teaching.* London; H.M.S.O.

Desbaumes, P. (1968). 'Intoxications mortelles par les gaz de fermentation de silos agricoles (oxyde de carbone et oxydes d'azote).' *Arch. Tox.* **23**, 160–164

de Villiers, A. J. and Windish, J. P. (1964). 'Lung cancer in a fluorspar mining community. I. Radiation, dust and mortality experience.' *Br. J. ind. Med.* **21**, 94–109

Doig, A. T. and Challen, P. J. R. (1964). 'Respiratory hazards of welding.' *Ann. occup. Hyg.* **7**, 223–229

Doll, R. (1958). 'Cancer of the lung and nose in nickel workers.' *Br. J. ind. Med.* **15**, 217–223

— (1972). 'The age distribution of cancer: implications for models of carcino-genesis.' *Jl R. statist. Soc.* **134**, 133–155.

Donaghue, J. K., Dyson, E. D., Hislop, J. S., Leach, A. M. and Spoor, N. L. (1972). 'Human exposure to natural uranium. A case history and analytical results from some postmortem studies.' *Br. J. ind. Med.* **29**, 81–89

Donaldson, A. W. (1969). 'The epidemiology of lung cancer among uranium miners.' *Hlth Phys.* **16**, 563–569

Dowell, A. R., Kilburn, K. H. and Pratt, P. C. (1971). 'Short term exposure to nitrogen dioxide.' *Archs intern. Med.* **128**, 74–80

Duggan, M. J., Howell, D. M. and Soilleux, P. J. (1968). 'Concentrations of radon-222 in coal mines in England and Scotland.' *Nature, Lond.* **219**, 1149

— Soilleux, P. J., Strong, J. C. and Howell, D. M. (1970). 'The exposure of United Kingdom miners to radon.' *Br. J. ind. Med.* **27**, 106–109

Duke, W. W. (1935). 'Wheat hairs and dust as a common cause of asthma among workers in wheat flour mills.' *J. Am. med. Ass.* **105**, 957–958

Ehrlich, R. and Henry, M. C. (1968). 'Chronic toxicity of nitrogen dioxide I. Effect on resistance to bacterial pneumonia.' *Archs envir. Hlth* **17**, 860–865

Engelbracht, F. M., Byers, P. D., Stacy, B. D., Harrison, C. V. and King, E. J. (1959). 'Tissue reactions to injected aluminium and alumina in the lungs and livers of mice, rats, guinea pigs and rabbits.' *J. Path. Bact.* **77**, 407–416

Farmer and Stockbreeder (1970). 'Check on poison gas in tower silos.' **84**, 11

Federal Radiation Council (1967). *Report No. 8 Revised.* Washington, D.C.; U.S. Government Printing Office

Finlay, G. R. (1950). In *Pneumoconiosis* (Sixth Saranac Symposium), pp. 493–497. Ed. by A. J. Vorwald. New York; Hoeber

Flake, R. E. (1964), 'Chlorine inhalation.' *New Engl. J. Med.* **271**, 1373

Flindt, M. L. H. (1969). 'Pulmonary disease due to inhalation of derivatives of *Bacillus subtilis* containing proteolytic enzyme.' *Lancet*, **2**, 1153–1157

Fowler, P. B. S. (1952). 'Printer's asthma.' *Lancet* **2**, 755–757

Frankland, A. W. and Lunn, J. A. (1965). 'Asthma caused by the grain weevil.' *Br. J. ind. Med.* **22**, 157–159

Frant, R. (1963). 'Formation of ozone in gas-shielded welding.' *Ann. occup. Hyg.* **6**, 113–125

Freeman, G. and Haydon, G. B. (1964). 'Emphysema after low-level exposure to NO_2.' *Archs envir. Hlth* **8**, 125–128

— Crane, S. C. and Furiosi, N. J. (1969). 'Healing in rat lung after subacute exposure to nitrogen dioxide.' *Am. Rev. resp. Dis.* **100**, 622–676

Friberg, L. (1957). 'Deposition and distribution of cadmium in man in chronic poisoning.' *Archs ind. Hlth* **16**, 27–29

— (1971). 'Cadmium, alloys, compounds.' In *Encyclopaedia of Occupational Health and Safety*, pp. 233–234. Geneva; International Labour Office

Gandevia, B. (1970). 'Occupational asthma. Part I.' *Med. J. Aust.* **2**, 332–335

Gleason, R. P. (1968), 'Exposure to copper dust.' *Am. ind. Hyg. Ass. J.* **29**, 461–462

Godbert, A. L. and Leach, E. (1970). *Research Report 265.* 'A preliminary survey of the pollution of mine air by nitrogen oxides from diesel exhaust gases.' Sheffield; Safety in Mines Research Establishment

Goldman, K. P. (1965). 'Mortality of coal-miners from carcinoma of the lung.' *Br. J. ind. Med.* **22**, 72–77

Goralewski, G. (1940). 'Zur Symptomatologie der Aluminium-Staublunge.' *Arch. Gewerbepath. Gewerbehyg.* **10**, 384–408

— (1947). 'Die Aluminiumlunge: eine neue Gewerbeerkrankung.' *Z. ges. inn. Med.* **2**, 665–673

— (1950). 'Die Aluminiumlunge. Eine klinische Studie.' *Arbeitsmedizin.* **26**

— and Jaeger, R. (1941). 'Zur Klinik, Pathologie und Pathogenese der Aluminiumlunge.' *Arch. Gewerbepath. Gewerbehyg.* **11**, 102–105

Gough, J. (1960). 'Emphysema in relation to occupation.' *Ind. Med. surg.* **29**, 283–285

— (1968). 'The pathogenesis of emphysema.' In *The Lung*, pp. 124–126. Ed. by A. A. Liebow and D. E. Smith. Baltimore; Williams and Wilkins

Gowdy, J. M. and Wagstaff, M. J. (1972). 'Pulmonary infiltration due to aerosol thesaurosis.' *Archs envir. Hlth* **25**, 101–108

Graham, J. I. and Runnicles, D. F. (1943). 'Nitrous fumes from shot-firing in relation to pulmonary disease.' In *Chronic Disease in South Wales Coal Miners*. Med. Res. Council Spec. Rep. Ser. No. 244, pp. 187–213

Grayson, R. R. (1956). 'Silage gas poisoning: nitrogen dioxide pneumonia, a new disease in agricultural workers.' *Ann. intern. Med.* **45**, 393–408

Greenburg, M. (1972). 'Respiratory symptoms following brief exposure to Cedar of Lebanon (*Cedra libani*) dust.' *Clin. Allergy* **2**, 219–224

Greenburg, M., Milne, J. F. and Watt, A. (1970). 'Study of workers exposed to dusts containing derivatives of *Bacillus subtilis*.' *Br. med. J.* **2**, 629–633

Gross, P., Westrick, M. L. and McNerney, J. M. (1960). 'Glass dust: a study of its biological effects.' *Archs ind. Hlth* **21**, 10–23

— Tuma, J. and de Treville, T. P. (1971). 'Lungs of workers exposed to fiber glass. A study of their pathologic changes and their dust content.' *Archs envir. Hlth* **23**, 67–76

Hagen, J. (1950). 'Ueber Lungenveränderungen be Korundschmelzern.' *Dt. med. Wschr.* **75**, 399–400

Hall, A. D. (1923). 'Can silage be substituted for roots?' *J. Fmr's Club*, March, 20–21

Hama, G. M. (1957). 'Symptoms of workers exposed to isocyanates.' *Archs ind. Hyg.* **16**, 232–233

Harding, H. E. (1950). 'Notes on the toxicology of cobalt metal.' *Br. J. ind. Med.* **7**, 76–78

Harris, D. K. (1951). 'Polymer-fume fever.' *Lancet* **2**, 1008–1011

— (1959). 'Some hazards in the manufacture and use of plastics.' *Br. J. ind. Med.* **16**, 221–229

Hatch, T. F. (1950). In *Pneumoconiosis* (Sixth Saranac Symposium), pp. 498–501. Ed. by A. J. Vorwald. New York; Hoeber

Haug, H. P. (1964). 'Zur Frage der Speicherkrankheit in der Lunge nach Gebrauch von Haarspray.' *Dt. med. Wschr.* **89**, 87–92

Hill, J. W., Whitehead, W. S., Cameron, J. D. and Hedgecock, G. A. (1973). 'Glass fibres: absence of pulmonary hazard in production workers.' *Br. J. ind. Med.* **30**, 174–179

Hirsch, E. F. and Russell, H. B. (1945). 'Chronic exudative and indurative pneumonia due to inhalation of shellac.' *Archs Path.* **39**, 281–286

Holden, H. (1965). 'Cadmium fume.' *Ann. occup. Hyg.* **8**, 51–54

Holt, P. F. (1957). *Pneumoconiosis*, p. 181. London; Arnold

Horáček, J. (1969). 'Der Joachimstaler Lungenkrebs nach dem zweiten Weltkreig (Bericht über 55 Fälle).' *Z. Krebsforsch.* **72**, 52–56

How, M. J. and Cambridge, G. W. (1971). 'Prick tests and serological tests in the diagnosis of allergic reactivity to enzymes used in washing products.' *Br. J. ind. Med.* **28**, 303–307

Huber, G. L., Mason, R. J., La Force, M., Spencer, N. J., Gardner, D. E. and Coffin, D. L. (1971). 'Alteration in the lung following the administration of ozone.' *Archs intern. Med.* **128**, 81–93

Hueter, F. G. and Fritzhand, M. (1971). 'Oxidants and lung biochemistry.' *Archs intern. Med.* **128**, 48–53

Hunter, D., Milton, R., Perry, K. M. A. and Thompson, D. R. (1944). 'Effect of aluminium and alumina on the lung in grinders of duralumin aeroplane propellers.' *Br. J. ind. Med.* **1**, 159–164

Hygienic Guide Series (1969). 'Uranium (natural) and its compounds. U. (Revised 1969).' *Am. ind. Hyg. Ass. J.* **30**, 313–317

International Commission on Radiological Protection (1959). *Report of Committee of Permissible Dose of Internal Radiation.* Publication 2. London; Pergamon

International Labour Office (1968). *Radiation Protection in the Mining of Radioactive Ores.* Geneva; I.L.O.

Jafafer, W. M. (1953). 'Health of workers in the chromate producing industry.' *Publ. Hlth Rep.* No. 192. Washington

Jenkins, H. M. (1884). 'Report on the practice of ensilage.' *Jl R. agric. Soc.* 2nd ser. **20**, 132–137

Jennings, G. H. and Gower, N. D. (1963). 'Thrombocytopenic purpura in toluene di-isocyanate workers.' *Lancet* **1**, 406–408

Jephcott, C. M. (1950). 'Chemical aspect of Shaver's disease.' In *Pneumoconiosis*. (Sixth Saranac symposium), pp. 489–493. Ed. by A. J. Vorwald. New York; Hoeber

Jesson, M. W. (1972). *Removal of Gases from a Forage Tower Prior to Entry.* Rep. No. 3. Silsoe, Beds.; National Institute of Agricultural Engineering

Jobs, H. and Ballhausen, C. (1940). Quoted by Bech, A. O., Kipling, M. D. and Heather, J. C. (1962). 'Hard metal disease.' *Br. J. ind. Med.* **19**, 239–252

John, H. H. (1963). 'Thesaurosis: a survey of those at risk.' *Med. Off.* **109**, 399–400

Jones, A. T. (1952). 'Noxious gases and fumes.' *Proc. R. Soc. Med.* **45**, 609–610

Joseph, M. (1968). 'Hard metal pneumoconiosis.' *Australas. Radiol.* **12**, 92–95

Kaltreider, N. L., Elder, M. J., Cralley, L. V. and Colwell, M. O. (1972). 'Health survey of aluminium workers with special reference to fluoride exposure.' *J. occup. Med.* **14**, 531–541

Kaplun, Z. S. and Mezencewa, N. W. (1960). 'Experimentellstudie über die toxische Wirkung von Staub bei der Erzengung von Sintermettallen.' *J. Hyg. Epidem. Microbiol. Immunol.* **4**, 390–399

Kazantzis, G., Flynn, F. V., Spowage, J. S. and Trott, D. G. (1963). 'Renal tubular malfunction and pulmonary emphysema in cadmium pigment workers.' *Q. Jl Med.* **32**, 165–192

Keane, W. T. and Zavon, M. R. (1966). 'Occupational hazards of pipe insulators.' *Archs envir. Hlth* **13**, 171–184

Kendrey, G. and Roe, F. J. C. (1969). 'Cadmium toxicology.' *Lancet* **1**, 1206–1207

Kleinfeld, M., Giel, C. and Tabershaw, I. R. (1957). 'Health hazards associated with inert-gas-shielded metal arc welding.' *Archs ind. Hlth* **15**, 27–31

Kowitz, T. A., Reba, R. C., Parker, R. T. and Spicer, W. S. (1967). 'Effects of chlorine gas upon respiratory function.' *Archs envir. Hlth* **14**, 545–558

Kramer, C. G. (1967). 'Chlorine.' *J. occup. Med.* **9**, 193–196

Kronenberger, F. L. (1959). 'Bronchiolitis after shot-firing in a colliery.' *Br. J. Dis. Chest* **53**, 308–313

Lane, R. E. and Campbell, A. C. P. (1954). 'Fatal emphysema in two men making a copper cadmium alloy" *Br. J. ind. Med.* **11**, 118–122

Lea, D. E. (1955). *Actions of Radiations on Living Cells*, 2nd edition, p. 25. London; Cambridge University Press

Lewis, C. E. and Kerby, G. R. (1965). 'An epidemic of polymer-fume fever.' *J. Am. med. Ass* **191**, 375–378

Lewis, G. P., Lyle, H. and Miller, S. (1969). 'Association between elevated hepatic water-soluble protein-bound cadmium levels and chronic bronchitis and/or emphysema.' *Lancet* **2**, 1330–1333

— Jusko, W. J., Coughlin, L. L. and Hartz, S. (1972). 'Contribution of cigarette smoking to cadmium accumulation in man.' *Lancet* **1**, 291–292

Lim, J., Balzer, J. L., Wolf, C. R. and Milby, T. H. (1970). 'Fiber glass reinforced plastics. Associated occupational health problems.' *Archs envir. Hlth* **20**, 540–544

Lloyd, R. D., Pendleton, R. C. and Downard, T. R. (1968). 'Radioactivity within a tunnel in granitic rock.' *Hlth Phys.* **15**, 274–276

Lloyd-Davies, T. A. and Harding, H. E. (1949). 'Manganese pneumonitis.' *Br. J. ind. Med.* **6**, 82–90

Lowry, T. and Schuman, L. M. (1956). ' "Silo-filler's disease"—a syndrome caused by nitrogen dioxide.' *J. Am. med. Ass.* **162**, 153–160

Ludewig, P. and Lorenser, E. (1924). 'Untersuchungen der Grubenluft in den schneeberger Gruben auf den Gehalt and Radiumemanation.' *Strahlentherapie.* **17**, 428–435

Lundgren, K. D. and Öhman, H. (1954). 'Pneumokoniose in der Hartmetallindustrie.' *Virchows. Arch. path. Anat. Physiol.* **325**, 259–284

Lundin, F. E., Jr., Lloyd, J. W., Smith, E. M., Archer, V. E. and Holaday, D. A. (1969). 'Mortality of uranium miners in relation to radiation exposure, hardrock mining and cigarette smoking—1950 through September 1967.' *Hlth Phys.* **16**, 571–578

Lunn, J. A. (1966). 'Mill-worker's asthma: allergic responses to the grain weevil (*Sitophilus grenarius*).' *Br. J. ind. Med.* **23**, 149–152

McAdams, A. J. (155). 'Bronchiolitis obliterans.' *Am. J. Med.* **19**, 314–322

McCann, J. K. (1964). 'Health hazard from flux used in joining aluminium electricity cables.' *Ann. occup. Hyg.* **7**, 261–268

McCullagh, S. F. (1968). 'Allergenicity of piperazine: a study in environmental aetiology.' *Br. J. ind. Med.* **25**, 319–325

McDermott, F. T. (1971). 'Dust in the cemented carbide industry.' *Am. ind. Hyg. Ass. J.* **32**, 188–193

McKerrow, C. B., Davies, H. J. and Jones, A. P. (1970). 'Symptoms and lung function following acute and chronic exposure to tolylene diisocyanate.' *Proc. R. Soc. Med.* **63**, 376–378

McLaughlin, A. I. G., Bidstrup, P. L. and Konstam, M. (1963). 'The effect of hair lacquer sprays on the lungs.' *Food Cosmet. Toxicol.* **1**, 171–188

McLaughlin, A. I. G., Kazantzis, G., King, E., Teare, R. J. and Owen, R. (1962). 'Pulmonary fibrosis and encephalopathy associated with inhalation of aluminium dust.' *Br. J. ind. Med.* **19**, 253–263

Malten, K. E. and Zielhuis, R. L. (1964). *Industrial Toxicology and Dermatology in the Production and Processing of Plastics.* Amsterdam; Elsevier.

Medical Research Council (1936). Industrial Pulmonary Disease Committee. *Br. med. J.* **2**, 1273–1275

Miller, C. W., Davies, M. W., Goldman, A. and Wyatt, J. P. (1953). 'Pneumoconiosis in the tungsten carbide tool industry.' *Archs ind. Hyg.* **8**, 453–465

Milne, J. E. H. (1969). 'Nitrogen dioxide inhalation and bronchiolitis obliterans.' *J. occup. Med.* **11**, 538–547

Mitchell, C. A. and Gandevia, B. (1971). 'Respiratory symptoms and skin reactivity in workers exposed to proteolytic enzymes in detergent dust.' *Am. Rev. resp. Dis.* **104**, 1–12

Mitchell, J., Manning, G. B., Molyneux, M. and Lane, R. E. (1961). 'Pulmonary fibrosis in workers exposed to finely powdered aluminium.' *Br. J. ind. Med.* **18**, 10–20

Morgan, A. (1970). 'Physical behaviour of radon and its daughters with particular reference to monitoring methods.' In *Pneumoconiosis. Proceedings of the International Conference, Johannesburg, 1969*, pp. 540–543. Ed. by H. A. Shapiro. Cape Town; Oxford University Press

Morichau-Beauchant, G. (1964). 'Pneumonies manganiques.' *J. fr. Méd. Chir. thorac.* **18**, 300–312

Morley, R. and Silk, S. J. (1970). 'The industrial hazard of nitrous fumes.' *Ann. occup. Hyg.* **13**, 101–107

Moskowitz, R. L., Lyons, H. A. and Cottle, H. R. (1964). 'Silo filler's disease.' *Am. J. Med.* **36**, 457–462

Mustafa, M. G., Cross, C. E., Munn, R. J. and Hardie, J. A. (1971). 'Effects of divalent metal ions on alveolar macrophage membrane adenosine triphosphatase activity.' *J. Lab. clin. Med.* **77**, 563–571

Nandi, M., Jick, H., Slone, D., Shapiro, S. and Lewis, G. P. (1969). 'Cadmium content of cigarettes.' *Lancet* **2**, 1329–1330

Newhouse, M. L., Tagg, B. B., Pocock, S. J. and McEwan, A. C. (1970). 'An epidemiological study of workers producing enzyme washing powders.' *Lancet.* **1**, 689–693

Nicaud, P., Lafitte, A. and Gros., A. (1942). 'Les troubles de l'intoxication chronique par cadmium.' *Archs Mal. prof. Méd. trav.* **4**, 192–202

Norwood, W. D., Wisehart, D. E., Earl, C. A., Adley, F. E. and Anderson, D. E. (1966). 'Nitrogen dioxide poisoning due to metal cutting with oxyacetylene torch.' *J. occup. Med.* **8**, 301–306

P'an, A. Y. S., Béland, J. and Jegier, Z. (1972). 'Ozone-induced arterial lesions.' *Archs envir. Hlth* **24**, 229–232

Parkes, H. G. (1970). 'Isocyanates in industry: environmental control.' *Proc. R. Soc. Med.* **63**, 368–370

Parrot, J., Hébert, R., Saindelle, A. and Ruff, F. (1969). 'Platinum and platinosis.' *Archs envir. Hlth* **19**, 685–691

Patterson, J. C. (1947). 'Studies on the toxicity of inhaled cadmium.' *J. ind. Hyg.* **29**, 294–301

Pattey, F. A. (1963). *Industrial Hygiene and Toxicology*, Vol. 11, pp. 919–923. New York and London; Interscience

Pepys, J. and Pickering, C. A. C. (1972). 'Asthma due to inhaled chemical fumes— amino-ethyl ethanolamine in soldering flux.' *Clin. Allergy* **2**, 197–204

Pepys, J., Pickering, C. A. C. and Hughes, E. G. (1972). 'Asthma due to inhaled chemical agents—complex salts of platinum.' *Clin. Allergy* **2**, 391–396

— — and Loudon, H. W. G. (1972). 'Asthma due to inhaled chemical agents— piperazine dihydrochloride.' *Clin. Allergy* **2**, 189–196

— Hargreave, F. E., Longbottom, J. L. and Faux, J. (1969). 'Allergic reactions of the lungs to enzymes of *Bacillus subtilis*.' *Lancet* **1**, 1181–1184

— Pickering, C. A. C., Breslin, A. B. X. and Terry, D. J. (1972). 'Asthma due to inhaled chemical agents—tolylene di-isocyanate.' *Clin. Allergy* **2**, 225–236

Peters, J. M. (1970). 'Cumulative pulmonary effects in workers exposed to tolylene di-isocyanate.' *Proc. R. Soc. Med.* **63**, 372–375

— Murphy, R. L. H. and Ferris, B. G. (1969). 'Ventilatory function in workers exposed to low levels of toluene di-isocyanate: a six months follow-up.' *Br. J. ind. Med.* **26**, 115–120

— Batten, J. C. and Pepys, J. (1972). 'Asthma due to inhaled wood dusts— Western red cedar and iroko.' *Clin. Allergy* **2**, 213–218

Pieters, H. A. J. and Creyghton, J. W. (1951). *Safety in the Chemical Laboratory.* London; Butterworths

Piscator, M. (1966). 'Proteinuria in chronic cadmium poisoning.' *Archs envir. Hlth* **12** 335–344

Posner, E. and Kennedy, M. C. S. (1967). 'A further study of china biscuit placers in Stoke-on-Trent.' *Br. J. ind. Med.* **24**, 133–142

Potts, C. L. (1965). 'Cadmium proteinuria—the health of battery workers exposed to cadmium oxide dust.' *Ann. occup. Hyg.* **8**, 55–61

Powell, M. (1961). 'Toxic fumes from shotfiring in coal mines.' *Ann. occup. Hyg.* **3**, 162–183

— and Lomax, A. (1960). 'The toxic effects of handling and firing explosives in coal mines.' *Ann. occup. Hyg.* **2**, 141–151

Prys-Roberts, C. (1967). 'Principles of treatment of poisoning by higher oxides of nitrogen.' *Br. J. Anaesth.* **39**, 432–438

Ramirez-R., J. and Dowell, A. R. (1971). 'Silo-filler's disease: nitrogen dioxide. induced lung injury.' *Ann. intern. Med.* **74**, 569–576

Reber, E. and Burckhardt, P. (1970). 'Über Hartmetallstaublungen in der Schweiz.' *Respiration* **27**, 120–153

Report of the Isocyanate Sub-committee of the British Manufacturers' Association Ltd Health Advisory Committee (1971). *Operating and Medical Codes of Practice for Safe Working with Toluene Di-isocyanate.* Birmingham; B.R.M.A. Health Res. Unit

Riddell, A. R. (1950). 'Clinical aspects of Shaver's disease.' In *Pneumoconiosis* (Sixth Saranac Symposium), pp. 459–482. Ed. by A. J. Vorwald. New York; Hoeber

Roberts, A. E. (1951). 'Platinosis.' *Archs ind. Hyg. occ. Med.* **4**, 549–559

Rock, R. L., Lovett, D. B. and Nelson, S. C. (1969). 'Radon-daughter exposure measurements with track etch films.' *Hlth Phys.* **16**, 617–621

Roe, J. W. (1959). 'Gases and fumes produced in fusion welding and cutting.' *Ann. occup. Hyg.* **2**, 75–84

Saccomanno, G., Archer, V. E., Saunders, R. P., James, L. A. and Beckler, P. A. (1964). 'Lung cancer of uranium miners in Colorado plateau.' *Hlth Phys.* **10**, 1195–1201

— — Auerbach, O., Kuschner, M., Saunders, R. P. and Klein, M. G. (1971). 'Histological types of lung cancer among uranium miners.' *Cancer, Philad.* **27**, 515–523

— Saunders, R. P., Archer, V. E., Auerbach, O., Kuschner, M. and Beckler, P. A. (1965). 'Cancer of the lung: the cytology of sputum prior to the development of carcinoma.' *Acta cytol.* **9**, 413–423

Sanders, C. L. and Park, F. J. (1971). 'Pulmonary distribution of alpha dose from $^{239}PuO_2$ and induction of neoplasia in rats and dogs.' In *Inhaled Particles and Vapours, III*, Vol. 1, 489–497. Ed. by W. H. Walton. Woking; Unwin

Sanderson, J. T. (1968). 'Hazards of the arc-air gouging process.' *Ann. occup. Hyg.* **11**, 123–133

Scheel, L. D., Dobrogorski, O. J., Mountain, J. T., Svirbely, J. L. and Stokinger,

H. E. (1959). 'Physiological, biochemical, immunological and pathological changes following ozone exposure.' *J. appl. Physiol.* **14**, 67–80

Schepers, G. W. H. (1955a). 'The biological action of particulate cobalt metal.' *Archs ind. Hlth* **12**, 127–133.

— (1955b). 'The biological action of particulate tungsten metal.' *Archs ind. Hlth* **12**, 134–136

— (1955c). 'The biological action of tantalum oxide.' *Archs ind. Hlth* **12**, 121–123

— (1961). 'The pathogenicity of glass-reinforced plastics.' *Archs envir. Hlth* **2**, 620–634

Scherer, M., Parambadathumalail, A., Bürki, H., Senn, A. and Zürcher, R. (1970). 'Drei Fälle von Hartmetallstaublunge.' *Schweiz. med. Wschr.* **100**, 2251–2255

Schwarz, L., Peck, S. M., Blair, K. E. and Markuson, K. E. (1945). 'Allergic dermatitis due to metallic cobalt.' *J. Allergy* **16**, 51–53

Shaver, C. G. (1948). 'Further observations of lung changes associated with the manufacture of alumina abrasives.' *Radiology* **50**, 760–769

— and Riddell, A. R. (1947). 'Lung changes associated with the manufacture of alumina abrasives.' *J. ind. Hyg. Toxicol.* **29**, 145–157

Sherwood, R. J. (1955). 'The hazards of Fluon (poly-tetrafluoroethylene). *Trans. Ass. ind. med. Offrs* **5**, 10–12

Shiel, O'M. F. (1967). 'Morbid anatomical changes in the lungs of dogs after inhalation of higher oxides of nitrogen during anaesthesia.' *Br. J. Anaesth.* **39**, 413–424

Shore, W., Greene, R. and Kazemi, H. (1971). 'Lung dysfunction in workers exposed to *Bacillus subtilis* enzyme.' *Arch. envir. Res.* **4**, 512–519

Šikl, H. (1930). 'Über den Lungenkrebs der Berglente in Joachimstal. (Tschechoslowakei).' *Z. Krebsforsch.* **32**, 609–613

Simon, G. (1972). Personal communication

Smith, J. P., Smith, J. C. and McCall, A. J. (1960). 'Chronic poisoning from cadmium fume.' *J. Path.* **80**, 287–296

Soap and Detergent Industry Association (1971). 'Recommended operating procedures for U.K. factories handling enzyme materials.' *Ann. occup. Hyg.* **14**, 71–87

Spencer, H. (1968). *Pathology of the Lung*, 2nd Edition, pp. 677–678. Oxford; Pergamon

Stacy, B. D., King, E. J., Harrison, C. V., Nagelschmidt, G. and Nelson, S. (1959). 'Tissue changes in rats' lungs caused by hydroxides oxides and phosphates of aluminium and iron.' *J. Path. Bact.* **77**, 417–426

Steel, J. (1964). 'Health hazards in the welding and cutting of paint-primed steel.' *Ann. occup. Hyg.* **7**, 247–251

— (1968). 'Respiratory hazards in shipbuilding and ship repairing.' *Ann. occup. Hyg.* **11**, 115–121

Steele, R. H. and Wilhelm, D. L. (1967). 'The inflammatory reaction in chemical injury II.' *Br. J. Exper. Path.* **48**, 592–607

Sterling, G. M. (1967). 'Asthma due to aluminium soldering flux.' *Thorax*, **22**, 533–537

Stevens, M. A. and Palmer, R. (1970). 'The effect of tolylene diisocyanate on certain laboratory animals.' *Proc. R. Soc. Med.* **63**, 380–381

Stokinger, H. E. (1965). 'Ozone toxicology: a review of research and industrial experience, 1954–1964.' *Archs envir. Hlth* **10**, 719–731

Taylor, G. (1970). 'Immune responses to tolylene diisocyanate.' *Proc. R. Soc. Med.* **63**, 379–380

Telescu, D. B. and Stănescu, D. C. (1970). 'Pulmonary function in workers with chronic exposure to cadmium oxide fumes.' *Int. Archs. Arbeitsmed.* **26**, 335–345

Thurlbeck, W. M. and Foley, F. D. (1963). 'Experimental pulmonary emphysema.' *Am. J. Path.* **42**, 431–441

Tolot, F., Girard, R., Dortit, G., Tabourin, G., Galy, P. and Bourret, J. (1970). 'Manifestations pulmonaires des "métaux durs": troubles irritatifs et fibrose (Enquête et observations cliniques).' *Archs Mal. prof. Méd. trav.* **31**, 453–470

Touey, G. P. and Mumpower, R. C. (1957). 'Measurement of the combustion-zone temperature of cigarettes.' *Tobacco N.Y.* **144**, 18–22

Townshend, R. H. (1968). 'A case of acute cadmium pneumonitis: lung function tests during a four-year follow-up.' *Br. J. ind. Med.* **25**, 68–71

Trapp, E., Rehzetti, A. D., Jr., Kobayashi, T., Mitchell, M. M. and Bigler, A. (1970). 'Cardiopulmonary function in uranium miners.' *Am. Rev. resp. Dis.* **101**, 27–43

Turiaf, J., Marland, P. and Tabart, J. (1966). 'L'asthme professionel des travailleurs de l'imprimerie.' *Poumon Coeur.* **22**, 539–554

Turner, C. (1953). 'Self-feeding of silage.' *Agriculture* **60**, 358–359

Turner-Warwick, M. (1971). 'Provoking factors in asthma.' *Br. J. Dis. Chest.* **65**, 1–20

Valand, S. B., Acton, J. D. and Myrvik, Q. N. (1970). 'Nitrogen dioxide inhibition of viral-induced resistance in alveolar monocytes.' *Archs envir. Hlth* **20**, 303–309

Vivoli, G. (1966). 'Richerche sperimentali sulle lesioni polmonari indotte dalla prolongata inalazione di lacche per capelli.' *Ig. mod.* **19**, 67–88

Wagoner, J. K., Miller, R. W., Lundin, F. E., Jr., Fraumeni, J. F., Jr. and Haij, M. E. (1963). 'Unusual cancer mortality among a group of underground metal miners.' *New Engl. J. Med.* **269**, 284–289

Webster, I. (1970). 'Bronchogenic carcinoma in South African gold miners.' In *Pneumoconiosis. Proceedings of the International Conference, Johannesburg, 1969*, pp. 572–574. Ed. by H. A. Shapiro. Cape Town; Oxford University Press

Weill, H., George, R., Schwarz, M. and Ziskind, M. (1969). 'Late evaluation of pulmonary function after acute exposure to chlorine gas.' *Am. Rev. resp. Dis.* **99**, 374–379

Wittich, F. W. (1940). 'The nature of various mill dust allergens.' *Lancet* **60**, 418–421

Wolfromm, R., Gervais, P. and Herman, D. (1966). 'Definitions et critéres de l'asthme professionel.' *Poumon Coeur.* **22**, 453–471

World Health Organization (1972). *Protection Against Ionizing Radiation: A Survey of Current World Legislation.* Geneva; W.H.O.

Wright, G. W. (1968). 'Airborne fibrous glass particles. Chest roentgenograms of persons with prolonged exposure.' *Archs envir. Hlth* **16**, 175–181

Wyatt, J. P. and Riddell, A. C. R. (1949). 'The morphology of bauxite fume pneumoconiosis.' *Am. J. Path.* **25**, 447–465

Young, W. A., Shaw, D. B. and Bates, D. V. (1964). 'Effect of low concentrations of ozone on pulmonary function in man.' *J. appl. Physiol.* **19**, 765–768

Appendix

In order that the features of normal and abnormal lung tissue may be accurately observed, standardized techniques of preparing and preserving the lungs are essential. Those available for routine purposes are not unduly time consuming but without them study of the lungs is incomplete and conclusions drawn liable to inaccuracy.

The basic principle of these techniques involves the injection of a fixative fluid or vapour into the bronchial tree until the lungs are expanded approximately to the position of maximum inspiration.

When removing the lungs from the thorax it is important that the visceral pleura should remain intact; emphysematous lungs are especially apt to puncture. Where there is symphysis of pulmonary and parietal pleurae the latter should be removed with the lung.

BRONCHIAL PERFUSION WITH LIQUID FORMALIN

After removal formol-acetate solution (10 per cent formalin in 4 per cent sodium acetate) is run through a cannula into both main bronchi from a reservoir placed at a height of about 120 cm, or delivered at this pressure by an electric pump. When perfusion is complete the lungs are placed in a large vessel containing the same solution for at least 48 hours. This is the method of Gough and Wentworth.

Another method, employing formalin vapour, is used for research purposes especially where quantitative studies of the lung or examination of bronchial mucus (which is unaffected) is to be made; but it is not appropriate for routine use and also tends to cause some shrinkage of the lungs.

Silverton (1964) has made a detailed survey and comparison of these and similar methods which should be referred to.

Lungs prepared by these methods are best examined by cutting serial slices 1 to 3 cm thick in the sagittal plane (in some cases the coronal plane may be preferable). The slices can then be studied in order and the observations recorded both in writing and diagrammatically. When the lung is inspected in this way discrete, non-fibrotic dust macules are indistinguishable to touch

503

from the surrounding lung and are not raised above the surface; by contrast, discrete, fibrotic dust lesions are firm, hard and 'nodular' to touch and are raised above the cut surface.

A *whole lung section* mounted on paper for permanent record is prepared by cutting 300 to 500 μm sections from slices about 4 cm thick and, after special processing which preserves the natural colours of the lung, attaching them to paper (Gough and Wentworth, 1960; Silverton, 1964). They are then covered with Cellophane or a layer of methacrylic resin. A modification of this method which permits more rapid preparation of sections has been described by Whimster (1969).

MICROSCOPY

Routine examination requires sections about 6 to 7 μm thick but when 'asbestos bodies' (or other ferruginous bodies) are sought, additional 30 μm sections greatly increase the chance of their being found.

Standard staining practice should include haemotoxylin and eosin and van Gieson methods and a silver impregnation method (such as that of Gordon and Sweet) demonstrating reticulin.

POLARIZED LIGHT MICROSCOPY

Polarized light is often used in routine microscopy of lung tissue to detect double refraction (birefringence) of non-cubic (anisotropic) crystalline particles and, on this evidence, it may be claimed that the nature of the crystals (for example, quartz) can be identified. It must be emphasized, however, that the successful application of this method of identification calls for the use of a properly equipped polarizing microscope with a graduated rotating stage for orientating the specimen with respect to the vibration direction of the incident light; or, alternatively, some means of rotating the polarizers in unison with respect to the specimen. Such instruments, which are not usually available in medical laboratories, have been used by petrologists for many years for identifying the mineral constituents of rocks. A knowledge of crystallography and crystals optics is also required to interpret the observations made with the polarizing microscope; simple rule-of-thumb tests are inadequate.

It is clear, therefore, that if the examination of lung sections is confined to simple observations with a 'medical' microscope to which crossed polars have simply been added, the demonstration of birefringent particles in the tissues establishes nothing more than the fact of birefringence; it does *not* by itself identify the nature of the crystals causing the birefringence. This point is fundamental. Of course, if the composition of the dust inhaled by the subject is known or suspected, it can be said that the birefringent particles *may* consist of, or at least include, this material; but it must always be borne in mind that particles of many different substances may be present as a result of exposure to a variety of dusts over the years. In some cases a clue as to the identity of the particles may be afforded by their shape. Thus the platy shape of crystals of talc and micaceous minerals is virtually characteristic, as is the fibrous character of fragments of textile materials and particles of commercial asbestos. A further clue may be given by the strength of the birefringence of the particles estimated qualitatively. The birefringence of the various substances which may be present in the lungs varies widely.

The maximum birefringences of some mineral substances of interest in the present context may be summarized as follow: quartz, weak; tridymite and chalcedony, very weak; cristobalite, virtually zero; crocidolite, weak; chrysotile and gypsum, moderate; talc, sericite, and muscovite mica, strong; calcite, dolomite, hematite, and magnesite, very strong. Most fibres exhibit some birefringence which varies from very weak, as is the case with cellulose acetate, to medium or strong with cotton, silk and nylon, and extremely strong with Terylene. It is evident from this list that some particles of high fibrogenic potential show feeble birefringence, while some non-fibrogenic particles are strongly birefringent.

POSITIVE IDENTIFICATION OF MINERAL PARTICLES IN THE LUNGS

Positive identification is usually only required for research purposes, but is sometimes needed in the investigation of obscure individual cases. Methods used include x-ray diffraction and emission spectrography after micro-incineration of lung tissue (although incineration has the drawback of altering the composition of some minerals), and electron microscopy, the scanning instrument being especially informative. An extraction replication technique with electron microscopy, which may prove valuable, has recently been introduced (Henderson, Gough and Harse, 1970). It must be remembered, however, that it does not necessarily follow from the identification of certain minerals that they are of pathogenic significance.

REFERENCES

Gough, J. and Wentworth, J. E. (1960). 'Thin sections of entire organs mounted on paper.' In *Recent Advances in Pathology*, 7th Edition. Ed. by C. V. Harrison. London; Churchill
Henderson, W. J., Gough, J. and Harse, J. (1970). 'Identification of mineral particles in pneumoconiotic lungs.' *J. clin. Path.* **23**, 104–109
Silverton, R. E. (1964). 'A comparison of formaldehyde fixation methods used in the study of pulmonary emphysema.' *J. med. Lab. Technol.* **21**, 187–217
Whimster, W. F. (1969). 'Rapid giant paper sections.' *Thorax* **24**, 737–741

Index

507

509